Fundamentals of General Surgery

Francesco Palazzo
Editor

Fundamentals of General Surgery

With Contribution by
Michael J. Pucci

Springer

Editor
Francesco Palazzo
Department of Surgery
Sidney Kimmel Medical College
Thomas Jefferson University
Philadelphia, PA
USA

ISBN 978-3-030-09289-4 ISBN 978-3-319-75656-1 (eBook)
https://doi.org/10.1007/978-3-319-75656-1

Printed on acid-free paper

This Springer imprint is published by the registered company Springer International Publishing AG part of Springer Nature
The registered company address is: Gewerbestrasse 11, 6330 Cham, Switzerland

To my wife, Silvia, and to my children Gaia, Giada, and Bruno;

to the many mentors who contributed to the field of General Surgery and to the Jefferson residents, present and past, for inspiring me to strive for clarity and excellence every single day.

Francesco Palazzo

To my family whom have supported me in every way to allow me to pursue my dream. To the masters and mentors of surgery whom have inspired me to continually strive for technical excellence. To the patients whom entrust me with their care, and provide endless learning opportunities for myself and our trainees. And finally, to the resident surgeons I have the opportunity to learn from and teach. Your endless thirst for knowledge and mastery of surgical skills inspires and drives me to continue to improve in all skills necessary for the transference of surgical ability.

Michael J. Pucci

Foreword: Why Another Textbook of Surgery?

So, why offer another textbook in the domain of Surgery? Certainly, there have been numerous surgical textbooks published over the last few centuries. New books continue to be added annually, as older textbooks cease to be revised. New areas of surgical specialty are developed, and textbooks are composed. In addition to books, we have journals, webcasts, audio guides, blogs, newsfeeds, and many other sources of information to assist the surgical learner. This book is designed to be different!

The intent of this book is to provide medical students, surgical physician assistants, surgical nurse practitioners, surgical residents, and surgical fellows with a novel resource—a place where they can find modern surgical knowledge upon which to base their surgical development. This book includes information that is typically transferred in the operating room setting, or at the bedside, but is frequently lost or limited during current training due to shorter work hours or due to the lesser amount of direct observation or interaction as part of teaching rounds, serving as a second assistant, etc. That is, much of what is contained herein is not typically contained in other textbooks, but rather has been transmitted verbally from the master to the learner.

So, enjoy the content of this textbook. There are many chapters on the operating room and its setup, patient positioning and skin preparation, retractors, and robotics. Contained here are useful discussions of gastrointestinal anastomoses, laparotomy for trauma, temporary abdominal wall closure, acceptable behavior in the operating room, and management of the operative catastrophe. Every topic is current, important, timely, and well discussed.

In the spirit of full disclosure, I must admit to a certain bias. The two editors of this textbook are young rising star members of our faculty at the Sidney Kimmel Medical College of Thomas Jefferson University. They both served as chief residents at Thomas Jefferson, and they both went on to fellowship training: Dr. Palazzo at the University of California—San Francisco

(UCSF) and Dr. Pucci here at Thomas Jefferson. I have scrubbed with both of these editors—they are superb surgeons and extraordinarily talented and caring physicians. Acknowledging this bias, I nonetheless enthusiastically recommend this textbook. I have learned much from the chapters I have read.

Charles J. Yeo
Samuel D. Gross
Professor and Chairman, Department of Surgery,
Senior Vice President and Chair,
Enterprise Surgery, Jefferson Health, Jefferson University Hospital,
Philadelphia, PA, USA

Preface

It is with great excitement that we present to you the first edition of *Fundamentals of General Surgery*. This book you hold in your hands—or more likely read on a computer screen—is the result of long conversations, reflections, and some degree of whining that have followed the many elective, urgent, and emergent procedures we have been lucky enough to bring to successful completion during our last several years in practice in Philadelphia.

While surgical education continues to rely on textbooks (or videos), oral transference of information at the bedside or in the operating room, and technical expertise demonstrated by and practiced with skilled mentors, it seems that current limitations have made it, at times, fragmented and not always uniformly delivered to all trainees. This book hopes to bridge the gap that exists between surgical education and the practice of surgery for novice and expert surgical trainees of all levels.

Herein you will find valuable information that is at times based on evidence, and other times based on years of practice in countless procedures. You will be able to use this when you need to take a patient to the operating room, when you first set foot in the operating room, when you need to independently position your first patient for a low anterior resection, but also for when you begin to construct your first gastrointestinal or vascular anastomoses. A sizeable portion of the book looks at sutures, knots, and instruments we use to make our procedures possible and safe (from retractors, to dissectors, to energy devices). Much focus is devoted to key concepts of trauma surgery which we believe any general surgeon should be familiar with; and an equally important portion of the book is dedicated to the frequently unaddressed concepts of progression from resident to independent surgeon, etiquette in the operating room, leadership and followership, and how to manage your time successfully. In each chapter we have asked the authors to provide a brief historical background, discuss some controversial areas, and present a list of recommended readings.

We are proud of the fact that this book should not be consulted frantically while preparing for the ABSITE or the American Board of Surgery qualifying exam. What can be found in these pages is not meant to be "swallowed whole and quick" but is meant to be carefully read, re-read, and slowly digested alternating practice, questions to your mentors, and review of this text (and many others) which is the only way to make knowledge easily retrievable and long lasting.

We are indebted to the many superb authors who contributed chapters to this book for their knowledge, their dedication, and willingness to invest their valuable time with a new editorial concept of surgical education. We have both read the chapters many times, have enjoyed them, and have learned much: our deepest thanks go to all of you!

A special acknowledgment goes to Jennifer Brumbaugh, MA, who is the medical illustrator and webmaster in the Department of Surgery at the Sidney Kimmel Medical College of Thomas Jefferson University, and who has worked with us on several of these chapters providing (once again) top-notch illustrations that complement and enrich the text.

We would also like to thank the production team at Springer UK and Springer Nature that have made this possible and deserve to be mentioned: Melissa Morton, Leo Johnson, Prakash Jagannathan, and many others.

We hope that this book will serve the many out there entering the fascinating world of General Surgery so that their journey can be easier and lead to the mastery we all seek. On the other hand, for those among us who have been navigating these waters for a few years this book may offer a new way to teach "young dogs some of the old tricks."

Philadelphia, PA, USA — Francesco Palazzo
Philadelphia, PA, USA — Michael J. Pucci

Contents

Contributors

Navid Ajabshir Mount Sinai Medical Center, Comprehensive Cancer Center, Miami Beach, FL, USA

Allison A. Aka Department of Surgery, Sidney Kimmel Medical College, Thomas Jefferson University, Philadelphia, PA, USA

Alexander F. Arriaga Department of Anesthesiology, Perioperative and Pain Medicine, Harvard Medical School, Brigham and Women's Hospital, Boston, MA, USA

Department of Anesthesiology and Critical Care, University of Pennsylvania Health System, Philadelphia, PA, USA

Alec C. Beekley Department of Surgery, Division of Acute Care Surgery, Division of Bariatric Surgery, Sidney Kimmel Medical College at Thomas Jefferson University, Philadelphia, PA, USA

Igor Belyansky Department of Surgery, Anne Arundel Medical Center, Annapolis, MD, USA

Kfir Ben-David Mount Sinai Medical Center, Comprehensive Cancer Center, Miami Beach, FL, USA

William R. Berry Ariadne Labs, Boston, MA, USA

Center for Surgery and Public Health, Boston, MA, USA

Department of Health Policy and Management, Harvard School of Public Health, Boston, MA, USA

Andrew M. Brown Department of Surgery, Sidney Kimmel Medical College, Thomas Jefferson University, Philadelphia, PA, USA

Guillaume S. Chevrollier Department of Surgery, Sidney Kimmel Medical College, Thomas Jefferson University, Philadelphia, PA, USA

Karen A. Chojnacki Department of Surgery, Sidney Kimmel Medical College, Thomas Jefferson University, Philadelphia, PA, USA

Daniel J. Deziel Department of Surgery, Rush University Medical Center, Chicago, IL, USA

Victoria G. Dodge Department of Surgery, Indiana University School of Medicine, Indianapolis, IN, USA

Katerina Dukleska Department of Surgery, Sidney Kimmel Medical College, Thomas Jefferson University, Philadelphia, PA, USA

Annie P. Ehlers Department of Surgery, University of Wisconsin, Madison, WI, USA

Robert D. Fanelli Department of Surgery, The Guthrie Clinic, Sayre, PA, USA

The Geisinger Commonwealth School of Medicine, Scranton, PA, USA

Albany Medical College, Albany, NY, USA

Idalid Franco Harvard Medical School, Boston, MA, USA

Giulio Giambartolomei The Bariatric and Metabolic Institute, Cleveland Clinic Florida, Weston, FL, USA

Selena G. Goss Department of Surgery, Sidney Kimmel Medical College, Thomas Jefferson University, Philadelphia, PA, USA

Samuel D. Gross Professor and Chairman, Department of Surgery, Senior Vice President and Chair, Enterprise Surgery, Jefferson Health, Jefferson University Hospital, Philadelphia, PA, USA

David L. Hepner Department of Anesthesiology, Perioperative and Pain Medicine, Harvard Medical School, Brigham and Women's Hospital, Boston, MA, USA

Ariadne Labs, Boston, MA, USA

William W. Hope New Hanover Regional Medical Center, University of North Carolina at Chapel Hill, Wilmington, NC, USA

Folasade O. Imeokparia Department of Surgery, The Ohio State University Wexner Medical Center, Columbus, OH, USA

Adam P. Johnson Department of Surgery, Sidney Kimmel Medical College, Thomas Jefferson University, Philadelphia, PA, USA

Deepika Koganti Department of Surgery, Sidney Kimmel Medical College, Thomas Jefferson University, Philadelphia, PA, USA

Jessica A. Latona Department of Surgery, Sidney Kimmel Medical College, Thomas Jefferson University, Philadelphia, PA, USA

Harish Lavu Jefferson Pancreas, Biliary and Related Cancer Center and the Department of Surgery, Thomas Jefferson University, Philadelphia, PA, USA

Sidney Kimmel Medical College, Thomas Jefferson University, Philadelphia, PA, USA

Chia-jung K. Lu Department of Surgery, Division of Acute Care Surgery, Sidney Kimmel Medical College at Thomas Jefferson University, Philadelphia, PA, USA

Amin Madani Department of Surgery, McGill University, Montreal, QC, Canada

Joshua A. Marks Department of Surgery, Sidney Kimmel Medical College, Thomas Jefferson University, Philadelphia, PA, USA

Niels D. Martin Trauma and Surgical Critical Care, University of Pennsylvania, Philadelphia, PA, USA

H. Mason Hedberg Department of Surgery, University of Chicago Medicine, Chicago, IL, USA

Neal S. McCall Department of Surgery, Sidney Kimmel Medical College, Thomas Jefferson University, Philadelphia, PA, USA

Robin S. McLeod Zane Cohen Centre, Lunenfeld-Tanenbaum Research Unit, Mount Sinai Hospital, Toronto, ON, Canada

Department of Surgery, The Institute of Health Policy, Management and Evaluation, University of Toronto, Toronto, ON, Canada

Cancer Care Ontario, Toronto, ON, Canada

Emanuele Lo Menzo Research Institute, The Bariatric and Metabolic Institute, Cleveland Clinic Florida, Weston, FL, USA

Tomoko Mizota Department of Surgery, Indiana University School of Medicine, Indianapolis, IN, USA

Carmen L. Mueller Department of Surgery, McGill University, Montreal, QC, Canada

Kenric Murayama Department of Surgery, John A Burns School of Medicine, University of Hawaii at Manoa, Honolulu, HI, USA

Nabeel R. Obeid Department of Surgery, Stony Brook Medicine, Stony Brook, NY, USA

Francesco Palazzo Department of Surgery, Sidney Kimmel Medical College, Thomas Jefferson University, Philadelphia, PA, USA

Emily A. Pearsall Zane Cohen Centre, Lunenfeld-Tanenbaum Research Unit, Mount Sinai Hospital, Toronto, ON, Canada

Department of Surgery, The Institute of Health Policy, Management and Evaluation, University of Toronto, Toronto, ON, Canada

Michael J. Pucci Department of Surgery, Sidney Kimmel Medical College, Thomas Jefferson University, Philadelphia, PA, USA

Marc Rafols Mount Sinai Medical Center, Comprehensive Cancer Center, Miami Beach, FL, USA

Shelby Resnick Trauma and Surgical Critical Care, University of Pennsylvania, Philadelphia, PA, USA

Ernest L. Rosato Department of Surgery, Sidney Kimmel Medical College, Thomas Jefferson University, Philadelphia, PA, USA

Francis E. Rosato Department of Surgery, Sidney Kimmel Medical College, Thomas Jefferson University, Philadelphia, PA, USA

Michael J. Rosen Cleveland Clinic, Cleveland, OH, USA

Raul Rosenthal Department of Surgery, The Bariatric and Metabolic Institute, Cleveland Clinic Florida, Weston, FL, USA

Dawn M. Salvatore Department of Surgery, Sidney Kimmel Medical College, Thomas Jefferson University, Philadelphia, PA, USA

Lawrence A. Shirley Department of Surgery, The Ohio State University Wexner Medical Center, Columbus, OH, USA

Udai S. Sibia Department of Surgery, Anne Arundel Medical Center, Annapolis, MD, USA

Christina Souther Department of Surgery, John A Burns School of Medicine, University of Hawaii at Manoa, Honolulu, HI, USA

Konstantinos Spaniolas Department of Surgery, Stony Brook Medicine, Stony Brook, NY, USA

Dimitrios Stefanidis Department of Surgery, Indiana University School of Medicine, Indianapolis, IN, USA

Adam Strickland Department of Surgery, Sidney Kimmel Medical College, Thomas Jefferson University, Philadelphia, PA, USA

Samuel Szomstein The Bariatric and Metabolic Institute, Cleveland Clinic Florida, Weston, FL, USA

Sami Tannouri Department of Surgery, Sidney Kimmel Medical College, Thomas Jefferson University, Philadelphia, PA, USA

Talar Tatarian Department of Surgery, Sidney Kimmel Medical College, Thomas Jefferson University, Philadelphia, PA, USA

Michael B. Ujiki Department of Surgery, Grainger Center for Innovation and Simulation, NorthShore University HealthSystem, Evanston, IL, USA

Michael E. Villarreal Department of Surgery, The Ohio State University Wexner Medical Center, Columbus, OH, USA

Adam S. Weltz Department of Surgery, Anne Arundel Medical Center, Annapolis, MD, USA

Andrew S. Wright Department of Surgery, University of Wisconsin, Madison, WI, USA

Charles J. Yeo Professor and Chairman, Department of Surgery, Senior Vice President and Chair, Enterprise Surgery, Jefferson Health, Jefferson University Hospital, Philadelphia, PA, USA

H. Reza Zahiri Department of Surgery, Anne Arundel Medical Center, Annapolis, MD, USA

Fundamentals of Patient Preparation for the Operating Room in the Twenty-First Century

1

Emily A. Pearsall and Robin S. McLeod

1.1 General Concepts

Modern surgery can be performed safely with low mortality and morbidity rates, even in patients having complex operations or who have significant comorbidities. However, to achieve excellent results, there must be thorough evaluation and preparation of patients. Even in patients having emergency surgery, it is important, if possible, to ensure that patients are in optimal condition. This requires a full preoperative assessment of their primary condition, as well as their comorbidities. In addition, patients may require preoperative imaging and appropriate laboratory testing. Depending on the urgency of their surgery, patients may need various interventions to optimize their condition. Finally, preoperative education is an important part of the preoperative work-up.

E. A. Pearsall
Zane Cohen Centre, Lunenfeld-Tanenbaum Research Unit, Mount Sinai Hospital, Toronto, ON, Canada

Department of Surgery, University of Toronto, Toronto, ON, Canada

R. S. McLeod (✉)
Zane Cohen Centre, Lunenfeld-Tanenbaum Research Unit, Mount Sinai Hospital, Toronto, ON, Canada

Department of Surgery, University of Toronto, Toronto, ON, Canada

Institute of Health Policy, Management and Evaluation, University of Toronto, Toronto, ON, Canada

Cancer Care Ontario, Toronto, ON, Canada
e-mail: robin.mcleod@cancercare.on.ca

1.2 Preoperative Assessment and Care

In all patients, a complete history and examination is essential. In addition to understanding the presenting condition, it is necessary to know if the patient has underlying comorbidities and what medications he/she is on. There are some fairly common drugs which patients are often taking such as anticoagulants, steroids, and diabetic medications which may need to be discontinued or modified prior to surgery. As well, diagnostic imaging should be performed to assist in the planning of the operation. Finally, it might be worthwhile in some situations to delay surgery to optimize the patient's condition. For instance, patients presenting with an abdominal abscess who do not require emergency surgery should have the abscess drained, antibiotics started, and surgery performed on a semi-elective basis. Similarly, in patients presenting with an obstruction due to a stricture, it might be possible to decompress the bowel prior to undertaking surgery.

With respect to imaging and laboratory tests to prepare patients for surgery, *Choosing Wisely* has made a number of specific recommendations for asymptomatic patients who are undergoing noncardiac low-risk surgery [1]. In these patients, it

F. Palazzo (ed.), *Fundamentals of General Surgery*, https://doi.org/10.1007/978-3-319-75656-1_1

is recommended that the following should not be done routinely but rather selectively utilized:

- Blood count, coagulation testing, and serum biochemistry tests
- ECG, chest x-ray, ECHO cardiogram, cardiac stress tests, and pulmonary function tests
- Type and screen for blood

1.2.1 Patient Education

Patient education is an essential component of preoperative care. Appropriate preoperative education has been shown to decrease patients' anxiety and fears about surgery, lessen the use of postoperative analgesia, reduce postoperative complications, and decrease the length of hospital stay [2–5]. Many patients view surgery as a threatening experience with many stressful components which elicit strong emotional responses [4, 5]. These responses can have negative repercussions for the patient in the postoperative period [3, 4]. Research, although limited, has shown that preoperative psychosocial interventions also have positive effects on postoperative psychological and physical functioning [4–6].

With the implementation of enhanced recovery after surgery programs, there is greater emphasis on self-management and early discharge [6]. This means that patients require more information about what the expectations of them are in hospital as well as after discharge, what they can expect with normal recovery, and finally how to identify complications and what they should do if they occur. Patients should receive this information both verbally and in written format. Ideally, this information should be provided prior to their preadmission visit to better prepare them for the appointment and be able to have questions ready. In addition, patients should be offered a second appointment with the surgeon because often they forget to ask questions at their first meeting, especially if they received unexpected recommendations. It is also essential that patients receive a consistent message from all healthcare providers and standardized messaging in all written materials. Additionally, patients should be encouraged to have a family member in attendance so they are well informed and can share information with the patient.

1.2.2 Nutritional Evaluation and Supplements

Malnutrition is a common problem for general surgery patients, as approximately 14% of elective GI surgical patients are at risk of malnutrition. Several studies have shown that patients at risk of malnutrition often have longer hospital stays as well as an increased rate of postoperative complications. The European Society for Clinical Nutrition and Metabolism released a guideline in 2017 on clinical nutrition in surgery [7]. In addition to recommending a shortened fast and carbohydrate drinks up to 2 h prior to surgery, they also recommend that the nutritional status of all patients should be assessed before and after surgery. The authors suggest that nutritional therapy, preferable by the enteral route, should be initiated in patients who are malnourished or those at nutritional risk. Additionally, patients who may not be able to eat or may have a low oral intake prior to surgery may also benefit from nutritional therapy.

A 2012 Cochrane review was undertaken to review the literature on preoperative nutritional support in patients undergoing gastrointestinal surgery. The authors found that immune-enhancing nutrition reduces the risk of complications; however, these studies included well-nourished surgical patients and excluded those at high risk of malnutrition. Thus, immune-enhancing nutrition has not been proven to be beneficial for malnourished surgical patients. Similarly, there was inconclusive evidence to support preoperative oral supplements and enteral nutrition. Lastly, parental nutrition appears to have an effect on total complications but not on infectious complications in malnourished patients [8].

With regards to nutritional screening, while the literature strongly recommends that screening should take place, there is limited information on the preferred screening method. Both Nutritional Risk Screening 2002 [see Editors' Corner at end of chapter] and Subjective Global Assessment are most commonly used [9].

1.2.3 Management of Patients with Diabetes Mellitus

With the increasing prevalence of obesity, diabetes is seen more frequently in patients having surgery. Depending on the surgical procedure, approximately 10–15% of patients will be diabetic. These patients are at higher risk for developing complications, having a longer length of stay, and dying postoperatively. The poorer outcomes may be due to the diabetes or the associated comorbidities.

Patients scheduled for elective surgery should be seen as soon as the date of surgery is determined so the patient's status can be assessed, and if necessary, interventions can be implemented to optimize the patient when he/she undergoes surgery.

Random glucose levels are of no value and should not be ordered in patients with diabetes mellitus. Instead, the patient should have their HbA1c measured. Generally, individuals with a HbA1c of less than 69 mmol mol^{-1} (i.e., 8.5% NGSP) can be managed with fasting and simple manipulation of their insulin. On the other hand, individuals with an elevated HbA1c will likely require careful monitoring and manipulation of their treatment. In addition to measuring HbA1c, diabetic patients should be assessed for comorbidities including ordering of serum electrolytes and an ECG [10].

Patients with a HbA1c below 69 mmol mol^{-1} usually can withstand fasting with minor changes in their insulin requirements or medication. On the other hand, individuals who have a HbA1c greater than 69 mmol mol^{-1}, have poorly controlled diabetes, are having emergency surgery, or will be unable to take a normal diet after surgery may require significant changes to their care and should be seen by a specialist consultant [10].

For all diabetic patients having surgery, it is important that there is careful monitoring to ensure there is normal glycemia and minimal disruption of their usual routine. To accomplish this, all efforts should be made for these patients to have a shortened fast, so diabetic patients undergoing elective surgery should be scheduled early in the day.

1.2.4 Smoking Cessation

Smokers who undergo surgery are at greater risk for developing pulmonary and surgical-related complications. This risk may be in the order of a three- to sixfold increase in intraoperative pulmonary complications [11]. There are a number of short-term and long-term risks related to smoking. *Short-term effects* are due to increased concentrations of carbon monoxide and nicotine in the blood. Carbon monoxide preferentially binds to hemoglobin over oxygen. Carbon monoxide also changes the structure of hemoglobin, so there is a shift in the oxygen hemoglobin curve. Together, these effects lead to decreased availability of oxygen. Nicotine increases blood pressure, pulse rate, and systemic vascular resistance. Thus, nicotine increases the work of the heart, while carbon monoxide decreases the availability of oxygen. These harmful effects may disappear after 48 h of stopping smoking.

The *long-term effects* of smoking are related to atherosclerosis and effects on pulmonary function including increased mucus which may increase the likelihood of infection [7]. Lastly, in addition to the effects on the cardiovascular and respiratory systems, smoking impairs wound healing. This may affect the surgical wound as well as increase the risk of anastomotic leaks [11].

A Cochrane Review which was published in 2014 included 13 studies looking at the effect of preoperative smoking cessation programs [11]. These studies were quite heterogeneous in regards to their interventions and intensity. The authors classified them as short and long intensive interventions based on the length of time before surgery they were instituted and the intervention. Generally, the intensive strategies were started 4–8 weeks before surgery and included weekly behavioral interventions as well as nicotine replacement therapy. Both the short and long intensive programs were effective in decreasing smoking rates, but the results were more favorable in the long intensive program and were also sustainable. In addition, only intensive programs were effective in decreasing surgical complications (RR 0.42, 95% CI 0.27–0.65) including wound complications (RR 0.31, 95% CI 0.16–0.62).

The authors concluded that the optimal preoperative intervention intensity remains unclear, but based on this review, they recommend interventions which are started 4–8 weeks before surgery and provide behavioral support as well as offering nicotine replacement therapy.

1.2.5 Prehabilitation

There is some evidence that there is an association between patients' fitness before surgery and their outcomes after surgery including complications, length of stay, and health-related quality of life [12, 13]. Several trials assessing whether preoperative exercise programs ("prehabilitation") have been performed and have shown mixed results. A recent systematic review and meta-analysis of nine studies [13] focusing on abdominal surgeries found that preoperative exercise was associated with a 41% decrease in postoperative complications and a 1.6-day reduction in LOS. However, the studies which were included were of "very low quality," due to improper allocation concealment, randomization strategies at high risk of bias, and biased outcome assessment. There are also other studies which have not shown a benefit including a study of patients over the age of 60 years having colorectal surgery [14].

While there may be some benefit to prehabilitation programs, there are some limitations to their adoption. In particular, these programs may delay surgery for 4–6 weeks. This may not be possible, particularly in patients who are having surgery for a cancer diagnosis where a delay might not be advantageous or patients who are receiving other treatments such as neoadjuvant therapy in that interval.

At the current time, there is insufficient evidence to recommend prehabilitation programs, but it is an area of interest. Not only may this increase patient physical well-being but also may alleviate anxiety and depression and give patients a sense of empowerment that they can improve their health.

1.2.6 Blood Conservation

The World Health Organization defines anemia as an insufficient number of red blood cells (RBC) to meet physiologic needs [15]. The most common indicator of anemia is a hemoglobin (Hb) concentration below the normal adult values, with thresholds of 12.0 g/dL in women and 13.0 g/dL in men [16]. In the general population, the prevalence of anemia is generally under 5%, but in the perioperative setting, anemia is more common. An observational study looking at data from the National Surgical Quality Improvement Program (NSQIP) identified 33.9% of 6301 non-cardiac surgical patients with preoperative anemia [17]. Perioperative anemia appears to be multifactorial. The most obvious causes can be associated with the disease for which surgery is required, such as gastrointestinal bleeding leading to chronic blood loss, nutritional deficiency from decreased oral intake, or hematologic toxicities from chemotherapy treatments. The anemia of chronic disease also plays an important role.

Perioperative anemia has been shown to have negative effects on surgical outcomes. In the NSQIP analysis, the postoperative infection rate increased from 2.6% to 5% with increasing degrees of anemia [17]. Overall, 92% of postoperative infections occurred in anemic patients. Low preoperative and postoperative hemoglobin levels were independent risk factors of increased mortality, postoperative pneumonias, and length of stay [17]. Furthermore, another meta-analysis found that allogeneic blood transfusion was significantly associated with a higher risk of postoperative infection (OR 3.45, 95% CI 1.43–15.15) [18].

A number of non-transfusion strategies have been suggested to correct preoperative anemia and hopefully lower its consequences. The perioperative use of erythropoietin in colorectal cancer surgery was summarized in a Cochrane Review in 2009 [19]. Four randomized controlled trials were included. No difference was observed in the proportion of patients requiring RBC transfusions. The authors concluded that there was insufficient evidence to recommend the use of erythropoietin in colorectal cancer surgery.

The use of perioperative iron supplementation has been shown to decrease the need for RBC transfusion either alone or in combination with erythropoietin or autologous blood donation. In a randomized controlled trial, 49 patients scheduled for colorectal surgery were randomized to ferrous sulfate or no supplements for 2 weeks prior to surgery. Preoperative iron led to higher hemoglobin and ferritin levels at admission and decreased likelihood of requiring blood transfusion, along with a 66% cost reduction [20]. Another study compared intravenous iron supplementation, and no difference was observed in either hemoglobin level at admission or the need for blood transfusion [21].

In an attempt to reduce transfusion-related morbidity by limiting the exposure to allogeneic blood, preoperative autologous donation has been used. A Cochrane Review included 14 trials. Preoperative autologous blood donation was associated with a reduction in the relative risk of receiving allogeneic blood transfusion by 68% (RR 0.32 [95% CI 0.22–0.47]). However, the risk of receiving any blood transfusion was increased (RR 1.24 [95% CI 1.02–1.510). The rate of postoperative infection was not different between autologous and allogeneic blood transfusion groups (RR 0.70 [95% CI 0.34–1.43]) [22]. Moreover, preoperative blood donation would appear to be difficult to use in gastrointestinal surgery where a significant proportion of patients present with anemia.

1.2.7 Mechanical Bowel Preparation

Mechanical bowel preparation (MBP) before elective colorectal surgery has been the standard in surgical practice for over a century. Surgeons believed that MBP decreases intraluminal fecal mass and presumably decreases bacterial load in the bowel. It is argued that a decrease in fecal load and bacterial contents reduces the rates of infectious postoperative complications such as surgical site infections, deep intra-abdominal infections, and anastomotic dehiscence. These theories, however, have been based largely on clinical experience and expert opinion.

In the recent years, the value for MBP in patients having elective colonic and rectal surgery has been challenged. MBP is generally safe but has been associated with serious complications in patients with existing cardiac and renal disease as well as previously healthy patients. Furthermore, most patients find taking a MBP to be unpleasant. A meta-analysis published by Slim et al. in 2009 included 14 trials in which 4859 patients were randomized to MBP or no MBP. The pooled results revealed no significant differences in anastomotic leakage rates (OR 1.12, 95% CI [0.824, 1.532], $p = 0.46$) or superficial SSI (9.5% in the MBP group vs. 8.3% in the no MBP group; OR 1.17, 95% CI [0.96, 1.44], $p = 0.11$) [23].

More recently, there has been laboratory evidence that the combination of oral antibiotics and intravenous antibiotics reduces the risk of anastomotic leaks as well as SSI. The WHO found moderate quality evidence for prescribing MBP and oral antibiotics to reduce SSIs in colorectal surgery [24]. Their systematic review of 11 RCTs compared MBP with oral antibiotics to MBP alone and found an OR 0.56 (95% CI 0.37–0.83). Numerous oral antibiotic regimens have been studied but usually a combination of an aminoglycoside (neomycin) with erythromycin or metronidazole is prescribed.

Thus, while more evidence is required, it is possible that MBP with a combination of oral and intravenous antibiotics may be the preferred option.

1.2.8 Stoma Siting

An ileostomy or colostomy is frequently required in patients having surgery for benign or malignant indications. The stoma may be permanent or temporary. Preoperative marking of the stoma is essential since how well the stoma functions may have a profound effect on outcome and the patient's acceptance of it. When siting a stoma, it should be placed away from scars and creases and in a location where the patient can visualize it adequately when he/she is sitting or lying. If not, the patient may have difficulty changing the appliance. Both stoma placement and siting of incisions are extremely important both in the short term as well as the long term since if the stoma is permanent, it may require revision in the future [25].

Siting of the stoma should be performed prior to surgery and should include education on how to look after the stoma. Optimally this should be given by a trained enterostomal therapist. While education has always been important, it has even more relevance now since patients' hospital stays are shorter, and thus, there is less time for them to get comfortable with a stoma [26].

1.2.9 Fasting

Despite many institutions still requiring patients to be "NPO after midnight," there is strong evidence that favors reducing preoperative fasting times and is supported by numerous worldwide guidelines. *The current guidelines all support a fast of 6 h following a light meal at night* [27–29]. The recommendations are based on the estimated physiologic gastric emptying time for healthy patients which is relatively short and thus will not increase the risk of pulmonary aspiration [30].

Furthermore, rather than prohibiting oral intake, *current guideline recommendations encourage patients to consume drinks high in carbohydrates up to 2–3 h prior to surgery* [30]. Clear fluids may include coffee and tea (without milk) but preferably should be drinks that are high in carbohydrates (i.e., apple juice and pulp-free orange juice). This may improve patient outcomes by minimizing the adverse effects of starvation and decreasing the effects of surgical stress. Additionally, it has been hypothesized that carbohydrate drinks may reduce insulin resistance and glycogen depletion and may attenuate loss of muscle mass, hunger, thirst, anxiety, nausea, as well as surgical complications leading to reduced length of hospital stay.

Early research in the role of preoperative fasting determined that for passive regurgitation and pulmonary aspiration to occur during anesthesia, a certain gastric volume must be present. It has been assumed that a minimum of 200 mL of residual volume is required for regurgitation [31, 32]. Numerous studies have reported that in most patients, the preoperative mean gastric fluid volume is in the range of 10–30 mL, and 120 mL is rarely exceeded irrespective of intake of clear liquids.

With regards to carbohydrate drinks, the majority of the evidence has shown no benefit, but some studies have shown modest effects for reduced length of stay, postoperative insulin resistance, return to GI function, and patient well-being [33]. As well, none of the studies found that carbohydrate drinks increased the risk of postoperative complications such as aspiration. Thus, they concluded that while there is no strong evidence to support its use in terms of improved surgical outcomes, there is no evidence for potential postoperative complications, and carbohydrate drinks may be encouraged as it may improve the tolerability of the presurgical period.

There is much debate regarding carbohydrate loading in diabetic patients. Unfortunately, there is limited evidence available to support or refute a recommendation on this. To date, only one study has assessed preoperative carbohydrate loading in type 2 diabetes patients [34]. This study was of low quality, comparing 25 patients with diabetes to 10 healthy controls. The patients in the experimental group were given a carbohydrate-rich drink (400 ml, 12.5% with 1.5 g of paracetamol). The authors found that peak glucose was higher in diabetic patients (13.4 ± 0.5 vs. 7.6 ± 0.5 mm; $P < 0.01$); however, glucose concentrations were back to baseline at 180 min for diabetic patients compared to 120 min in the control group ($P < 0.01$). Gastric half-emptying time (T50) was also significantly different with it occurring at 49.8 ± 2.2 min in diabetics compared to 58.6 ± 3.7 min in the control ($P < 0.05$). *Despite these differences, the authors concluded that type 2 diabetic patients showed no signs of delayed gastric emptying suggesting that the use of carbohydrate drinks may be safely administered prior to surgery.*

Despite the lack of evidence, preoperative assessment of individuals for gastroesophageal reflux disease, dysphagia symptoms, or other gastrointestinal motility disorders is recommended because these individuals might be at higher risk for reflux and aspiration [29].

1.3 Preparation on the Day of Surgery

1.3.1 Surgical Checklist

Surgical checklists have been adopted by most hospitals. Checklists include items which are essential to all parts of the work load in the operating room. The goal is to increase communication among all individuals who are part of the surgical team including anesthesiologists, nurses, and surgeons and optimize the care and safety of patients. There are three phases to the checklist including the "sign in" phase which should occur before the patient is anaesthetized, the "time out" phase before the incision is made, and the "sign out" phase before the patient leaves the operating room. Haynes et al. were able to show a significant reduction in mortality (1.5% vs 0.8%) and complications (11% vs 7%) following the implementation of the checklist in eight hospitals across the world [35].

In the Haynes study, hospitals in developing nations had the greatest improvement in outcomes which may be the reason why a subsequent study in Ontario, Canada, did not identify any improvement following the adoption of the checklist [36]. The checklist consists of a list of items which pertain to all aspects of the operation. Simply confirming that these items are in place may not lead to improved outcome. Rather, the value of the checklist may be that it fosters improved communication among all members of the surgical team. In addition, the checklist has three phases, and in many instances, not all phases are completed which may decrease its utility. In particular, there may not be compliance with the sign out phase. The handoff of patients has been shown to be important especially in patients who have had a complex procedure or have multiple comorbidities. In a follow-up study, Haynes and colleagues surveyed providers and found that the attitudes of the individuals correlated with the degree of improvement in care [37].

1.3.2 Surgical Site Infection Prevention

Surgical site infections (SSIs) are the most common and expensive healthcare-associated infections leading to increased morbidity and mortality and increased hospital stays. However, evidence-based initiatives have been shown to prevent more than 50% of SSIs [38]. There are four essential components which have strong evidence to support their use to decrease surgical site infections: antibiotic prophylaxis, maintenance of normothermia before and throughout the surgical procedure, adequate skin preparation, and avoidance of shaving.

1.3.2.1 Antibiotic Prophylaxis

Table 1.1 outlines the preferred choice of antibiotics for different general surgical procedures. The benefit of antimicrobial prophylaxis varies depending on the procedure. Antibiotics are often not recommended for clean surgeries unless postoperative infections would have severe consequences. When choosing a regimen, the narrowest antimicrobial spectrum should be used to minimize the risk of *Clostridium difficile* infections and the emergence of antibiotic resistance.

While cephalosporins are the preferred antibiotics for many procedures, another drug is often substituted if the patient has a history of a penicillin allergy. Instead, a detailed allergy history as outlined in the Cefazolin Safety Checklist (Fig. 1.1) should be obtained because in most instances, cephalosporins can be prescribed without significant risk. Severe anaphylactic type 1 reactions are not common in patients receiving antibiotics: 0.01–0.05% in patients receiving penicillin and 0.0001–0.1% for cephalosporins.

Table 1.1 Considerations in the preoperative assessment and management of patients undergoing general surgery procedures

A. Preoperative assessment should include the following:
1. History and physical examination
2. Appropriate imaging and diagnostic tests
B. Preoperative interventions that should be considered depending on the patient status and surgical procedure
1. Smoking cessation
2. Prehabilitation
3. Blood conservation
4. Nutritional assessment
5. Management of the diabetic patient
6. Mechanical bowel preparation
7. Stoma siting (in patients where a stoma may be required)
8. Preoperative fasting
C. Patient education
D. Preparation on the day of surgery
1. Surgical checklists
2. Strategies to decrease the risk of surgical site infections (SSI)
3. Venous thromboembolic prevention

A significant allergy is defined as a prior allergic reaction (or positive skin testing) with resultant hospitalization or anaphylaxis (hypotension, laryngeal edema, wheezing, angioedema, urticaria). If the patient did suffer this type of reaction, he/she should not receive the same drug or another penicillin. The rate of cross-reactivity between penicillin and cephalosporins is approximately 10%, so if the patient has a history of a severe reaction, an alternative antibiotic should be prescribed such as vancomycin. However, non-severe reactions/side effects such as mild maculopapular rash and gastrointestinal upset are not reasons for prescribing clindamycin or vancomycin.

To reduce surgical site infections, antibiotic prophylaxis must attain adequate tissue concentration at the time of incision and be maintained during the procedure. To achieve this objective, antibiotics directed against the most common contaminating bacteria must be administered within 60 min before incision at the correct dose. Vancomycin and fluoroquinolones require a longer infusion time and need to be initiated earlier to ensure completion within 60 min of incision.

Additionally, re-dosing of antibiotics for prolonged procedures is necessary to maintain adequate tissue concentration (Table 1.2). Thus, additional intraoperative doses are recommended at intervals approximating two times the half-life of the antibiotic or if there is significant blood loss (>1.5 L). Finally, antibiotics should not be routinely continued postoperatively. They do not decrease the risk of a SSI but can increase the risk of *Clostridium difficile* infections (Table 1.3).

1.3.2.2 Normothermia

General and neuraxial anesthesia impair thermoregulatory control. As a result, nearly all unwarmed surgical patients become hypothermic if active measures are not taken to maintain normothermia. The typical rate of heat loss leads to a drop in body temperature of 1–1.5 °C during the first hour of general anesthesia. Hypothermia increases the risk of surgical site infections through one of two mechanisms. First, thermoregulatory vasoconstriction reduces subcutaneous oxygen tension, and secondly, mild core hypothermia impairs immune function through impairment of T-cell-mediated antibody production and neutrophil oxidative killing. Mild perioperative hypothermia has also been causally linked to numerous complications including increased blood loss, adverse cardiac events, and prolonged post-anesthetic recovery and hospitalization. In the review by the WHO guidelines, pre- and intraoperative body warming significantly reduced SSIs compared to no warming (OR, 0.33; 95% CI, 0.14–0.62) [26]. Normal core temperature should be maintained during surgery through the use of active measures including warmed intravenous fluids, inspired gases, forced air warming, and ensuring that irrigation fluids used in a surgical procedure are at or slightly above body temperature before use. The OR should be kept in the range of 20 °C, a compromise between what is acceptable for the patient and tolerable for the surgical team. In addition, measures should be taken preoperatively to maintain the patient's temperature at 36 °C or above. This may require warmed blankets while patients wait in the holding area and ensuring they are covered in the operating room prior to induction.

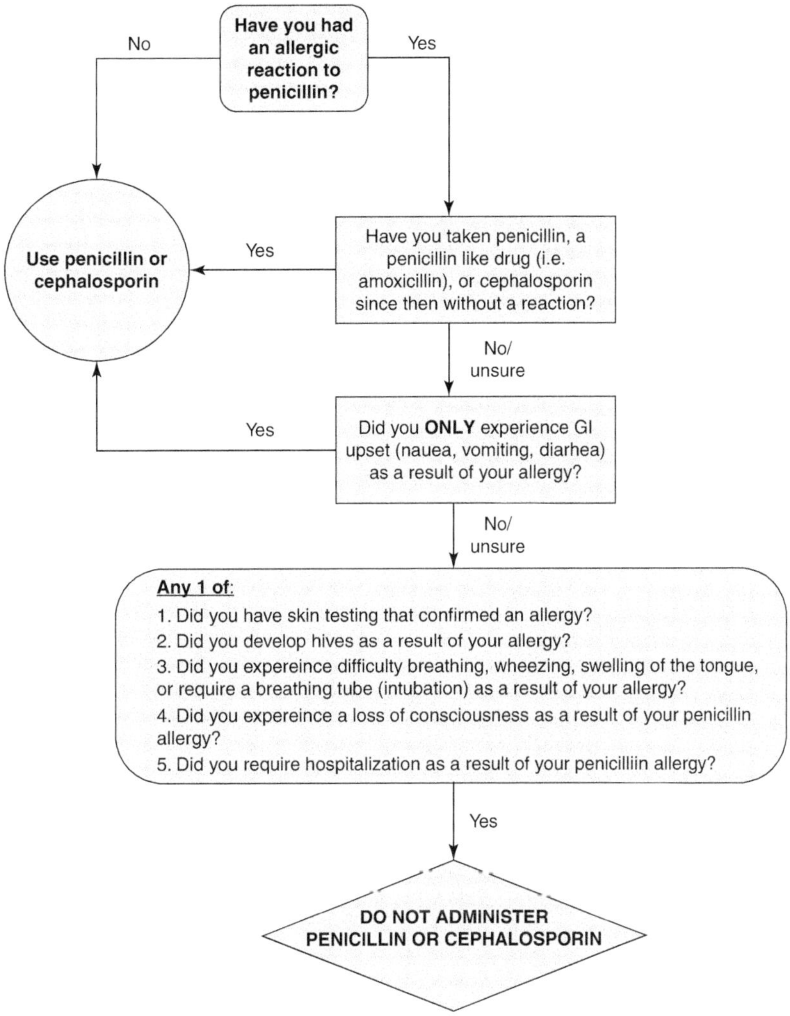

Fig. 1.1 Cefazolin safety checklist

1.3.2.3 Preoperative Skin Preparation

Chlorhexidine alcohol should be used to clean the skin in most patients [see Chap. 4]. The exceptions are procedures where there is contact with the eyes, the middle ear, mucous membranes, and meninges (including lumbar puncture). In addition, it should be avoided in infants less than 2 months old.

A 2010 meta-analysis of 6 studies containing 5031 patients undergoing clean-contaminated general or gynecological surgery showed that chlorhexidine alcohol was more effective than povidone-iodine in reducing the risk of SSIs (pooled odds ratio 0.68, 95% CI 0.50–0.94, $p = 0.019$) [39]. A more recent large, multicenter trial which included 849 patients who underwent clean-contaminated surgery (colorectal, small intestinal, gastroesophageal, biliary, thoracic, gynecologic, urologic) confirmed these results: SSI rates of 9.5% in the chlorhexidine alcohol group vs 16.1% in the povidone-iodine group. However, while this solution is more effective, there is a small risk of fire with the 70% alcohol which can be mitigated by ensuring there is no pooling of the alcohol and time is left for it to dry [40].

Bathing or showering prior to surgery to clean the skin is considered good clinical practice. However, there is no definitive evidence to support the use of antimicrobial soap (chlorhexidine) compared to plain soap to reduce SSIs.

Table 1.2 Recommended antibiotics for prophylaxis of general surgery procedures[a]

Surgical procedure	Recommended agents	B-lactam allergy recommended agents
Breast surgery	Cefazolin	Vancomycin
Gastroduodenal/esophageal/distal pancreatic resection	Cefazolin	Vancomycin + aminoglycoside
Percutaneous endoscopic gastrostomy (PEG)	Cefazolin	Vancomycin + aminoglycoside
Biliary tract—laparoscopic procedure—elective low risk	None	None
Biliary tract—laparoscopic procedure—high-risk emergency, inserting prosthetic device, diabetes, risk of intraoperative gallbladder rupture/conversion to open, age >70 years, ASA ≥3, reintervention within 1 month, acute cholecystitis, obstructive jaundice, CBD stones, nonfunctional GB, pregnancy, immunosuppression	Cefazolin	Vancomycin + aminoglycoside
Biliary tract—open procedure		
Liver resection		
Colorectal, small bowel, appendectomy	Cefazolin + metronidazole	Vancomycin + aminoglycoside + metronidazole
Pancreaticoduodenectomy	If risk of Gram-negative resistance, add aminoglycoside	
Hernia repair—hernioplasty, herniorrhaphy	Cefazolin	Vancomycin
Low-risk anorectal procedures: hemorrhoidectomy, fistulotomy, sphincterotomy	None	None
Head and neck procedures: clean with no incision through oral/nasal/pharyngeal mucosa (e.g., parotidectomy, thyroidectomy, and submandibular gland excision)	None	None
Head and neck procedures: clean with placement of prosthetic material (excludes tympanostomy tubes)	Cefazolin	Vancomycin + metronidazole
Head and neck procedures: clean-contaminated (incision through oral/pharyngeal mucosa): cancer surgery and other clean-contaminated procedures with the exception of tonsillectomy and functional endoscopic sinus procedures	Cefazolin + metronidazole	Vancomycin + aminoglycoside + metronidazole

[a]Adapted from Best Practice in Surgery http://www.bestpracticeinsurgery.ca

Table 1.3 Recommended dosing and re-dosing of antimicrobial prophylaxis[a]

Agent	Adult dose	Pediatric dose (max dose should not exceed the recommended adult dose)	Intraoperative re-dosing normal renal function
Cefazolin	2 g	30 mg/kg IV (max dose: 2 g)	q4 h if CrCl >30 mL/min (Max 6 g/24 h)
	3 g if weight ≥120 kg		
Aminoglycoside:[b] gentamicin or tobramycin	1.5–2 mg/kg (round to nearest 20 mg)	2.5 mg/kg	Repeat once at 3 h if CrCl >60 mL/min
Metronidazole	500 mg	15 mg/kg Neonates <1200 g: 7.5 mg/kg	8 h
Vancomycin[c,d]	15 mg/kg round nearest 250 mg (max 2 g/dose)	15 mg/kg (max dose: 1 g)	8 h, if CrCl >50 mL/min
	Administer ≤1 g over 60 min		
	>1 g–1.5 g over 90 min		
	>1.5 g over 120 min		

[a]Adapted from Best Practice in Surgery http://www.bestpracticeinsurgery.ca

[b]Dose based on actual body weight (ABW) unless obese. If ABW >20% above ideal body weight (IBW), use Dosing Weight = IBW + 0.4*(ABW – IBW); IBW Men: 50 kg + 2.3 kg (× inches above 60 in.); IBW Women: 45.5 kg + 2.3 kg (× inches above 60 in.)

[c]Dose should be based on total body weight

[d]If tourniquet is used, entire dose should be infused prior to inflation

1.3.2.4 Preoperative Hair Removal

Preoperative preparation for surgery has traditionally included the removal of body hair from the intended surgical site. However, several lines of evidence have challenged this practice, and current data suggest that hair removal might increase SSI rates [41–43]. A Cochrane Review conducted by Tanner et al. included six trials totalling 972 participants comparing hair removal (shaving, clipping, or depilatory cream) with no hair removal and found no statistically significant difference in SSI rates. However, three trials with 1343 participants compared clipping to shaving and showed significantly more SSIs associated with shaving (RR 2.09, 95% CI 1.15–3.80). Thus, the authors concluded that when it is necessary to remove hair, clippers are associated with fewer SSIs than razors [44].

1.3.3 Venous Thromboembolic Prophylaxis

Patients undergoing surgery are at risk for developing deep venous thrombosis (DVT) following surgery. Several factors make patients prone to develop DVT including prolonged stasis during the procedure and possibly postoperatively if the patient cannot or does not ambulate and increased coagulability. It is estimated that between 15% and 30% of patients having a general surgical procedure will develop asymptomatic DVTs in the absence of prophylaxis [44–47]. The more sinister complication, pulmonary embolism, is said to occur in 1–3% of patients [48]. Factors which further increase the risk include age, obesity, history of varicose veins and thromboembolism, cancer diagnosis, inflammatory bowel disease, and medications including hormone replacement.

In 1975, a randomized controlled trial demonstrated that low-dose heparin significantly reduced the rates of asymptomatic DVT, symptomatic DVT, and fatal PE [48]. Since then, hundreds of randomized controlled trials, meta-analyses, systematic reviews, and guidelines on thromboprophylaxis in major abdominal general surgery have been published [45–47]. Despite the overwhelming evidence that thromboprophylaxis is an essential component of the postoperative care of general surgery patients, there is evidence that prophylaxis is not used as consistently as recommended nor as often as surgeons think it is being used in their patients. An audit of 123,000 patients hospitalized in the United States found that the majority received no prophylaxis [49]. Among general surgical patients, 78% received no prophylaxis, and 83% did not receive a prophylaxis option recommended by the sixth American College of Chest Physicians (ACCP) Consensus Guidelines on the Prevention of Venous Thromboembolism [49].

There are a number of options for decreasing the risk including intermittent pneumatic compression, low dose unfractionated, and low-molecular heparin. Which intervention is chosen depends on the risk of developing a VTE. In addition, all patients having surgery should be encouraged to ambulate as soon after surgery as possible and frequently thereafter. Thromboprophylaxis is not required in low-risk patients (<0.5%). This includes all patients having outpatient surgery and minor procedures such as anorectal procedures, inguinal hernia repairs, and laparoscopic cholecystectomy, unless patients have other risk factors. In addition, patients having breast procedures do not require prophylaxis and, in fact, should not receive prophylaxis unless there are other risk factors because of the risk of wound hematomas [46, 47].

Other general surgery patients having elective or emergency abdominal surgery, whether it is performed open or laparoscopically and their disease is benign or malignant and are at moderate risk (3%), should receive low-molecular-weight heparin, unfractionated heparin, or mechanical prophylaxis with intermittent pneumatic compression. For individuals receiving unfractionated or low-molecular heparin, thromboprophylaxis should be started preoperatively at the time of the "time out" and continued until discharge. This recommendation is based on evidence from numerous RCTs and meta-analyses in patients undergoing major abdominal surgery over a 40-year period which have demonstrated a consistent 70% or greater relative risk reduction in DVT as well as a similar decrease in PE [46, 47].

While most patients should receive a preoperative dose of heparin, the American Society of Regional Anaesthesia and Pain Medicine (ASRA) guidelines recommend delaying administration of prophylaxis for 6–8 h (post-insertion of an epidural catheter) [50]. The ASRA also recommends that VTE prophylaxis may be given 2 h after removal of an epidural catheter. In obese patients, in whom the BMI is less than 50, the above recommendations can be followed. However, for individuals with a BMI greater than 50, the dose should be increased. There is no Level 1 evidence on the effectiveness of thromboprophylaxis in bariatric surgery. However, the American Society for Metabolic and Bariatric Surgery recommends that perioperative thromboprophylaxis should be given [51]. Furthermore, indirect evidence suggests that dosing should be weight based. In patients with renal dysfunction, dose modification also is required.

Patients with cancer undergoing major abdominal or pelvic surgery and are at high risk (6%) should receive unfractionated or low-molecular heparin plus mechanical prophylaxis. In addition, there is evidence that asymptomatic DVT can be reduced by extending prophylaxis to about 1 month after surgery [50].

Editors' Comments

- The preparation of the patient for the day of surgery has undergone significant changes during the last several years and since we were in training. The implementation of ERAS pathways has dramatically affected the way patients are educated for what expects them in the perioperative period; additionally, the way that fluids and pain medications (NSAIDS and opiates) are managed perioperatively has determined a significant reduction in length of stay and faster return to regular activities of daily living.
- Several calculators are in existence to help the medical practitioner estimate risk preoperatively. These apply to the overall risk of the surgical intervention (ACS-SQIP risk calculator: https://riskcalculator.facs.org/RiskCalculator/), to potential risk of developing a DVT in the perioperative period (Caprini risk score: http://venousdisease.com/dvt-risk-assessment-online/).

- Pain management continues to evolve, and many studies have now identified how useful NSAIDS (acetaminophen, ibuprofen, celecoxib) and gabapentinoids can be in decreasing opioids utilization and overall pain scores, when started preoperatively.

Selected Readings

Choosing Wisely. http://www.choosingwisely.org/.

Thomsen T, Villebro N, Møller AM. Interventions for preoperative smoking cessation. Cochrane Database Syst Rev. 2014;3:CD002294.

Hathaway D. Effect of preoperative instruction on postoperative outcomes: a meta-analysis. Nurs Res. 1986;35:269–75.

McLeod RS, Aarts MA, Chung F, Eskicioglu C, Forbes SS, Conn LG, McCluskey S, McKenzie M, Morningstar B, Nadler A, Okrainec A, Pearsall EA, Sawyer J, Siddiqui N, Wood T. Development of an enhanced recovery after surgery guideline and implementation strategy base on the knowledge-to-action cycle. Ann Surg. 2015;262:1016–25.

References

1. Choosing Wisely. http://www.choosingwisely.org/.
2. Zargar-Shoshtari K, Hill AG. Optimization of perioperative care for colonic surgery: a review of the evidence. ANZ J Surg. 2008;78(1–2):13–23.
3. Kiecolt-Glaser JK, Page GG, Marucha PT, MacCallum RC, Glaser R. Psychological influences on surgical recovery: perspectives from psychoneuroimmunology. Am Psychol. 1998;53(11):1209–18.
4. Devine EC. Effects of psychoeducational care for adult surgical patients: a meta-analysis of 191 studies. Patient Educ Couns. 1992;19(2):129–42.
5. Hathaway D. Effect of preoperative instruction on postoperative outcomes: a meta-analysis. Nurs Res. 1986;35:269–75.
6. Sibbern T, Bull Sellevold V, Steindal SA, Dale C, Watt-Watson J, Dihle A. Patients' experiences of enhanced recovery after surgery: a systematic review of qualitative studies. J Clin Nurs. 2017;26(9–10):1172–88.
7. Weimann A, Braga M, Carli F, Higashiguchi T, Hübner M, Klek S, Laviano A, Ljungqvist O, Lobo DN, Martindale R, Waitzberg DL, Bischoff SC, Singer P. ESPEN guideline: clinical nutrition in surgery. Clin Nutr. 2017;36(3):623–50.
8. Burden S, Todd C, Hill J, Lal S. Pre-operative nutrition support in patients undergoing gastrointestinal surgery. Cochrane Database Syst Rev. 2012;11:CD008879.
9. Karateke F, Ikiz GZ, Kuvvetli A, Menekse E, Das K, Ozyazici S, Atalay BG, Ozdogan M. Evaluation of nutritional risk screening-2002 and subjective global assessment for general surgery patients: a prospective study. J Pak Med Assoc. 2013;63(11):1405–8.
10. Association of Anaesthetists of Great Britain and Ireland. Peri-operative management of the surgical patient with diabetes 2015. Anaesthesia. 2015;70:1427–40.
11. Thomsen T, Villebro N, Møller AM. Interventions for preoperative smoking cessation. Cochrane Database Syst Rev. 2014;3:CD002294.
12. Santa Mina D, Clarke H, Ritvo P, et al. Effect of total-body prehabilitation on postoperative outcomes: a systematic review and meta-analysis. Physiotherapy. 2014;100(3):196–207.
13. Moran J, Guinan E, McCormick P, Larkin J, Mockler D, Hussey J, Moriarty J, Wilson F. The ability of prehabilitation to influence postoperative outcome after intra-abdominal operation: a systematic review and meta-analysis. Surgery. 2016;160(5):1189–201.
14. Loojaard SM, Slee-Valentijn MS, Otten RH, Maier AB. Physical and nutritional prehabilitation in older patients with colorectal carcinoma: a systematic review. J Geriatr Phys Ther. 2017. https://doi.org/10.1519/JPT.0000000000000125.
15. de Benoist B, McLean E, Egli I, editors. Worldwide prevalence of anaemia 1993–2005: WHO global database on anaemia. Geneva: World Health Organization; 2008.
16. WHO. Haemoglobin concentrations for the diagnosis of anaemia and assessment of severity. Vitamin and mineral nutrition information system. Geneva: World Health Organization; 2011. http://www.who.int/vmnis/indicators/haemoglobin.
17. Dunne JR, Malone D, Tracy JK, Gannon C, Napolitano LM. Perioperative anemia: an independent risk factor for infection, mortality, and resource utilization in surgery. J Surg Res. 2002;102(2):237–44.
18. Hill GE, Frawley WH, Griffith KE, Forestner JE, Minei JP. Allogeneic blood transfusion increases the risk of postoperative bacterial infection: a meta-analysis. J Trauma. 2003;54(5):908–14.
19. Devon KM, McLeod RS. Pre and peri-operative erythropoeitin for reducing allogeneic blood transfusions in colorectal cancer surgery. Cochrane Database Syst Rev. 2009;1:CD007148.
20. Lidder PG, Sanders G, Whitehead E, Douie WJ, Mellor N, Lewis SJ, Hosie KB. Pre-operative oral iron supplementation reduces blood transfusion in colorectal surgery - a prospective, randomised, controlled trial. Ann R Coll Surg Engl. 2007;89(4):418–21.
21. Edwards TJ, Noble EJ, Durran A, Mellor N, Hosie KB. Randomized clinical trial of preoperative intravenous iron sucrose to reduce blood transfusion in anaemic patients after colorectal cancer surgery. Br J Surg. 2009;96(10):1122–8.
22. Henry DA, Moxey AJ, O'Connell D, Brown T, Fergusson DA, Carless PA. Pre-operative autologous donation for minimising perioperative alloge-

neic blood transfusion. Cochrane Database Syst Rev. 2010;1:CD001888.
23. Slim K, Vicaut E, Launay-Savary M, Contant C, Chipponi J. Updated systematic review and meta-analysis of randomized clinical trials on the role of mechanical bowel preparation before colorectal surgery. Ann Surg. 2009;249(2):203–9.
24. World Health Organization. Global guideline on the prevention of surgical site infection, November 2016. http://www.who.int/gpsc/ssi-prevention-guidelines/en/.
25. Salvadalena G, Hendren S, McKenna L, Muldoon R, Netsch D, Paquette I, Pittman J, Ramundo J, Steinberg G. WOCN society and ASCRS position statement on preoperative stoma site marking for patients undergoing colostomy or ileostomy surgery. J Wound Ostomy Continence Nurs. 2015;42(3):249–52.
26. Miller D, Pearsall E, Johnston D, Frecea M, McKenzie M. Ontario provincial ERAS enterostomal therapy nurse network. Executive summary: enhanced recovery after surgery: best practice guideline for care of patients with a fecal diversion. J Wound Ostomy Continence Nurs. 2017;44(1):74–7.
27. Merchant R, Chartrand D, Dain S, Dobson G, Kurrek MM, Lagace A, Stacey S, Thiessen B, Canadian Anaesthesiologists Society. Guidelines to the practice of anaesthesia-revised edition 2015. Can J Anaesth. 2015;62:54–67.
28. Smith I, Kranke P, Murat I, Smith A, O'Sullivan G, Soreide E, Spies C, In't Vedl B, European Society of Anaesthesiology. Perioperative fasting in adults and children: guidelines from the European Society of Anaesthesiology. Eur J Anaesthesiol. 2011;28:556–69.
29. American Society of Anaesthesiologists. Practice guidelines for preoperative fasting and the use of pharmacologic agents to reduce the risk of pulmonary aspiration: application to healthy patients undergoing elective procedures: updated report. Anesthesiology. 2011;114:495–511.
30. Brady MC, Kinn S, Stuart P, Ness V. Preoperative fasting for adults to prevent perioperative complications. The Cochrane Collab. 2003;4:CD004423.
31. Tryba M, Zenz M, Mlasowsky B, Huchzermeyer H. Does stomach tube enhance regurgitation during general anaesthesia? Anaesthesist. 1983;32:407–9.
32. Plourde G, Hardy JF. Aspiration pneumonia: assessing the risk of regurgitation in the cat. Can Anaesth Soc J. 1986;33:345–8.
33. Pre-operative carbohydrate loading or hydration: a review of clinical and cost-effectiveness, and guidelines. Ottawa: Canadian Agency for Drugs and Technologies in Health; 2016. Available from https://www.ncbi.nlm.nih.gov/books/NBK362272/.
34. Gustafsson UO, Nygren J, Thorell A, Soop M, Hellström PM, Ljungqvist O, Hagström-Toft E. Pre-operative carbohydrate loading may be used in type 2 diabetes patients. Acta Anaesthesiol Scand. 2008;52:946–51.
35. Haynes AB, Weiser TG, Berry WR, Lipsitz SR, Breizat AH, Dellinger EP, Herbosa T, Joseph S, Kibatala PL, Lapitan MC, Merry AF, Moorthy K, Reznick RK, Taylor B, Gawande AA, Safe Surgery Saves Lives Study Group. A surgical safety checklist to reduce morbidity and mortality in a global population. N Engl J Med. 2009;360(5):491–9.
36. Urbach DR, Govindarajan A, Saskin R, Wilton AS, Baxter NN. Introduction of surgical safety checklists in Ontario, Canada. N Engl J Med. 2014;370(11):1029–38.
37. Haynes AB, Weiser TG, Berry WR, Lipsitz SR, Breizat AH, Dellinger EP, Dziekan G, Herbosa T, Kibatala PL, Lapitan MC, Merry AF, Reznick RK, Taylor B, Vats A, Gawande AA, Safe Surgery Saves Lives Study Group. Changes in safety attitude and relationship to decreased postoperative morbidity and mortality following implementation of a checklist-based surgical safety intervention. BMJ Qual Saf. 2011;20(1):102–7.
38. Umscheid CA, Mitchell MD, Doshi JA, Agarwal R, Williams K, Brennan PJ. Estimating the proportion of healthcare-associated infections that are reasonably preventable and the related mortality and costs. Infect Control Hosp Epidemiol. 2011;32(2):101–14.
39. Noorani A, Rabey N, Walsh SR, Davies RJ. Systematic review and meta-analysis of preoperative antisepsis with chlorhexidine versus povidone-iodine in clean-contaminated surgery. Br J Surg. 2010;97(11):1614–20.
40. Darouiche RO, Wall MJ Jr, Itani KM, Otterson MF, Webb AL, Carrick MM, Miller HJ, Awad SS, Crosby CT, Mosier MC, Alsharif A, Berger DH. Chlorhexidine-alcohol versus povidone-iodine for surgical-site antisepsis. N Engl J Med. 2010;362(1):18–26.
41. Hypothermia: prevention and management in adults having surgery Clinical guideline [CG65]: National Institutes for Health and Care Excellence; 2008.
42. Forbes SS, Eskicioglu C, Nathens AB, Fenech DS, Laflamme C, McLean RF, McLeod RS, Best Practice in General Surgery Committee, University of Toronto. Evidence-based guidelines for prevention of perioperative hypothermia. J Am Coll Surg. 2009;209(4):492–503.e1.
43. Madrid E, Urrútia G, Roqué i Figuls M, Pardo-Hernandez H, Campos JM, Paniagua P, Maestre L, Alonso-Coello P. Active body surface warming systems for preventing complications caused by inadvertent perioperative hypothermia in adults. Cochrane Database Syst Rev. 2016;4:CD009016.
44. Tanner J, Norrie P, Melen K. Preoperative hair removal to reduce surgical site infection. Cochrane Database Syst Rev. 2011;11:CD004122.
45. Geerts WH, Pineo GF, Heit JA, et al. Prevention of venous thromboembolism: the seventh ACCP conference on antithrombotic and thrombolytic therapy. Chest. 2004;126(3 Suppl):338S–400S.
46. Geerts WH, Bergqvist D, Pineo GF, et al. Prevention of venous thromboembolism: American college of chest

physicians evidence-based clinical practice guidelines (8th edition). Chest. 2008;133(6 Suppl):381S–453S.
47. Douketis JD, Spyropoulos AC, Spencer FA, Mayr M, Jaffer AK, Eckman MH, Dunn AS, Kunz R. Perioperative management of antithrombotic therapy: antithrombotic therapy and prevention of thrombosis, 9th ed: American college of chest physicians evidence-based clinical practice guidelines. Chest. 2012;141(2 Suppl):e326S–50S.
48. Kakkar VV, Corrigan TP, Fossard DP. Prevention of fatal postoperative pulmonary embolism by low doses of heparin. Lancet. 1975;2:45–51.
49. Yu HT, Dylan ML, Lin J, Dubois RW. Hospital's compliance with prophylaxis guidelines for venous thromboembolism. Am J Health Syst Pharm. 2007;64:69–76.
50. Horlocker TT, Wedel DJ, Rowlingson JC, Enneking FK, Kopp SL, Benzon HT, Brown DL, Heit JA, Mulroy MF, Rosenquist RW, Tryba M, Yuan CS. Regional anesthesia in the patient receiving antithrombotic or thrombolytic therapy: American society of regional anesthesia and pain medicine evidence-based guidelines (3rd edition). Reg Anesth Pain Med. 2010;35(1):64–101.
51. ASMBS. Prophlyactic measures to reduce the risk of venous thromboembolism in bariatric surgery patients. Surg Obes Relat Dis. 2007;3:494.

Fundamentals of Operating Room Setup and Surgical Instrumentation

2

Katerina Dukleska, Allison A. Aka, Adam P. Johnson, and Karen A. Chojnacki

2.1 Introduction

Caring for a patient in the operating room requires an integrated system of healthcare professionals with the primary goal to safely bring the patient through a surgical procedure. This is a principle that is initiated in the preoperative setting and is carried through the operation and to the postoperative setting. The goal of this chapter is to introduce the reader to basic information about the operating room and the operating team. We will also discuss fundamental concepts and the proper use of equipment related to open, laparoscopic, and endoscopic surgery.

2.1.1 Introduction to the Operating Room Team

The operating room (OR) is one of the most dynamic locations in a hospital. Those who enter into this atmosphere must be well trained and prepared for any potential emergent situation that may arise. The main OR team is made up of physicians, nurses, and technicians who all play essential roles in order to achieve a safe and efficient operation for the patient. However, it is important to remember that there are a number of other staff that support the flow of the OR, including those responsible for sterilizing equipment, the environmental staff, etc. The focus in this section will be to provide an overview of the staff in the OR and to define the sterile field.

2.1.1.1 Sterile Versus Non-sterile Members of the OR Team

In general, team members who are sterile during an operation include:

1. The surgeon who will be performing the procedure, along with his or her assistants. These assistants could be residents, physician's assistants, medical students, or nurse practitioners.
2. The scrub nurse or scrub technician who is in charge of the sterile instruments.

The non-sterile group includes:

1. The anesthesia team, made up of an anesthesiologist who may be supervising a resident or certified registered nurse anesthetist. They are responsible for airway management and intraoperative life support.
2. A circulating nurse who oversees OR documentation, obtaining needed equipment, and overall nursing care for the patient undergoing the procedure.

K. Dukleska · A. A. Aka · A. P. Johnson
K. A. Chojnacki (✉)
Department of Surgery, Sidney Kimmel Medical College, Thomas Jefferson University, Philadelphia, PA, USA
e-mail: Karen.Chojnacki@jefferson.edu

F. Palazzo (ed.), *Fundamentals of General Surgery*, https://doi.org/10.1007/978-3-319-75656-1_2

2.1.1.2 The Sterile Field

The importance of a sterile field is paramount, as it prevents surgical site infections. Multiple steps are utilized in an effort to minimize surgical site infections, including patient evaluation and their overall risk, sterilization of OR instruments, environmental cleaning, the use of antibiotic prophylaxis, and the use of aseptic technique. The goal of aseptic technique is to minimize pathogenic contamination by isolating the operative field from the non-sterile environment. Once properly gowned and gloved, or "scrubbed," a sterile OR team member is theoretically void of pathogen colonization. Furthermore, sterile surgical drapes are used to establish an aseptic barrier to minimize the passage of pathogens from the non-sterile areas of the operating room. Only individuals that are "scrubbed" can handle the sterile drapes, which should not be rearranged once placed. Only the top of the draped area is considered sterile. Similarly, instruments that are opened onto the sterile field are done so by methods that maintain sterility. All members of the operative team are tasked with maintaining the sterile field. If contamination is identified, it is everyone's duty to speak up and identify appropriate actions to maintain sterility [1, 2].

2.1.2 Introduction to Operating Room Equipment

The basic physical layout of the OR is dependent on the specific requirements of the operation at hand. There are common components that are present in essentially all instances. These include the OR table, anesthesia machine for the provision of oxygen and inhaled anesthesia, intraoperative hemodynamic monitors, illumination, electrocautery, suction, back table, Mayo stand, kick bucket, instrumentation, etc. (Fig. 2.1). The setup of all of these components is driven by the requirements for patient positioning and need for any additional specialized equipment.

2.1.2.1 Anesthesia Setup

The anesthesia machine and anesthesia team are typically positioned at the head of the OR table. This allows for the team to have an unobstructed view of the patient's airway, easy access to the anesthesia machine, access to monitoring equipment, etc. The determination on the type of anesthesia is highly case specific, and the anesthetic plan should be discussed preoperatively.

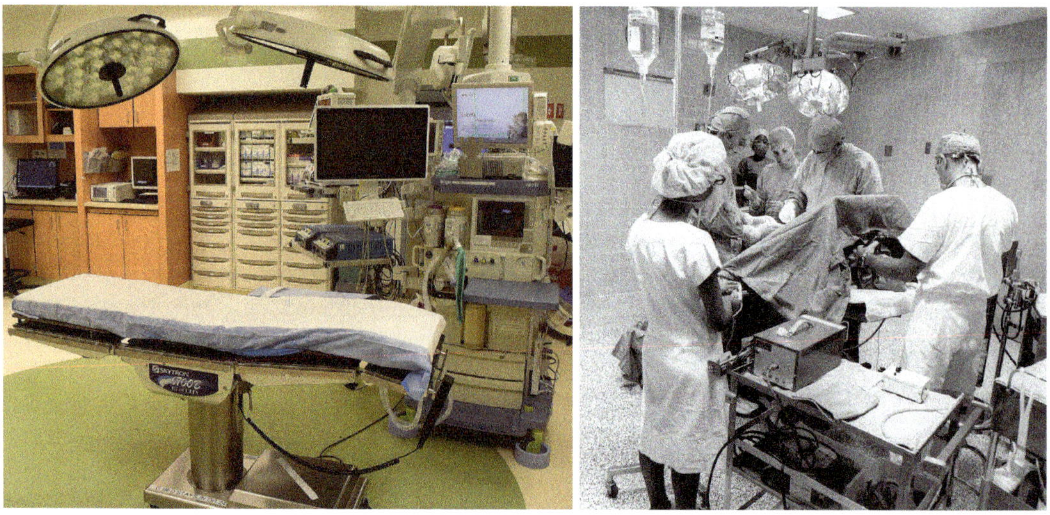

Fig. 2.1 Typical OR components include OR table, light sources, anesthesia machine, etc. A historical picture from the 1960s shows that some of the equipment in the OR hasn't changed

2.1.2.2 Operating Room Table

Upon entry into the OR room, patients typically start in a supine position and are safely secured to the OR table with arms extended, thus allowing the anesthesia team to then safely secure the airway. For operations that are long and require specialized patient positioning, knowledge of how to maneuver the OR table is essential. Moreover, the OR table can be broken into modular parts, and additional extensions can be added as needed. In the event of the need to use specialized equipment, such as X-ray or fluoroscopy during an operation, it is important to understand the location of the bed stand. For example, when fluoroscopy is used for intraoperative cholangiography, it is oftentimes necessary to flip the bed in the opposite direction. This allows for the bottom hand of the C-arm to safely be placed under the bed to allow the surgeon to maneuver the patient and C-arm in order to successfully perform a cholangiogram (Fig. 2.2). Some OR tables have the ability to be automatically adjusted where they can slide up or down on the base of the bed. This is another way to successfully perform cholangiography without having to change the direction of the bed.

It is important to be mindful where the base of the bed is for all operations, especially in instances as mentioned above or in foregut or colorectal procedures. For example, for laparoscopic foregut surgery, such as during laparoscopic paraesophageal hernia repair, the patient is typically placed in a lithotomy position, and the operating surgeon stands in between the patient's legs. Therefore, it is imperative to be mindful of the location of the base of the OR table so as to not interfere with the operation at hand.

After successful induction of anesthesia, it is essential to further position the patient safely and appropriately for the specific case at hand. General principles to keep in mind while positioning a patient include:

- Avoiding hyperextension of the arms to avoid brachial plexus injury
- Care when positioning the patient in lithotomy to avoid peroneal nerve injury
- Adequately securing the patient to the bed when extreme table positions are expected, such as in bariatric or some laparoscopic cases

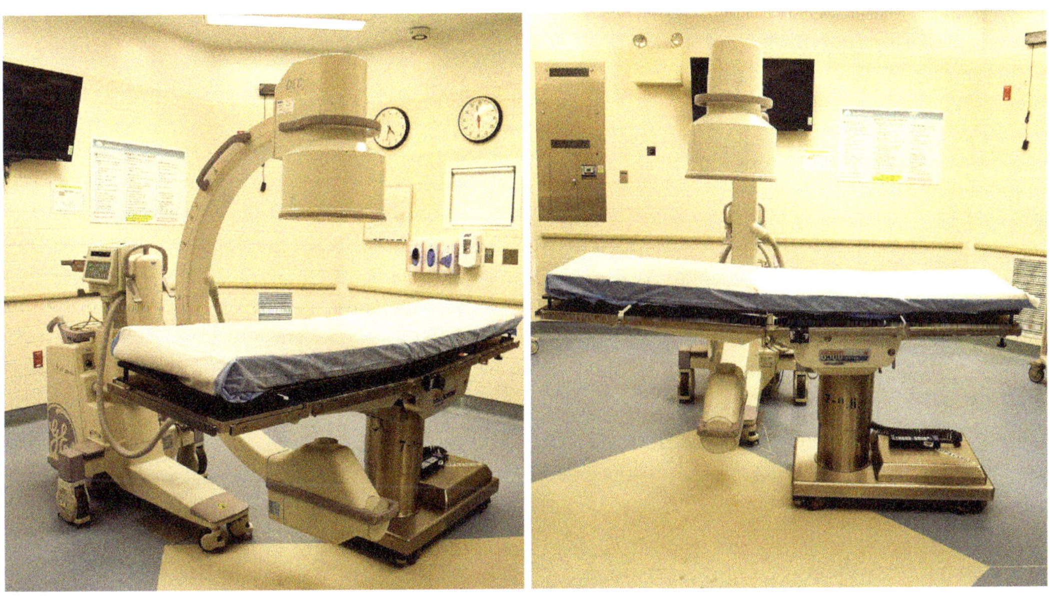

Fig. 2.2 Positioning of the OR table base in relation to how the C-arm is positioned for a laparoscopic cholecystectomy. Note the base of the OR bed does not obstruct the bottom of the C-arm and allows the movement of the equipment to be unobstructed

More specific details regarding patient positioning can be found in the *Fundamentals of Patient Positioning and Skin Prep* chapter (Chap. 4).

2.1.2.3 Electrosurgical and Powered Devices

Most operating rooms are equipped with electrosurgical devices and other powered devices. Care should be taken to avoid injury to the patient and staff when using this equipment.

The most commonly utilized electrosurgical device in the OR is the "electrocautery" device, commonly known as the Bovie. Electrosurgical units work by generating heat and vaporization of intracellular contents, which results in coagulation and hemostasis. The Bovie requires close supervision since it has been associated with patient injury and even surgical fires. This risk increases when alcohol-based skin preparation products are used or the dispersive electrode is not appropriately placed. The purpose of the dispersive electrode is to ground the patient, and it should be attached on dry, hairless skin on a location over large muscle mass (e.g., patient's thigh) and not be adjacent to metal. More details on energy devices in the operating room can be found in the *Fundamentals of Energy Utilization in the Operating Room* in (Chapter 9).

Powered devices include drills and powered saws. For example, when performing lower extremity amputations, the bone saw is commonly used. These devices must be very carefully used so as to avoid injury to the patient or staff. Powered saws and drills aerosolize body fluids; therefore, one must be cautious and wear appropriate personal protective equipment to minimize potential infectious exposure.

2.1.2.4 Additional OR Components

During the operation, the sterile instruments that are required for the case are stored on the back table. The Mayo stand is an extension of the back table. The surgical scrub utilizes the Mayo stand to place instruments and equipment commonly used during the operation at hand for easy and quick access. The kick bucket is used to place soiled lap pads and to remove them from the sterile field.

Illumination during surgery is provided by overall illumination, which is generally attached to the OR ceiling to allow for movement of the overhead lights. This allows for the lights to be adjusted during the procedure.

2.1.2.5 Specialized Equipment

The ability to perform certain cases in an OR may require specialized equipment. For example, it is important to have equipment specifically tailored to laparoscopic surgery as such components may not typically be part of every OR. The operation at hand will guide the team in determining what needs to be available.

Additional specialized equipment includes an endoscopy tower when it is required intraoperatively. The location of the endoscopy tower will depend on what it will be used for (i.e., EGD versus colonoscopy) and the patient's positioning. For example, when performing an EGD as in the case for a percutaneous endoscopic gastrostomy tube, the endoscopy tower should be located on the operating surgeon's right side.

When the use of the C-arm is necessary, as in during intraoperative cholangiography, in the beginning of the procedure, it should be located at the patient's feet. During the preparation stage, the surgeon should be mindful to securely and safely tuck the patient's right arm and to ensure the bed stand is flipped or the patient is on a sliding bed. This will allow for the C-arm to be placed in the appropriate position in a way that it is not obstructed by the patient or other OR equipment.

2.1.3 Basics of Personal Protective Equipment

The American College of Surgeons released a statement in 2016 regarding appropriate operating room attire [3]. The goal was to balance surgeon comfort, professionalism, and infection control. The following recommendations are most important for those new to the operating room:

- OR scrubs should be changed at least daily.
- OR scrubs should not be worn at any time outside of the hospital perimeter.
- Scrubs and hats worn during dirty or contaminated cases should be changed prior to subsequent cases even if not visibly soiled.
- Masks should not be worn dangling at any time.
- OR scrubs should not be worn in the hospital facility outside of the OR area without a clean lab coat or appropriate cover over them.

The use of personal protective equipment is required not only to prevent contamination of the sterile surgical field but also to protect clinicians from contact with patient bodily fluids [4]. Full sterile attire includes:

- Surgical cap/bouffant—This should be worn at all times in the OR and any other designated areas.
- Surgical mask—Different masks are often available for the OR. Selection of a mask varies based on personal preference and level of risk of airborne pathogens. While wearing a mask, the air flow is directed posteriorly; thus it is not recommended to turn one's back on the sterile field.
- Surgical gown—In order to maintain sterility, gowns are often donned with assistance. They must be properly secured prior to participation in the surgical procedure.
- Eye protection—The eyes are a surgeon's most important tools. Corrective lenses are not sufficient protection without the addition of side guards. Masks with eye shields or disposable visors are highly recommended.

Additional protective equipment possibly utilized in specialized procedures includes:

- Body exhaust suit—A full body suit and hood sometimes used in orthopedic procedures, such as joint replacements.
- Lead gown—The use of lead is highly recommended during procedures that implement ionizing radiation, such as plain X-ray or fluoroscopy.

2.2 Technical Considerations

2.2.1 Basics of Instrumentation and Equipment for Open Operative Technique

Being a successful and efficient surgeon requires training and knowledge about foot positioning, hand movements, and efficient use of instruments. In general, an ergonomic position for open surgery is with the shoulders and elbows relaxed, elbows in a flexed position, and the wrists should not be bent. For most major open abdominal operations, the surgeon stands on the patient's right side; however, this can vary depending on the type of surgery and the required exposure.

There are numerous instruments that are utilized during open surgery to assist with dissection, exposure, and suturing, some of which are highly specialized for certain operations. The appendix of this book includes the most commonly utilized instruments during open surgery along with a description of their proper use and handling.

Personal special equipment, in addition to the personal protective equipment, utilized by surgeons in open surgery includes:

- Headlights provide additional illumination to the operative field, particularly focused within the line of sight of the surgeon. The proper use of a headlight can provide improved visualization, particularly in deep surgical areas, such as the pelvis. Improper positioning or body ergonomics can result in fatigue and injury during lengthy cases; therefore, practice outside of the operating room or with short procedures is recommended prior to prolonged use.
- Surgical magnification can either be achieved via surgeon eyewear (i.e., loupes) or through a free-standing microscope. These are particularly useful for delicate operations or microsurgery that requires fine anastomoses, such as during vascular procedures. Loupes are custom fit to a surgeon's visual acuity and focal

length, and using another surgeon's equipment is not recommended. The use of magnification severely limits a surgeon's peripheral vision and visual field. The surgeon and the OR team need to be aware of these limitations in the surgeon's visual field, especially when passing instruments and sharps (needles and scalpels).

For most open abdominal cases, the patient is positioned on the operating room table in the supine position with both arms out. In addition to the surgeon being on the patient's right, the assistant is located on the patient's left side. In these instances, the scrub assistant is located on the right side along with the surgeon and ensures sterility of the instruments, and the operative field is maintained. For major abdominal cases, the Mayo stand and scrub assistant are generally located to the right of the operating surgeon.

2.2.2 Basics of Setup for Laparoscopic and Robotic Surgery

When positioning a patient for laparoscopic surgery, one has to be mindful of appropriate patient positioning and of ideal positioning of the equipment that will be used. For example, when performing laparoscopic appendectomy, both the surgeon and assistant are located on the patient's left side. This means that the left arm must be safely and securely tucked to allow for two individuals to comfortably stand on the same side. Conversely, when performing a diagnostic laparoscopy and there is an intent to inspect the entire small bowel and large bowel, it is ideal to tuck both arms to allow for any positioning of the surgeon and assistant. For operations that will require extreme patient positions, for example, in morbidly obese patients who undergo a laparoscopic Roux-en-Y gastric bypass, safely securing the patient is of paramount importance in order to avoid any injury. A similar approach needs to be employed during robotic surgery. The surgeon must be mindful of the position of the OR table, the robot itself, and the console.

In regard to the location of the equipment, the monitors should always be placed in a way that they are ergonomic and allow for the surgeon and assistant to have an unobstructed view. When the use of energy devices is necessary, it is important to be mindful of where the equipment is placed. For example, during a laparoscopic cholecystectomy, if using a foot pedal to control the cautery, it needs to be located on the patient's left side where the primary surgeon is located. This equipment should be placed in the appropriate place prior to prepping the patient and establishing the sterile field.

As with open surgery, specialized equipment is required to gain entry into the abdomen along with specific instruments to perform the procedure. The appendix of this book contains information about some general concepts pertinent to laparoscopic surgery and commonly used instruments.

2.3 Future Directions

Surgery is an ever-evolving field with surgical innovation driving development of new equipment and instrumentation. Surgeons are always looking for ways to best utilize the operating room using minimally invasive techniques—laparoscopic, endoscopic, robotic, natural orifice, or hybrid approaches. However, despite this focus on advancing surgery while minimizing trauma to the patient, the fundamental goal of surgery continues to be rooted in its beginnings: to provide safe and effective care to patients.

Take-Home Points

- The operating room is a dynamic environment, and, in order to safely bring the patient through an operation, a team approach is required.
- Understanding of commonly found equipment in the OR and its proper use is important to ensure there is no harm to the patient or staff.
- Maintaining the sterile field is the responsibility of the entire OR team, especially of the "scrubbed" personnel.
- Proper use of instruments for open surgery is necessary to ensure integrity of the tissue that is handled.

- Understanding laparoscopic instruments and their proper use allows for increased efficiency and safety during laparoscopic surgery.
- Surgical endoscopy is becoming increasingly utilized and becoming an integrated component in many general surgical procedures.

OR Instrument Appendix: OR Instruments for Open Surgery

Scalpels (Fig. 2.3)

The scalpel is one of the synonymous instruments that is associated with surgery. Perhaps the most important decision to make prior to using the scalpel is the decision for where the incision will be placed. This should be a deliberate decision with the goal of the operation in mind. Essentially, the location of the incision should allow you to perform the operation safely and should provide you with adequate exposure. In general, reusable scalpels include a handle and blade. First, the blade. It comes in different sizes, with the most common sizes used in surgery being the 10, 11, 15, and rarely the 20 blade. The belly of the blade should be in contact with the surface that is being cut. As a general rule, when making an incision, one always cuts away from oneself or from the nondominant to the dominant side. The handle which safely holds the blade also comes in different sizes. The size of the handle used is dependent on the location where the incision will be made. Of note, some surgeons sometimes use the scalpel for sharp dissection which necessitates the use of a longer handle (as in abdominal cases).

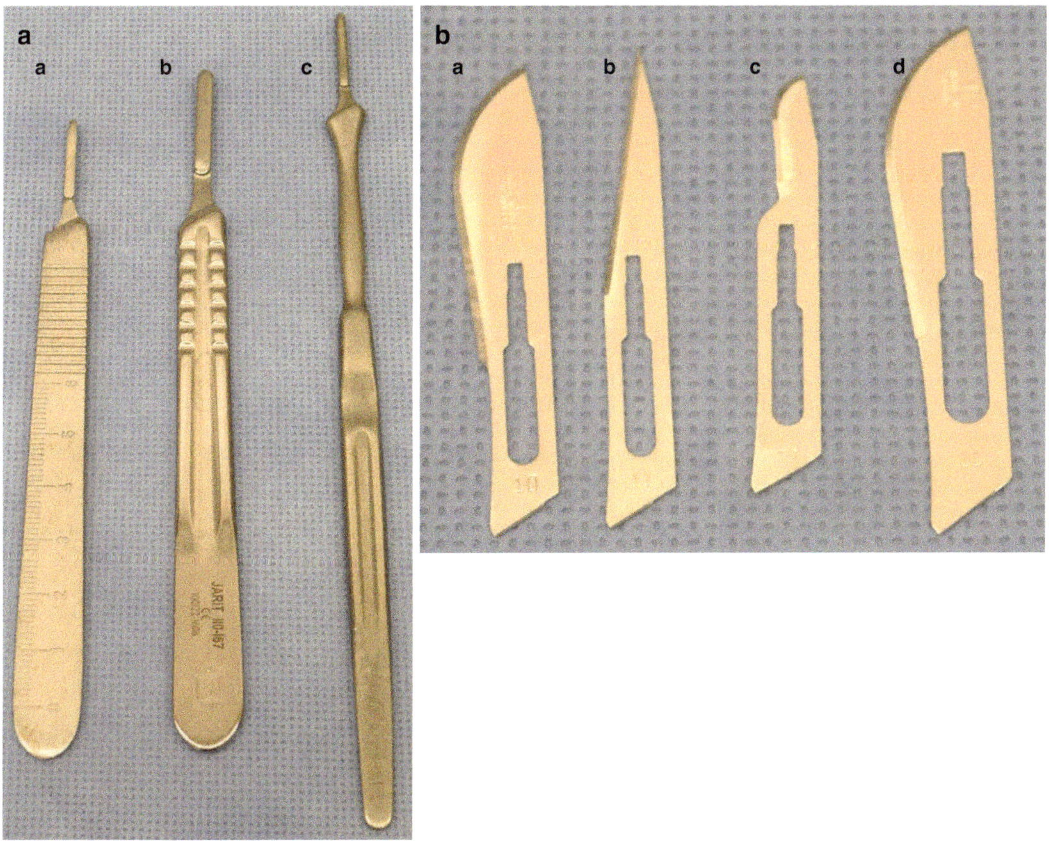

Fig. 2.3 (**a**) *Left to right*, different varieties of knife handles: **A**, Bard-Parker knife handle #3; **B**, Bard-Parker knife handle #4; **C**, Bard-Parker knife handle #7. (**b**) *Left to right*, different varieties of blade numbers: **A**, number 10 blade; **B**, number 11 blade; **C**, number 15 blade; **D**, number 20 blade

Scissors (Figs. 2.4 and 2.5)

Scissors come in multiple varieties, and depending on the type, they are used in various settings. They have a bias for right-handed individuals. When using a scissor, place only about a half of the distal phalanx of your thumb and ring finger, and attempt to use your dominant hand if possible. Scissors used for dissection include the Metzenbaum scissor, which can be used for sharp dissection as in lysis of adhesions. Potts scissors are generally used in vascular surgery to extend

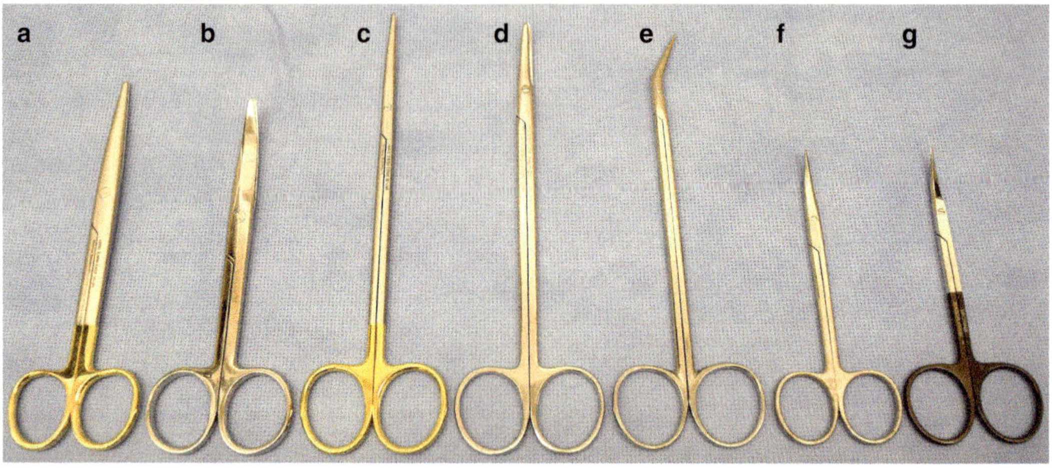

Fig. 2.4 *Left to right*, (**a**) Mayo scissor, straight; (**b**) Mayo scissor, curved; (**c**) Metzenbaum dissecting scissor, straight; (**d**) Metzenbaum dissecting scissor, curved; (**e**) Potts scissor; (**f**) tenotomy scissor; (**g**) Iris scissor

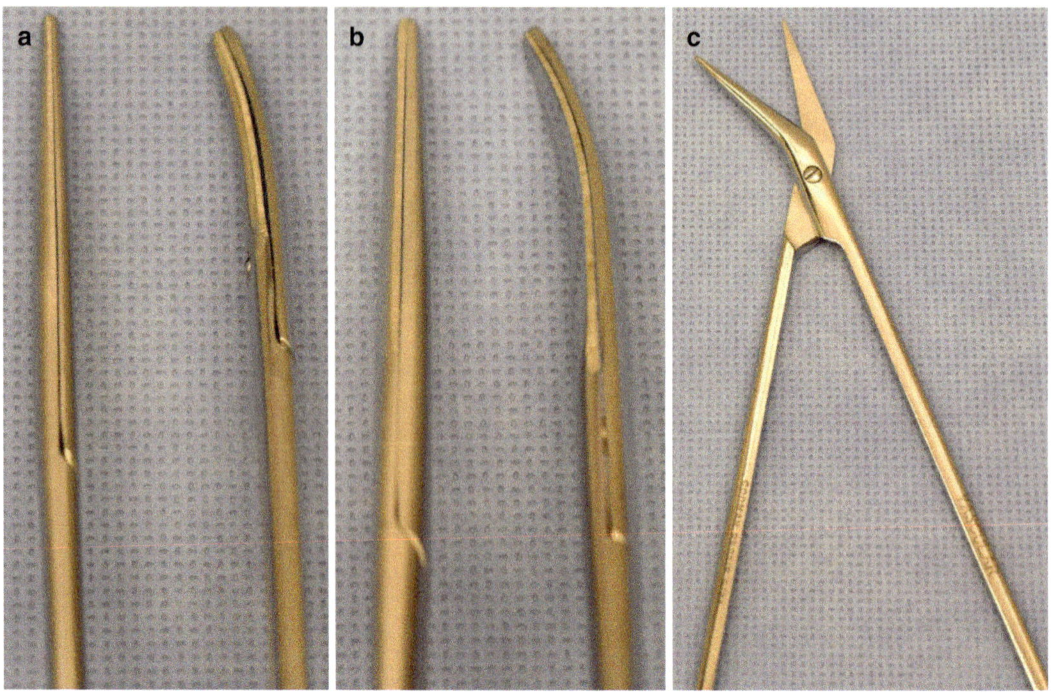

Fig. 2.5 *Left to right*, (**a**) straight versus curved Mayo scissor; (**b**) straight versus curved Metzenbaum scissor; (**c**) Potts scissor, open

the arteriotomy or venotomy. In contract, scissors, such as the straight and curved Mayo, are used for cutting suture or bowel during gastrointestinal anastomoses. One should avoid the use of finer instruments, such as the Metzenbaum scissor, to cut suture as it will dull the instrument.

Forceps (Figs. 2.6 and 2.7)

The general principle for how forceps work is by grasping tissue in between two opposing surfaces. Deciding on which forceps to use depends on the task at hand. In general, forceps come in two varieties, smooth and toothed. Forceps that are smooth cause crushing tissue trauma, and in instances as such, the use of toothed forceps is preferable. An example is when handling skin, toothed Adson forceps are preferred so as to minimize tissue trauma.

Needle Holders (Fig. 2.8)

The type, size, and weight of the needle holder are determined by the needle and suture. For example, larger and heavier needle holders are required for large needles, such as the ones used for fascial closure. Conversely, small needles that are used for vascular anastomoses require finer and lighter needle drivers, such as the Castroviejo. When loading the needle on to the needle holder, it is important to remember that a circular motion requires pronation and supination of the surgeon's wrist. This is necessary in order to prevent tissue trauma at the site of the needle point's entry.

Retractors (Figs. 2.9 and 2.10)

Much like other instruments, retractors come in different varieties, and their use is determined by

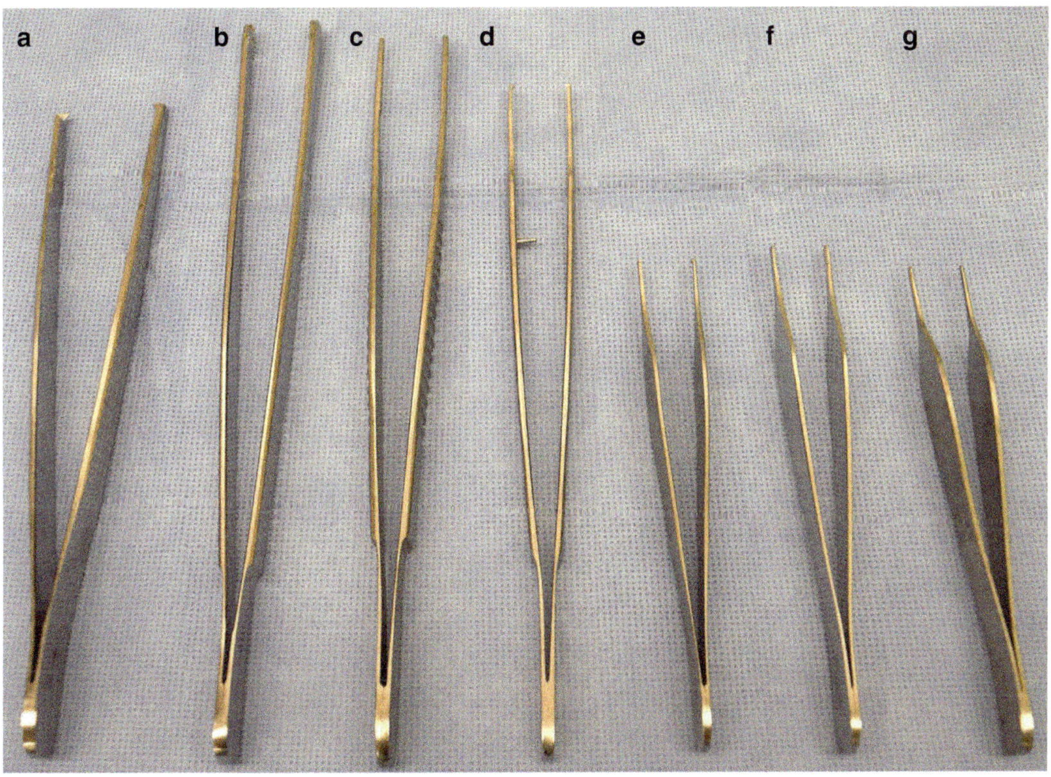

Fig. 2.6 *Left to right*, commonly used tissue forceps or pickups: (**a**) Bonney tissue forceps; (**b**) Russian tissue forceps; (**c**) DeBakey forceps; (**d**) Gerald tissue forceps; (**e**) Adson tissue forceps with teeth; (**f**) Adson tissue forceps without teeth; (**g**) Adson-Brown tissue forceps

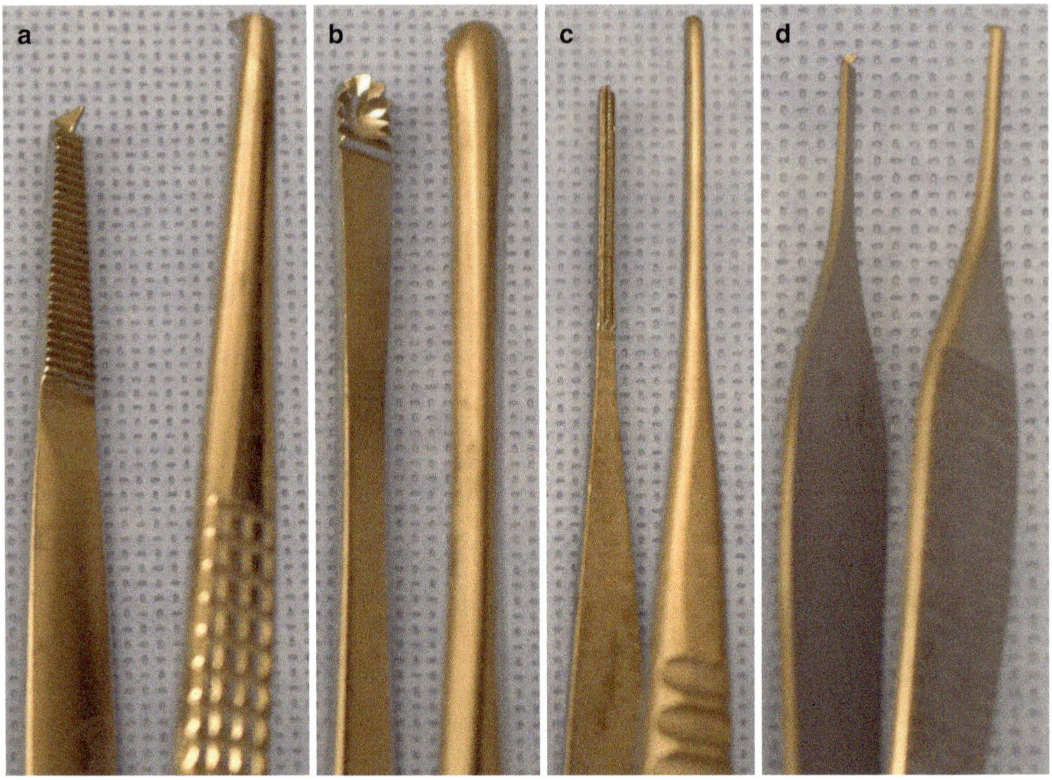

Fig. 2.7 *Left to right*, (**a**) Bonney tissue forceps; (**b**) Russian tissue forceps; (**c**) DeBakey tissue forceps; (**d**) Adson tissue forceps

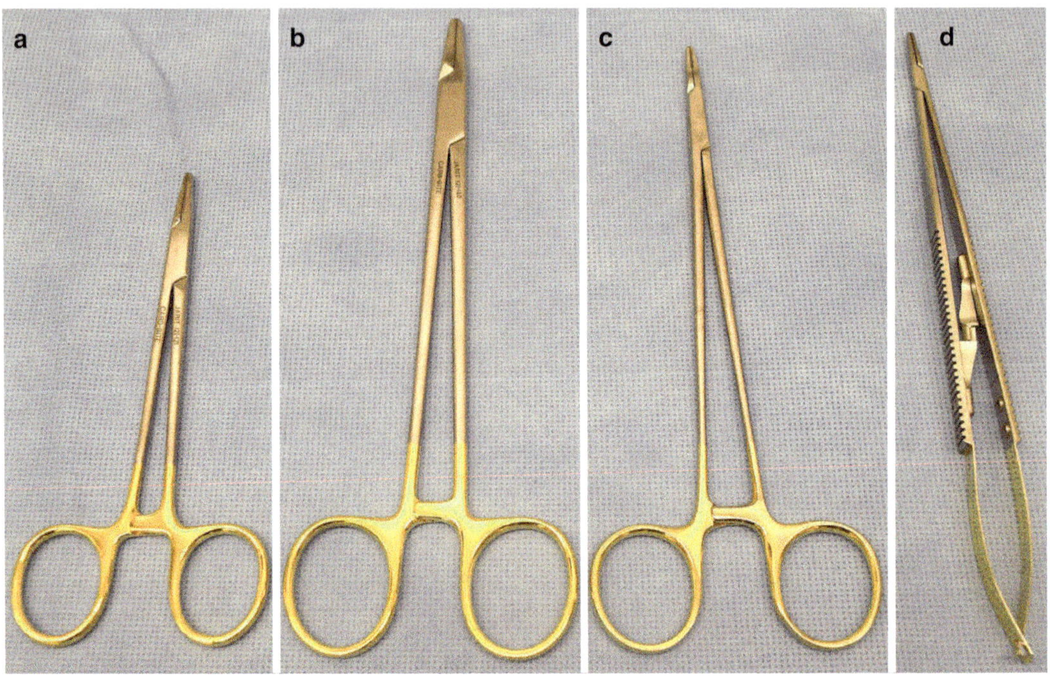

Fig. 2.8 *Left to right*, (**a** and **b**) Mayo-Hegar needle driver, two different sizes; (**c**) Ryder needle driver; (**d**) Castroviejo needle driver

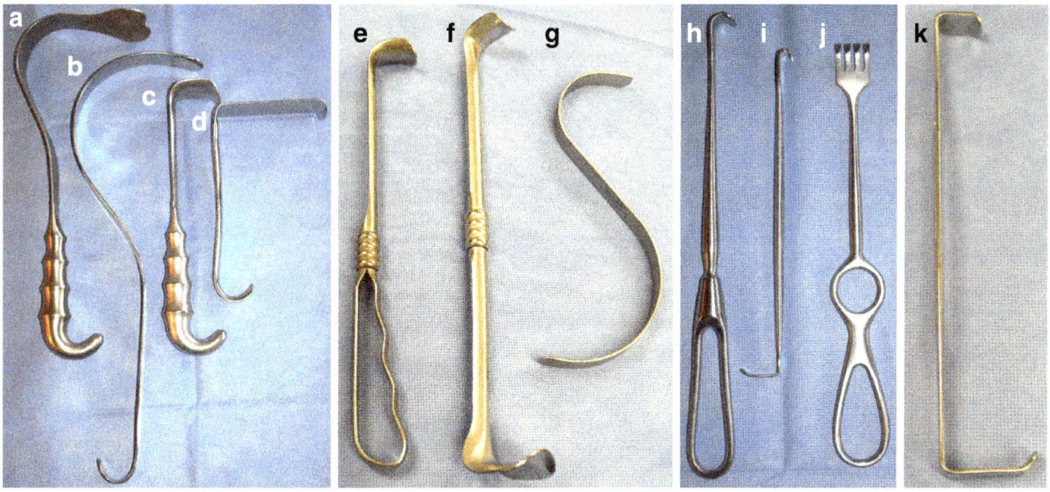

Fig. 2.9 *Left to right*, different varieties of handheld retractors. (**a**) Harrington or Sweetheart retractor, (**b**) Deaver, (**c**) Kelly retractor, (**d**) Eastman, (**e**) Richardson retractor, (**f**) Richardson-Eastman retractor, (**g**) S-retractor, (**h**) Cushing vein retractor, (**i**) Senn retractor, (**j**) Rake retractor, (**k**) Army-Navy

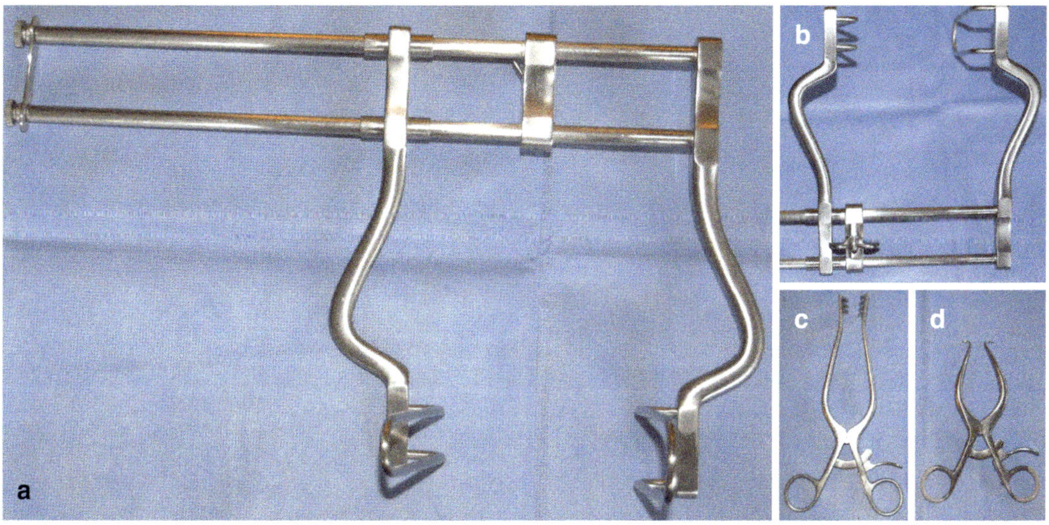

Fig. 2.10 *Left to right*, (**a** and **b**) Balfour self-retraining retractor, (**c**) Weitlaner self-retaining retractor, (**d**) Gelpi

the task at hand. They can be handheld or self-retaining retractors. An example of commonly utilized handheld retractors that are utilized in general surgery include the Army-Navy and Richardson retractors. Similarly, self-retaining retractors, such as the Bookwalter and Balfour, are commonly utilized during large abdominal procedures. There are also smaller self-retaining retractors, such as the Weitlaner, which are used during open procedures, such as an inguinal hernia repair.

Suction (Fig. 2.11)

Visualization of the operative field is important, which is accomplished through the use of suction devices. Sizes of the suction tip depend on the area and type of tissue being worked on. The commonly used Yankauer aspirates through the tip end and is either disposable plastic or reusable metal. A Poole sucker has multiple ports all along the side and is used to quickly aspirate a large

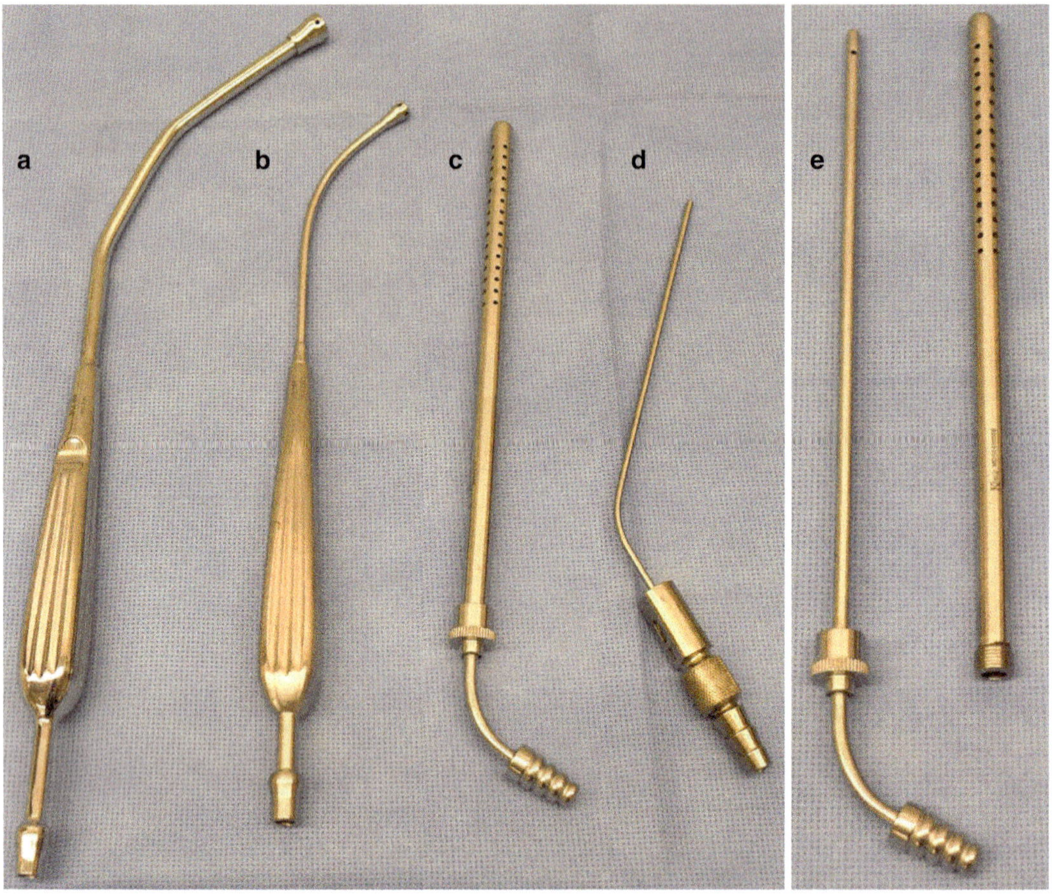

Fig. 2.11 *Left to right*, (**a**) Yankauer suction; (**b**) Andrews suction; (**c**) Poole suction; (**d**) Frazier suction; (**e**) Poole suction broken down into its components

volume of fluid, such as after irrigating the abdominal cavity with liters of saline. Smaller tips include the Andrews or Frazier, usually used in pediatric or vascular cases. Suction on Frazier tips are controlled by a small hole on the handle.

Clamps (Figs. 2.12, 2.13, 2.14, 2.15, 2.16, and 2.17)

Clamps are used to hold objects in place and/or to maintain control of tissue, such as cutting off blood flow to an area of interest. They can be either straight or curved, perforating or non-perforating, fine-tipped for more precise clamping or broad for thicker or more generalized areas, and with or without teeth depending on the power of the grip desired. Tissue type and desired outcome are some of the factors that determine clamp choice. Babcocks are used to grasp bowel firmly while causing the least amount of damage, whereas a Kocher has multiple serrations that allow for strong grasping of fascia.

Basics of Instrumentation and Equipment for Laparoscopic Surgery

Laparoscopic procedures require surgical skills that include dexterity, efficiency, and the ability to operate in a three-dimensional environment

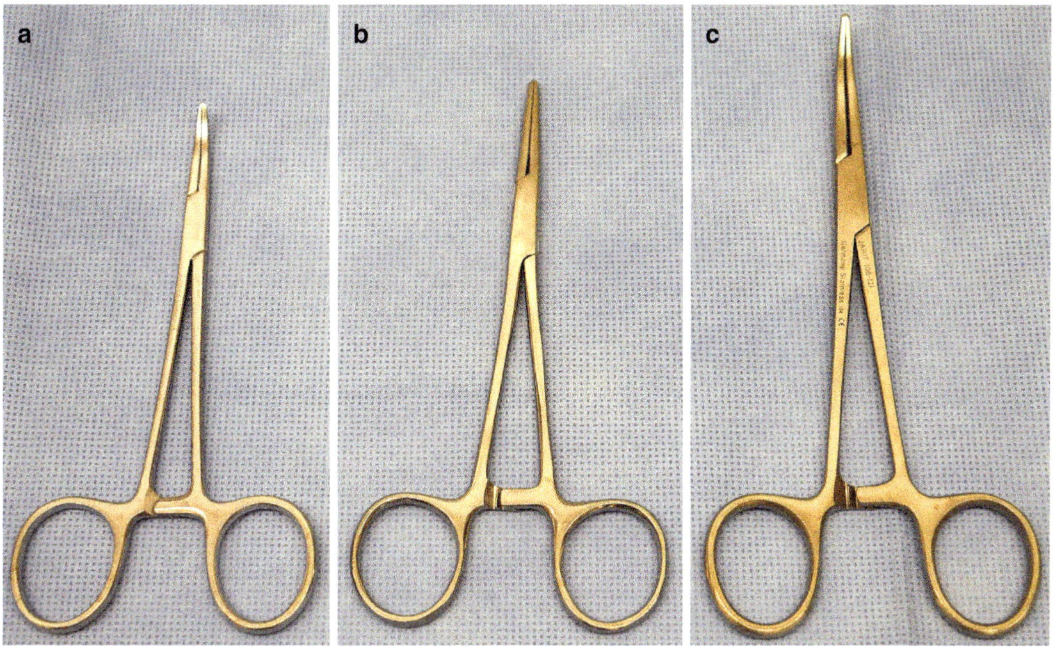

Fig. 2.12 *Left to right*, (**a**) curved Crile; (**b**) straight Crile; (**c**) mosquito

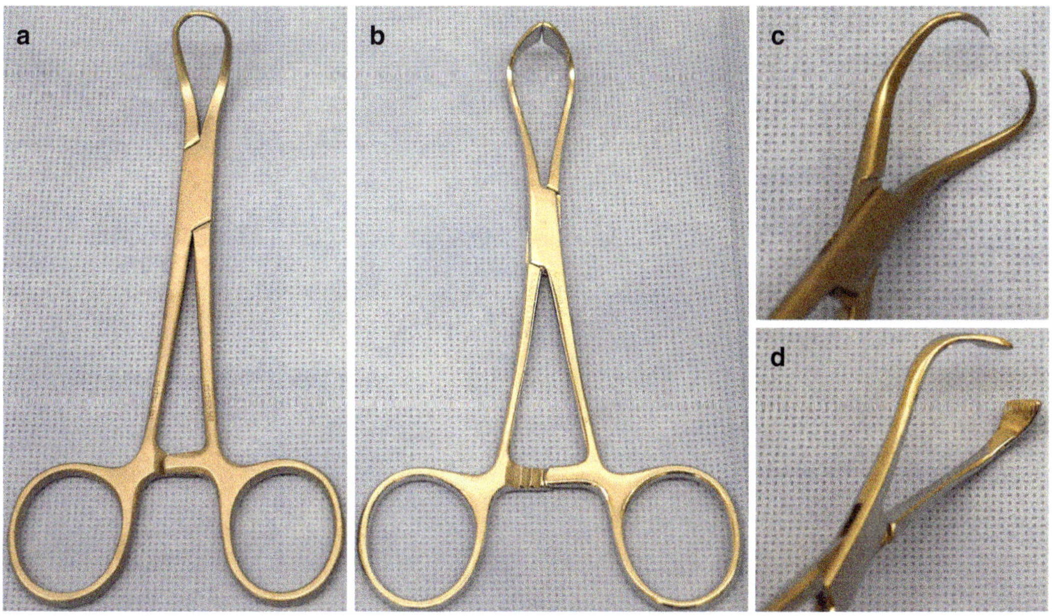

Fig. 2.13 (**a** and **c**) Perforating towel clip; (**b** and **d**) non-perforating towel clip

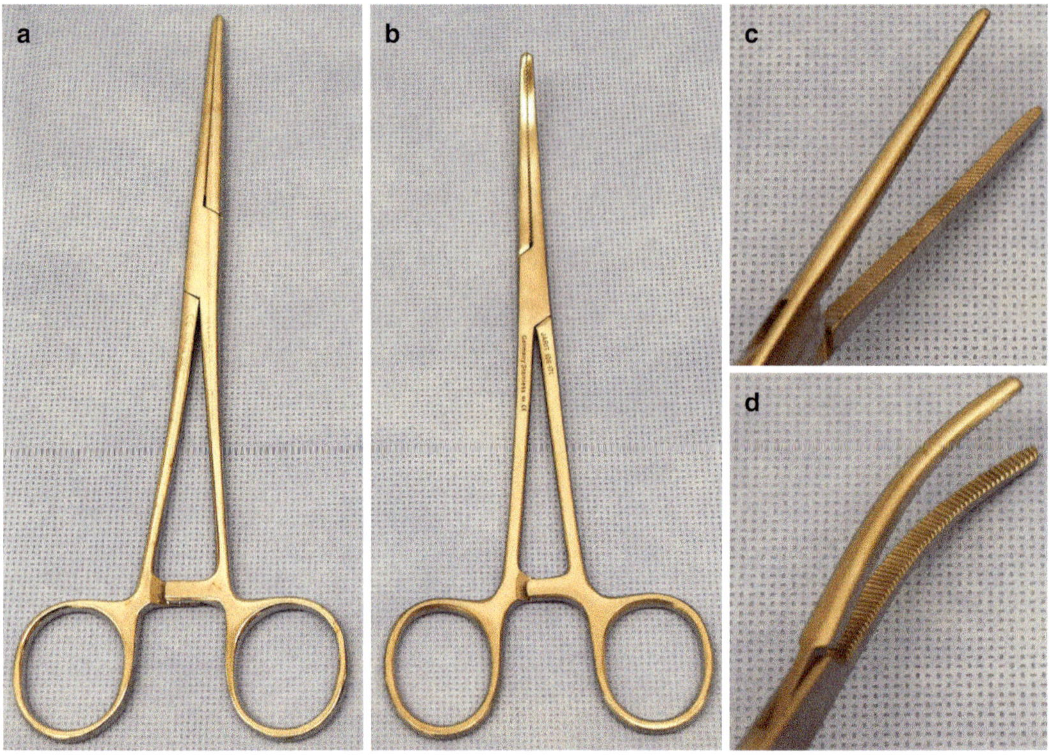

Fig. 2.14 (**a** and **c**) Straight Kelly clamp; (**b** and **d**) curved Kelly clamp

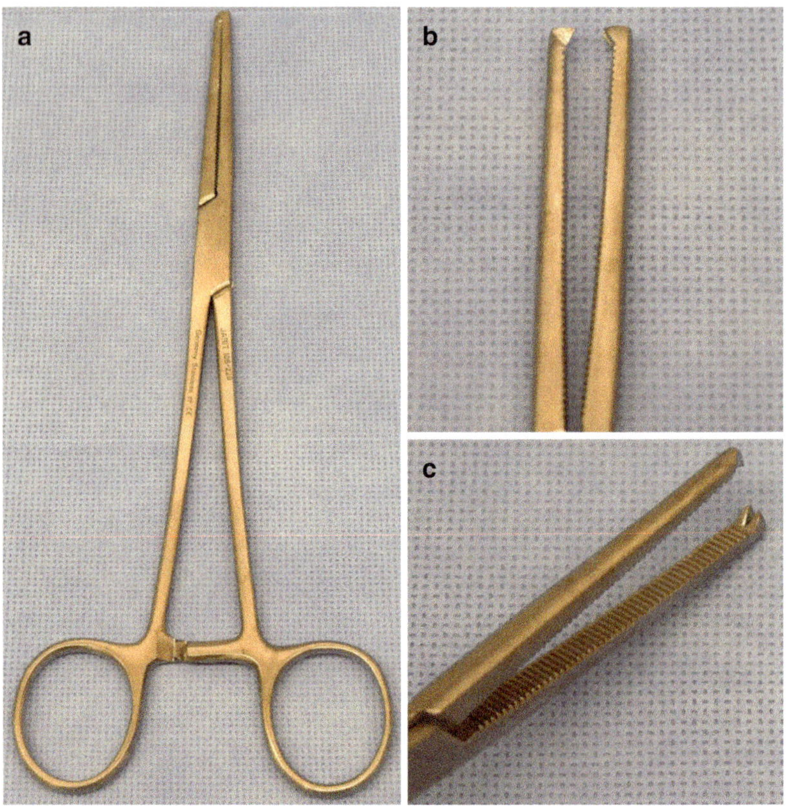

Fig. 2.15 (**a**) Kocher clamp; (**b** and **c**) Kocher clamp details

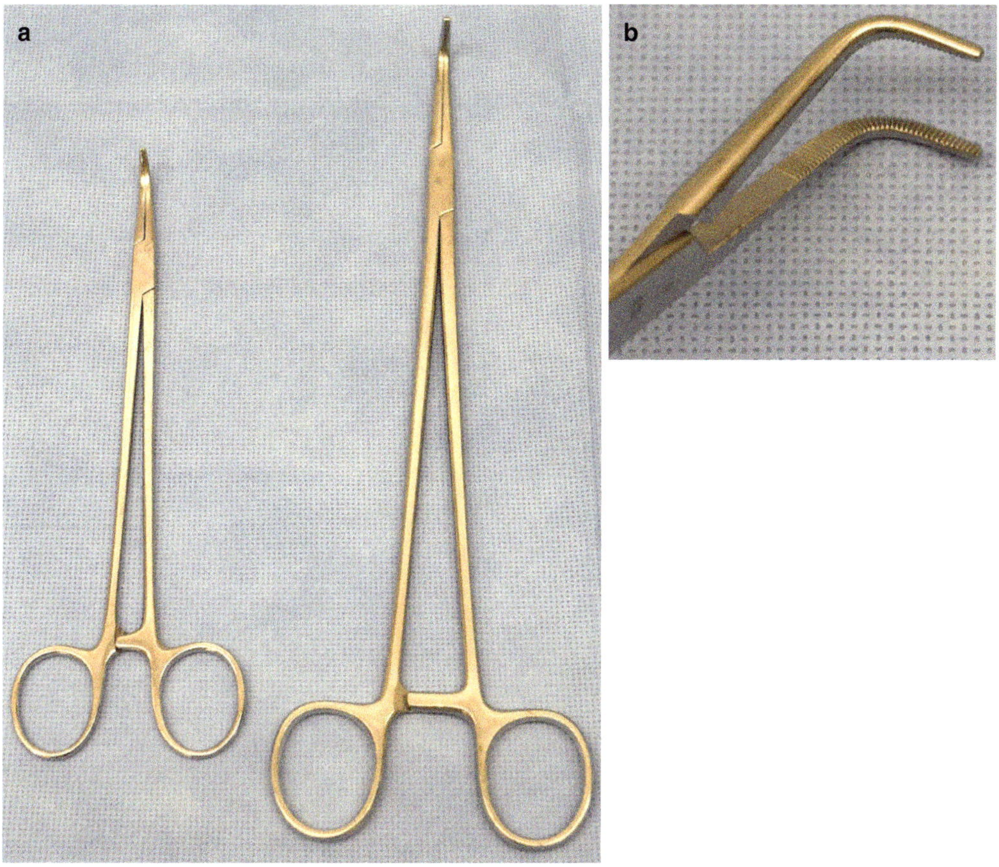

Fig. 2.16 (**a**) Right angle, two different sizes, (**b**) right angle details

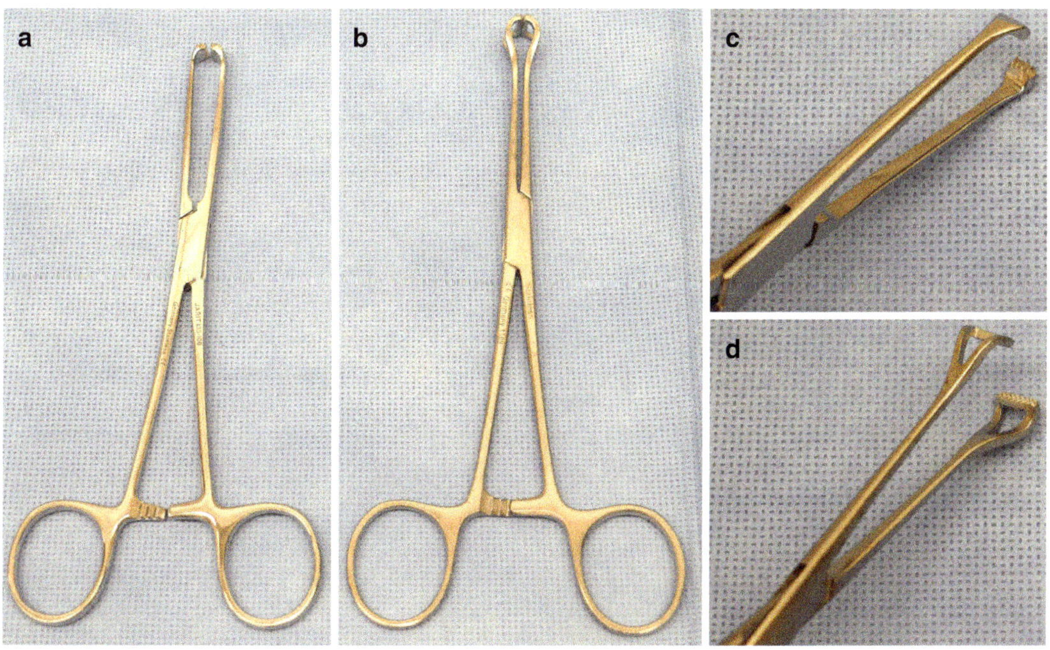

Fig. 2.17 *Left to right*, (**a** and **c**) Allis clamp; (**b** and **d**) Babcock clamp

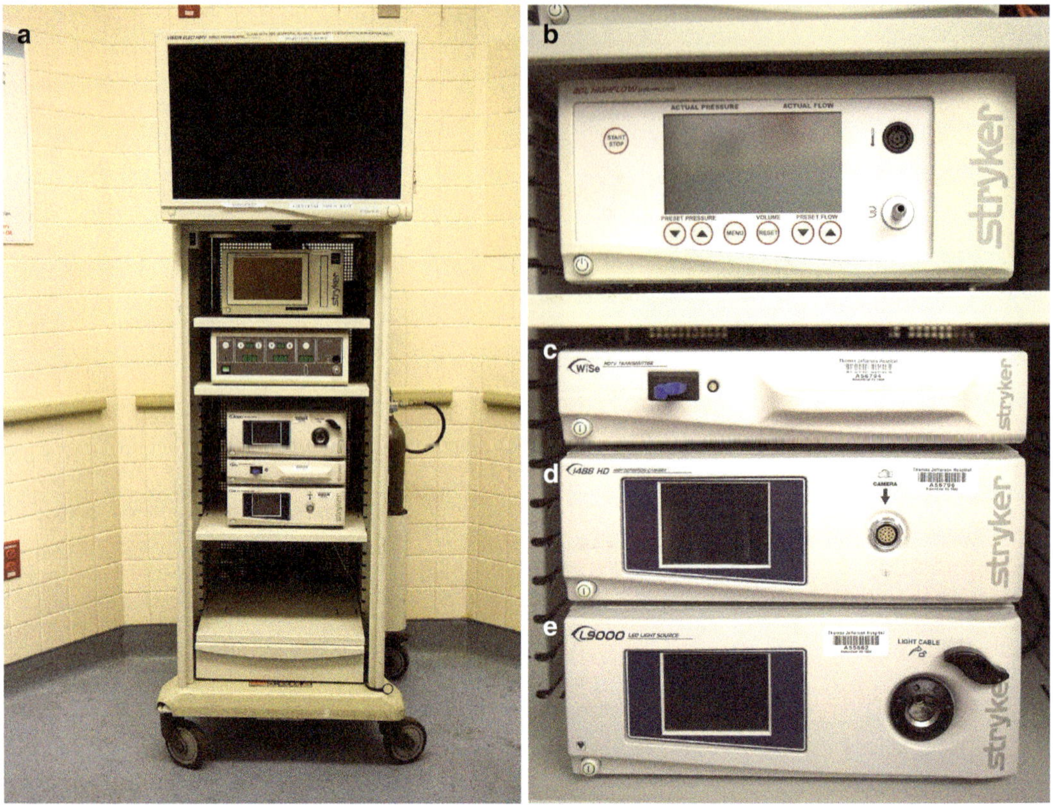

Fig. 2.18 Laparoscopic tower that includes the necessary hardware during a laparoscopic case. (**a**) Broad overview of components located on the tower. (**b**) Insufflator measures the pressure and the flow of gas that is provided during the case. The surgeon can vary the insufflation pressure by adjusting the preset pressure. (**c**) Transmitter that allows for signal to be sent to other monitors in the room. (**d**) Camera connection. (**e**) Light source connection

that is usually visualized in two dimensions. In addition to patient and surgeon positioning, one must be cognizant of equipment positioning in order to facilitate the expeditious progression of the operation. The equipment that is required to carry out a laparoscopic case, such as the components of the imaging system or insufflator, is oftentimes located on a laparoscopic tower (Fig. 2.18). For the remainder of this section, basic laparoscopic equipment and the fundamentals of proper use will be discussed. A more detailed overview of instruments used in laparoscopic surgery can be found in the appendix of this book.

Imaging System

The imaging system consists of the laparoscope, camera, video monitor(s), and light source. In general, the sterile components of this system include the laparoscope, camera, and fiber-optic cord that connects the laparoscope to the light source.

Most modern laparoscopes utilize a rod-lens system that was initially discovered by Harold H. Hopkins in the late 1950s. This was coupled with fiber-optic transmission technology by Karl Storz in the 1960s. Since then, the rod-lens system has revolutionized laparoscopy [5, 6]. Significant advances have been made that allow for a number of laparoscope options, and therefore, not surprisingly, laparoscope selection is largely surgeon dependent. The ultimate goal when selecting a laparoscope is to maintain adequate visualization of the operative field. Laparoscopes can vary in a number of ways, as described below.

- Size—The diameter (or size) of the laparoscope can vary from 0.88 mm to 12 mm. The larger the diameter of the laparoscope, the better the visualization. The most commonly utilized laparoscopes are 5 mm and 10 mm.
- Angle—The angle of laparoscope can vary from 0 to 70°. A laparoscope that is 0° allows for a panoramic view, i.e., provides a view of the field that is directly ahead. In contrast, an angled laparoscope allows one to view a structure from different viewpoints without the necessity to change between ports. The most commonly utilized angles are 30° and 45°. An important tip to remember when using an angled laparoscope is to point the angle *away* and not *toward* the area of interest [7].

Significant advances in camera designs have occurred as laparoscopy has become more popular. Perhaps the most notable advance in enhanced imaging in laparoscopy has been the introduction of the charged-coupled device (CCD) chip camera and digital video imaging (i.e., high-definition imaging). In the future, improvements in three-dimensional imaging will address depth perception, which is lost with two-dimensional imaging. There are a number of features and controls that one must be familiar when it comes to the laparoscopic camera. Controls present on the camera are manufacturer specific but, in general, include:

- White balance allows for the color that is produced by the camera to be adjusted to the color of the light source. It is important to white balance the camera against a white object, such as a lap sponge, prior to use.
- Focus allows for a clear image to be viewed. Prior to inserting the camera into the abdominal cavity, the camera is held 5 cm away from a target object, and the camera is focused to the clearest image.
- Illumination adjustments allow for the intensity of the light to be increased or decreased.
- Optical zoom allows for closer viewing of the operative field without loss of resolution of the image.

Monitors come in a variety of sizes and resolutions. Using a high-resolution monitor with a camera with similar capabilities optimizes the quality of the image.

The light source can vary by type and voltage. The current industry standard is a Xenon lamp with an output of 300 W. The laparoscope is connected to the light source through a fiber-optic cable. Any breakage in the fiber-optic cable results in decreased light transfer from the light source to the laparoscope, which results in decreased light being transferred to the operative field. Always be mindful of the fiber-optic cable once the illumination is turned on, regardless of whether or not it is connected to the laparoscope. It generates a significant amount of heat that has been known to start fires or burn holes through the sterile drapes and can lead to patient injury.

Other necessary equipment for laparoscopic surgery includes:

- Insufflator—The insufflator is necessary to obtain pneumoperitoneum that allows for a successful laparoscopic case to be carried out. Several options are available for the type of gas used to insufflate, the most common being carbon dioxide. Carbon dioxide is preferentially used since it is nonflammable, colorless, and odorless. And, in general, it is safely absorbed and excreted. Insufflator tubing connects the insufflator to the instrument (i.e., trocar or Veress needle) that will facilitate the delivery of the gas into the abdominal cavity.
- Trocars or ports are used to pierce the abdominal wall and serve as a conduit that allows for the entry of laparoscopic instruments into the abdominal cavity. They can vary in size and be either cutting or blunt. Trocars can have

additional features, such as a side port, which allows for pneumoperitoneum to be maintained if the insufflator tubing is changed between ports [7].

Instrumentation for Obtaining Access to the Abdominal Cavity

When initially planning the location for initial access for an abdominal laparoscopic procedure, first, survey the abdomen for scars from prior surgery or for any masses. Second, keep the planned operation and the operative field in mind. The most common site for initial entry and trocar placement is the umbilicus. The amount of soft tissue between the skin and the fascia is less compared to other areas in the abdomen in this location. It is also possible to hide a scar in an existing skin crease for improved cosmesis. Another common entry location is in the left upper quadrant in a location known as Palmer's point, which is located 3 cm below the left subcostal border in the midclavicular line [8]. Instruments commonly used to obtain access for laparoscopic surgery will be briefly described next. For more specific details, refer to Chap. 14—*Fundamentals of Laparoscopic Surgery*.

First described by Dr. Harrith M. Hasson in the 1970s, the open technique for laparoscopic access is preferred by some as it is believed to minimize complications such as gas embolism, major vessel or visceral injury, or insufflation of the preperitoneal space [9]. The cannula itself is usually fitted with a cone-shaped sleeve and an outer secondary sleeve that allows for stay sutures to be placed to secure the port. It is primed with a blunt obturator to prevent injury to underlying structures. The Hasson cannula is inserted into the abdomen with the blunt obturator in place, and stay sutures secure the cannula to the fascia on either side to seal the opening in the abdominal wall and to prevent gas leak during the procedure [10].

The Veress is used to obtain access to the abdominal cavity during laparoscopic surgery with the closed technique. The Veress needle was first discovered in the 1930s by Janos Veres, and it was Raoul Palmer who introduced the use of the Veress needle in laparoscopic surgery to establish pneumoperitoneum in the 1940s [8, 11]. It is a spring-loaded needle that is 12–15 cm long with an external diameter of 2 mm. It consists of a two-cannula system. The outer cannula has a beveled needle that is sharp to cut through the abdominal wall. The inner cannula is nested within the outer cannula and has a spring-loaded stylet with a dull tip. When the Veress needle is passed through tissue, direct pressure on the tip of the needle pushes the dull stylet into the outer cannula. Once the needle tip enters a space, such as the peritoneal cavity, the dull inner stylet springs forward and protects any underlying tissue.

Optical trocars are a relatively new technique that utilizes the conventional trocar and cannula push-through design. These units are designed in such a way that the trocar is hollow and allows for a 0° laparoscope to be inserted and locked along with the trocar. It can then be used to visualize entry into the abdominal cavity as the trocar pierces sequential abdominal wall layers. This system is generally used after the abdominal cavity has been insufflated [10, 12].

Tips for "Driving" the Camera During Laparoscopic Surgery

All of the components of the imaging system are put together to allow the visualization of an image. Once access to the abdominal cavity is obtained, proper use of the imaging equipment to provide adequate visualization during the operation is of paramount importance. Here are a few pearls for proper handling of the camera and laparoscope and for effective "driving" of the camera:

- Practice holding the camera. In general, the non-dominant hand should cradle the camera and laparoscope. The buttons of the camera should always point up.
- The light cord is attached to the laparoscope, and in the neutral position, it points up. This is especially important to remember when using an angled laparoscope, since the direction of the light cord corresponds to the direction of the viewing angle.

- When "driving" the camera, a good rule to keep in mind is the rule of opposites. To view an image to the right, the camera is moved to the left. Or to view an image that is up, the camera is pointed down. Moreover, the camera should be moved toward the object of interest to provide a closer view. Movement of the camera out (or into the trocar) will result in the ability to get a panoramic view of the field.
- When using an angled laparoscope, movement of the light handle results in a change of the angle. Therefore, when the light handle is in the neutral position, i.e., pointing up, the viewing angle is down. When the light handle points up, the viewing angle points down.
- The lens can fog once the laparoscope is inserted into the abdominal cavity. This occurs due to the temperature difference between the outside environment and the intra-abdominal cavity. This can be avoided by warming the lens tip in warm water or with the use of antifog solutions [12].

Basics of Instrumentation and Equipment for Endoscopy

Endoscopy in general surgery has many applications and can be used in abdominal or thoracic procedures. This section will provide a brief overview of the common components of endoscopes used for upper and lower endoscopy.

The Endoscope

The endoscope is comprised of three main parts:

The handpiece is used to control the direction the tip of the insertion tube is facing, which aids in visualization as well as maneuvering the scope as it traverses a lumen. A large and small wheel is used to either maneuver the tip up-down or left-right, respectively. Turning of the wheel leads to tip angulation in the opposite direction on the monitor. For example, turning the large wheel up causes the endoscopic tip to be directed downward and vice versa. The wheels can be locked in a desired position to aid in diagnostic or therapeutic maneuvers, such as obtaining a biopsy. Buttons on the handpiece control different capabilities. The blue button has two features: covering the port will insufflate air, while pushing the button infuses water. Pushing the red button provides suction. A biopsy port allows for the passage of biopsy forceps or other instruments through the insertion shaft. Camera buttons allow the operator to obtain pictures or videos.

The insertion tube is a flexible cord that is manually manipulated by the operator by pushing, pulling, and torqueing. The deflectable tip at the distal end of the cord has the capability of flexing side to side and up and down via controls on the handpiece. The tip also contains the port sites for multiple applications, including a water nozzle for irrigation, an air nozzle for insufflation, a suction channel, a light source, and objective lens.

The umbilical cord is a flexible tube that contains all of the channels (air/water, suction, and light source) that connect to the tower that houses the video processor and displays screen. The proximal end of this cord is directly inserted to the tower. A video processor cord connects the umbilical cord to the image processor. A water bottle and suction tubing are connected to the umbilical cord to allow for irrigation and aspiration.

The Endoscopy Tower

The endoscopy tower consists of an image processor and display screen, a light source and air insufflator, water irrigation, and energy source. Once all equipment is positioned and connected appropriately, check that the insufflation, irrigation, and suction are working properly before beginning the procedure [13].

OR Instruments Used in Laparoscopic Surgery

Laparoscopes (Fig. 2.19)

Laparoscopes come in many varieties, as discussed in the *Fundamentals of operating room setup and surgical instrumentation* chapter. Illustrated here are 10 mm laparoscopes, both at various angles.

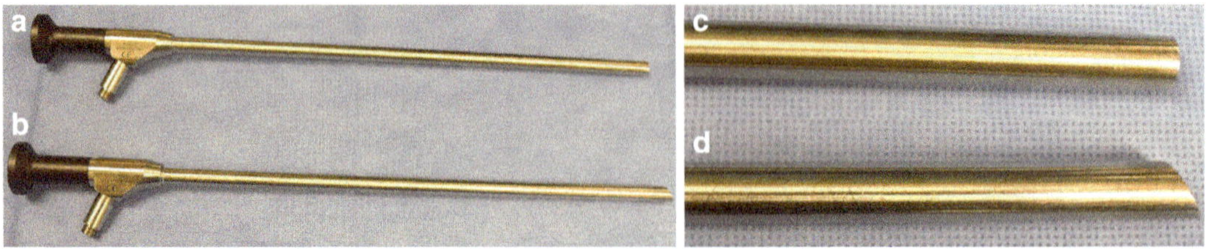

Fig. 2.19 *Top to bottom*, (**a** and **c**) 0° laparoscope, (**b** and **d**) 30° laparoscope

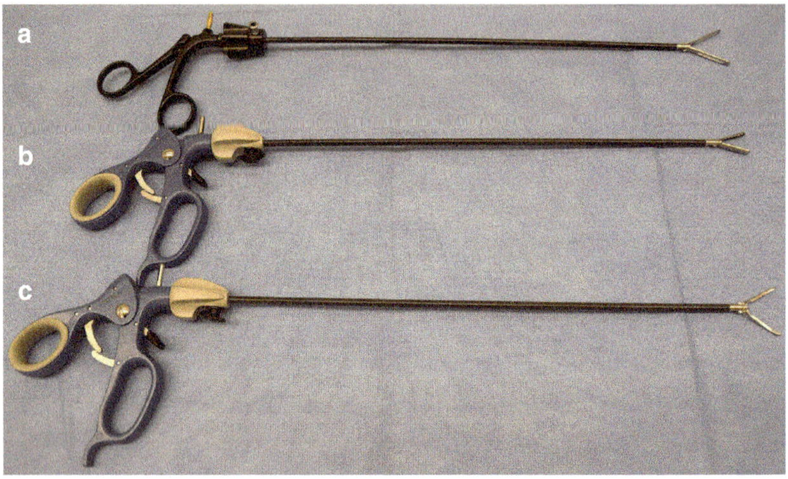

Fig. 2.20 *Top to bottom*, laparoscopic graspers; (**a**) bowel grasper; (**b**) Clinch grasper; (**c**) Maryland dissector

Laparoscopic Graspers (Figs. 2.20 and 2.21)

Most laparoscopic instruments have a 360° rotating knob to turn the tip of the instrument in order to maintain the wrist in the most ergonomically neutral position. Electrocautery sources can be plugged into the metal port on the handle, which are usually controlled via a foot pedal. The atraumatic bowel grasper is used to handle more delicate tissue, such as when running the bowel. One should use the majority of the jaw to grasp the anti-mesenteric side to minimize damage. Using just the tip of the grasper can cause more damage secondary to the increased pressure exerted by the smaller surface area. A hand-to-hand or hand-over-hand technique can be utilized to accomplish this task. Clinch graspers are usually toothed and ratcheted, with a locking mechanism. This could be used to grasp and retract thicker or heavier tissue, such as omentum. The Maryland dissector that has a pointed tip can be utilized to dissect through more fine tissues and is commonly used when dissecting around the cystic duct and artery during a laparoscopic cholecystectomy.

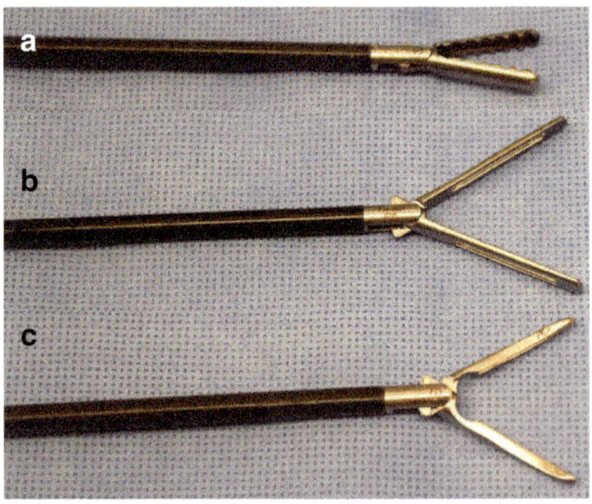

Fig. 2.21 *Top to bottom,* (**a**) Cinch grasper; (**b**) atraumatic bowel grasper; (**c**) Maryland dissector

Suction Devices and Cautery (Fig. 2.22)

There are a variety of instruments that exist that allow for the utilization of electrocautery during laparoscopic procedures. Illustrated here is the spatula, in which the metal shaft is insulated so as to protect the surrounding tissue. Suction cannulae come in variety of sizes. The tip doubles as a suction and irrigator when connected to the appropriate adaptor and tubing. This adaptor usually has two buttons: red for suction and blue for irrigation. The combination of suction and the blunt tip can also be utilized to dissect tissue.

Trocars and Obturator (Fig. 2.23)

Once inserted through the abdominal wall, trocars (commonly referred to as ports) are left in place to allow for the passage of laparoscopic instruments. Once this first port is placed, either through open or Veress technique, the laparoscope can be introduced intra-abdominally to help visualize the placement of subsequent ports. To place a port, a twisting motion along with constant, steady pressure is applied to the trocar with the obturator insert. This allows the pointed obturator tip to dissect through the abdominal wall layers. The tip should be visualized with the

Fig. 2.22 *Top to bottom*, (**a**) insulated spatula cautery with suction cannula; (**b**) insulated spatula cautery with suction cannula separated in individual components; (**c**) laparoscopic suction cannula in two different sizes

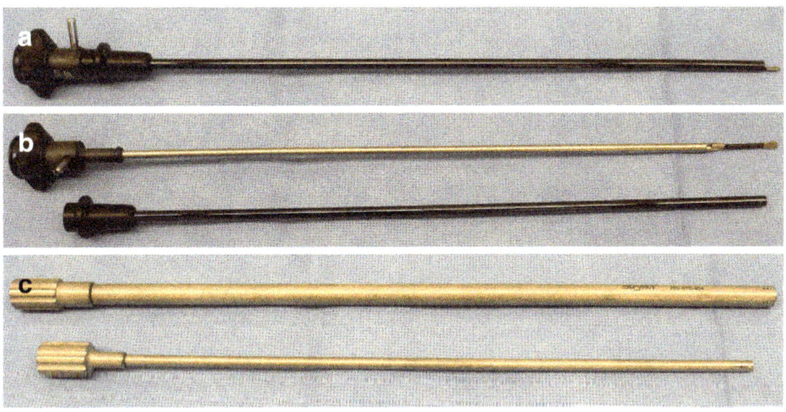

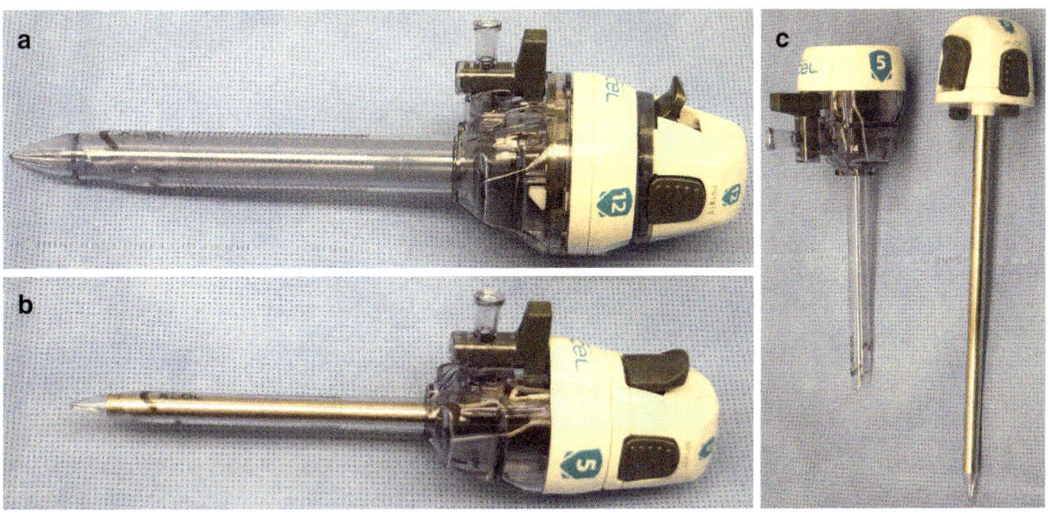

Fig. 2.23 *Top to bottom*, laparoscopic trocars; (**a**) 12 mm trocar with obturator; (**b**) 5 mm trocar with obturator; (**c**) 5 mm trocar and obturator

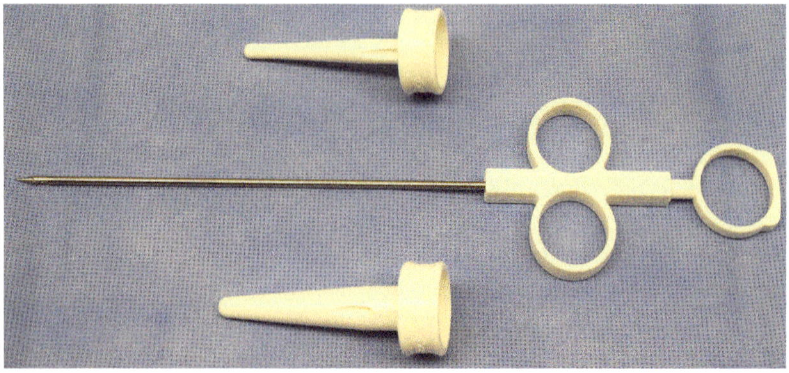

Fig. 2.24 Carter-Thomason laparoscopic port closure device with cone-shaped guides in two different sizes

laparoscope as it enters into the abdominal cavity so as to avoid injury to organs, such as the bowel, liver, or spleen. The obturator is removed once the trocar is in place, and a laparoscopic instrument can then be introduced. Ideally, the trocar should be able to freely move in any direction so as to allow for an optimal operative field.

Port Closure Device (Fig. 2.24)

Large port sites, particularly 10 mm or greater, usually require that the fascia be closed after port removal. Port closure devices are particularly useful when it would be difficult to close the fascial defect by hand, such as in an obese patient. The Carter-Thomason system uses a cone-shaped obturator that is placed into the port site. A free suture is grasped by the tip of the suture passer and then introduced into one of the two holes in the cone. The laparoscope is used to visualize the sharp suture passer as it pierces one side of the fascial defect. Once the sharp tip is in the abdomen, the suture is released, and the suture passer is removed and then placed into the opposite hole in the cone. Again, the sharp tip is visualized as it pierces the opposite side of the defect and grabs the free suture to pull it back out so the free ends of the suture can be tied down to close the fascial defect.

Suggested Readings

Scott-Conner CEH. The Sages manual: fundamentals of laparoscopy, thoracoscopy and GI endoscopy. New York: Springer; 2006.

Marks JM, Dunkin B. Principles of flexible endoscopy for surgeons. New York: Springer; 2013.

Vilos GA, et al. Laparoscopic entry: a review of techniques, technologies, and complications. J Obstet Gynaecol Can. 2007;29(5):433–65.

ACS. Statement on operating room attire. Bulletin of the American College of Surgeons. 2016.

References

1. Kennedy L. Implementing AORN recommended practices for sterile technique. AORN J. 2013;98(1):14–26.
2. Schulmann K, et al. The patient with multiple intestinal polyps. Best Pract Res Clin Gastroenterol. 2007;21(3):409–26.
3. ACS. Statement on operating room attire. Bulletin of the American College of Surgeons. 2016 [cited 2017 April 17].
4. Spruce L, Wood A. Clinical issues – December 2016. AORN J. 2016;104(6):593–600.
5. Morgenstern L. Harold Hopkins (1918–1995): Let there be light.... Surgical Innov. 2004;11(4):291–2.
6. Lau WY, Leow CK, Li AKC. History of endoscopic and laparoscopic surgery. World J Surg. 1997;21:444–53.
7. Mishra RK, Mishra R. Textbook of practical laparoscopic surgery. New Delhi: Jaypee Brothers; 2013.
8. Palmer R. Safety in laparoscopy. J Reprod Med. 1974;13(1):1–5.
9. Hasson HM. A modified instrument and method for laparoscopy. Am J Obstet Gynecol. 1971;110(6):886–7.
10. Vilos GA, et al. Laparoscopic entry: a review of techniques, technologies, and complications. J Obstet Gynaecol Can. 2007;29(5):433–65.
11. Szabó I, László A. Veres needle: in memoriam of the 100th birthday anniversary of Dr János Veres, the inventor. Am J Obstet Gynecol. 2004;191(1):352–3.
12. Scott-Conner CEH. The Sages manual: fundamentals of laparoscopy, thoracoscopy and GI endoscopy. New York: Springer; 2006.
13. Marks JM, Dunkin B. Principles of flexible endoscopy for surgeons. New York: Springer; 2013.

Fundamentals of Sutures, Needles, Knot Tying, and Suturing Technique

3

Jessica A. Latona, Sami Tannouri, Francesco Palazzo, and Michael J. Pucci

3.1 Sutures and Needles

3.1.1 Historical Background/Introduction

3.1.1.1 Suture History

Sutures were used by Egyptians and Syrians as far back as 2000 BC. The materials used as suture have evolved through the years and continue to evolve today. Some of the historical materials used for suture include linen, cotton, hemp, flax, tree bark, wire made of gold, silver, or steel, animal or human hair, vegetable fibers, animal tendons and intestines [1]. Today, suturing material is so refined that there are even suture and needles designed for a singular purpose!

Catgut has been used since the fifteenth century. It was named after the string chords of a musical instrument called a "kit" [1]. By the twentieth century, cotton, linen, and silk were used regularly. Historically, silk was established as the premier suture material because it was noted to heal quickly with few disadvantages, the result of security even with a small knot. The main problem with silk was its persistence in wounds and tendency to cause suppuration. With the advent of antisepsis, Joseph Lister applied this system to suture material. Believing that germs embedded in the silk suture were responsible for infection, he began sterilizing the strands in carbolic acid. When he continued finding evidence of inflammation at surgical sites, he began to believe that it was the rough material that made up the fiber and he searched for a better material [2].

It was Lister who reintroduced catgut reinforced with chemical coating and antisepsis into practice and is responsible for the development of sterile absorbable sutures. He studied and wrote about the properties and outcomes of his innovation extensively. Due to his work, catgut suture gained popularity for its strength, flexibility, and absorbability toward the end of the nineteenth century [2].

Catgut suture had numerous properties that were problematic: variability in strength, unpredictable rate of absorption, intense inflammatory reaction, a nidus for infection, tendency to fray, and weakening of knots. William Halstead spoke out strongly against using catgut and by the early twentieth century, silk had once again become the suture material of choice even for vascular anastomoses [1].

It wasn't until 1960 that experimentation with synthetic materials began in order to develop a suture with more desirable properties. The first synthetic suture material (Dexon) was introduced

J. A. Latona · S. Tannouri · F. Palazzo
M. J. Pucci (✉)
Department of Surgery, Sidney Kimmel Medical College, Thomas Jefferson University, Philadelphia, PA, USA
e-mail: michael.pucci@jefferson.edu

F. Palazzo (ed.), *Fundamentals of General Surgery*, https://doi.org/10.1007/978-3-319-75656-1_3

in 1970. Dexon was a polyglycolic acid polymer similar to catgut, but with better performance with respect to tissue reactivity and a more uniform response to tissue, strength, and rate of absorption. The second absorbable suture to be introduced in 1974 was polyglactin (more commonly known as Vicryl) [1].

3.1.1.2 Needle History

Much like suture material, needles are not specific to surgery and are one of man's oldest tools. Eye needles were first recorded in use in 50,000–30,000 BC and there are remnants of needles made of bone, antlers, and tusks dating from as far back as 20,000 BC. Needles manufactured from metals emerged around 4000 BC, but the application of needles in surgery began in 600 BC. Initially, suture needles were straight and generally hand-held. Because anatomic structures had to be deformed to allow for entry and exit of the needle, they were primarily used for skin closure [1].

As one could imagine, needle puncture was not uncommon. It was the simultaneous realization that transmission of infection could occur with needle puncture and Lister's introduction of aseptic technique that prompted a need for "no-touch" needles [1]. Ambroise Paré designed curved needles. His hand-held needle was further refined by Jacques-Louis Reverdin in the nineteenth century and was popular for over a hundred years. In the 1920s, it was discovered that a strong connection between the suture and needle could minimize tissue trauma [3]. This led to the development of "atraumatic" needles that form the basis for the modern needle used today. The variety of needle sizes, shapes, points, and eyes grew tremendously and expanded the functionality of the needle in surgery.

Suture and needles are the most basic surgical equipment. Our aim is to provide information on the physical properties of suture and needles so that residents feel comfortable calling for the proper suture for a task.

3.1.2 General Concepts

3.1.2.1 Anatomy of/Dissecting a Suture Package

Looking at a suture package can be confusing to the new-comer. Figure 3.1 diagrams representative suture packages from the major manufacturers. The information contained on a suture package includes suture material, construction, strand size, strand length, suture color, needle

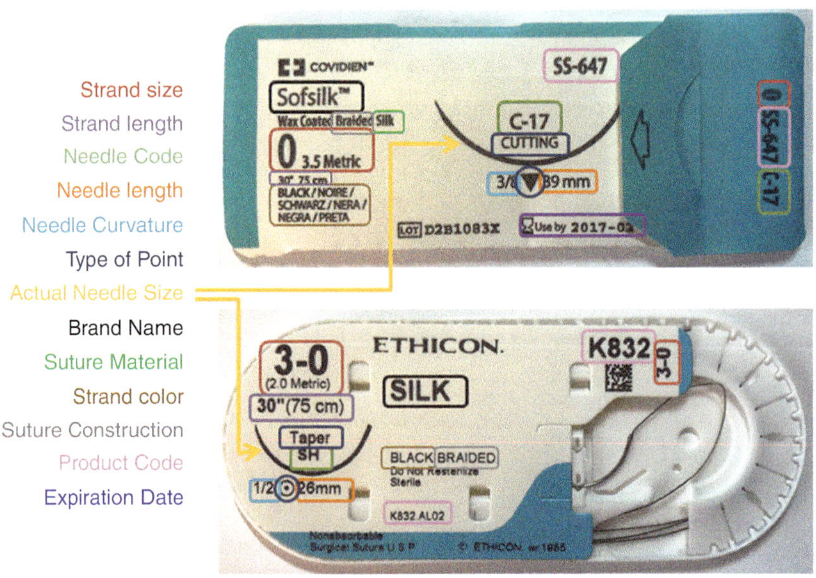

Fig. 3.1 Representative suture packages from major manufacturers. The properties of each suture are outlined in the color corresponding to each element listed on the left

point type, needle curve, needle length, and needle color. These properties will be described in detail in the following sections. By the time you finish reading this chapter, you should be equipped with the knowledge to not only navigate this information, but also to confidently select an appropriate suture and needle combination for use.

3.1.2.2 Suture

Suture materials differ based on their construction, size, and ability to be "absorbed" or undergo degradation after a certain amount of time within the body. When thinking about absorbability, ask yourself "How long do I need the suture to keep its strength?" Absorbable sutures are broken down by one of two mechanisms and lose a majority of their tensile strength within 60 days [4, 5]. The two mechanisms by which suture material is absorbed are proteolysis and hydrolysis. Natural materials like chromic catgut are degraded by proteolytic enzymes and this process occurs quickly. Synthetic materials like polyglycolic acid, polyglactin, polydioxanone, and poliglecaprone (just to name a few) are broken down by hydrolysis, which occurs more slowly. Absorbable suture is useful for tissue that requires wound support from a few days (skin, subcutaneous tissue, muscle) to weeks or months (fascia). Table 3.1 contains details regarding the tensile strength and time to absorption for the most commonly used/available absorbable suture materials [5].

Non-absorbable materials are not biodegradable. They remain where they are placed and ultimately are walled off by fibroblasts. They should be used when suturing collagenous tissues that are strong and heal slowly (tendon) and when long-term stability is required (prosthetic grafts). Table 3.2 contains details regarding the properties of the most commonly used/available non-absorbable suture materials [5]. The disadvantage of non-absorbable suture is that it can form chronic draining sinuses and suture granulomas. For this reason, avoid using it above the fascial layer.

The next common subdivision of suture materials is construction. Construction refers to the number of strands that each suture is made from. Monofilament suture is made of a single strand compared to multifilament suture which is created from multiple strands being twisted or braided together. Monofilament construction generates less tissue reaction and harbors fewer bacteria. It can be more difficult to handle because of its elasticity (more likely to return to original shape and length after being stretched) and memory (the ability to return to its original shape after tying). Monofilament suture also possesses less knot strength and loses tensile strength at any point that it is grasped by an instrument.

Multifilament or braided suture is more difficult to pass through tissue and more likely to cause tissue injury. For all types of suture, but especially for multifilament suture, it is best practice when "running" a suture to draw the strand through the tissue as much as possible to limit *en masse* movement through multiple entry and exit points. Braided suture is liked for its ease of handling and tying. Suture construction is single handedly the most important property to determine the number of knots that should be created to secure the suture (see Tables 3.1 and 3.2) and the length of suture that should be left attached to the knot when cutting suture. In general, a 4–5 mm tail should be left for monofilament suture and 2–3 mm should be left for silk or braided synthetic suture.

A third grouping of suture material is natural versus synthetic. It answers the question: "How much tissue reaction is this material going to cause?" Regardless of its composition, all suture material is a foreign body and may elicit an inflammatory reaction. However, synthetic materials are less reactive compared to natural fibers, which tend to produce an intense inflammatory reaction. The amount of inflammation generated by a suture can either promote or hinder the healing process.

Suture size is another important physical property. Sizing is standardized according to U.S. Pharmacopeia (U.S.P.) regulations and based on the diameter necessary to generate a certain tensile strength. Table 3.3 details the U.S.P. suture size and the corresponding diameters in millimeters. It varies somewhat with material absorbability and whether it is natural or synthetic. The conventional nomen-

Table 3.1 Physical properties of absorbable suture and common uses

Name	Trade names	Tensile strength	Absorption time	Common uses	Construction	Knots	Natural or Synthetic
Chromic catgut	Ethicon and Covidien = Chromic gut	Lost within 10–15 days	90 days	Splenorrhaphy, hepatorrhaphy, suture ligature of vessels, mucosal layer of GI anastomosis	Monofilament	4–6	Natural
Polyglactin	Ethicon = Vicryl	75% at 14 days, 25% at 28 days	56–70 days	Approximate soft tissue, GI anastomosis (mucosal layer)	Braided	4	Synthetic
Lactomer	Covidien = Polysorb			Soft tissue approximation, ligation	Braided	5–6	Synthetic
Polygytone	Covidien = Caprosyn	60% at 5 days, 20 –30% at 10 days	56 days	Skin closure	Monofilament	5–6	Synthetic
Poliglecaprone	Ethicon = Monocryl	50–60% at 7 days, 30–40% at 14 days, complete by 21 days	91–119 days	Skin closure	Monofilament	4–5	Synthetic
Glycomer 631	Covidien = Biosyn	75% at 2 weeks, 40% at 3 weeks	90–110 days	Soft tissue approximation and/or ligation	Monofilament	5–6	Synthetic
Polyglycolic acid	Syneture = Dexon	5% at 28 days	90–120 days	Soft tissue approximation and/or ligation	Braided	4	Synthetic
Polydioxanone	Ethicon = PDS	70% at 14 days, 58% at 28 days, 25% at 6 weeks	183–238 days	Soft tissue approximation, fascial closure	Monofilament	6–10	Synthetic
Glycolide Polytrimethylene carbnoate	Covidien = Maxon	75% at 14 days, 65% at 3 weeks, 50% at 4 weeks, 25% at 6 weeks	180–210 days	Soft tissue approximation and/or ligation, pediatric CV tissue, peripheral vascular surgery	Monofilament	6–10	Synthetic

Table 3.2 Physical properties of non-absorbable suture and common uses

Name	Trade names	Tensile strength	Common uses	Construction	Knots	Natural or Synthetic
Silk	Ethicon = Silk Covidien = Sofsilk		Secure surgical drains, ligation of large blood vessels, outer layer in GI anastomosis	Braided	3	Natural
Stainless steel	Ethicon = surgical stainless steel		Closure of median sternotomy, abdominal wound closure, hernia repair	Monofilament	3	Natural
Polyester	Ethicon = Ethibond Covidien= Surgidac, TiCron		Cardiovascular surgery, for vessel anastomosis, and placement of prosthetic materials	Braided	4–5	Synthetic
Nylon	Ethicon = Ethilon Covidien = Monosof, Dermalon	89% at 1 year, 72% at 2 years, 66% at 11 years	Interrupted skin closure, secure surgical drains, repair of lacerated nerves or blood vessels	Monofilament	6–7	Synthetic
Nylon	Ethicon= Nurolon Covidien = Surgilon	89% at 1 year, 72% at 2 years, 66% at 11 years	Soft tissue approximating and/or ligation	Braided	4–5	Synthetic
Polypropylene	Ethicon = Prolene Covidien = Surgipro	89% at 1 year, 72% at 2 years, 66% at 11 years	Vascular anastomosis	Monofilament	6–7	Synthetic
Expanded polytetra-fluoroethylene	Gore-Tex		Creation of cardiac or vascular graft anastomosis, securing Gore-Tex patch	Monofilament	5–8	Synthetic
Polybutester	Covidien = Novafil, Vascufil		Lacerations from blunt trauma	Monofilament	4–7	Synthetic

Table 3.3 U.S.P. suture sizes

Suture U.S.P. size	Diameter (mm)
8-0	0.040–0.049
7-0	0.050–0.069
6-0	0.070–0.099
5-0	0.100–0.149
4-0	0.150–0.199
3-0	0.200–0.249
2-0	0.300–0.339
1-0 or 0	0.350–0.399
1	0.400–0.499

clature is *number*—zero and pronounced “*number*, Oh.” Size ranges from 1 to 12-0 where more zeroes indicate a smaller size. The smaller the suture size, the less tensile strength it has. Tensile strength refers to the maximal stress that a strand can withstand before breaking. While breaking suture is undesirable, it is better to break the suture when it is in your direct focus so that you can replace it rather than have it break later and having it go unnoticed.

The loss of tensile strength over time should not be confused with the rate of absorption. Loss of tensile strength occurs upon implantation of suture, with tying (knotted sutures have two-thirds the strength of unknotted sutures), and with exposure to tissue environment (4–13% reduction after being soaked in sodium chloride solution for 24 hours). Tables 3.1 and 3.2 list loss of tensile strength for commonly used suture [6–11].

The final elements found on the suture package that describe the suture material are length and color. Length is important when you are working in a deep space because you want the strands to be long enough to be manipulated outside the cavity or when running along the length of an incision because you don’t want to run out of suture before you reach the end. A good rule to guide the length needed for a "running" closure is to have a suture that is 4 times the length of the incision that you are closing. Sutures come in various colors, but other than knowing you should not use dyed suture at the skin level, it is not of much consequence.

3.1.2.3 Needles

Needles are necessary for carrying suture material through tissue. The goal is to achieve this with as little trauma to the tissue as possible. Needles must be sharp to avoid resistance within the tissue, rigid enough to resist bending, and ductile to allow for bending before breakage. To expand on these points, grasping the tip of a needle with forceps or a needle holder should be avoided as this dulls the point and increases the resistance on your next pass through the tissue. A needle that is too weak will bend easily resulting in decreased control of the needle once it is inserted into tissue and possibly damage the surrounding tissue. If a needle is bending, it means too much force is being applied or that the size of the needle driver is too large relative to the needle.

The basic anatomy of all surgical needles (depicted in Fig. 3.2) is the same; they each have a point, a body, and a swage (the end which is attached to suture material). The types of needle points are tapered, cutting, reverse cutting, taper-cut, and blunt. Tapered needles (Fig. 3.3a) are

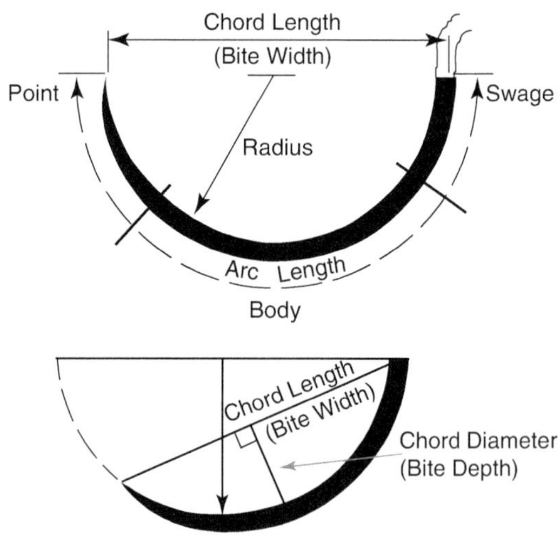

Fig. 3.2 Anatomy of a surgical needle. The three main parts of a surgical needle are the swage, body, and point. The swage is attached to the suture and the body is the portion grasped by the needle driver. The chord length is the distance between the swage and the point and determines the bite width. The chord diameter determines the bite depths and varies with the curvature of the needle

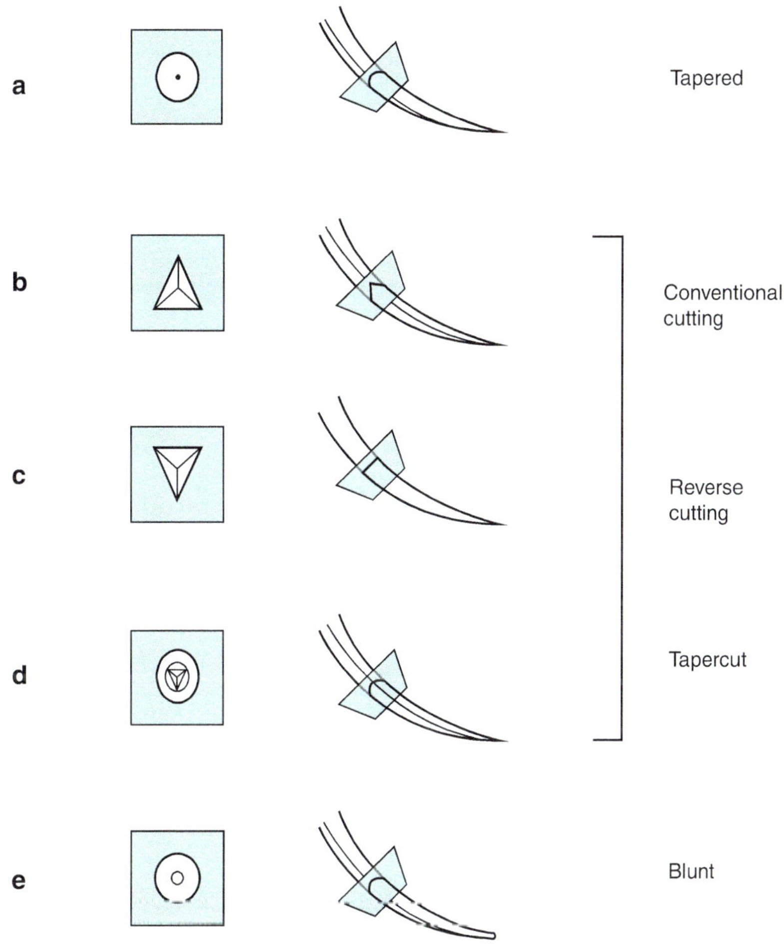

Fig. 3.3 Types of needle points. Each needle point is designed for a specific function. Namely, tapered needles (**a**) are appropriate for suturing bowel, blood vessels, and fascia, whereas cutting needles (**b**–**d**) are suited for skin, and blunt needles (**e**) are used on highly vascularized organs

cone shaped and suitable for sewing soft tissues (fat, muscle, blood vessels, gastrointestinal viscera, and fascia). Cutting needles (Fig. 3.3b) have a triangular body with a sharpened cutting edge on the inside curve. A reverse cutting needle (Fig. 3.3c) has a sharp edge on the outside of the needle curve. Generally, cutting needles are suitable for inserting sutures in the skin. They create holes in the tissue that are larger in diameter than the suture itself which precludes their use in tissue where leakage can occur. Reverse cutting needles are stronger than a conventional cutting needle and are preferentially used when minimal tissue trauma is desired. Blunt needles (Fig. 3.3e) are dull and are reserved for suturing highly vascularized solid organs (i.e. liver).

Most modern surgical needles are affixed to suture via a swage. The swage is the thickest but weakest part of the needle and holding it here often results in distortion of the needle. It also causes more tissue trauma because the swage is wider than the suture material itself. The other type of needle end is an eye where the suture must be manually secured to the needle. Unlike a swaged needle, an eyed needle causes minimal trauma to the tissue. Swaged sutures can be permanent or controlled released. Compared to a permanent suture, which must be cut from the needle, controlled released sutures can be detached with a quick, straight tug on the needle while holding the suture strand taut. In this way, the needle "pops-off" the strand. This feature allows for efficient interrupted suturing.

The needle body is the portion designed for grasping the needle with a needle holder. Several important properties of the needle body are gauge, curvature, and chord length. The size of the needle is a function of gauge and chord length. The gauge is the diameter or thickness of the needle and varies from thousandths of an inch to hundredths of an inch. The chord length (Fig. 3.2) is the arc distance between swage and point and determines the bite width. Needle curvature is measured by what proportion of a circle is completed and ranges from 0 (straight) to 5/8 (Table 3.4). A more curved needle requires less lateral movement for advancement. This feature can be taken advantage of when suturing two edges as the exposure of a wound decreases because a more curved needle requires less rotation to exit tissue [6–11].

The specific needle types that are available through the major manufacturers are pictured in Fig. 3.4 to illustrate various curves and relative sizes [12]. To gain familiarity with the characteristics of various needle sizes, arrange two columns of dots at varying widths on a cloth. The dot in the right column serves as the entry point and the dot in the left column serves as the exit point. The goal is to improve the accuracy with which the needle exits as one improves their "needle tip consciousness."

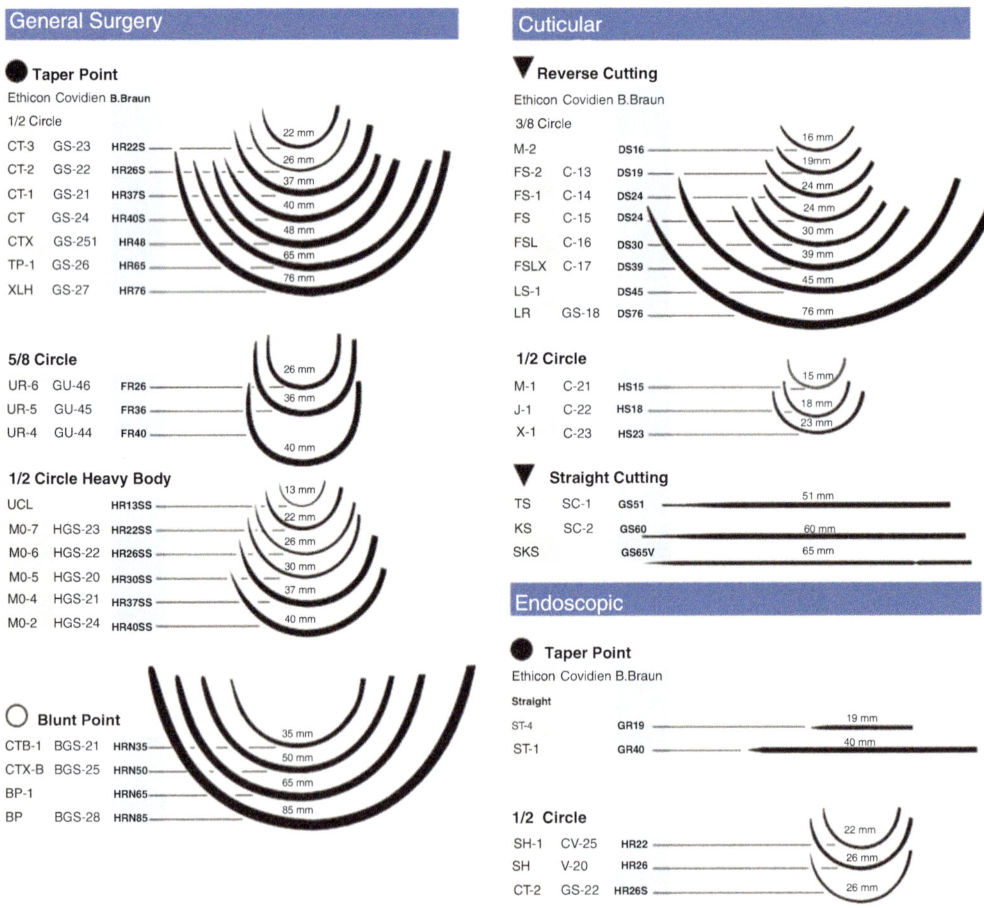

Fig. 3.4 Needle comparison chart. The specific needle types that are available through the major manufacturers are grouped according to point type and arranged by size for comparison. Modified from https://www.aesculapusa.com/assets/base/doc/DOC571RevC-AesculapNeedleComparisonChart-3-foldBrochure.pdf

Table 3.4 Various needle curves and their uses

Curvature	Common uses
Straight	Skin, laparoscopy
Half-curved/ski	Laparoscopy
¼ circle	Eye
3/8 circle	Skin closure, small blood vessels
½ circle	Closure below the skin
5/8 circle	Trocar site fascia, bladder

3.1.3 Technical/Practical Considerations/Safety Precautions

There is no ultimate suture that will work under any circumstance, but guiding principles will allow you to choose the best option. Suture selection should be based on knowledge of the physical and biologic characteristics of the material (which you are now an expert on), the rate of tissue healing, and patient factors (infection, frailty, obesity, etc.). Ultimately, suture selection depends on surgeon training and preference, as well as institutional factors.

Let us talk about specific situations in which suture and needle selection comes into play.

Scenario A: You are the surgical intern and are paged to the trauma bay to see a patient who tripped and fell through a glass door. He/she has multiple lacerations on his/her extremities. These wounds are contaminated, as are most traumatic wounds. In addition to thoroughly irrigating the lacerations, your goal is to reapproximate the tissues. Inert (monofilament) suture should be used when tissue is contaminated as they cause less tissue inflammation and reaction.

Scenario B: You are about to begin the proximal anastomosis of a femoral to popliteal bypass when the surgical attending is paged to an emergency. On their way out of the operating room the surgeon tells you to start the anastomosis as the vascular clamps have already been applied and the leg is now ischemic. In this situation, the size of the suture you choose has great implications. If the suture size is too large, it will traumatize the vessels and you will have difficulty controlling needle hole bleeding. If the suture size is too small, the tension of the anastomosis may cause your sutures to tear through the tissue. Your needle selection matters here as well. Cutting and reverse cutting needles leave triangular cross sectional holes in tissue, but your suture has a circular cross section. This additional space also may lead to increased needle hole bleeding and inadvertently can weaken the tissue and your sutures may saw through the vessel wall. Tapered needles have a circular cross section which better approximate the cross section of your suture, and should be used in these situations.

Scenario C: You have been rotating on a colorectal service and just finished an open colectomy where you closed fascia with heavy suture such a PDS™ or Maxon™. Your very next case is a hemorrhoidectomy. After resecting the hemorrhoid, you notice bleeding at the apex of your incision and want to suture ligate this point. You ask for chromic suture. This is an example where you cannot just use the same suture you used in your last case to close fascia. Different tissues vary greatly in healing time. Fascia takes weeks to reach its full strength, and thus requires a very slow absorbing or even permanent suture to close. Mucosa, whether it is oral, rectal, or otherwise, is a very rapidly healing tissue and makes a highly absorbable suture desirable for approximation.

Scenario D: You perform a melanoma excision right along the edge of one of your patient's shoulder blades. The skin is thick here, and of course you realize that every time your patient moves their arm that the wound closure will be tested. Here tensile strength of the suture you choose will matter. Bigger (thicker) suture has higher tensile strength than finer suture, as well as braided suture typically has a higher tensile strength that of a similar monofilament. For tendon repairs, which are highly mobile and tough tissues, large braided sutures are often used due to their extremely high tensile strength.

Scenario E: You have just finished a panniculectomy and have two drains underneath the abdominal flap. You are asked by the circulating nurse which suture you would prefer to secure the drains to the skin. Suture has memory meaning that different suture materials have variable ability to resist changes in configuration. You can think of this as how stubborn the suture is to remaining in the position where you place it. Silk and other braided sutures typically have less memory and are easily manipulated. Some synthetic monofilaments and even nylons are stiffer, and have greater memory. You must be aware that these sutures do not as easily give up their shape. It is easier to tie around a drain with a suture with less memory. You choose your suture and begin tying knots, knowing that these drains may remain in place for weeks and your knots must not slip. Braided suture, due to the higher contact surface area on itself allows for fewer knots to hold securely than monofilaments. You can tie down the drain using only three or four throws of a silk knot, but you may need to place six or more knots in a nylon suture as this knot has a higher tendency to unravel since it is a monofilament suture.

Scenario F: It's the middle of the night and you have just performed an emergent perforated colectomy on a morbidly obese patient who had five prior laparotomies. The attending hurriedly leaves the room as soon as you finish irrigating the abdomen, leaving you to close the incision. You confidently, but inattentively take the needle driver from the scrub tech and turn your attention to the wound edge. You are met with a thick wall of tissue resembling ground beef and lacking discernable layers. In this scenario, it may be appropriate to perform a "mass closure" of the abdominal wall, taking a bite that goes through all layers of the abdominal wall, regardless of your ability to distinctly identify them. This cannot be accomplished with a small needle. The chord length (distance of the straight line between the tip and the tail of the needle) will need to slightly over-approximate the thickness of all the layers of tissue you are trying to close. If the chord length in inadequate, you will not be able to push the needle through the thick mass of tissue, and instead lose the needle within the tissue. Likewise, when you are sewing through thinner tissue, such as bowel or blood vessels, make sure that the chord length is not too long or else you will have difficulty maneuvering your needle in and out of the lumen that you are trying to sew.

Scenario G: You decided to use an open Hasson technique to enter the abdomen on a laparoscopic case. The case is done and you now turn your attention to closure of the fascia at this port. Your patient's anterior fascia is 5 cm below the surface of a 1 cm long incision. This scenario requires taking advantage of highly curved needles (5/8th Curvature, or 5/8th of the way around a circle). First your chord length must be small enough such that the needle will fit *inside* this incision. Needles that are not as highly curved (3/8th or ½ curvature) can be used when sewing tissues that are more accessible and shallower in the operative field as they require a larger arc of motion to smoothly pass them through the tissue. A 5/8th curvature needle can almost be completely rotated through tissue from a fixed fulcrum, allowing you to get an adequate bite of tissue while deep in a hole, all by rotating your wrist.

Scenario H: It is Sunday morning and a patient who was walking to their grandmother's house sustained a gunshot wound to their abdomen. You take the patient to the operating room and notice a large laceration in the liver as well as a colotomy. You begin frantically asking for suture to repair these injuries. The liver and the colon have quite different consistencies and the purpose of your suturing on each organ will be different. Suturing a highly vascularized, soft, and friable organ requires a special needle, one with a blunt tip. This will allow the needle to pass through the tissue without causing further lacerations, and the tip pushes small blood vessels out of the path of the needle, without puncturing them or causing bleeding. Needles that are used to sew tendon, skin, or other soft tissues often have sharp or "cutting" tips to allow the needle to enter and pass through the tissue smoothly. Blunt needles can be used on organs such as the lung, liver, or spleen.

Now you turn your attention to the colotomy. You believe the hole is small enough to repair primarily. You are given a needle and look carefully at the tip when you notice that the cross section of the tip is a triangle with sharp points. This is called a cutting needle and this leaves a triangular hole in the tissue that you are sewing. The cross-sectional shape of suture is circular, so you can imagine that a circular suture sitting inside a triangular hole will not be as watertight as a circular suture passing through a circular hole. You will need to use a "taper" point needle in this scenario, where the body of the needle gradually tapers to a circular point, without any sharp edges. Tapered needles are used on blood vessels, bowel, bladder, or in any situation where a watertight closure is important. Taper points have less of a tendency for suture to tear through the tissue because the hole in the tissue is round, as opposed to triangular where the apices act as a lead point for suture to tear through.

3.1.4 Current Controversies/Future Directions

Antibiotic-coated material was recently introduced as a novel method for fascial closure with a specific application to decrease surgical site infections (SSIs). Triclosan is a bacteriostatic agent that interferes with microbial lipid synthesis. Triclosan-impregnated suture types ranging from absorbable monofilament to braided are commercially available. Data from animal and *in vivo* studies support that when triclosan-coated suture is used to close wounds there is inhibition of bacterial colonization. A number of non-randomized studies and randomized controlled trials have been performed to assess the effectiveness of decreasing SSIs when midline fascial closure is performed with triclosan-coated suture [13–17]. One single-center randomized trial examining outcomes after closure of general and abdominal vascular procedures showed a significant reduction in SSIs from 11.3% to 6.4% with the introduction of PDS Plus (antibiotic-coated suture) compared to non-coated PDS suture [14]. The PROUD trial studied midline closure of all midline laparotomies in well matched control and study groups and found that the rate of SSIs did not differ between the PDS Plus group (14.8%) and the non-coated PDS II group (16.1%) [16]. Similarly, no differences were found in surgical site infection rates when examining closure in colorectal procedures only [13, 17]. In a meta-analysis, the overall risk of surgical site infection in the antibiotic-coated group was 10.4% compared to 13.0% in the control group [18]. Two meta-analyses have been inconclusive, in large part because of variability in patient demographics, the type of suture material used, and closing technique [19, 20]. Future studies are necessary to determine the utility and define a clinical application for this innovation.

Barbed suture is another innovation in suture material that is gaining popularity. Its design has linear nicks along its length which allows the suture only to be pulled in one direction. As a concept, barbed suture can be traced back to 1956 when Dr. John H. Alcamo patented his idea. Clinically, barbed suture was first used in 1967 by Dr. A.R. McKenzie for tendon repair in human cadavers and *in vivo* in dogs. Physical characteristics of the early suture design limited the application of barbed suture. From 1967 to 1999, a variety of techniques were presented. Dr. Harry J. Buncke (a microsurgeon) is credited for patenting the modern design of one-way sutures with exterior barbs and either a uni- or bi-directional needle. This design was ultimately acquired by Quill Medical in 2002, commercialized as Quill™ Knotless Tissue-Closure Device and FDA approved in 2004 [21].

Currently, there are three types of barbed suture commercially available [18, 21]:

1. Quill SRS™ (Quill Self-Retaining System; Angiotech Pharmaceuticals, Vancouver, British Columbia, Canada)—this is a bidirectional barbed suture
2. V-Loc™ Absorbable Wound Closure device (Covidien, Mansfield, MA, USA)—this is a unidirectional barbed suture that has only one needle and a loop at the opposite end for anchoring the suture in tissue
3. Stratafix™ (STRATAFIX Knotless Tissue Control Devices, Ethicon Inc., Somerville, NJ, USA)—this suture has a unique spiral distribution of the barbs and anchors

Barbed suture is used frequently by plastic surgeons and is gaining attractiveness in robotic surgery (see Fundamentals of Knot Tying, Ligatures, and Suturing).

Take-Home Points

- Precise knowledge of suture materials and needles is required to be a competent surgeon.
- The process of suture selection may also depend on surgeon training and preference as well as the type of suture material that is available at a particular location.
- No one suture will have all desirable characteristics, but selection can be guided by patient factors, the type of tissue, and suture properties.
- Needle selection depends on the type, location, and accessibility of the tissue to be sutured, as well as the size of the suture.
- Select your needle such that you minimize trauma to the tissue you are sewing. Remember: the tissue you are sewing should not realize what is happening to it.

3.2 Knot Tying, Ligatures, and Suturing

3.2.1 Historical Background/Introduction

3.2.1.1 Knots and Knot Tying

The practice of using knots to secure ropes or cables is as old as human history. There are many types of knots that have been employed as part of daily life and were necessary for survival in ancient times. Before knots were adopted for use in surgery, intricate knots were developed and utilized by other trades such as sailors and tackle makers. Proprietary knots are not unique to surgery and some are still in use in surgical specialties today. For example, the miller's knot which is used to secure the opening of a sac (usually containing grains) has been adopted for use in ligating vascular pedicles particularly in veterinary medicine.

The earliest accounts of surgical knots are from the first century. A Greek physician Herakles wrote about tying 16 knots and nooses used to apply traction when reducing dislocations and setting broken bones or to hold patients in position when performing surgery. Interestingly, the "Hercules" knot which he described but did not provide any particular use resembles the current surgeon's knot which is extensively used by all sorts of surgical disciplines today [1, 2].

3.2.1.2 Ligatures

Ligating refers to tying a ductal structure with a suture thread. Ambroise Paré is credited for introducing the concept of ligatures as a method to control hemorrhage in modern surgery. He designed an instrument called the bec de corbin (which can be likened to a hemostat) to control the bleeding while the vessel was handled. Although Paré's suggested technique was not initially readily accepted, this practice became a turning point in the evolution of surgery [3].

3.2.1.3 Suturing

Like knot tying, the technique of sewing is thousands of years old and evolved from a civilian skill that was necessary for survival. In the Stone Age, needles made from bone, antler, horn, or ivory were used to punch holes in animal hides and then thread was drawn through the holes. As a method for closing cutaneous wounds, an Indian physician Sushruta wrote in the first detailed description of surgical suturing in 500 B.C. Ancient Egyptians also wrote about the use of medical sutures to join separated wound edges, incisions, and mummies [1, 2].

Suturing remains the fundamental technique for closing spaces, reducing infection, speeding healing, and minimizing scarring. Modern suturing is no longer limited to simple techniques for cutaneous closure. Methods have been developed for application in every type of tissue and all organ systems. Perhaps the most diverse methods are those that have been described for use in the gastrointestinal tract.

Knot tying and suturing form the foundation for more advanced surgical techniques. Mastery of these basic skills is imperative. Unlike many other surgical skills which are difficult or require sophisticated simulation, these techniques can be easily practiced with little equipment required other than your own two hands. Our aim in this section is to provide explanations on the proper application of various knots and types of stitches with a focus on describing the subtleties of suturing and knot tying that are often not found in textbooks and typically transferred verbally from mentor to mentee.

3.2.2 General Concepts

3.2.2.1 Knot Tying

Knot Security

Knots serve to secure two ends of suture as a ligature or to anchor suture in tissue. Knot strength is defined as the force necessary to cause slippage. Knot slippage can have postoperative consequences from thicker scar formation to more serious complications including hemorrhage or leaks. Knot strength depends on the area of contact, suture construction (braided versus monofilament), knot tightness, and length of suture projecting from the knot. Certain principles apply to all types of suture materials:

- Knots should be tied quickly, but speed should not substitute for accuracy (i.e., creating a square knot).
- Friction between the strands should be avoided.
- Choose the simplest knot for the suture material and make the knots as small as possible. Extra knots do not add strength, but rather weaken the suture material and just add bulk.
- The completed knot should be firm so that it holds securely, but not too tight that the suture breaks, cuts through tissue, or decreases circulation.

Square Knot by One-Hand and Two-Hand Techniques

The basic maneuver for knot tying involves crossing the strands to create a loop and passing one end through the loop to emerge on the opposite side. It does not matter if initial strand crossing is right over left or left over right. What is more critical is the direction in which each strand is pulled when tightening the knot as this determines whether the knot "lies flat" and the direction of the second-hitch which determines whether the knot will "be square." This will be discussed in more detail in the next section "Types of knots."

Knots can be tied two-handed or one-handed. The two-handed tie is the easiest and most reliable method for tying even the most stubborn suture materials like surgical steel. In a two-handed tie, both hands are actively involved in forming the crossing of strands and tightening the knot. For this reason, it provides a better sense of the tension on both suture ends and makes for tying a much safer knot. If you want to be a surgeon, master this technique. The one-handed tying technique is advantageous because it is more efficient; it can be performed with the left hand while still holding an instrument in the right hand. The main challenge is in creating square knots. When in doubt about which to use, the two-handed tie should be used by default and most certainly should be used when tying important structures.

Tips for Practicing Knot Tying

Whether employing a one- or two-handed technique, the suture ends should always be under complete control. This requires practice to gain familiarity with the optimal suture length for each strand based on your hand size. In general, the working strand (the one being passed through the loop) should be at a length that prevents redundancy of the strands within the loop, avoids interference with other instruments in the environment, and reduces the incidence of the knot being prematurely pulled up and thus loosening. A resident even at the most junior level should feel comfortable crossing the strands and passing suture through the loop with either hand. This is a mandatory skill because you will be asked to tie when you are standing on different sides of the operating room table in relation to the structure to be tied and handed ties that are already crossed in a particular arrangement. A good target for practice is being able to tie 50 knots per minute both two- and one-handed with each hand taking the dominant role.

Instrument Tie

Knots can also be created with the aid of an instrument. An instrument tie is most commonly used when suture is too short to be hand tied, tying in a deep cavity, or to secure cutaneous stitches with greater efficiency. To perform an instrument tie, the suture should be pulled through the tissue so that there are two ends (one short about 2–3 mm and a longer end attached to needle). Holding the needle driver over the center of the wound, the long end of the suture is wrapped clockwise around the needle holder tip twice. The short end of the suture can then be grasped with the needle driver and pulled through the looped suture. The knot is tightened by crossing hands. For subsequent knots, the needle driver should again maintain a central position relative to the wound. The suture should be wrapped counterclockwise once around the needle driver and tightened by grasping the short end, pulling it through the loop, and pulling the ends in opposite directions from the first knot to create a square knot. This can be repeated until an adequate number of knots are placed and the suture should be cut no longer than distance between interrupted stitches to prevent the suture tails from being caught in the subsequent knot.

3.2.2.2 Types of Knots

There are several different types of surgical knots: simple knot, slip knot (also known as a Granny knot), square knot, and surgeon's knot (Fig. 3.5). A simple knot is also referred to as a half-hitch. It involves only one revolution of one strand around the other. All surgical knots require two half-hitches. The orientation of the second half-hitch dictates the type of knot. More specifically, if two identical half-hitches are tied in a row as occurs when the suture strands are inadvertently pulled in the same direction, a slip or Granny knot is created. Looking down on the knot, the ends are at right angles to the standing part (Fig. 3.5b) which allows for slippage of the strands. This feature which allows for tightening of the knot has advantages and disadvantages. It can be used initially to generate the desired tightness of a knot, but should not be the only type of knot used because it has a tendency to slip and can open up spontaneously.

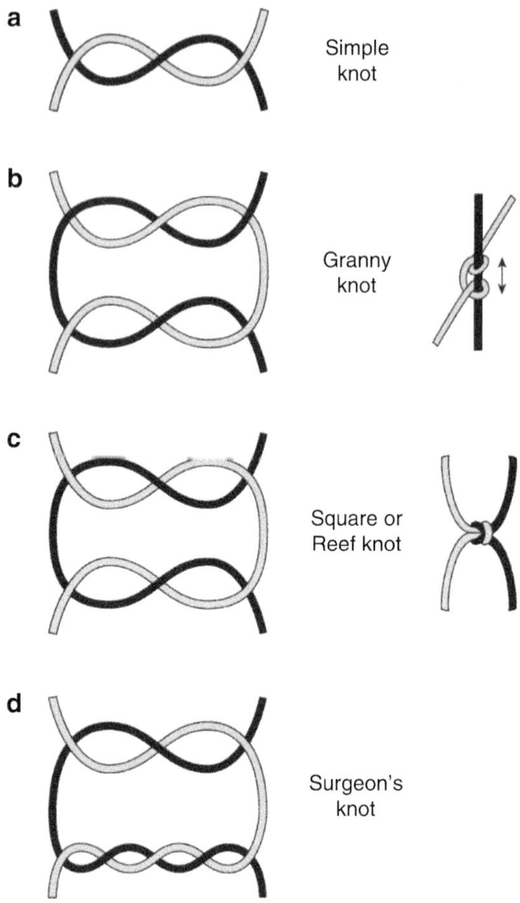

Fig. 3.5 Types of surgical knots. (**a**) A simple knot is one half-hitch. (**b**) A slip or Granny knot is made with two half-hitches of the same throw. This allows for slippage of the strands and adjustment of tension on the knot. (**c**) A square or reef knot is made with two-half hitches of opposite throws. It does not allow for slippage and locks the strands in place at the knot. (**d**) To make a Surgeon's knot, one end of the suture makes two passes through the loop on the first hitch prior to locking the first throw with an opposite half-hitch

The most common surgical knot is the square or reef knot (Fig. 3.5c). Compared to a granny knot, the second half-hitch is made by crossing the strands in the direction opposite to that of the first one. In this knot, the first hitch sets the tension on the tissue and the second secures the knot. As alluded to previously, the square knot is the most secure and it is best to develop a habit of throwing square knots whenever possible. To facilitate creation of a square knot when using the two-handed technique, alternate between using your thumb and index finger on the same hand to create the loop. For the one-handed technique, alternate between a forehand (leading with the index-finger) and a backhand (leading with a middle-finger) throw.

The proper placement of a knot requires the left hand grasping one end of the suture, the structure being ligated, and the right hand grasping the opposite end all positioned in a straight line to avoid traction on the tissue when the knot is being tightened. The hands controlling the ends of suture must cross to guarantee that a knot lies flat. It is preferable to cross in the sagittal plane to prevent obscuring view of the knot. This often requires adjustment of posture. A surgeon once told me that tying square knots is like a dance and that he could tell from outside of the operating room if knots were square based on whether or not the tying surgeon's shoulders were moving back and forth.

Another strategy that works to limit the amount of hand-crossing is to exchange the end of suture at the beginning of knot formation. Alternatively, you can change which hand forms crossing of strands based on the orientation of the two suture strands. If the passing end of the suture is closer to you than the other end, use the index finger hitch first (for a two-handed tie) or the middle finger hitch first (for a one-handed tie) to create the first half-hitch. If the tying end of the suture is far from you, use the thumb hitch first (for a two-handed tie) or the index finger hitch first (for a one-handed tie) to create the first half-hitch.

When tightening or securing a knot, the index finger should be used to push or slide the knot down. The key here is that the finger aims into empty space, slightly off to the side of the knot rather than down into the tissue you are tying. This technique is demonstrated in Fig. 3.9c, d.

The surgeon's knot (Fig. 3.5d) will be discussed in a later section in the context of tying under tension.

3.2.2.3 Suturing Technique

With few exceptions, the basic techniques of needle holding and needle driving are the same regardless of the specific suture and needle that are chosen and the type of tissue that is being brought together. In this section, we will describe these techniques and concentrate on specific points that are troublesome.

Basics of Needle Holding

The two main components of needle holder are the jaw and the handle. The jaws of the needle holder should match the needle size. The needle should be stable within the jaws when the needle driver is tightened with just one catch of the ratchet. The handle of the needle driver must be appropriate for the depth needed for the suture placement. If you are stitching in a deep space, a long-handled needle driver is necessary to prevent your hand from blocking your view of the operative site. You should always ask for the needle on a proper needle holder in order to maximize your efficiency.

Figure 3.6 depicts how to hold the needle holder and properly "load" or position a needle within the jaws of a needle holder. When holding the needle holder, distal tips of the thumb and ring fingers should be positioned in the rings with index and middle finger on shaft to provide stability (Fig. 3.6a). To load the needle, it should be situated at the tips of the instrument and oriented at a 45° angle from the line of the instrument (Fig. 3.6b), pointing away from the surgeon as shown in Fig. 3.6a. Whether one loads the needle midway along its curve, close to the tip, or closer to the swage depends on the distance of tissue that surgeon would like the needle to travel. Placing a needle too far back on the needle holder or failure to follow a needle's curve as it passes through tissue can result in distortion of the needle. For most common uses, the needle should be loaded 1/3 to 2/3 of the distance from the swage (Fig. 3.6c).

Proper Use of Needle Driver

"Driving" a needle through tissue requires knowledge and respect for the fact that needles are curved and will only pass through tissue in a circular motion. This requires the acquisition of a steady rotational wrist movement from a pronated to supinated position. Lateral movement of a needle caused by pushing a needle straight for-

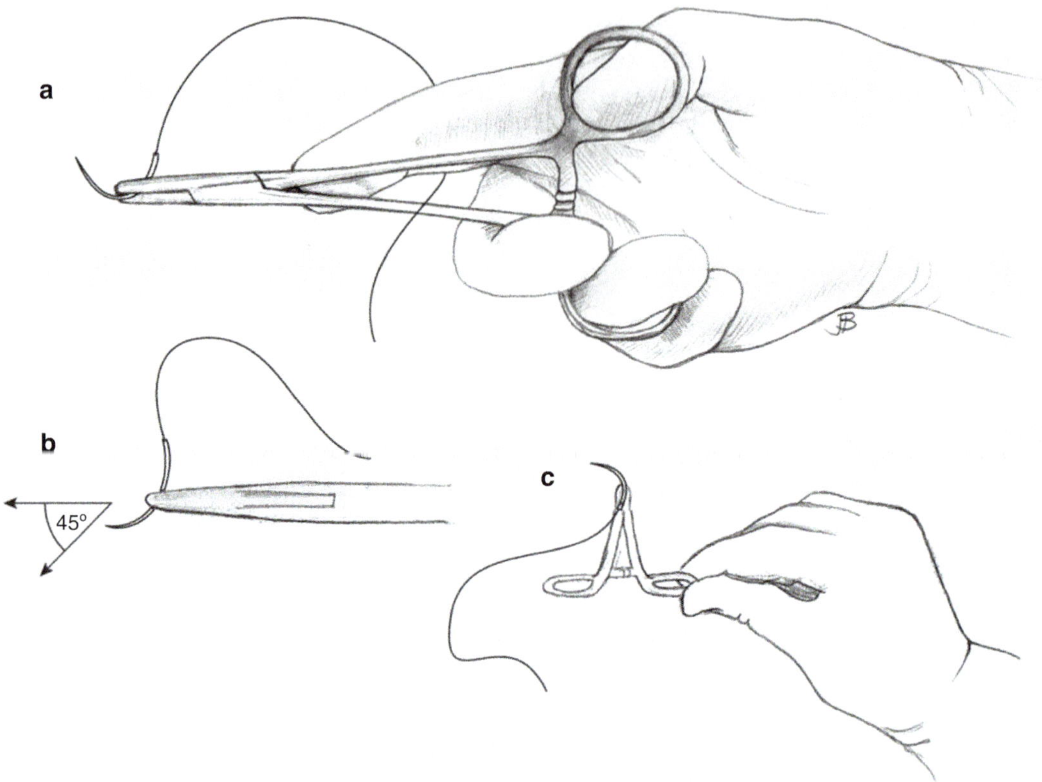

Fig. 3.6 Holding and loading a needle driver. The proper way to hold the needle driver with the thumb and ring finger is demonstrated in panel a. When positioning the needle within the jaws, the needle should be loaded halfway between the needle's tip and swage at the very ends of the jaws (**a**), at a 45° angle from the line of the instrument (**b**) and perpendicular to the short axis of the driver (**c**)

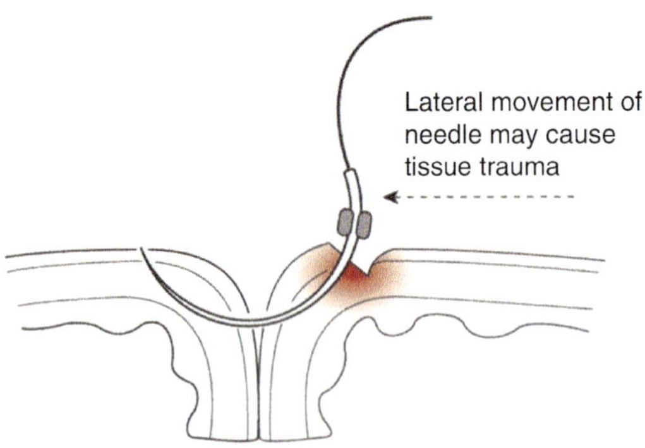

Fig. 3.7 Needle "driving." The correct technique of advancing a needle requires rotating the needle through tissue. Pushing the needle through tissue in a straight line (rather than rotating along the axis of the curvature of the needle) causes trauma to the tissue at the needle entry point

ward while it is inserted in tissue can result in trauma to the tissue at the entrance wound (Fig. 3.7). This should be particularly emphasized if one desires to complete a bite through both ends of tissue in one pass. In this case, the surgeon must pick up the opposing segment and bring it toward the needle rather than torquing the needle and dragging it to the opposing segment of tissue.

With this in mind, proper technique for tissue entry involves entrance into the tissue perpendicularly (Fig. 3.8a) with the wrist pronated and supinating the wrist until the needle exits the wound or the needle holder makes contact with tissue (Fig. 3.8b). For the needle to completely exit the tissue, one can use a forceps to rotate the needle through the tissue or re-engage the needle driver in a pronated position on the portion of the needle exiting the tissue (Fig. 3.8c). At times, the needle tip will not emerge from the tissue enough to completely exit. This can hap-

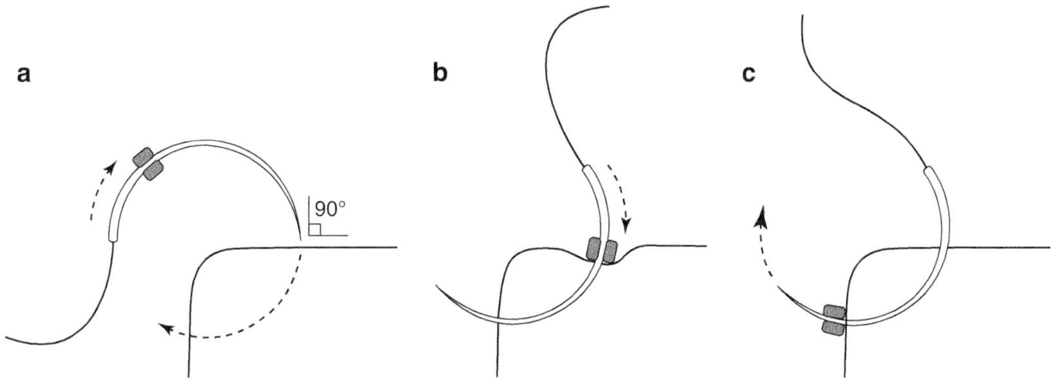

Fig. 3.8 Needle entry and exit. The needle enters the tissue perpendicular to the tissue (**a**) and rotates through the tissue along the axis of the curvature of the needle until the needle exits the wound or the needle holder makes contact with the tissue (**b**). Reengage the needle in a pronated position near the needle tip's exit site of the tissue and continue along the needles natural rotation (**c**) to ensure the needle completely exits without causing undue trauma

pen for several reasons—the bite can be too big for the needle, the needle was loaded too close to the tip, etc. If this occurs, rather than removing the needle and creating a new entrance wound, forceps can be used to apply counter pressure on the tissue near the anticipated point of emergence to expose more of the needle and avoid grasping the needle tip.

Tips for Practicing Handling a Needle Driver

When possible, residents should strive to remove the needle from tissue in the proper orientation for the next bite as this allows for efficient, one-handed continuous suturing. One can practice the movements necessary for properly advancing and loading a needle by using a "push, push, pull" method. For this exercise, a piece of cloth (OR towels work well), needle holder, suture, and forceps are needed. The resident should begin by "pushing" or passing the needle through the cloth until the tip is exposed and the needle holder is in contact with the towel. The needle holder should then be repositioned toward the swage of the needle and "pushed" to advance the needle tip even farther out of the cloth. The needle can then be removed from the cloth by positioning the needle in the proper orientation for the next bite within the jaws and then "pulling" or drawing the needle outward. Of note, when positioning the needle holder for the final movement, the operator's hand should be situated so that the palm is facing down such that rotating the needle does not result in an uncomfortable and awkward over-twisting of the wrist and forearm.

An extension of this practice is an advanced maneuver of adjusting the needle orientation without the use of a second hand. It can be accomplished by resting the needle tip on a stationary object (surgical drapes or nearby soft tissue), opening the ratchet on the needle driver slightly while maintaining grasp of the needle body, and using the tip of the needle driver as a fulcrum to turn the needle slightly in the desired direction.

Maximize Utilization of Body Positioning

Your attending surgeons will never miss a chance to point out whenever you appear awkward during an operation. For the right-handed surgeon, an easy way to avoid this criticism is to sew (with the needle tip pointing) toward yourself whenever possible. Occasionally, certain stitches require you to point the needle away from your body or "sew away from yourself," but normally it is not necessary. In general, your dominant hand should be moving toward your non-dominant hand, but exactly how this looks will vary depending on your body position as well as the orientation of the wound. As with knot tying, get used to adjusting your body positioning to give yourself the best leverage. Some specific examples to illustrate this concept include turning your body perpendicular to the OR table and taking your first bite on the opposite side when closing a longitudinal fascial incision. When you are unsure of which end to start with a running stitch, it can be helpful to image that you are sewing towards your left foot.

Suture Bite Size

The size of the bite depends on the needle size, the distance of the needle insertion site from the wound edge, and depth of the bite taken. It is yet another spatial skill that must be learned, but once it is understood it can be leveraged for various applications. Generally, bites should be symmetric on each side to allow for an equal distribution of tension. If a wound is asymmetrical, different sized bites can be used to correct the appearance of the defect. Smaller bites are employed when a more precise closure is desired (i.e., ends of incision that is not uniform in length to prevent dog-earing). Larger bites are used when less wound tension is desirable.

Tips for Practicing Proper Bite Size

The spatial awareness skill can be honed through an exercise nicknamed "needle tip consciousness." This exercise can be performed using an OR towel marked with two columns of dots of various widths. The purpose is to enter at one dot and emerge at the other with accuracy. It requires knowledge of the needle and attention to way the needle is loaded and the depth of entry.

Suture Tail Control

As a final point, the concept of suture tail control is an important one that is often forgotten until it becomes a problem. Suture material has a tendency to get caught around the handles of surgical instruments or any other projection along its path. This can be extremely detrimental when needle movement is hindered or exaggerated by any subsequent manipulation of the strands. Techniques to combat this occurrence are the intentional setting of the tail opposite the direction of sewing which can be done by dragging the tail across the wound and flicking the instrument so that the tail is cast away from you, removing unnecessary instruments, and covering projections with towels. It also helps to limit the tail to the least length necessary for tying a knot.

3.2.3 Technical/Practical Considerations/Safety Precautions

3.2.3.1 Knotting Under circumstances

Just when you think you've mastered tying knots, you will find yourself in a situation that makes you think again. This section will describe techniques for approaching the following circumstances: tying under tension, tying into a body cavity, passing ties around a hemostat, and passing ties into a deep cavity.

Tying Under Tension

Tying knots under tension should be avoided because they have a tendency to slip. However, certain circumstances (i.e., fascial closure, drawing together two structures that are at a distance) require it. Using specialized knots such as a surgeon's or a fisherman's knot is one way to help avoid slippage of the first knot. To create a surgeon's knot, one end of the suture makes two passes through the loop on the first hitch prior to squaring the knot (Fig. 3.5d). While this type of knot decreases the likelihood of wound separation as the second hitch is being formed, it should be note that it offers no additional strength and generates a bulkier knot which can be difficult to tie and more prone to breakage. It is primarily used for heavy monofilament suture.

Other techniques for tying under tension require the participation of an assistant. First, the assistant can compress tissue together to relieve the tension. If the tissue is not compressible, the strands must be kept taut after the first half-hitch is formed and tightened. To keep hold of the first hitch, the strands can be rotated 90°. Then, the assistant can place a finger to compress the first half-hitch which the second hitch is formed. The assistant's finger can be released as the knot is tightened.

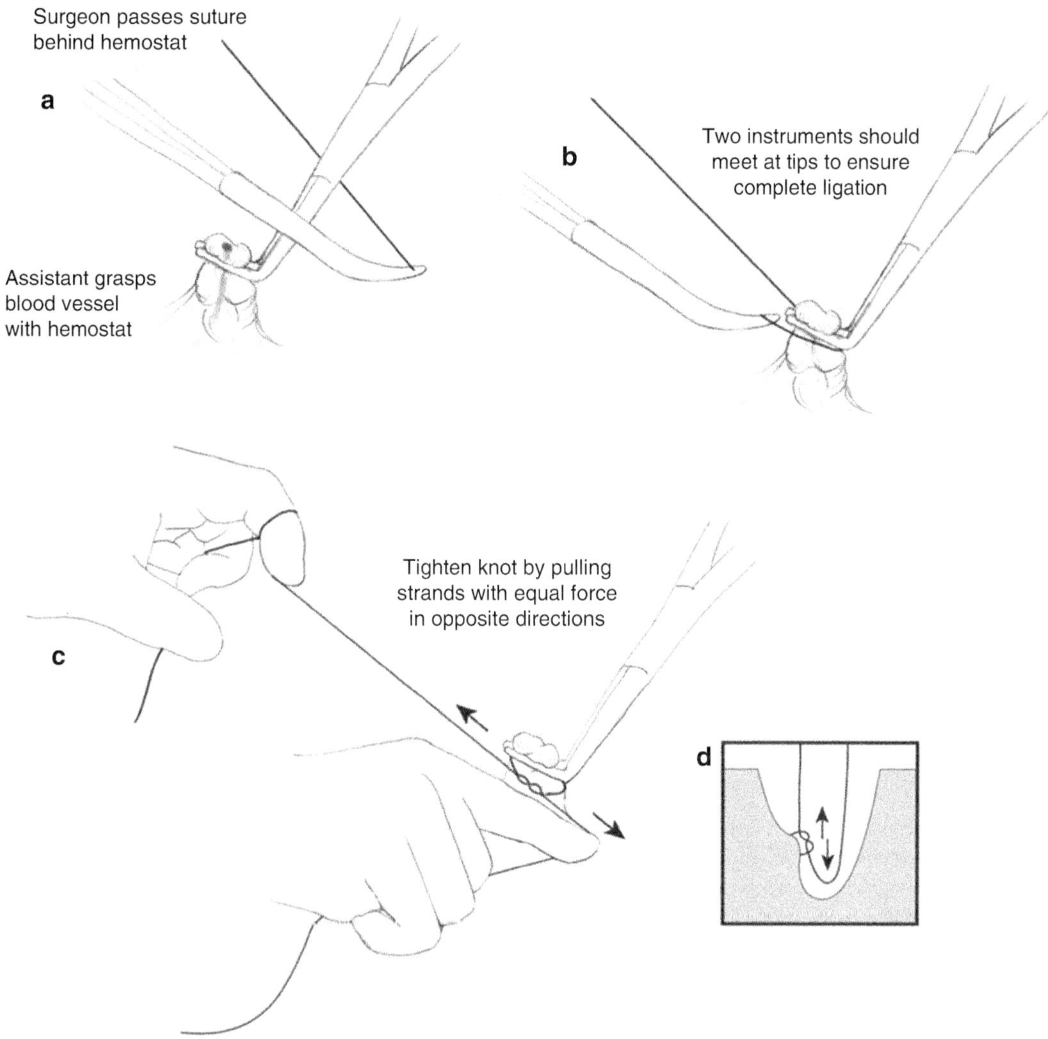

Fig. 3.9 Ligation around hemostatic clamp. Panel a demonstrates how to properly pass a suture ligature around a clamp. The suture within the passer should be brought around the tissue to be tied by passing the tip of the passing clamp directly facing the tip of the tissue clamp tips (**a**). The clamp and passing instrument should meet "tip-to-tip" (**b**). As the knot is being tightened, the clamp is slowly released to allow for the tie to compress the tissue within the clamp (**c**). Tying in a hole may require pulling up on one strand of suture while simultaneously pushing down the other strand of suture with your index finger with equal tension in both directions (**d**)

Tying in a Body Cavity

Tying a *good* knot in a deep space is difficult. It presents a challenge for a number of reasons. First, the resident must manipulate the strands gently to avoid undue upward tension because even minor movements can be amplified over the distance and result in tearing or avulsion of the tissue. Second, due to limited space, pulling the ends of strands in opposite directions in the horizontal plane is not always possible. The key to forming a square knot becomes dependent on pulling both strands with equal force in opposite directions. Unless one is acutely aware, the natural tendency is to pull one of the sutures with unopposed force. This converts a square knot into a slip knot which can loosen spontaneously or give way to internal pressure.

Essential habits to develop proficiency with this skill include ensuring an adequate length of suture material, using a two-handed technique, and forming half-hitches outside of the cavity. An adequate length of suture material is long enough to be manipulated outside of the cavity. Using a two-handed technique prevents generating excessive torque on the structure being tied. A helpful exercise for recognizing the degree of tension that is exerted on tissue is tying knots on the tab of an empty can. This exercise teaches residents through tactile feedback. With the goal of minimal to no movement of the can during the forming or setting of the knot, residents can develop the "soft hands" necessary for tying delicate structures.

It is important to advance the knot into the cavity before securing it. Pulling the two ends of the suture outside of the body often advances the crossing of the strands to the point that there will be appropriate length to secure the knot. If it does not, you may have to manually push the preformed knot into the deep space prior to setting yourself up to tighten the knot.

To tighten the knot, the movement is a pushing down on one end with a simultaneous matched pulling on the other end from within the body cavity with the same force (Fig. 3.9d). Sometimes it is necessary to use forceps to position and manipulate a knot into a very deep space. Under these circumstances, the forceps act as an extension of your fingers, but this comes with a loss of tactile feedback on the degree of tension being applied and the potential to damage or break the suture. Tightening a knot in a cavity is another skill that is easily practiced outside of the operating room. There are pre-fabricated practice boards with cylinders of various sizes, but empty canisters that are found commonly around the hospital or house also do quite well to simulate a deep, narrow working space.

Ligation Around Hemostatic Clamp

Ligating a blood vessel or tissue that is grasped by a hemostatic clamp (hemostat, Kelly clamp, or right angle) is a common technique for achieving hemostasis. Sufficient tissue around the vessel should be cleared away. The assistant should position the clamp with its tips turned upward and with the tissue near the end of the clamp, but ensure that the very tip of the clamp is free (Fig. 3.9a). The suture can be held with a forceps or on a hemostat in the right hand of the surgeon. The loose end of the suture is passed behind the assistant's instrument (Fig. 3.9a). The two instruments should meet at the tips to ensure that the ligature is entirely around the tissue contained in the clamp and positioned just below the jaws of the clamp (Fig. 3.9b). As the first throw is tightened, the assistant should be given a cue to begin opening the clamp just as the knot is being cinched.

3.2.3.2 Methods of Suturing

The primary goals of suturing are to close dead space, support and strengthen wounds until healing increases their tensile strength, approximate skin edges for cosmesis and functional result, and/or minimize bleeding and infection.

Stitching can be classified broadly according to the number or layers (one or multiple), number of rows (typically only one), or technique (interrupted versus continuous). Interrupted suturing is safer because the tension on each suture can be adjusted individually and if one suture comes undone, the integrity of the entire closures is not affected. For continuous suturing, the integrity depends on just one knot, but for the same reason, it can be carried out rapidly because less knot tying is required.

Approximating Skin and Soft Tissues

The goal of subcutaneous closure is to reapproximate and evert the skin edges. The subcutaneous tissues themselves are not typically sutured closed, but instead brought together by closing the deeper layers of tissue as well as the dermal and subcuticular layers above. The most commonly used stitches to accomplish this are: simple, vertical mattress, continuous subcuticular, and inverted-U stitch. The principal differences in these suturing methods is whether the sutures are placed in an interrupted fashion or use one continuous suture and the orientation of the knot (above or below the skin).

Simple Interrupted

A simple interrupted is the workhorse stitch. You can never go wrong using this stitch to close any wound. One disadvantage of the stitch is that is leaves marks at the entry and exit points. Another is that for longer incisions it can be time consuming and it can be uncomfortable for patients to have these stitches removed. For stellate lacerations, it is useful for aligning angulated skin flaps. In cases where you are concerned about contamination, it is preferable because the entire wound will not come apart if one stitch is removed in order to allow for drainage or packing. A vertical mattress is a variation of the simple interrupted that can be used when the tissue is fragile. The placement of the suture takes tension off the suture line. When placing this stitch, load your needle as far back on the needle holder as possible without positioning on the needle swage to allow for a large bite. For the reverse bite, load the needle in a backhanded position. Be careful when setting the knot to avoid excessive tension; this results in puckering of wound edges and makes for difficulty removing.

Continuous Subcuticular Stitch

One of the most popular, but misunderstood cosmetic stitches is the continuous subcuticular stitch (Fig. 3.10). The purpose of the stitch is to invisibly align two skin edges. Most likely you have seen this stitch incorrectly result in a serpentine appearing wound. If done properly, this stitch should make your incision disappear. The key principals to this stitch are shown in Fig. 3.10. First, ensure that the suture runs continuously and precisely within the same horizontal plane. Second, there must be direct opposition of the suture exit point on one side and entry point on the other side. Any deviation from this plane results in scalloping of the wound. Third, the bites should maintain the same depth from the surface throughout the length of the wound.

The proper technique to ensure a good closure is called "sewing straight with a curved needle." Ninety percent of this technique relies on utilization of the retracting (left-hand) forceps. The wound edge should be grasped sufficiently far away from the predicted exit point of the nee-

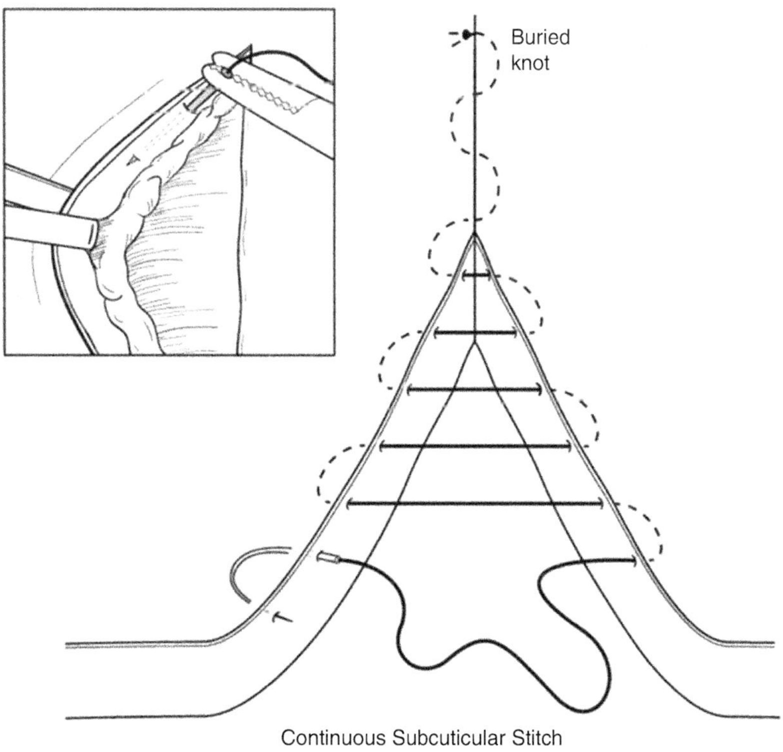

Fig. 3.10 Continuous subcuticular stitch. This stitch is most commonly used to close skin. Ensure the plane the needle travels is completely parallel with the surface of the skin (inset). When you cross the suture to the opposite side of the wound, it is essential that you enter the tissue directly opposite of the last stitch making sure that you do not travel forward at all and that you maintain the same depth from the surface throughout the length of the wound

dle and pulled to tension in line with the wound (Fig. 3.10 inset). Imagine laying your needle on the skin along the wound; this is the desired orientation that your needle should be in as it passes through the tissue. When you enter the tissue, pronating your wrist will cause your needle to advance farther laterally from the wound edge than necessary, warping the closure. The proper motion is a simple pushing of the needle through the tissue without any supination of the wrist.

Inverted U-Stitch

An inverted u-stitch is often employed to close laparoscopic port sites. All too often, when one is done placing this stitch, it appears as though the wound is still open. The primary reason for this failure is that the curve of the U is not superficial enough. The superficial entry and exit point should be at the exact cell layer that the knife cuts the skin. The forehand portion of the stitch is generally not problematic, but one should take the time to ensure that the needle exits as close to the surface of the wound as possible. When starting the superficial bite, it is often difficult to find the correct depth. Use your forceps to reach inside the wound and pull the dermis into the middle of the wound. While using your needle tip to push back the epidermis, you can then drive the needle straight through the dermis.

Stitches for Fascial Closure and Hemostasis

Continuous Running

The continuous over and over stitch is sometimes called a baseball stitch or a running whipstitch. It is used to quickly close long incisions. There are two techniques that you can practice for efficiency. First, practice releasing and reloading the needle while it is in the tissue. You will find that after reloading the needle, it is in a back-handed configuration and you will need to turn the needle holder 180° in your hand prior to taking the next bite. An alternative technique can be liked to a "pitch and catch" motion. This involves passing the needle through the tissue with rotational wrist movement and releasing the needle to be grasped and rotated through the remaining tissue using the forceps.

Suture Ligature

Suture ligatures and figure-of-eight can be used for achieving hemostasis. The suture ligature, colloquially known as a stick tie, should be used when a vessel can be identified and clamped or prior to division. On the other hand, when a vessel is not clearly identifiable, has retracted into tissue, or the surrounding tissue is friable and dissection is prohibitive, the figure of eight stitch is the preferred technique. In performing this technique, after the first bite on one side of the suspected bleeding point, pull up on both ends of the suture to ensure that the bleeding has stopped. This simultaneously helps to maneuver the tissue for the second bite.

Continuous Running Locking Stitch

A continuous running locking stitch (Fig. 3.11) resists unraveling when you are sewing a long wound. This technique is most efficiently per-

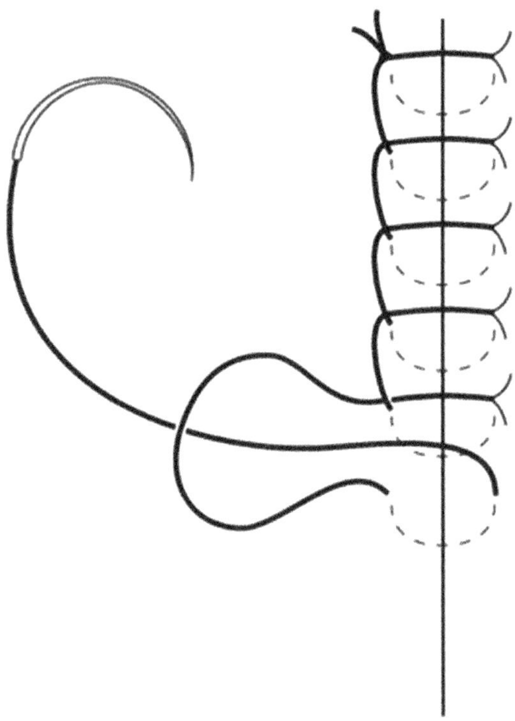

Fig. 3.11 Continuous running locking stitch. This fast suturing technique will help close longer wounds and maintain tension on the incision by mechanism of the "locking" loop, which is formed by passing the needle and suture through the last placed loop

formed with an active assistant who will present the loop of suture after each bite for the surgeon to pass the needle under. Otherwise, this stitch can be cumbersome and time consuming for a solo surgeon.

Stitches for Gastrointestinal Anastomosis

The next series of stitches are for sewing on bowel. They hinge on the concept of a seromuscular bite which effectively inverts and approximates two ends of bowel [22].

Lembert Suture

The Lembert suture is the quintessential stitch that includes a bite of serosa and submucosa about 2.5 mm from cut edge and exits just proximal to cut edge of bowel (Fig. 3.12). It should be stressed that more so than for any other stitch, the needle must enter perpendicularly to the tissue. A helpful way of thinking about this is that the needle tip should be pointed straight down to the floor and rotated sharply just after the needle is felt popping through the serosa. If done correctly and the bite is of an appropriate thickness, the suture should not be visible through the bowel wall. It is the safest and most useful stitch in constructing a GI anastomosis because the mucosal surface is inverted and the fibromuscular layer is incorporated. It can be used in an interrupted fashion where the tension can be set on each individual suture or in a continuous fashion.

Purse-String Suture

A purse-string suture is essentially a continuous Lembert suture around a circular opening. The size of the opening dictates the number of sutures to complete the circle. If the opening is large, it may require reversal of the needle for a backhanded stitch. One way to quickly switch between a forehand and backhand is by loosely grabbing just proximal to the point of the needle with Debakey forceps and either tapping the tail of the needle toward or away from you to change the orientation of the needle.

Connell Stitch

The Connell stitch is typically used for the anterior mucosal layer of two-layer anastomosis because it is more fluid tight and slightly hemostatic. The suture should be placed loose enough to avoid ischemia of the bowel wall. Depicted in Fig. 3.13, the stitch is often remembered as "the bar crawl." First, take a full thickness bite from

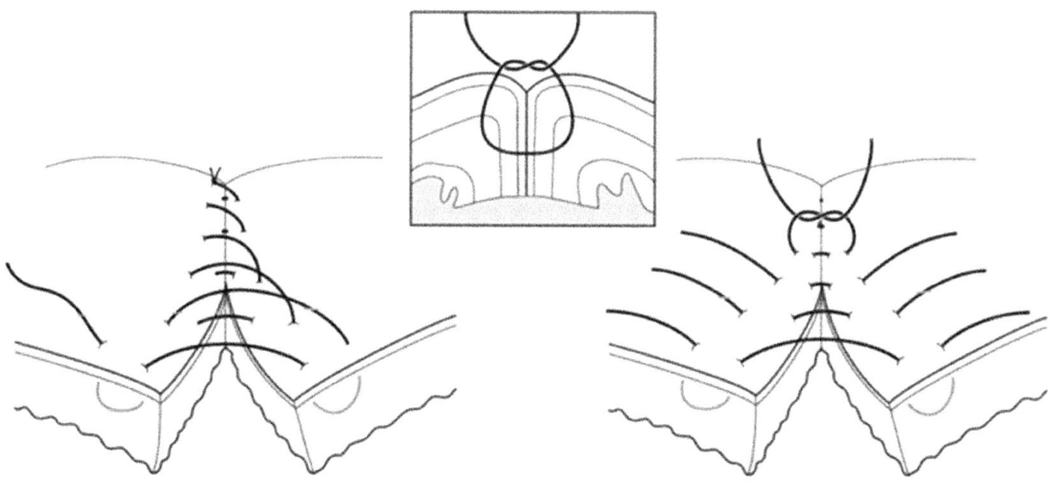

Fig. 3.12 Lembert stitch. These seromuscular bites predominate when creating a gastrointestinal anastomosis. The needle must enter the serosa perpendicularly about 2.5 mm from the cut edge. The suture must be at the depth of the submucosal plane, and thus not visible through the bowel wall. Always take these stitches in two bites to ensure that you are truly entering the tissue at a 90° angle

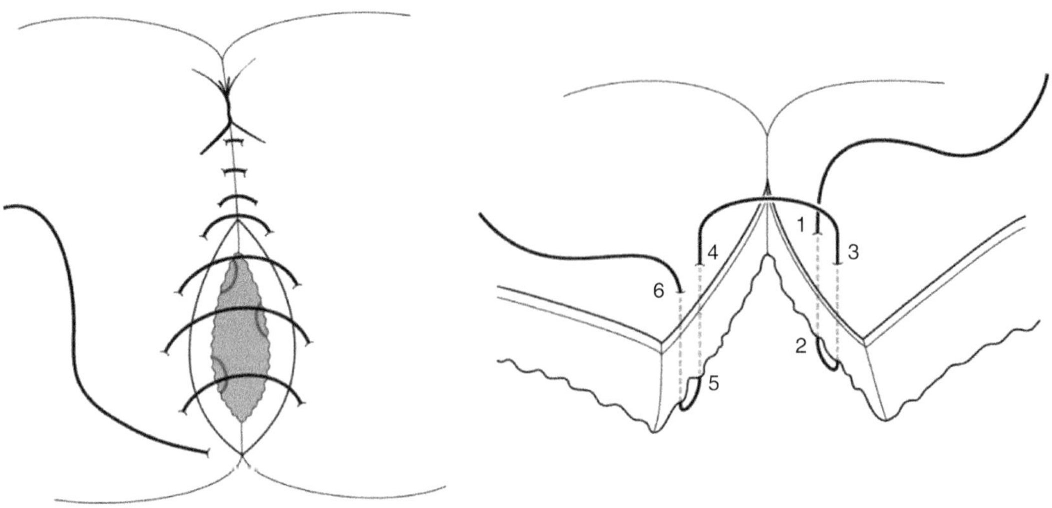

Fig. 3.13 Connell stitch. This stitch is used to invert mucosa so that the serosa is opposed. Each bite must be full thickness through serosa and mucosa. Traveling along the cut edge is always done within the lumen of the bowel. Traveling to the other side is done directly in line with the exit point of your last stitch

serosa to lumen about 4–5 mm from the cut edge of the bowel or "enter the bar" (#1). After traveling a short distance (about 3 mm) parallel to the cut surface (#2), exit the lumen to serosa or "leave the bar" (#3). Then, cross to the opposite edge of the enterotomy or "go across the street" (#4) and repeat the same out to in (#5) and then in to out (#6) sequence.

Modified Gambee Stitch

The Gambee stitch allows for apposition of two layers (mucosa and serosa) with a single stitch. This allows you to use a single suture to mimic a two-layer anastomosis. It can be useful in creating an anastomosis when two cut edges are mismatched in size. When performing a modified Gambee stitch (Fig. 3.14), enter serosa 6–8 mm from cut edge (#1) and penetrate the mucosa into the lumen but immediately exit by taking a bite through the mucosa and submucosa 2–3 mm from edge (#2). The second part of the stitch follows a mirror image: enter the submucosa 2–3 mm from the edge (#3), penetrate the mucosa and immediately return through the mucosa to exit the serosa 6–8 mm from the cut edge (#4).

3.2.4 Current Controversies/Future Directions

3.2.4.1 Knotless Suturing

Knots have several inherent and acquired limitations. They reduce a suture's tensile strength, distribute tension unequally along a wound, can extrude from a wound, serve as a potential nidus for infection, and can come undone as a result of human error. Barbed suture was developed and allows for knotless suturing where knot tying would affect cosmetic outcome because of unequal tension or extrusion.

Barbed suture has linear nicks along its length which allows the suture only to be pulled in one direction. It was first introduced as a concept in 1956. It was first used clinically in 1967. From 1967 to 1999, a variety of designs were trialed. The modern design of one-way sutures with exterior barbs has been employed since 2004 and there are currently three types available commercially (see Sect. 3.1).

Barbed suture allows for knotless suturing and as a result is appealing to surgeon's who encounter circumstances where tying knots is quite frankly difficult. For example, laparo-

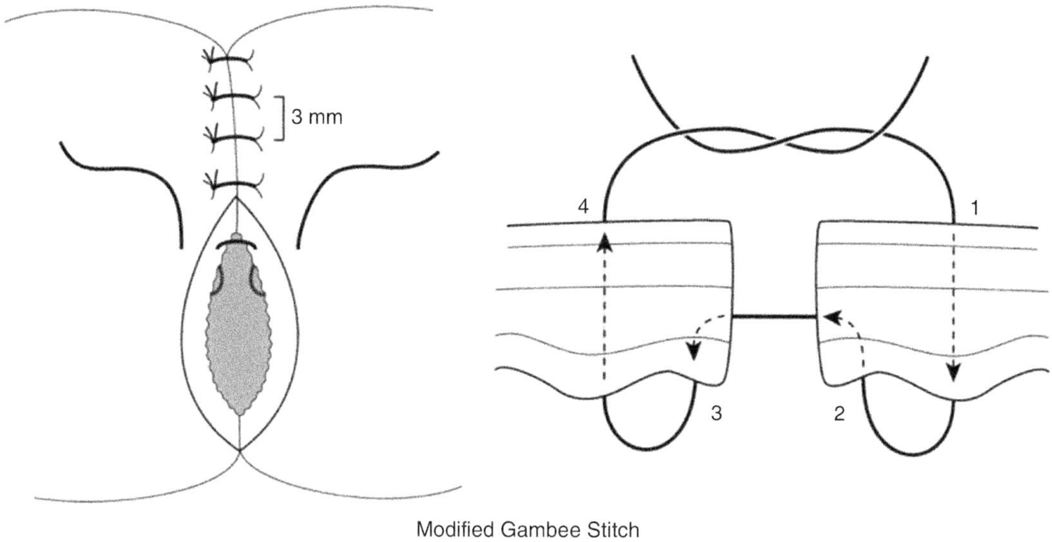

Fig. 3.14 Modified Gambee stitch. This stitch allows you to perform a "two layer" closure that inverts the mucosa and apposed the serosa using one stitch

scopic knot tying is considered to be one of the most technically challenging surgical skills. The ability to properly and efficiently tie surgical knots requires extensive rehearsal. This challenge remains for robotic suturing. As minimally invasive techniques predominant and robotic techniques gain momentum in general surgery practice, the use of barbed suture is becoming more commonplace.

To date, there have been 17 RCTs in various surgical disciplines (cosmetic surgery, bariatric surgery, urology, gynecology, and orthopedic surgery) to evaluate outcomes with barbed suture versus conventional suture. Outcomes that have been studied include suture time, operative time, and post-operative complications. And, although there are theoretical advantages of this technique (i.e., stronger closure), no studies have comprehensively examined the benefits and clinical trials have only consistently shown a reduction in suture or operative time [23].

Take-Home Points

- Basic techniques of needle holding, needle driving, and knot placement are the same regardless of the specific suture and needle that are chosen.
- It is not sufficient to learn simply how to form knots. Just as important is how to tighten and place knots.
- You must become proficient tying one and two-handed knots, using both your left and right hands. Furthermore these skills must be practiced to the point where you automatically use the most efficient technique to tie each knot presented to you.
- Needle tip consciousness (the knowledge of the position of the tip of the needle as it passes through tissue) is an ability that needs to be acquired in order to safely and efficiently suture.
- Mastery of suturing is essential to all aspects of surgery, from achieving hemostasis to restoring proper function of various organ systems.
- Knowing various methods of suturing can help you choose the most appropriate for each situation.
- Practice knot tying every single day.

Suggested Readings

Dunn DL. Wound closure manual. Somerville: Ethicon; 2005.

Boros M, editor. Surgical techniques: textbook for medical students. Szeged: Innovariant; 2006.

Knot Tying Videos http://www.bumc.bu.edu/surgery/training/technical-training/basic-knots-sutures/.

ACS/APDS Surgery Resident Skills Curriculum.

References

1. Kirkup J. The history and evolution of surgical instruments. V Needles and their penetrating derivatives. Ann R Coll Surg Engl. 1986;68:29–33.
2. Barr J. Lister's ligatures. J Vasc Surg. 2014;60:1383–5.
3. Rutkow I. The rise of modern surgery: an overview. In: Townsend CM, Beauchamp RD, Evers BM, Mattox KL, editors. Sabiston textbook of surgery: the biological basis of modern surgical practice. 20th ed. Philadelphia: Elsevier; 2017. p. 2–19.
4. Knot Tying Manual. Ethicon http://surgsoc.org.au/wp-content/uploads/2014/03/Ethicon-Knot-Tying-Manual.pdf.
5. Surgical Knot Tying Manual, 3rd ed. Covidien http://www.covidien.com/imageServer.aspx?contentID=11850&contenttype=application/pdf.
6. Boros M, editor. Surgical techniques: textbook for medical students. Szeged: Innovariant; 2006.
7. "Basic Knots" http://www.ruralareavet.org/PDF/Surgery-Knot_Tying.pdf. Accessed 26 Aug 2017.
8. Cooper P. Observations on surgical training and technique. In: unknown editors. The craft of surgery. 1st ed.: Boston; year unknown. p. 3–18.
9. Deitch E, editor. Tools of the trade and rules of the road: a surgical guide. Philadelphia: Lippincott -Raven; 1997.
10. Kirk RM. Handling instruments and handling threads. In: Kirk RM, editor. Basic surgical technique. 6th ed. Amsterdam: Elsevier Health Sciences; 2010. p. 21–46.
11. Unknown. Dissecting and suturing. In: Scott-Conner C, editor. Chassin's operative strategy in general surgery: an expositive atlas. 3rd ed. New York: Springer; 2002. p. 26–37.
12. "Needle Comparison Chart." https://www.aesculapusa.com/assets/base/doc/DOC571RevC-AesculapNeedleComparisonChart-3-foldBrochure.pdf. Accessed 12 Sep 2017.
13. Baracs J, Huszár O, Sajjadi SG, Horváth OP. Surgical site infections after abdominal closure in colorectal surgery using triclosan-coated absorbable suture (PDS Plus) vs. uncoated sutures (PDS II): a randomized multicenter study. Surg Infect. 2011;12:483–9.
14. Justinger C, Slotta JE, Ningel S, Gräber S, Kollmar O, Schilling MK. Surgical-site infection after abdominal wall closure with triclosan-impregnated polydioxanone sutures: results of a randomized clinical pathway facilitated trial. Surgery. 2013;154:589–95.
15. Nakamura T, Kashimura N, Noji T. Triclosan-coated sutures reduce the incidence of wound infections and the costs after colorectal surgery: a randomized controlled trial. Surgery. 2013;153:576–83.
16. Diener MK, Knebel P, Kieser M. Effectiveness of triclosan-coated PDS Plus versus uncoated PDS II sutures for prevention of surgical site infection after abdominal wall closure: the randomised controlled proud trial. Lancet. 2014;384:142–52.
17. Mattavelli I, Rebora P, Doglietto G. Multi-center randomized controlled trial on the effect of triclosan-coated sutures on surgical site infection after colorectal surgery. Surg Infect. 2015;16:226–35.
18. "STRATFIX™ Knotless Tissue Control Devices." http://www.ethicon.com/healthcare-professionals/products/wound-closure/stratafix-knotless-tissue-control-devices. Accessed 12 Sep 2017.
19. Wang ZX, Jiang CP, Cao Y, et al. Systematic review and meta-analysis of triclosan sutures for prevention of surgical-site infection. Br J Surg. 2013;100:465–73.
20. Elsolh B, Xhang L, Patel SV. The Effect of antibiotic-coated sutures on the incidence of surgical site infections in abdominal closures: a meta-analysis. J Gastrointest Surg. 2017;21:896–903.
21. Matarasso A, Ruff GL. The history of barbed sutures. Anesthet Surg. 2013;33:12S–6S.
22. Zuidema GD, Shackelford RT. Gastrointestinal Suturing. In: Zuidema GD and Shackelford RT, editors. Surgery of the Alimentary Tract, 2nd ed. Saunders (W.B.) Co Ltd; 1986. p. 556–78.
23. Lin Y, Lai S, Huang J, et al. The efficacy and safety of knotless barbed sutures in the surgical field: a systematic review and meta-analysis of randomized controlled trials. Sci Rep. 2016;6:23425. https://doi.org/10.1038/srep23425.

4 Fundamentals of Patient Positioning and Skin Prep

Giulio Giambartolomei, Samuel Szomstein, Raul Rosenthal, and Emanuele Lo Menzo

4.1 Introduction

The evolution of surgery from being performed only through an open incision to being completed with minimally invasive techniques has required several changes to the traditional operating room setup but also mandated new and—at times—extreme positions to be kept during the procedure at hand. These have required the surgeons to become even more attuned to paying special attention to the positioning of patients prior to any surgical procedure since a mistake at this stage may result in poor or inadequate exposure and possibly in injury. Also the increased utilization of surgical implants on one hand, and the growing prevalence of multidrug-resistant bacteria on the other, demanded the manufacturing and utilization of new and more potent skin prepping compounds. The surgical resident is an integral part of the team and has to be familiar with the most up-to-date strategies for safe conduct in the operating room, including the utilization of team huddles, preoperative checklists, and time-out.

G. Giambartolomei · S. Szomstein · R. Rosenthal
E. Lo Menzo (✉)
Department of Surgery, The Bariatric and Metabolic Institute, Cleveland Clinic Florida, Weston, FL, USA
e-mail: lomenze@ccf.org

4.2 General Concepts

4.2.1 OR Environment

Modern operative room's design results from an evolution of technology and evidence-based studies on potential patient's injuries due to improper surgical positioning. However, despite newly engineered materials built to protect pressure vulnerable areas, careful patient positioning by the surgical team is paramount in order to safely and successfully complete an operation. While surgeons have traditionally focused on proper positioning to ensure appropriate exposure of a target organ, at times, safety considerations have been overlooked.

4.2.2 Postsurgical Injuries and Epidemiology

Although not extensively discussed in surgical programs, a thorough knowledge of the pathophysiology and etiology of potential position-related injuries should be part of a well-rounded surgeon.

The possible complications of patient positioning in the operating room can be summarized

F. Palazzo (ed.), *Fundamentals of General Surgery*, https://doi.org/10.1007/978-3-319-75656-1_4

as follows: falls, ocular injuries, peripheral neuropathies, pressure ulcers, and general anesthesia-related.

4.2.2.1 Falls

Unfortunately, hospital falls remain a current problem, and it is extensively reported in the literature. No accurate data have been published about the perioperative frequency of falls, except for anecdotal episodes resulted in patient's death. Thus an assessment of fall risk is advisable when admitting the patient to the operating room.

4.2.2.2 Ocular Injuries

The frequency of ocular injuries is usually low (<0.1%), but the range of severity could vary from mild discomfort to corneal abrasions and to permanent loss of vision. Simply taping the eyelids more than ointment application during general anesthesia can prevent minor damages secondary to anesthesia-related reduction of tears. Instead retinal ischemia and consequent unilateral or bilateral loss of vision could be a result of low optic artery inflow and venous outflow secondary to high ocular pressure in the prone position [1].

4.2.2.3 Peripheral Neuropathies

Peripheral neuropathies are the second most common complication in the American Society of Anesthesiologist's closed claim database, occurring in 16% of the cases [2]. The severity of the symptoms and expected recovery vary depending on the mechanism and extent of the injury [3]. Neuropraxia is the most common situation when the injury involves the endoneurial capillaries, resulting in perineural edema and conduction block. The main symptom of neuropraxia is paresthesia. A complete resolution of symptoms is usually achieved within 1 week since there is no axonal damage. Whenever the insult is intense enough to generate segmental demyelinization, the functional recovery will take a few months. More severe damages are axonotmesis and neurotmesis that involve complete axonal rupture within an intact nerve sheath and complete nerve disruption, respectively, which are unlikely to resolve spontaneously.

Ulnar neuropathy is the most common peripheral neuropathy and is more frequent in males [4]. It was previously thought to be a consequence of stretch and compression of the nerve due to its superficial course around the medial epicondyle of the elbow. Observed symptoms usually are hypoesthesia of the fourth and fifth fingers, hypothenar eminence's muscle atrophy, and claw hand. Warner et al. retrospectively analyzed 414 patients with a diagnosis of perioperative ulnar neuropathy and found that factors other than patient incorrect positioning are involved in developing this condition, such as male gender, BMI less than 24 or higher than 38, and length of hospitalization higher than 14 days. Their conclusions were supported by a delayed onset of neuropathy, usually 24 h after the procedure, suggesting mechanisms other than simple compression or stretch. However, they found that 53% of the patients regained motor function and sensation within 1 year and those patients who did not regain full function presented only minor disability from pain and weakness (Fig. 4.1).

Brachial plexus injuries are extensively reported as a complication due to malpositioning of the patient and can potentially be irreversible depending on the mechanism of nerve injury.

In general, they are associated with median sternotomy, in which the brachial plexus can be damaged during sternal separation, and with head-down position when the arm is hyperextended over the trunk due to arm-board incorrect placement or shoulder brace compression [5]. A lower incidence of brachial plexus injury is found in the prone position. Also, an exaggerated rotation of the neck or hyperextension of the arm may favor a brachial plexus injury (Fig. 4.2).

Related symptoms will vary from decreased sensation around the shoulder area to motor impairment in arm abduction and usually resolve within 6–8 months depending on the severity.

Lower limb nerve injuries are usually secondary to a compression of the common peroneal nerve at the head of the fibula and in 80% of the cases are encountered when the patient is placed in lithotomy position [6]. Thin patients who smoke are more susceptible to this kind of injury

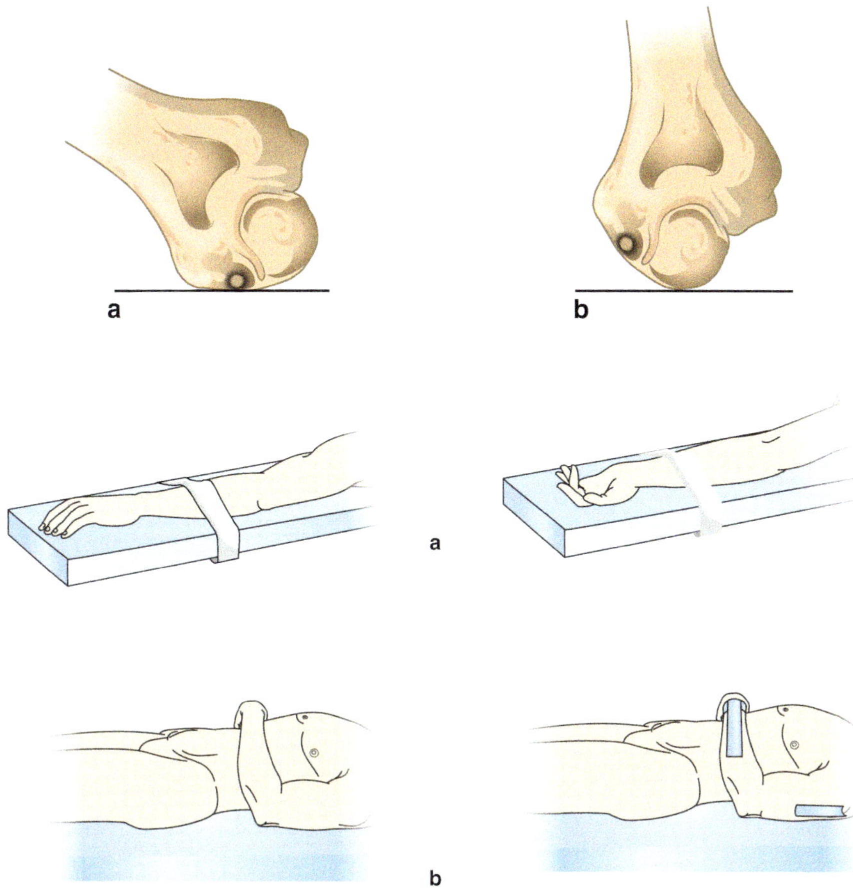

Fig. 4.1 Ulnar nerve injury. (**a**) Potentially nerve threatening position. (**b**) Correct positioning (taken from web)

that may result in foot drop and loss of sensation over the lateral aspect of the leg and dorsum of the foot [3] (Fig. 4.3).

Up to 15% of lower limb peripheral nerve injuries are related to the sciatic nerve, especially with hyperflexion of the hip and extension of the knee in exaggerated lithotomy position. This will result in loss of extension and flexion of the foot and decreased sensation along the anterior and posterior aspects of the leg and foot.

Femoral neuropathy comprises 4% of the cases and is usually caused by continuous compression from intraabdominal retractors on iliopsoas muscle and external iliac artery, resulting in ischemic or mechanical damage to the femoral nerve. Clinical symptoms of femoral nerve injury are sensory loss along the area covered by the anterior and lateral femoral cutaneous nerves and will resolve spontaneously in 94% of the cases.

4.2.2.4 Pressure Ulcers

According to the Agency for Healthcare Research and Quality, 2.5 million patients are affected by pressure ulcers every year, of which 60,000 die from direct consequences.

The surgical patient is more vulnerable to pressure effect because the anesthesia itself induces vasodilation that leads to a decrease in blood pressure and perfusion. In addition, the typically cooler operating room environment,

Fig. 4.2 Brachial plexus injuries. (**a**) Incorrect extension of the arm board more than 90°. (**b**) Correct position of the arm board. (**c**) Inadequate arm padding resulting in a sagging arm board. The dorsal extension of the arm stretches the brachial plexus. (**d**) Correct leveling and padding of the arm board to minimize brachial plexus stretch and ulnar nerve compression at the wrist (taken from web). From Winfree CJ, Kline DG. Intraoperative positioning nerve injuries. Surg Neurol. 2005 Jan;63(1):5-18; discussion 18. Review. Figs. 1 and 2 page 8. Permission not requested

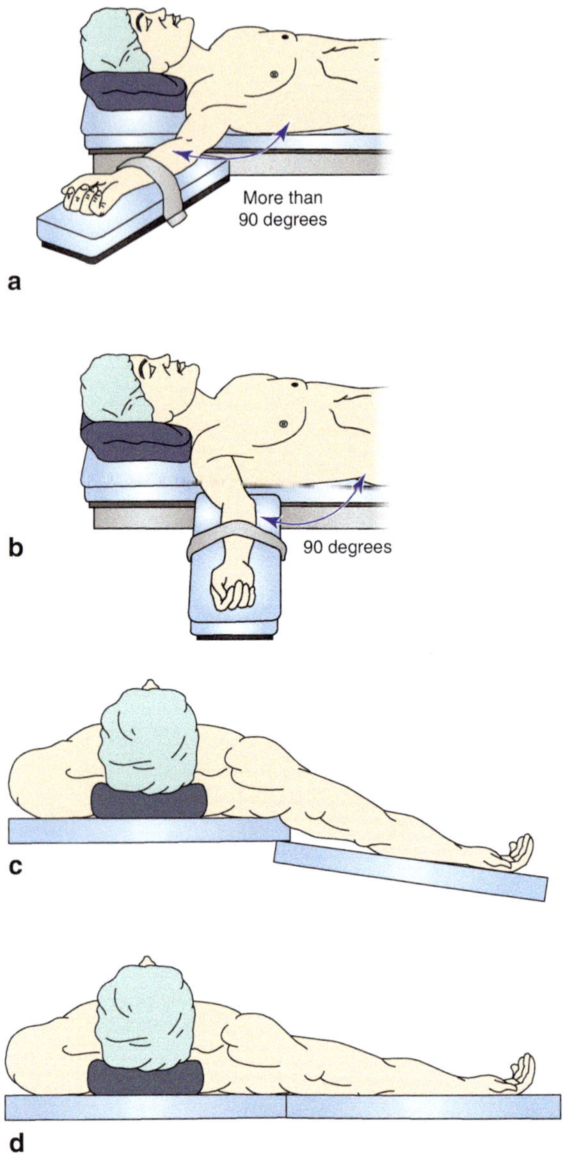

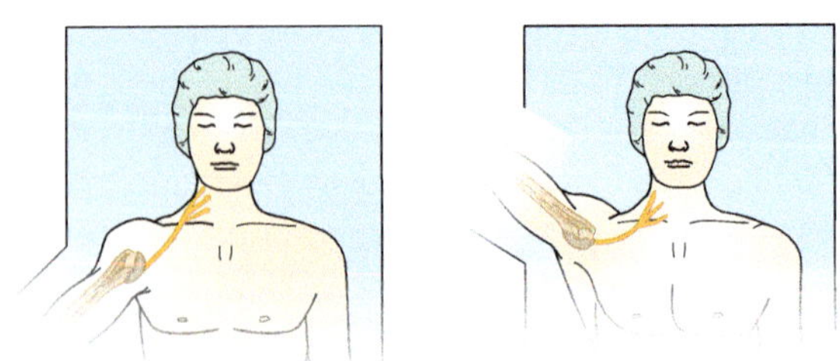

a b

and the use of vasopressors and diuretics, may result in additional decrease in tissue perfusion.

It has been shown that a pressure greater than 32 mmHg, which is the capillary filling pressure, will result in occlusion of blood flow and tissue ischemia. Skin and underlying tissues can tolerate high pressure for short amount of time and low pressures for prolonged time, so that the surgical patient is predisposed to develop ischemic injuries anyway. The duration of pressure over 2 h is associated with an increased risk of development of pressure ulcers [7]. These occur more likely over bony prominences covered by skin and small amounts of muscles and subcutaneous tissue (Fig. 4.4).

Identified risk factors associated with the development of perioperative pressure ulcers can be divided into intrinsic or patient-related, extrinsic, and operating room related.

Patient-related risk factors comprise of the ability to maintain an adequate tissue perfusion. These factors include malnutrition (serum albumin $\leq$3 g/dl), older age, ASA score $\geq$3, decreased mental status, immobility, infection, incontinence, impaired sensory perceptions, and comorbidities such as diabetes, peripheral vascular disease, pulmonary disease, BMI, and altered hemodynamic status.

Extrinsic and operating room-related factors include the type of anesthesia, use of vasopressors, length of surgery, room temperature, type of table and pads, positioning and warming devices, retractors, intraoperative blood pressure fluctuations, and all the factors that affect shear forces, moisture, and friction. The most meaningful risk

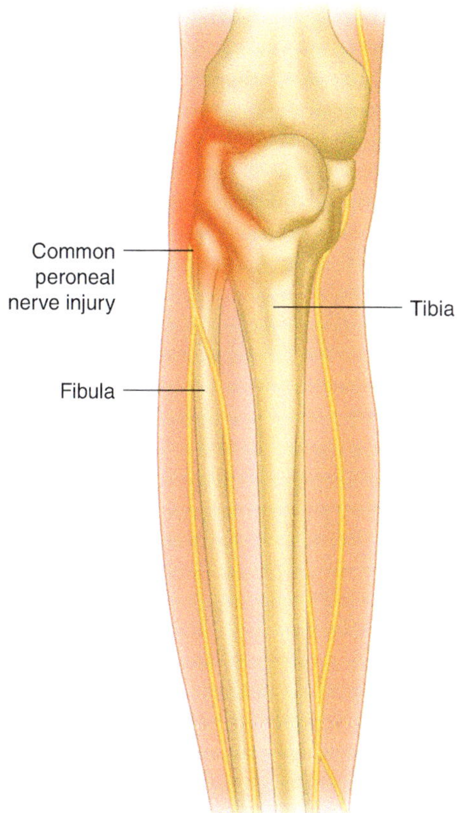

Fig. 4.3 Common peroneal nerve injury (taken from web)

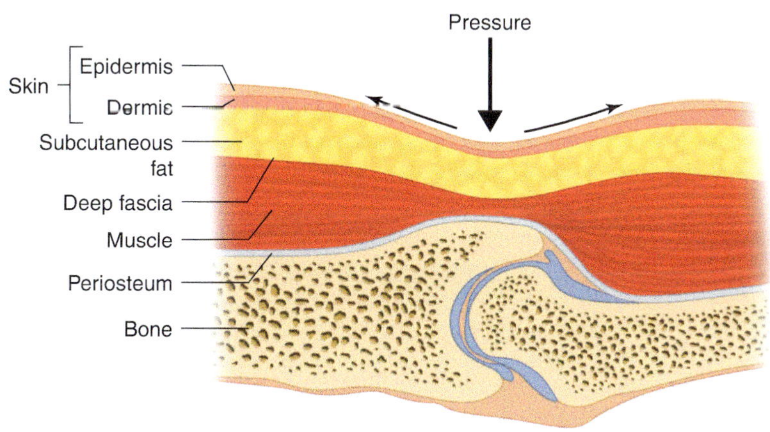

Fig. 4.4 Pressure exerted over bony prominences

factor is the duration of the procedure, with increased risk of developing pressure ulcers after 2.5–3 h.

Rhabdomyolysis is a syndrome caused by crush injury to the skeletal muscles that might occur intraoperatively. The mechanism is related to an ischemia-reperfusion syndrome that compromises sarcolemmal membrane integrity. Skeletal muscle is able to tolerate up to 2 h of ischemia with a complete recovery, but the inflammatory response that follows the reperfusion may be more detrimental for the evolution of the syndrome, due to its increase in capillary permeability, delivery of oxygen-derived free radicals leading to sarcolemmal disruption, and spreading into circulation of intracellular components like myoglobin and potassium ions [8]. The resulting syndrome is characterized by hyperkalemia, hypocalcemia, and high serum creatine kinase (CK), which might lead to acute renal failure, severe arrhythmias, and disseminated intravascular coagulation. Clinical presentation could vary from numbness to pain and motor deficit of the interested area and dark urine. The extended lithotomy position is mostly involved in this type of complication, followed by lateral decubitus position. Obese patients are at particularly high risk for developing this syndrome.

4.3 Technical/Practical Considerations/Safety Precautions

4.3.1 Patient Positioning

The goals of a correct patient positioning can be summarized as follows: ensuring optimal surgical exposure while protecting anatomical structures and ensuring patient comfort and dignity. This must be accomplished while still guaranteeing adequate access for the anesthesia team to the airway and to intravenous medication administration.

It is therefore preferable to ensure a comfortable position to the patient when he/she is still conscious.

4.3.2 Basic Positions

Every surgical subspecialty requires a different position in order to provide ideal exposure of the surgical site. Also, every surgeon might adjust the basic position according to his/her technical needs.

4.3.3 Supine

This position is widely applied in surgical procedures, including abdominal surgery, urology, orthopedic surgery, otorhinolaryngology, and plastic surgery or whenever the surgical site is located on the anterior aspect of the body.

The operative table is horizontally flat; the patient lies on his/her back, hips and knees extended and arms positioned along the trunk or abducted on arm boards. If the arms are positioned along the patient's sides, the palm should be facing the thigh; if placed on arm board, proper padding should be provided together with supination and slight flexion in order to minimize ulnar nerve compression injuries (Fig. 4.5).

The pressure points more susceptible to potential injury are the occiput, the spinous processes of the thoracic vertebrae, the sacrum and coccyx, the scapulae, the olecranon, and the calcaneae. It is a standard practice to use pink foam and pads to protect these pressure points. The routine use of such adjuncts should be included in the surgical checklist.

Abduction of an arm could make an access to IVs and peripheral veins for the administration of drugs and blood draws easier for the anesthesiologist. However, this position could result in less work-space for the surgeon, especially if there is reduced range of motion of the patient's shoulder. Moreover, extra care must be taken not to hyperextend the upper limbs more than 90° from the trunk (Fig. 4.2). Also, the arm boards should be at the same height of the table, in order to avoid brachial plexus injuries. Brachial plexus injuries are extensively reported as a complication due to malpositioning of the patient and can potentially be irreversible depending on the mechanism of nerve injury, as previously described.

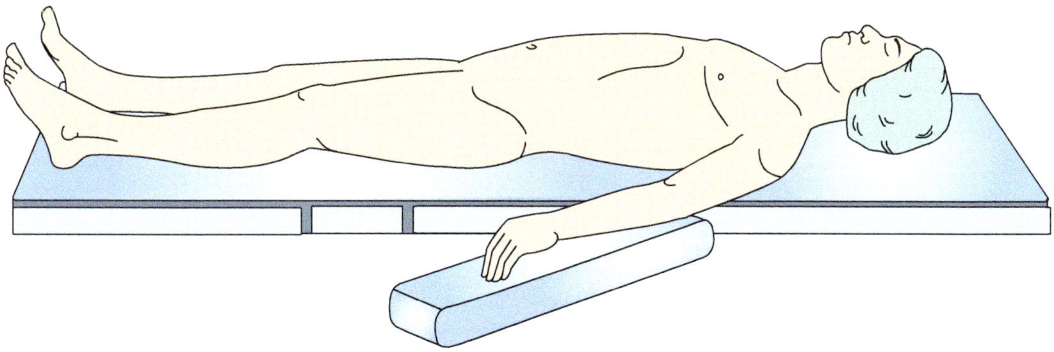

Fig. 4.5 Supine position (taken from web)

The patient must be thoroughly secured to the table with restraining straps or belts, surrounding the thighs, the arms, and sometimes the chest. These precautions are necessary to ensure stability of the patient even in steep positions (such as the head-down tilt (Trendelenburg), and the head-up tilt (reverse Trendelenburg) without exerting excessive pressure on the limbs that might impair blood flow or stretching injuries to the brachial plexus. Securing the patient at the wrist level is then contraindicated (Fig. 4.6). This is particularly important for obese patients, as the weight shifts can cause compression injuries, limbs to falls from table and arm board, and even torso to fall from the operating table. For steep reverse Trendelenburg position, foot plates can be utilized to prevent patients from sliding (Fig. 4.7). However, careful foot padding and knee alignment are paramount to prevent compression injuries.

These principles are particularly important in laparoscopic surgery. In fact, because of the reduced ability of retraction, the exposure of the operative field is often achieved by the use of gravity of steep table tilts. Vacuum beanbags can be utilized as an adjunct to improve patient stability on the operating room table. It is important to avoid direct contact of the beanbag to the patient's skin, in order to avoid skin burns and lacerations. The use of shoulder braces during steep head-down tilt positions could result in potential compression of the brachial plexus. Hence, when used they should be well padded and away from the neck. Finally, in head-up tilt positions, a footboard can be used, after providing optimal padding to the heels.

4.3.4 Lateral

This position is usually used in neurosurgery, thoracotomies, and total hip replacement, as well as in urology and vascular surgery when retroperitoneal structures are approached directly. In general surgery this position is utilized for the laparoscopic approach to the spleen and adrenal gland.

The patient is usually transferred from a supine to a lateral position when secure endotracheal anesthesia has been already established. During the rolling maneuver, a correct spinal alignment should be maintained, and shearing and friction injuries should be avoided. A pillow or headring should be placed to support the head and maintain correct alignment with the neck and the rest of the body.

The patient lies on one side, usually at 90° angle between the patient's back and the table. The lower limb resting on the table should be flexed with an angle of 90° between the thigh and the leg, while the other lower limb should be extended. A pillow should be placed between the legs to prevent damage to peroneal and saphenous nerves.

To protect the axillary nerve bundle and artery of the arm resting on the table, an axillary roll

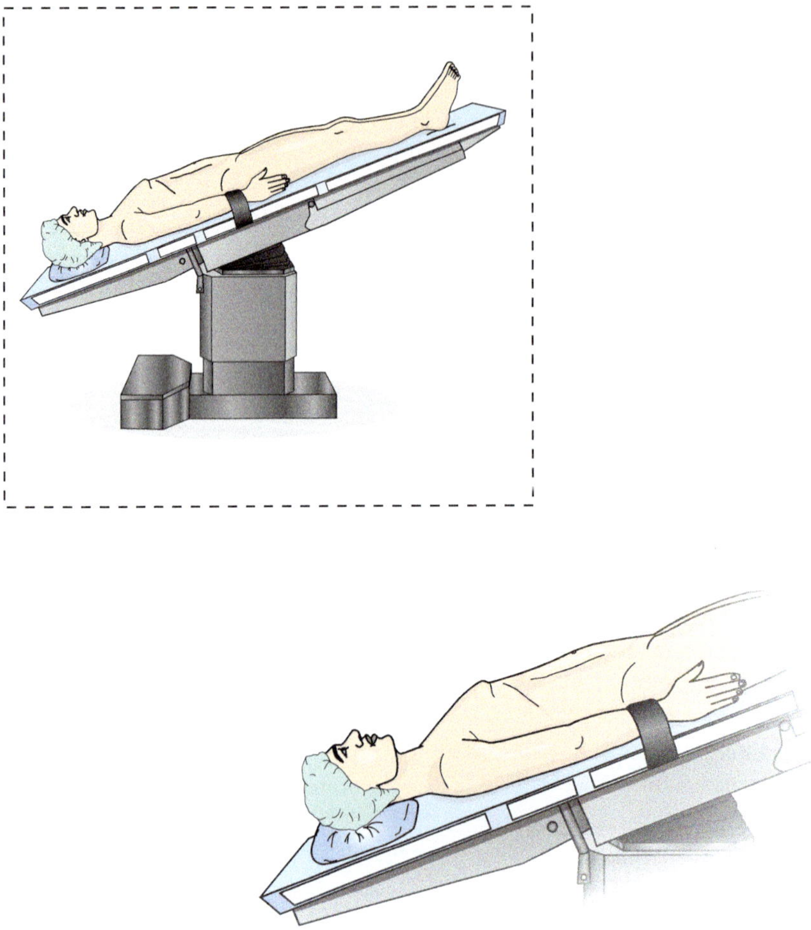

Fig. 4.6 A Trendelenburg position with the patient secured at the wrists determines a downward pull of the humerus head and stretching injury of the brachial plexus. From Cooper DE, Jenkins RS, Bready L, Rockwood CA Jr. The prevention of injuries of the brachial plexus secondary to malposition of the patient during surgery. Clin Orthop Relat Res. 1988 Mar;(228):33-41. Fig. 5-A page 37. Permission not requested

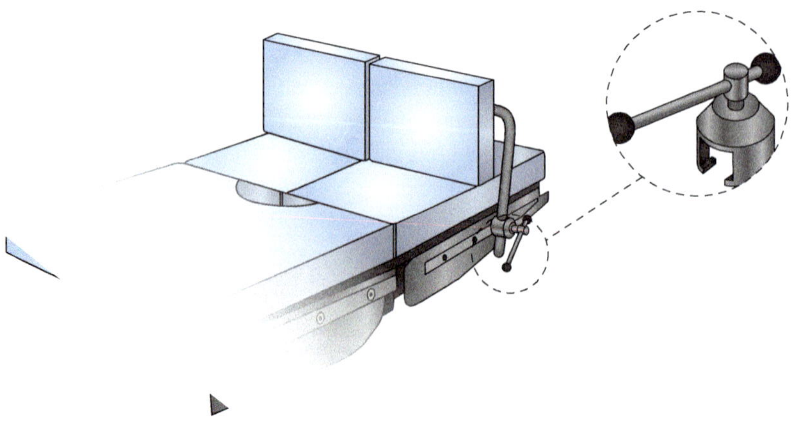

Fig. 4.7 Adjustable foot plate for reverse Trendelenburg positions. From the web

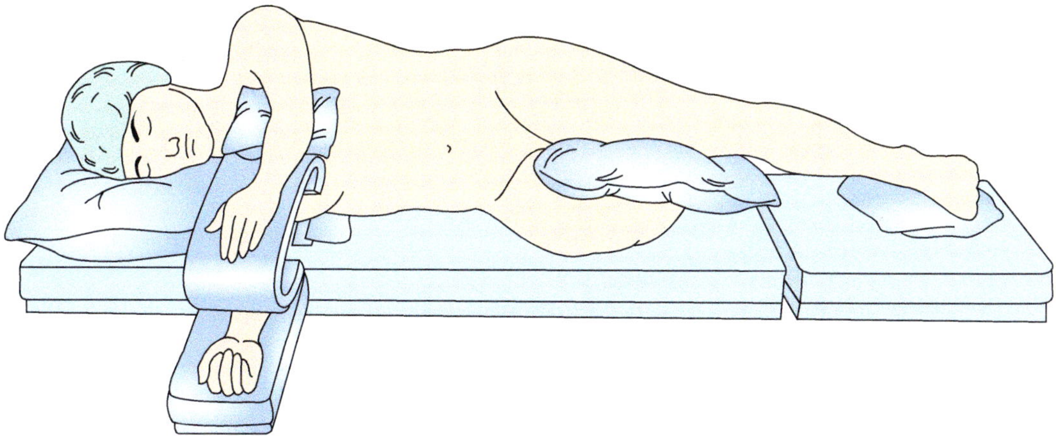

Fig. 4.8 Lateral decubitus position (taken from web)

should be positioned just under the axilla to relieve direct lateral pressure on the shoulder and avoid perfusion impairment. However, there are few old reports of complications of axillary rolls secondary also to compression of the axillary vessels, nerves, and even bronchus ("axillary" compression syndrome) [9]. For this reason, some authors suggest to use a rubber foam under the upper chest just inferior to the tip of the scapula, instead of an axillary roll. It is also advisable to check the radial pulse of the dependent arm to confirm a proper perfusion.

The upper arm should be kept horizontal by the use of a pillow or by an arm board. The horizontal position of the arm will also allow for a more reliable and precise blood pressure measurements. The palm of the inferior hand is positioned upward, and the palm of the superior hand is positioned downward.

Proper padding should be provided to pressure points such as the downside ear, the acromion process, the olecranon, the rib cage, the iliac crest, the greater trochanter, the medial and lateral condyles of the knee, and the medial and lateral malleoli (Fig. 4.8).

4.3.5 Lithotomy

This position is widely used in gynecological, urological, and colorectal/proctologic surgery, as it provides direct access to the perineal area [10].

In the lithotomy position, the patient lies on the back; inferior limbs are positioned on leg holders, unforcedly abducted about 30–45° from the midline; and thighs are flexed over the hips with an angle of about 80–100° on the trunk, with the knees being flexed until the legs are parallel to the frontal plane of the torso (Figs. 4.9 and 4.10). In order to prevent traction of the obturator nerve, the leg should be abducted and aligned with the contralateral shoulder (Fig. 4.11).

The patient's buttock should be positioned at the edge of the lower table break, to reduce lordosis, and the external rotation of the hips should be minimal (Figs. 4.10 and 4.11). The legs and feet should be positioned on stirrups with a popliteal support and a calf rest, avoiding unnecessary pressure points and minimizing movements within the stirrups (Fig. 4.12). For this reason stirrups with a foot and ankle support are preferred to decrease pressure on the calf (Fig. 4.13). Also appropriate padding should be provided to the head of the fibula to avoid common peroneal injuries, excessive hip flexion can stretch sciatic and obturator nerves, and the femoral nerve can be compressed under the inguinal ligament (Fig. 4.14). Legs should be raised simultaneously and slowly to avoid a progressively increasing venous return impairing cardiovascular function, especially in poor heart-compliant patients. Also when raising legs above heart level, peripheral pulses should be checked because local ischemia to neuromuscular structures can occur, resulting

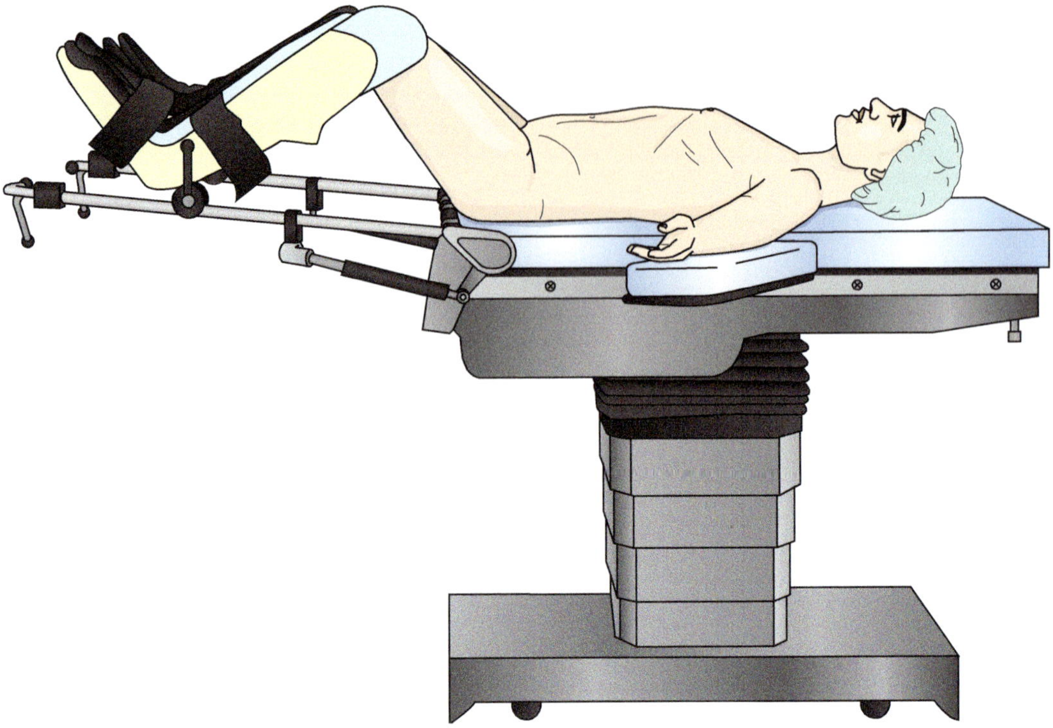

Fig. 4.9 Lithotomy position (taken from web)

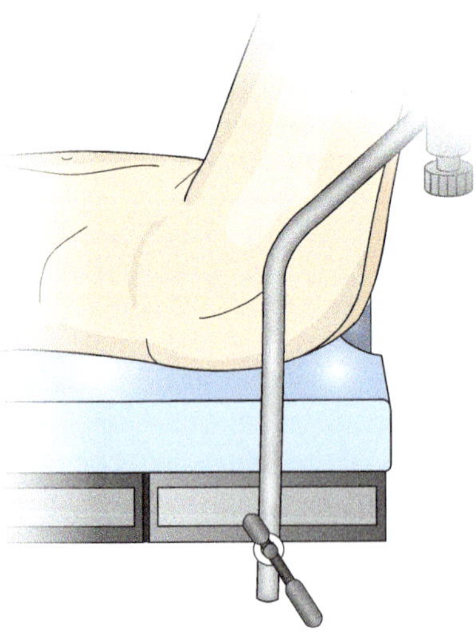

Fig. 4.10 Correct position of the sacrum (from the Prevention of Positioning Injuries during Gynecologic Operations. Guideline of DGGG. M. C. Fleisch, D. Bremerich, W. Schulte-Mattler, A. Tannen, A. T. Teichmann, W. Bader, K. Balzer, S. P. Renner, T. Römer, S. Roth, F. Schütz, M. Thill, H. Tinneberg, and K. ZarrasGeburtshilfe Frauenheilkd. 2015 Aug; 75(8): 792–807. doi: 10.1055/s-0035-1557776). Permission not requested

in a compartment syndrome [9]. Similarly, at the end of the procedure, legs should be simultaneously and slowly lowered to avoid spine torsion and to allow the vessels to progressively refill minimizing the risk of hypotension due to relative hypovolemia.

The upper limbs should be positioned on padded arm boards, abducted no more than 90°, or over the abdomen. Placing the arms to the patient's side could result in finger injury when the lower table section is elevated.

Critical pressure points in the lithotomy position are the occiput, the spinous processes of the thoracic vertebrae, the sacrum, the medial and lateral epicondyles, the olecranon, the scapulae, the femoral condyles, and the medial and lateral malleoli and calcaneae, so proper padding should be provided.

4.3.6 Prone

The prone position is frequently used for surgical access to the posterior spine and thorax and the posterior cranial fossa. Since the patient lies on the ventral aspect of the torso, unfavorable cardiorespiratory mechanics occurs. In fact, abdominal compression causes an increase in intraabdominal pressure that might lead to a compression of the vena cava and ultimately in a decrease in venous return and cardiac output. Also epidural veins could be engorged and result in increased surgical bleeding. It is therefore mandatory to allow diaphragmatic excursion using chest and pelvis support or using a specialized prone operating table (Jackson table).

Arms can be either raised beside the head on padded arm boards or retained along the sides of the body; when raised bedside the head, forearms should be lower than the head to avoid brachial plexus stretching (Fig. 4.15).

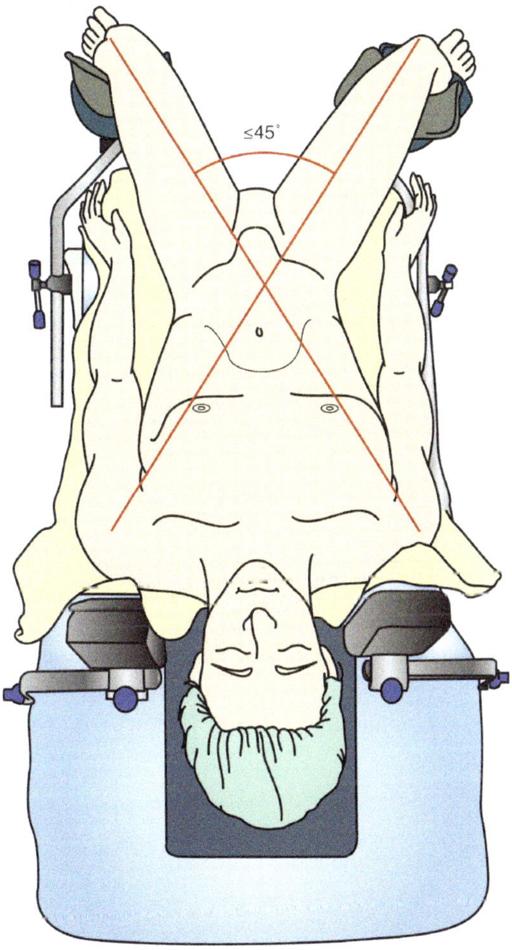

Fig. 4.11 Correct angulation and abduction of the lower extremities to prevent traction of the obturator nerve (from the Prevention of Positioning Injuries during Gynecologic Operations. Guideline of DGGG. M. C. Fleisch, D. Bremerich, W. Schulte-Mattler, A. Tannen, A. T. Teichmann, W. Bader, K. Balzer, S. P. Renner, T. Römer, S. Roth, F. Schütz, M. Thill, H. Tinneberg, and K. ZarrasGeburtshilfe Frauenheilkd. 2015 Aug; 75(8): 792–807. doi: 10.1055/s-0035-1557776). Permission not requested

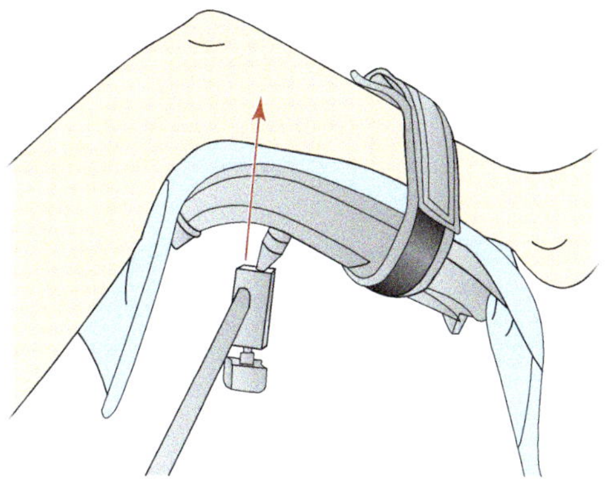

Fig. 4.12 Avoid pressure to the popliteal fossa with the ankle suspended (from the Prevention of Positioning Injuries during Gynecologic Operations. Guideline of DGGG. M. C. Fleisch, D. Bremerich, W. Schulte-Mattler, A. Tannen, A. T. Teichmann, W. Bader, K. Balzer, S. P. Renner, T. Römer, S. Roth, F. Schütz, M. Thill, H. Tinneberg, and K. ZarrasGeburtshilfe Frauenheilkd. 2015 Aug; 75(8): 792–807. doi: 10.1055/s-0035-1557776). Permission not requested

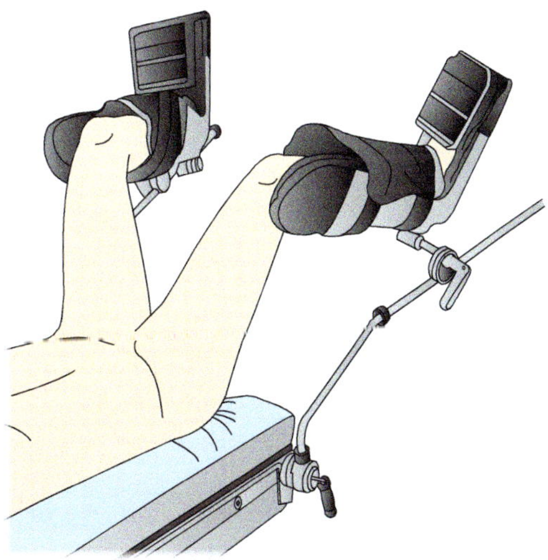

Fig. 4.13 Stirrups with foot and ankle support to avoid pressure on the calf. From the web. Permission not requested

Extra caution should be taken when moving the patient from supine to prone, especially to endotracheal tube, vascular access, and shearing of the skin that could result in injuries.

The head should be placed on a supporting device and gently turned laterally to provide airway access. In females with large breasts, these should be positioned laterally; in males, genitalia should be appropriately placed to avoid compression or torsion.

Ankles and feet should be placed in the neutral position with the aid of a padded footboard; hips and knees should be slightly flexed.

Important pressure points in the prone position are ears, eyes, cheeks, acromion processes, iliac crests, patellae, and toes, which should be adequately padded.

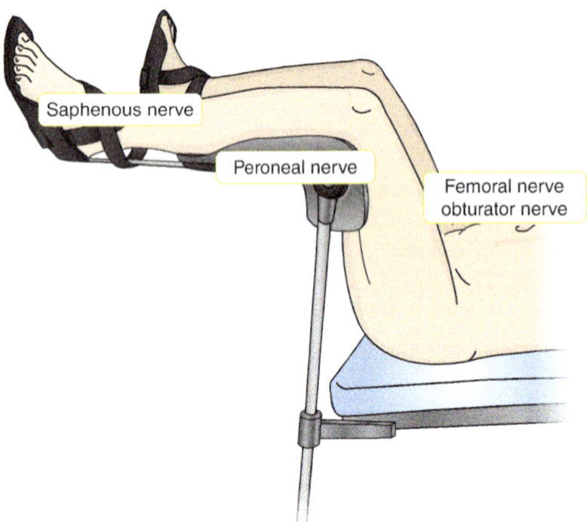

Fig. 4.14 Nerves potentially affected by incorrect lithotomy position. From the web. Permission not requested

Common complications occurring after prone interventions are facial swelling, chemosis, and temporary blurred vision. Other rare complications are corneal abrasions, ischemic optic neuropathy, and central retinal artery thrombosis which could result in permanent loss of vision, as already discussed.

4.4 Skin Prep

Since 1867, the year of Lister's "Antiseptic principle of the practice of Surgery" publication, great efforts have been employed in ensuring an increasing rate of sterility of the surgical field.

The introduction of sterile gloves and hand scrubbing certainly reduced the incidence of healthcare-associated surgical site infections (SSIs). However, according to WHO, the burden of this preventable complication is of 20,196 SSIs out of 2,417,933 surgical procedures performed in the USA in 2014, accounting for about an extra 900 billion US$ [11]. There is no clear-cut level of bacterial skin load that should be removed before surgery; however 80% of bacteria in surgical site infections derive from the skin of the patient. In order for a product to be approved to use as disinfectants, the Food and Drug Administration requires a reduction of colony-forming units (CFU) by more than two log10 at dry sites (e.g.,

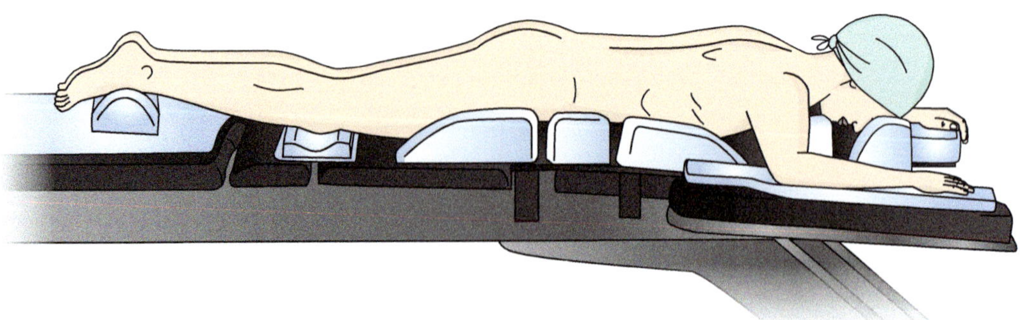

Fig. 4.15 Prone position (taken from web)

abdominal skin) and by three log10 at moist sites (e.g., groin), when tested at both 10 min and 6 h.

Besides hand hygiene and sterile gloves and instruments, proper patient's skin preparation contributes to reduce the risk of surgical wound contamination. The first antiseptic agent used from Lister was phenol, promptly replaced by cresol which was ten times more active and less corrosive on living tissues.

Respectively, in 1950 and 1955, chlorhexidine gluconate and povidone-iodine solutions were introduced into commercial use, and they are still widely used as antiseptic agents in the surgical field.

4.4.1 Preoperative Home Shower/Bath

Preoperative home showering with antiseptic agents is considered a well-accepted procedure for reducing skin microflora, but its efficacy in ultimately reducing surgical site infection is debated.

The most used antiseptic for this purpose is by far chlorhexidine gluconate.

Chlebicki et al. selected 16 prospective randomized or quasi-randomized trials comparing preoperative chlorhexidine baths versus non-antiseptic soap baths or no baths, focusing on surgical site infection outcomes [12]. They found the incidence of developing a surgical site infection to be statistically nonsignificant between the two groups, as 6.8% of the patients developed SSIs in the chlorhexidine group versus 7.2% in the control group.

The authors also concluded that these results could be biased by different antibiotic prophylaxis and/or by patients' lack of bathing instructions.

In fact, Paulson et al. showed that a daily 4% chlorhexidine gluconate for 5 days progressively reduced the microbial load of abdominal and inguinal region [13].

Chlorhexidine is found to have a cumulative antibacterial effect that lasts longer than other antiseptic agents.

Despite this findings, WHO's global guidelines for the prevention of surgical site infections still advise to bathe or shower with either plain or antimicrobial soap before surgery [14].

4.4.2 Hair Trimming

According to WHO, hair should not be removed from the patient's surgical field. If necessary, they should be trimmed with a clipper preoperatively or in the operative room, as shaving is strongly discouraged at all times. In fact, in a review from 2011, the authors identified three trials that compared shaving with clipping and showed that the incidence of SSIs was significantly higher in the shaving groups (RR 2.09). Probably this evidence could be elucidated by less skin trauma caused by the clipper compared to the razor [15]. However, the same review showed no statistically significant difference in SSI rates between hair removal and no hair removal [14].

4.4.3 Surgical Site Preparation

The purpose of the presurgical treatment of intact skin in the OR is to reduce as much as possible the load of skin bacteria before incision of the skin barrier. The three important variables contributing to a surgical site infection are the dose of bacterial contamination, the virulence of the bacteria, and the resistance of the host. Surgical skin preparation can affect only the first of such variables [16]. It has been shown how the risk for surgical site infection increases significantly if the wound is contaminated with more than 10^5 microorganisms per gram of tissue. Whenever a foreign body is present at the surgical site, however, this amount is much lower however (100 staphylococci per gram of tissue on braded suture).

The skin is not a sterile surface; bacteria tend to colonize the deeper layers of the stratum corneum and therefore cannot be shed by simple desquamation. Antiseptics bind to the stratum corneum to prolong their chemical action, together with a mechanical action, in order to kill and inhibit contaminating and colonizing flora. Commensal flora comprises *Staphylococci*, *Pseudomonas*, *Propionibacteria*, and diphtheroid organisms which can lead to harmful infection if they are allowed to grow and overcome host's defenses.

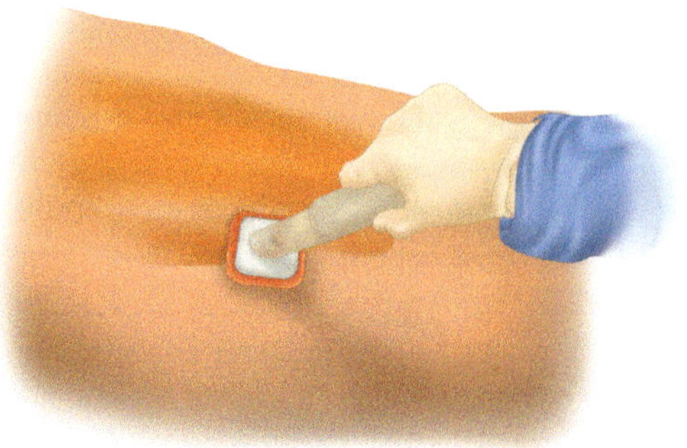

Fig. 4.16 Surgical site preparation (taken from web)

A thorough preoperative skin preparation is thus recommended routinely, and its efficacy is thought to be dependent to the antiseptic used and the method of application. According to the Center for Disease Control and Prevention (CDC), the patient's surgical site should be prepped as follows [17]:

- The skin must be primarily cleaned from gross contamination (dirt, soil, etc.).
- The site of the area prepared should be sufficient to include any potential incision different from the main incision site, including drains.
- The solution should be applied in concentric circles.
- A dedicated instrument should be used (sponge, swab), and the applicator should be discarded once the periphery has been reached.
- Time should be allowed for the solution to dry, as alcohol-based solutions are flammable, and to achieve a complete antimicrobial effect, as per manufacturer.

Also the Association of periOperative Registered Nurses (AORN) stated that the applicator used should be sterile and the solution should be applied with friction and extend from the incision site to the periphery (Fig. 4.16) [18]. In fact, friction increases the antibacterial effect of an antiseptic. For instance, alcohol applied without friction reduces bacterial counts by 1.0–1.2 log10 CFU, as compared with 1.9–3.0 log10 CFU when friction is used.

4.4.4 Antiseptic Solutions

The ideal antiseptic agent should have the following properties:

- Kill all bacteria, fungi, protozoa, viruses, tubercle bacilli, and spores.
- Nontoxic.
- Hypoallergenic.
- Safe to use in all body regions.
- Not be absorbed.
- Present residual activity.
- Safe for repetitive use.

Lately two kinds of antiseptics have been utilized for surgical skin preparation:

- Iodine-/iodophor-based solutions: effective against a wide spectrum of Gram-positive and Gram-negative bacteria, tubercle bacillus, viruses, and fungi. The mechanism of action comprises free iodine molecules bound to a polymer (povidone) that can penetrate cell walls and oxidize microbial contents. It is soluble in both water and alcohol. The risk of side effects, such as staining, tissue irritation, and iodine absorption, is lower with iodophors than with aqueous iodine. Increased serum iodine levels have been found in patients, so other products should be considered for patients with thyroid dysfunction. The efficacy of iodophors is reduced in the presence of organic material such as the blood. They are, however, preferred for antisepsis of mucous membranes and open wounds.
- Chlorhexidine gluconate-based solutions: aqueous or alcoholic; it is effective against a wide range of Gram-positive and Gram-negative bacteria, yeasts, and some viruses. It is most commonly formulated as a 4% aqueous solution, but the alcoholic version seems to result in having a superior antimicrobial activity. Chlorhexidine gluconate destroys the bacterial cell membrane, resulting in a bactericidal effect, especially for vegetative Gram-positive and Gram-negative bacteria. In addition, it has a durable antimicrobial action

for up to 6 h. However, chlorhexidine has little activity against bacterial and fungal spores. The alcoholic compounds are not suitable for use at or in close proximity to mucous membranes or the eyes.

A recent Cochrane review (2015) highlighted how 0.5% chlorhexidine in methylated spirit was superior to povidone-iodine paint only in one study [15] out of 13 clinical trials where it achieved a statistically significant result in terms of SSI rate [15]. They recruited 542 patients undergoing clean surgery classified as "hernia, genitalia, veins and other clean operations" and showed a 13% of SSI rate in the povidone-iodine versus 6.3% in the chlorhexidine group. It is important to note, though, that they did not report the concentration of povidone-iodine paint.

All other trials reported in the review were based on comparison either of two different antiseptics or different concentrations of the same antiseptic, and no statistical significance in term of SSI rate was found.

However, the WHO global guidelines for the prevention of SSI strongly recommend the utilization of alcohol-based antiseptic solutions with chlorhexidine gluconate for surgical site skin preparation in patients undergoing surgical procedures, in spite of low to moderate level of evidence.

Ostomies and open wounds require special consideration. First of all, no chlorhexidine products can be used. Sponges used to prep open wounds, and intestinal stomas, should be used once and then discarded. The intact skin should be prepped first, before open wounds and ostomies.

For intestinal ostomies that are not part of the surgical field, seal off the ostomy with a sterile adhesive drape, prior to the surgical site preparation. If the ostomy is in the surgical field, place a soaked sponge over the stoma before the intact skin is prepped, and then discard at the end of the prep. The mucin and organic matter can inhibit the effectiveness of antiseptic agents, and it should be mechanically removed along with the residual of the adhesive material of the ostomy bag. Some surgeons elect to close the skin of the mucocutaneous junction with running sutures to avoid spillage, using a separate prep and surgical tray. This is especially helpful during ostomy takedown during the dissection around the ostomy itself. Urostomies can be gently cannulated with red rubber catheters secured with sterile adhesive drapes. Prepare the ostomy gently in order to avoid mucosal injuries.

Open wounds, especially if traumatic, should be mechanically debrided using normal saline with a drip sheet under the wound. The surrounding area should be prepped first, while the open wound is packed with sterile gauze. The gauze should then be discarded, and the open wound prepped last.

4.4.5 Antiseptic-Related Fires

A general concern regarding alcohol-based solutions has always been their potential flammability, which is highly increased in the presence of other two components such as oxygen and heat that are largely present in the operative room [19]. These concepts will be further expanded upon in Chap. 25.

As clearly illustrated in the surgical triangle of fire showed below (Fig. 4.17), there are many factors that contribute to initiate a fire in the operating room, and all must be taken into considerations. Alcohol preparations account for the fuel aspect, especially when they are pooled or are not allowed to dry correctly or are spilled largely over drapes and gowns.

Vo et al. reported their own case of a third-degree burn occurred in a urologic procedure, which required the intervention of a plastic surgeon afterward [20]. The solution used was 2% chlorhexidine in 70% isopropyl alcohol. They also reported other six cases of accidental fires occurred during surgery, and they finally proposed best practice recommendations:

1. Before the application of chlorhexidine, the surgeon should ensure that no absorptive materials are present or should remove them after the patient has been prepped.
2. A sufficient amount of visibly dyed chlorhexidine should only be used to prevent pooling. Application of chlorhexidine-soaked sponges should be avoided.

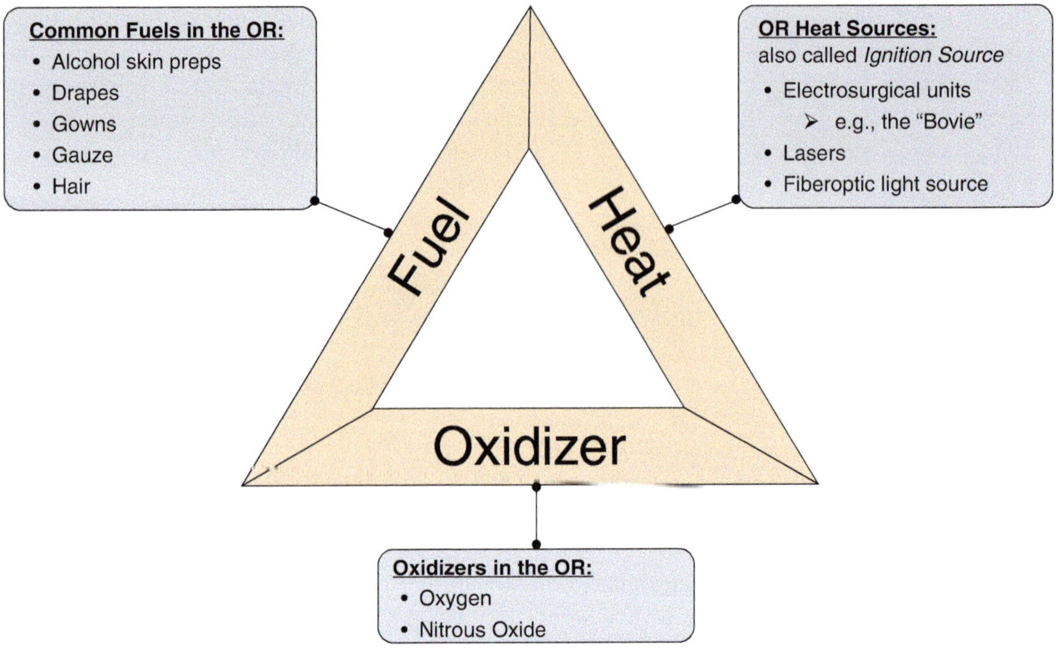

Fig. 4.17 Surgical triangle of fire (taken from web)

3. Ensure complete evaporation of chlorhexidine by allowing a longer drying time than what is recommended by the manufacturer (2 min to 3 min); 5 min is preferred.
4. Residual chlorhexidine should be dried with a surgical towel.
5. Surgical drapes should only be applied once chlorhexidine has completely evaporated. Adhesive drapes should be used and arranged so that residual chlorhexidine vapor is directed away from the surgical field.
6. The electrocautery unit should be used with the lowest possible setting and should be placed in its quiver when it is not being used.

4.4.6 Preoperative Sterilization

Sterilization is a process aimed to eliminate all microorganisms and spores from an instrument or device. There are different levels of sterilization based on the different degrees of resistance of the microorganisms. The capacity of the microorganism to resist sterilization depends, in terms, on the presence, composition, and thickness of the cell wall or viral envelope, the ability to form spores, and the sensitivity to heat, chemicals, and disinfectants. Since the bacterial spores are among the most difficult to eliminate, the process capable of eliminating such spores is considered sufficient to eliminate other infectious agents. If bacterial spores are not eliminated, the process cannot be named sterilization but "high-level disinfection."

The process of sterilization is composed of several phases.

Initially the instruments have to be cleaned by mechanically removing the gross contamination of organic and inorganic matter. This process is called decontamination. In fact, the presence of mechanical matter can decrease the efficacy of microbicidal agents.

The next step is the inspection to assure that the gross matter has been effectively removed.

The instruments are then assembled in trays and packed specifically to allow the sterilizing agents to be effective. The packaging system should be permeable to the sterilizing agent but resistant to traction and manipulation.

Table 4.1 summarizes the different types of sterilizing agents with their advantages and limitations.

Table 4.1 Summary of the different sterilizing agents with their advantages and limitation

Method	Advantages	Limitations
Heat (steam sterilization)	• Short exposure	• Not compatible with thermolabile items
	• Effective for prions	• Does not eliminate pyrogens
	• Not toxic for humans or the environment	• Cannot be used for oils or powders
	• Easy certification	
	• Low cost	
	• Widely available	
	• Easy to operate	
Heat (dry air)	• Not corrosive	• Long exposure
	• Deep penetration	• Not compatible with thermolabile items
	• Not toxic for humans or the environment	• Hard to certify
	• Easy to operate	• High cost
	• Widely available	• Efficacy against prions not known
Ethylene oxide	• Compatible with thermolabile items	• Long exposure
	• Penetrates certain plastics	• Not effective for prions
	• Easy to operate	• Toxic for humans and
		• the environment
Hydrogen peroxide plasma	• Compatible with thermolabile items	• Not all materials are compatible
	• Short exposure	• Not effective for prions
	• Not toxic for humans or the environment	• Does not reach the center of long lumens effectively
	• Easy to operate	
Liquid peracetic acid in automatic equipment	• Short exposure	• Useful only for materials that can be immersed
	• Easy to operate	• In existing equipment, few containers can be processed
	• Not toxic for the environment	• Not effective for prions
		• Processed items must be used immediately
Formaldehyde	• Compatible with thermolabile items	• Not all materials are compatible
	• Short exposure	• Not effective for prions
	• Easy certification	

From WHO Library Cataloguing-in-Publication Data WHO guidelines for safe surgery: 2009: safe surgery saves lives. ISBN 978 92 4 159855 2 (NLM classification: WO 178) © World Health Organization 2009. Requests for permission to reproduce should be addressed to WHO Press, World Health Organization, 20 Avenue Appia, 1211 Geneva 27, Switzerland (tel.: +41 22 791 3264; fax: +41 22 791 4806; e-mail: permissions@who.int). Permission not requested

Take-Home Points

- The patients' safety in the OR is guaranteed via a systematic approach by the entire operative team.
- The utilization of team huddles and preoperative checklists and time-out has become the standard approach currently followed in operating rooms.
- A thorough knowledge of the pathophysiology and etiology of potential position-related injuries should be part of a well-rounded surgeon.
- Simply taping the eyelids during general anesthesia can prevent minor damages secondary to anesthesia-related reduction of tears.
- Ulnar neuropathy is the most common peripheral neuropathy.
- Besides hand hygiene and sterile gloves and instruments, proper patient's skin preparation contributes to reduce the risk of surgical wound contamination.
- Antiseptics bind to the stratum corneum to prolong their chemical action, together with a mechanical action, in order to kill and inhibit contaminating and colonizing flora.

Editors' Comments

- Appropriate patient positioning is a critical part of any operation. Residents should be

knowledgeable about the benefit and risks associated with having any patient rest on the operating room table in a specific position for any given time. A surgical trainee should study the specific position required for a procedure with the same focus they use with any other step of the operation.
- The operating room table—with its several additional components—is a part of the operating room the surgical trainee needs to be familiar with it to allow for maximum benefit to be derived from its use.

Suggested Readings

Warner MA. Perioperative neuropathies. Mayo Clin Proc. 1998;73(6):567–74.

O'Connell MP. Positioning impact on the surgical patient. Nurs Clin North Am. 2006;41(2):173–92, v

Dumville JC, McFarlane E, Edwards P, Lipp A, Holmes A, Liu Z. Preoperative skin antiseptics for preventing surgical wound infections after clean surgery. Cochrane Database Syst Rev. 2015;4:CD003949.

Mangram AJ, Horan TC, Pearson ML, Silver LC, Jarvis WR. Guideline for prevention of surgical site infection, 1999. Hospital Infection Control Practices Advisory Committee. Infection control and hospital epidemiology. 1999;20(4):250–78; quiz 79–80.

References

1. Manfredini M, Ferrante R, Gildone A, Massari L. Unilateral blindness as a complication of intraoperative positioning for cervical spinal surgery. J Spinal Disord. 2000;13(3):271–2.
2. Cheney FW, Domino KB, Caplan RA, Posner KL. Nerve injury associated with anesthesia: a closed claims analysis. Anesthesiology. 1999;90(4):1062–9.
3. Warner MA. Perioperative neuropathies. Mayo Clin Proc. 1998;73(6):567–74.
4. Warner MA, Warner ME, Martin JT. Ulnar neuropathy. Incidence, outcome, and risk factors in sedated or anesthetized patients. Anesthesiology. 1994;81(6):1332–40.
5. O'Connell MP. Positioning impact on the surgical patient. Nurs Clin North Am. 2006;41(2):173–92.
6. King CA, Bridges E. Comparison of pressure relief properties of operating room surfaces. Perioper Nurs Clin. 2006;1(3):261–5.
7. Primiano M, Friend M, McClure C, et al. Pressure ulcer prevalence and risk factors during prolonged surgical procedures. AORN J. 2011;94(6):555–66.
8. Slater MS, Mullins RJ. Rhabdomyolysis and myoglobinuric renal failure in trauma and surgical patients: a review. J Am Coll Surg. 1998;186(6):693–716.
9. Furnas H, Canales F, Buncke GM, Rosen JM. Complications with the use of an axillary roll. Ann Plast Surg. 1990;25(3):208–9.
10. Graling PR, Colvin DB. The lithotomy position in colon surgery. AORN J. 1992;55(4):1029–39.
11. Global guidelines for the prevention of surgical site infection. Geneva: World Health Organization; 2016. Available from: https://www.ncbi.nlm.nih.gov/books/NBK401132/.
12. Chlebicki MP, Safdar N, O'Horo JC, Maki DG. Preoperative chlorhexidine shower or bath for prevention of surgical site infection: a meta-analysis. Am J Infect Control. 2013;41(2):167–73.
13. Paulson DS. Efficacy evaluation of a 4% chlorhexidine gluconate as a full-body shower wash. Am J Infect Control. 1993;21(4):205–9.
14. Byrne DJ, Napier A, Cuschieri A. Rationalizing whole body disinfection. J Hosp Infect. 1990;15(2):183–7.
15. Tanner J, Norrie P, Melen K. Preoperative hair removal to reduce surgical site infection. Cochrane Database Syst Rev. 2011; (11):Cd004122.
16. Dumville JC, McFarlane E, Edwards P, Lipp A, Holmes A, Liu Z. Preoperative skin antiseptics for preventing surgical wound infections after clean surgery. Cochrane Database Syst Rev. 2015;(4):CD003949.
17. Mangram AJ, Horan TC, Pearson ML, Silver LC, Jarvis WR. Guideline for prevention of surgical site infection, 1999. Hospital Infection Control Practices Advisory Committee. Infection control and hospital epidemiology 1999; 20(4): 250–78; quiz 79–80.
18. Girard NJ. Standards, recommended practices, and guidelines. AORN J. 2006;83(2):307–8.
19. WHO guidelines for safe surgery: 2009: safe surgery saves lives. ISBN 978 92 4 159855 2 (NLM classification: WO 178) © World Health Organization. 2009.
20. Vo A, Bengezi O. Third-degree burns caused by ignition of chlorhexidine: a case report and systematic review of the literature. Plast Surg (Oakville, ON). 2014;22(4):264–6.

Fundamentals of Incisions and Skin Closures

5

Folasade O. Imeokparia, Michael E. Villarreal, and Lawrence A. Shirley

5.1 Introduction

Every operation is punctuated by what may appear to be the most basic of surgical actions, the creation and closure of the incision. Basic as these may seem, a sound understanding of anatomy and physiology for the creation and re-approximation of wounds is required to successfully complete the operation planned, allow the patient the best opportunity for wound closure, and avoid costly, physically, and/or mentally burdening postoperative morbidities.

The general concepts of modern-day incision and closure were first described in the mid- to late nineteenth century. The Austrian anatomist, Karl Langer, is credited with the description of scar orientation based on local collagen configurations. Known as "Langer lines," these orientation patterns served as unofficial guidelines for surgical incisions (Fig. 5.1a). However, Langer's descriptions were largely applicable to the cadaveric tissue he studied. In practice, in vivo wounds and scars varied from the anticipated results predicted with "Langer lines." Austrian-born plastic surgeon, Cornelius Kraissl, was later attributed with describing the more optimal placement of incisions along tissue folds. This orientation allowed for an individual's natural folds to act as a guideline for incisions given that the perpendicular muscle contractions in relation to the skin would create folds unique to an individual (Fig. 5.1b). The use of skin folds minimizes the less appealing scarring from following "Langer lines" in live tissue. Consequently, the modern-day verbiage "Langer lines" is often conflated with the more optimal orientation described by Kraissl.

While the tenets of successful incisions and closure have evolved since the days of Langer and Kraissl, a strong understanding of anatomy, wound behavior, and healing still applies. This chapter will address the principles of incision and closure of routine general surgery procedures.

5.2 General Concepts

The anatomic considerations of incisions and closures begin with an understanding of the skin structure and properties. The largest organ of the body, the skin, oversees several functions: protection of the internal organs from the environment (e.g., trauma and pathogens), temperature regulation, as well as neurosensory interface (pain, temperature, pressure).

F. O. Imeokparia · M. E. Villarreal • L. A. Shirley (✉)
Department of Surgery, The Ohio State University Wexner Medical Center, Columbus, OH, USA
e-mail: Lawrence.Shirley@osumc.edu

F. Palazzo (ed.), *Fundamentals of General Surgery*, https://doi.org/10.1007/978-3-319-75656-1_5

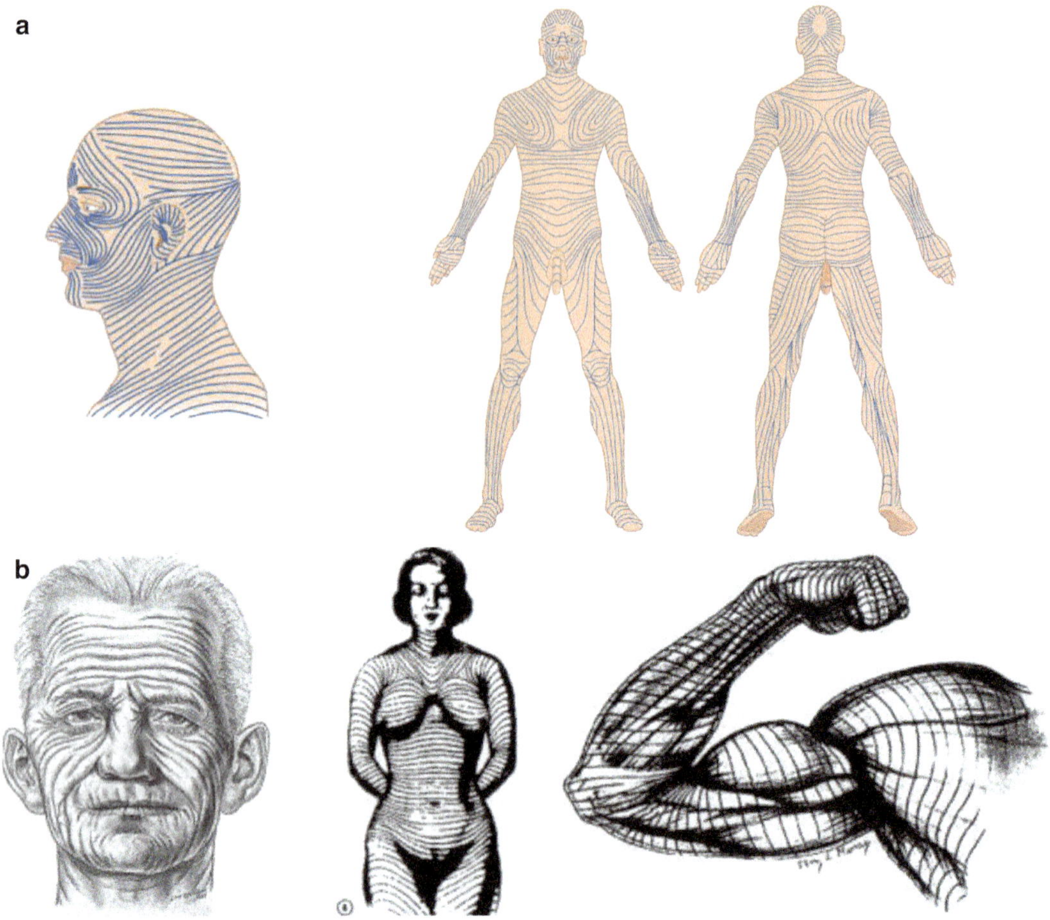

Fig. 5.1 (**a**) Langer lines (via Basic Techniques in Pediatric Surgery. Carachi R, Agarwala S, Bradnock TJ (Eds). Springer-Verlag Berlin Heidelberg 2013. Chapter A7: Skin Lines and Wound Healing; pg 34-35). (**b**) Kraissl lines (via Borges AF, Alexander JE. Relaxed skin tension lines, Z-plasties on scars, and fusiform excision of lesions. Br J Plast Surg. 1962;15:242-254)

The skin is divided into three main layers: the (a) epidermis, (b) dermis, and (c) subcutaneous tissue (Fig. 5.2).

The epidermis consists of four layers (from deepest to superficial): stratum basale, stratum spinosum, stratum granulosum, and stratum corneum. Some regions of the skin contain an additional layer known as the stratum lucidum that lies between the stratum granulosum and corneum. This is most commonly found in areas of the body with dense thickness, such as the bottom of the feet and the palms of the hands. The stratum basale houses the melanocytes that give the skin its pigmentation. Within the epidermis, there are no blood vessels.

The dermis hosts blood vessels, nerve receptors, sweat and sebaceous glands, as well as hair follicles. This layer is known for its protective function. The dermis contains abundant fibroblast cells that produce collagen. Collagen creates the strong tensile strength of the skin. *The subcutaneous tissue* has two components, a superficial fatty layer (Camper's fascia) and a membranous deep layer (Scarpa's fascia).

The physiologic considerations pertaining to incisions and closures center around wound healing. This process involves three phases: inflammatory, proliferative, and remodeling. The inflammatory period is characterized by epithelialization. The proliferative period is notable for collagen deposition, granulation deposition, and neovascularization. Lastly, the remodeling period consists of collagen cross-link formation.

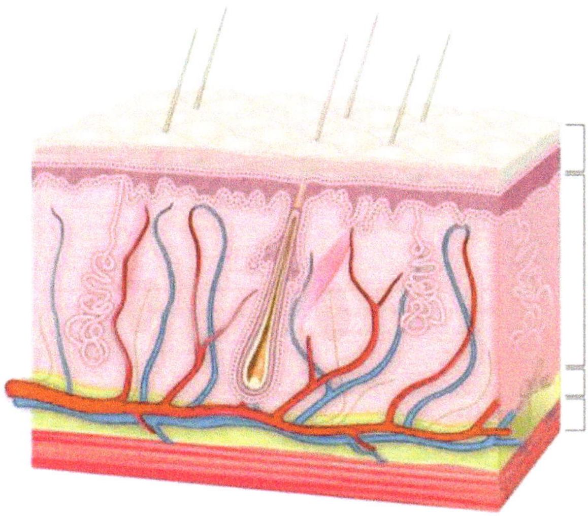

Fig. 5.2 Layers of the skin (via Plastic and Reconstructive Surgery. Siemionow, M, Eisenmann-Klein, M (Eds.). Springer-Verlag London Limited 2010. Chapter 7: Grafts, Local and Regional Flap; pg 69)

Factors that inhibit wound healing include desiccated environments, hypoxemia or frank ischemia, and the presence of devitalized or necrotic tissue. With these concepts in mind, creation and closure of an incision require attention to confirming hemostasis, preserving surrounding structural integrity, and maintaining sterility.

The process of wound healing begins in the first 24 h after a wound is created and lasts for up to 1 year. During this time, the tensile strength of a wound will increase as collagen is formed. At approximately 3 weeks after an incision or wound is created, the tissue has about 20% of the original strength of the tissue. Between 6 and 8 weeks, the tissue will have about 70% of the original strength of the tissue. Through the remainder of the healing process, *the wound will only increase to a maximum of 80% of the original strength of the tissue.*

5.3 Technical/Practical Considerations/Safety Precautions

5.3.1 Incisions: General Considerations

The major goal in choosing the optimal surgical incision is assuring adequate exposure. Simply identifying the most advantageous access point for the specific target organ while keeping in mind potential additional components to the procedure is an essential piece to selecting the right incision; for example, a pathology's lateral position within a cavity may alter the benefit of certain incisions; similarly planned or potential stomas should be considered for preoperative marking. Given the breadth of general surgery, there is a wide range of possible operative sites and incisions.

Careful handling of tissue is also important during incision. The use of tools that result in crushing of the skin should be avoided as this may lead to unsightly scarring from damage to the epidermis. The least damaging method for handling or retraction of the skin should be employed such as that achieved with fine skin hooks or Adson forceps. If pursuing exploration or a planned procedure on a prior surgical site, it is recommended to follow the scar of the previous incision. Parallel or adjacent incisions should be avoided because the intervening tissue between the previous scar and the new incision is susceptible to ischemia and/or necrosis from interrupted blood supply. Moreover, it is ideal to avoid creating multiple defects, knowing that each defect only achieves 80% of the original tissue strength.

5.3.2 Incisions: Technical and Practical Considerations

When making an incision, one should stretch and apply tension to the skin at the starting point with the non-dominant hand and, with the belly of the blade (if using sharp dissection), draw the scalpel perpendicular along the line of the planned incision with the dominant hand. If possible, this should be accomplished with a single sweep of the scalpel. Multiple sweeps will result in detached or ragged edges of the skin and subcutaneous tissue at different levels within the incision that may result in delayed wound healing or necrosis. The pressure utilized should be enough to incise through the epidermal and dermal layers. Once through the dermal layer, the additional tissue may be further dissected sharply with the scalpel or with electrosurgical energy.

Whether sharp dissection with a scalpel or electrosurgical energy is used for the creation of a skin incision has been a question posed and investigated over many years. A meta-analysis of these randomized controlled trials by Ly showed no difference in wound complication rates or pain scores between the two modalities but did find electrosurgical energy to result in less blood loss and shorter incision time [1].

The following content will highlight common incisions of the abdomen, retroperitoneum, neck, and breast.

5.3.3 Incisions: Abdomen

After incising through the skin and subcutaneous fat, the abdominal fascia is encountered: a small incision created sharply with knife, scissors, or electrosurgical energy should be used to begin opening of this layer. Once the fibers of the fascia are divided, the opposing sides can then be gently grasped with clamps and then lifted upward while concurrently being pulled slightly apart by an assistant. This maneuver will bring the peritoneum into view so that it may be sharply incised exposing a small window into the peritoneal cavity. This window should be spread or further incised so it is wide enough to fit two fingers inside the intra-abdominal space. Using electrosurgical energy or sharply with scissors, the length of the remainder of fascia can be opened using an assistant's hands or the surgeon's opposite hand to guide and gently lift the abdominal tissue upward for direct visualization and avoid injury to structures in the abdominal cavity. If possible, extending the incision a short distance superiorly or inferiorly will allow for entrance into the intra-abdominal space through an area where adhesions are less likely to be encountered. Many incisions can be used to access the peritoneal and retroperitoneal spaces of the abdomen (Fig. 5.3).

5.3.3.1 Vertical Midline

Abdominal pathologies of the upper and lower intraperitoneal cavity are generally suitable for a vertical midline incision. This incision should follow the linea alba through its length. The linea alba is the band of connective tissue separating the bilateral muscle pairings of the rectus abdominis in the anterior abdominal wall. A true midline vertical incision will avoid entrance into muscle or damage to major vessels or nerves and is a convenient avascular plane. Two anatomic structures to be aware of in the entry through a midline incision include the falciform ligament superiorly and the bladder inferiorly. Superiorly, the falciform ligament may require ligation to accommodate visualization in the upper abdominal structures, while incisions extending to the suprapubic region should include careful visualization or palpation of the bladder to avoid inadvertent injury in the suprapubic space. As a midline incision extends caudally, the umbilicus can be followed with a slight curvilinear deviation to either the left or the right and brought back to midline. When pathologies are anticipated in the upper abdominal cavity such as with the distal esophagus, stomach, proximal duodenum, liver, and pancreas, the incision can be limited to superior to the umbilicus. Similarly, when the target organ is in the lower abdominal cavity such as with the sigmoid, rectum, or bladder, the incision can be kept inferior to the umbilicus. Although midline incisions are the mainstay for abdominal operations, several other incisions hold specific benefits (Table 5.1).

5.3.3.2 Paramedian

The less often-used paramedian abdominal incision is created 2 to 5 centimeters lateral from the midline. The incision remains vertical through its

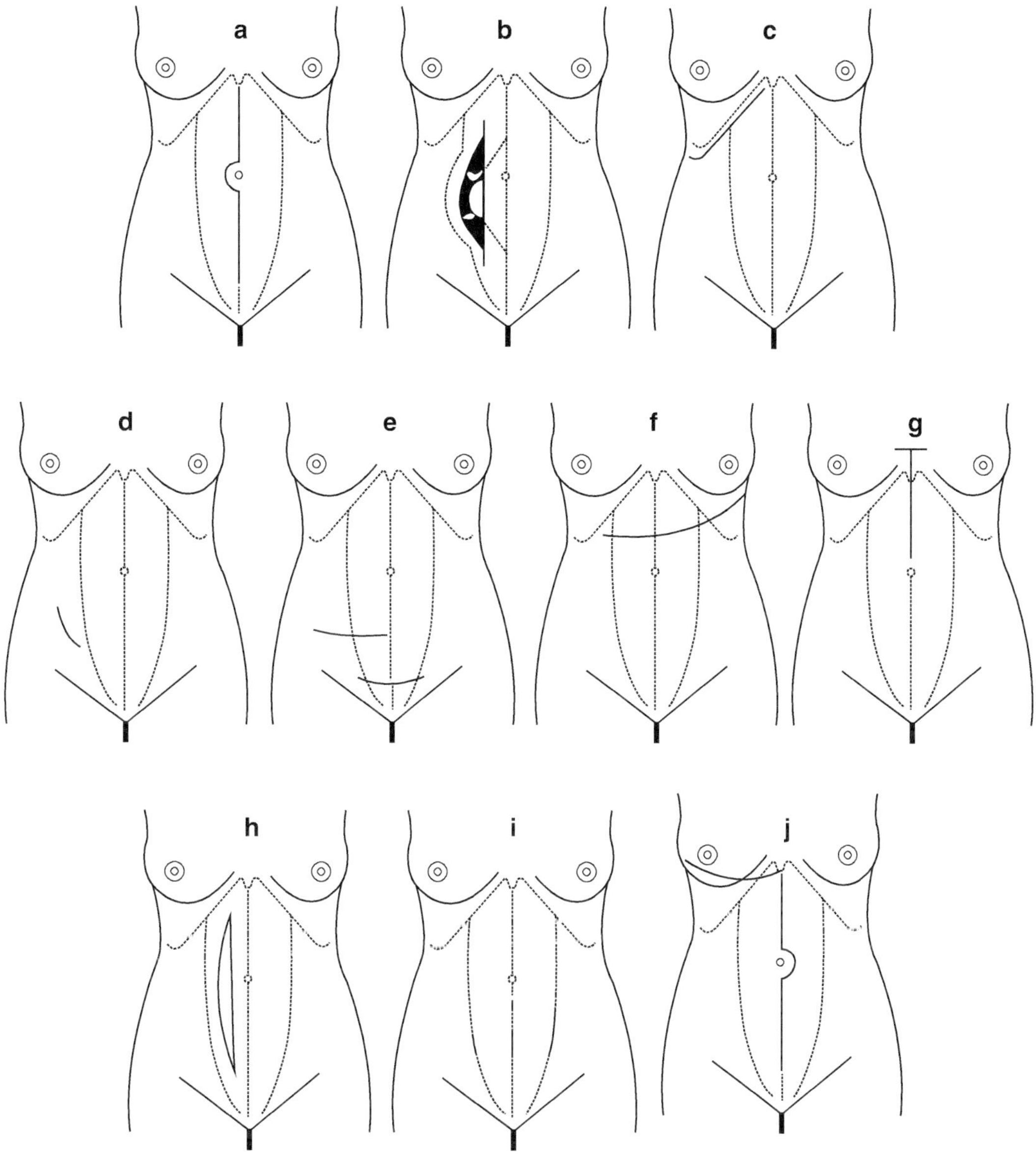

Fig. 5.3 Abdominal incision types. (**a**) Midline vertical. (**b**) Paramedian (muscle retraction). (**c, d**) Oblique. (**e**) Transverse. (**f, g**) Thoracoabdominal. (**h**) Paramedian (muscle splitting). (**i**) Pararectus. (**j**) "Hockey stick" (thoracoabdominal) (via JE Skandalakis, SW Gray, and JR Rowe. Anatomical Complications in General Surgery. New York: McGraw-Hill, 1983)

length. If one's interest lies in lateral structures such as the spleen, this can provide useful incision. More so, when interest lies in retroperitoneal structures such as the kidneys, adrenal, inferior vena cava, or aorta (as is needed for anterior spine exposure), the paramedian incision provides ample exposure. Care should be taken to plan the length and placement of the incision based on the structures or disc spaces of interest. Planning for this incision begins with proper patient positioning. While this incision can be utilized with the patient in the supine position, occasionally a gentle rotation of 30–40 of the torso may be beneficial. Depending on the laterality of the site of

Table 5.1 Abdominal incision advantages/disadvantages

Incision	Advantage	Disadvantage
Vertical midline	• Avascular • Expeditious opening, closure • Easily extended • Wide visualization	• Highest risk of herniation • Cosmetically unappealing
Paramedian	• Access to lateral structures • Buttressed closure	• Well-vascularized—risk of structural damage on entrance • Highest risk of infection • Cosmetically unappealing
Transverse	• Ideal for infants, small children, hepatobiliary surgery	• Well-vascularized • Limited exposure
Oblique	• Cosmetically appealing—may lie with skin folds	• Multiple-layered closure • Limited exposure
Thoracoabdominal	• Exposure of more than one cavity	• Well-vascularized—risk of structural damage on entrance • Painful incision

interest, the patient can be positioned with the lateral side of interest up. The free arm is placed at 90° from the long axis of the body in flexion and abduction. The contralateral leg and hip are placed in slight flexion. Pressure points should be appropriately padded.

The incision can either be carried down through the muscle fibers of the rectus abdominis or lateral to the fibers of the rectus abdominis and thus through the linea semilunaris. When the incision is carried down through the fibers of the rectus abdominis, the dissection does not proceed through an avascular plane. Namely, the superficial or deep epigastric vessels may be encountered in this dissection. Thus, care must be taken when incising through the abdominal wall to preserve and avoid injury to these structures. If inadvertently transected, one should be prepared to isolate and ligate these vessels. As such, the latter technique is the more commonly employed of the two. Many practitioners find the paramedian incision advantageous when the rectus is retracted medially because the re-approximation of the rectus over the posterior sheath at closure is thought to buffer or strengthen the closure.

5.3.3.3 Transverse

The transverse incision, although largely supplanted in modern general surgery with the vertical midline incision, is useful in specific instances, such as in infants, small children, obese patients, or hepatobiliary diseases. Unlike with vertical incisions, transverse incisions divide the tissue through a well-vascularized plane including muscle fibers; thus, care must be taken through dissection into the peritoneal cavity. It has been widely debated whether transverse incisions or vertical incisions are superior to the other. Mostly replete with non-randomized, non-blinded trials, there is not sufficient data to advocate consensus on the optimal choice between the two [2, 3]. Limited exposure of the extreme upper and lower abdomen reduces the more widespread value of the transverse incision.

5.3.3.4 Oblique

Oblique abdominal incisions, much like transverse, may be advantageous in instances of very specific areas of pathology or interest. For example, the McBurney incision is an oblique incision in the right lower quadrant that runs parallel to the external oblique muscle at a point about one-third the distance from the anterior superior iliac spine to the umbilicus. The incision is readily employed for open appendectomies. A variation to the McBurney incision is the Rockey-Davis incision that is also positioned in the right lower quadrant but employs a less severe oblique angle, orienting with a patient's skin folds for a theoretically improved aesthetic result. Furthermore, the Kocher incision is an oblique subcostal right upper quadrant incision utilized for upper abdominal procedures, such as open cholecystectomy or adrenalectomy.

A pre-peritoneal oblique incision is performed for renal transplantation. These incisions are oriented much like an oblique incision for an open inguinal hernia repair—medial to the anterior superior iliac spine extending toward the pubic symphysis. Unlike the inguinal hernia repair incision, this incision is often superior to the inguinal ligament and extends closer to the midline, as the bladder will need to be identified for the ureteral anastomosis. During the dissection for this incision, the peritoneum is not entered but can be closed with absorbable suture if done so accidentally. The external oblique and internal oblique aponeuroses are encountered and incised. The epigastric vessels, spermatic cord, or round ligament should be spared and is retracted medially. After this retraction, the external iliac artery and vein are exposed for the planned anastomoses.

5.3.3.5 Thoracoabdominal

Thoracoabdominal incisions are generally employed to simultaneously address a pathology spanning both the thoracic and abdominal cavities. For example, the various types of thoracoabdominal aneurysms, distal esophageal and stomach lesions, as well as unique liver or splenic processes can be adequately dealt with via a thoracoabdominal incision. With the patient positioned in a lateral position with the hip flexed, a curvilinear, subcostal paramedian incision can be extended continuously from the abdomen onto the thorax. The incision should be traced up to the level of the most appropriate intercostal space for the identified pathology of interest. Incising the thoracic structures will usually include some muscle splitting and division of the latissimus dorsi, serratus anterior, and the external oblique. At the intercostal rib space, the intercostal muscle is divided traversing as flush to the superior edge of the rib as possible. This maneuver will help to avoid injury to the intercostal vessel bundle. The costal cartilage can be excised if necessary during this incision. It is also possible to incise the diaphragm sharply or with electrocautery but care must be taken to avoid injuring the phrenic nerve.

5.3.4 Incisions: Retroperitoneal

Closely related to the abdominal incisions described are retroperitoneal incisions. These incisions are typically undertaken for management of retroperitoneal structures. This approach was largely described in the *paramedian* incision section. Additionally, the thoracoabdominal approach, just described, can be kept extraperitoneal if needed.

5.3.5 Incisions: Neck

Neck incisions need to achieve the three goals common to any incision: allow adequate exposure of anatomy, allow for potential extension, and allow for successful, safe, and cosmetic closure. Just as with the abdominal cavity, many incisions can be used to access the structures of the head and neck, and knowledge of the surgery being performed and the complications that may arise can help one plan a safe and cosmetic incision. The most common general surgery operations of the neck include tracheostomies, thyroidectomies and parathyroidectomies, and excisional lymph node biopsies.

A tracheostomy incision is often performed using a midline vertical incision extending from the cricoid cartilage down to the level of the fourth or fifth tracheal ring. This exposure does not follow the circumferential skin fold of the neck, but such a vertical incision allows for better access and can be extended if needed for added visualization and used in the emergent setting.

Thyroid and parathyroid incisions should follow the natural folds of a patient's skin (Fig. 5.4). Thus, this incision is typically curvilinear and made approximately two fingerbreadths above the sternal notch. At the time of skin marking, the surgeon should evaluate the natural skin creases of the patient by gently flexing and extending the patient's neck, opting to use a natural crease to allow the scar to be hidden when fully healed. These incisions can extend laterally for additional exposure. About 4–5 cm is the most common length of incision; however larger lesions may require extension.

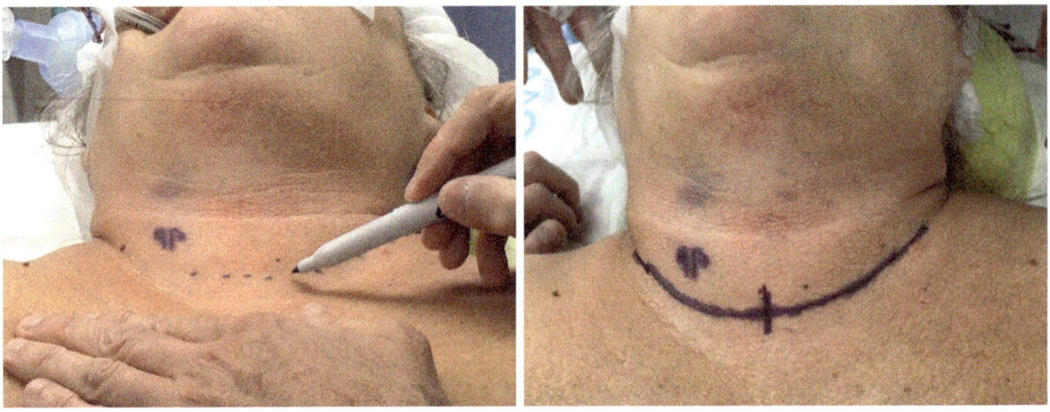

Fig. 5.4 Operative planning for midline cervical incision prior to thyroidectomy

A general surgeon may be referred to patient diagnosed with persistent cervical lymphadenopathy, and an incisional or excisional lymph node biopsy may be needed. The incisions for excisional biopsies tend to be more free form, but in general, a few rules can be followed. First, the site must be identified. This is typically done on physical exam with palpation, using preoperative imaging or even intraoperative ultrasound guidance. Once identified, the anatomy of that region of the neck should be deeply considered. For example, cervical zones 2, 3, and 4 are positioned in proximity to the carotid sheath and zone 5 to the accessory spinal nerve. Finally, once identified and potential hazards or underlying structures accounted for, the incision can be marked in relation to skin folds or other landmarks such as the sternocleidomastoid muscle. For cosmetic reasons, pain control, and recovery purposes, the incision can be planned small enough to accommodate excision of the lymph node and extended, if necessary.

5.3.6 Incisions: Breast

A general surgeon is expected to have a level of comfort in surgical management of benign and malignant breast diseases. Central to this management are excisional biopsies, lumpectomies, and mastectomies. Details to the approach of axillary lymph node management are beyond the scope of this chapter and will not be addressed. However, incision choice for these techniques will be discussed below. The principles behind the ideal breast incision can be applied to the management of breast abscesses and will be touched on briefly.

When percutaneous, ultrasound-guided, or stereotactic biopsy results are discordant with concerning imaging findings, it is often prudent to pursue excisional biopsy for a more adequate sample of tissue for thorough pathological review. The first principle in choosing the incision for an excisional biopsy is to identify the site of the pathology. Lesions are most commonly identified with radiologic-assisted wire localization or on physical exam with palpable lesions. In the operating room, after on-table exam and review of preoperative imaging, the next step is to assure that the site is in a location where healthy, uninvolved breast tissue margins will be obtained. The final principle to consider in the choice of incision on the breast is cosmesis.

Considering the quadrants of the breast, the most ideal incision in any quadrant is a curvilinear peri-areolar incision if the pathology is amenable. In the medial and lateral central quadrants, radial incisions are ideal choices. At the 5–7 o'clock position, many consider a radial incision to also be a good choice. And lastly, in the superior and inferior aspects of the outer and inner quadrants, curvilinear incisions following skin folds are ideal [4].

Simple mastectomies should include the nipple areolar complex (NAC). With a marking pen, an ellipse encompassing the NAC should be drawn with the patient supine after induction of anesthesia. The extent of the elliptical incision is made as follows: two points should be marked in line with the NAC. The first point is medial at the border of the sternum. The second point is marked lateral at the anterior axillary line. With the non-dominant hand, the breast tissue is manipulated downward, and a straight line is drawn from the medial point to the lateral point. Once the line is drawn, the breast tissue is released, and a curvilinear line will result. A second line is drawn delineating the inferior aspect of the incision by manipulating the breast tissue upward. These two lines will result in an ellipse. Adjustments to the lines may be required in order to assure that when brought together, the remaining skin can be brought together without undue tension.

The medial perforating vessels are the critical perfusion to the skin which should be carefully considered when planning the incision and during dissection.

A few final pearls on breast incisions are to keep in mind that a patient may require reoperation for additional excision of tissue or a mastectomy after lumpectomy, so placement of incisions should always bear this caution in mind. Additionally, one should forgo upper/inner quadrant incisions as they tend to be the most cosmetically unappealing [5]. Lastly, as mentioned, the complete discussion of the management of malignant breast disease is not covered here, but the NCCN Guidelines for breast cancer are easily accessible [6].

Modified radical mastectomy (MRM) incisions are similar to those of simple mastectomies. An important variation compared to simple mastectomies is that MRM incisions will encompass axillary lymph node levels 1 and 2 and so should be extended or angled further toward the axillary tail for sufficient dissection.

5.4 Closures

The principles of wound closure can be summarized into three major components: achieving primary skin closure, minimizing wound-healing complications, and optimizing cosmesis. This chapter will not cover the methods to securely and safely approximate abdominal fascia, as this topic is covered in a different section in this textbook.

Primary closure of the skin requires healthy, well-vascularized tissue. To this end, if there is any concern that the vascular supply to the skin edges is compromised or that there is contamination from the procedure performed, debridement when able is recommended. Delayed closure, after an initial period of granulation, may also be employed.

The wound class can aid in determining the risk to developing a surgical site infection (SSI) with primary closure. Contributors to SSI include wound class of the site, seroma or hematoma formation, and patient-based factors. SSI can prolong healing times and burden patients with further costs of care that may include dressing supplies, durable medical equipment, and skilled nursing care. The risk to develop a SSI is linked to the wound class. There are four wound class types: clean wounds carry a risk of SSI at 2%, clean contaminated at 3–5%, contaminated at 5–10%, and gross contaminated wounds have the highest risk of SSI at 30%. The Joint Commission on Accreditation of Healthcare Organizations created national patient safety guidelines that include recommendations to limit SSI. Major perioperative recommendations include the use of prophylactic antibiotics that are administered within 1 h of surgical incision, the use of chlorhexidine surgical bath preoperatively, and the clipping of hair when appropriate [7].

Closure of dead space is a simple but essential concept that can help reduce infection risk. Closure of dead space begins with careful inspection and evacuation of tissue space fluid collections. Retained hematomas and seromas can serve as energy-rich reservoirs for bacteria and accumulation of oxygen free radicals that weaken the strength of a closure. Thus, closure of dead space begins with identification and control of fluid sources, including meticulous hemostasis of the wound bed. Using an absorbable suture, the Scarpa's fascia and reticular dermis are the ideal layers to re-approximate to markedly reduce dead space. Generally speaking, the subcutaneous fat should not be re-approximated given the tendency that re-approximation strangulates blood supply which results in fat necrosis, another nidus for bacteria. Notably, closed suction drainage may be used per surgeon preference.

A final principle of closure is cosmesis. Whatever technique of closure is utilized, all attempts should be made to recreate the patient's natural contour and symmetry. Furthermore, following skin folds, in accordance with the concept of Kraissl lines, should help minimize tension to avoid inadvertent skin separation and unsightly scars. Some closures may be beset by abnormal scar formation including keloid and hypertrophic scarring. Keloids are the result of granulation tissue overgrowth at the site of skin injury that may extend beyond the borders of the original skin insult. Although considered a benign disorder, it can often lessen the quality of life for the patient in regards to poor cosmesis, pain, and pruritus. Hypertrophic scars are similar to keloids, as they are also raised lesions, but they do not extend beyond the boundaries of the original wound. The best treatment for keloid scarring is prevention, but if unable to do so, other treatment options are available, such as pressure therapy or triple therapy with corticosteroids, 5-fluorouracil, and pulsed dye laser. Prior unappealing scars, either hypertrophic or atrophic, can be considered for complete excision at the time of closure.

Wounds can be closed with glues or adhesives, staples, or sutures. When closing the skin with suture, one may decide between absorbable versus nonabsorbable forms (Table 5.2). Absorbable sutures degrade and lose their tensile strength within 60 days. When choosing the optimal suture for closure, important aspects include the inherent behavior of the suture material, predicted course of wound healing, and how the suture will interact with the tissue. Ideally, when a wound achieves maximal strength, suture is no longer needed for reinforcement. Therefore, slowly healing tissue, including skin, fascia, and tendon, is often closed with nonabsorbable suture or absorbable suture with extended wound support, whereas rapidly healing tissue, gastrointestinal tract and bladder, may be closed with absorbable suture. The details of primary suture closure material and techniques are numerous and referenced in Chap. 3.

Occasionally, a secondary line of sutures, retention sutures, is needed to reinforce the primary suture line. This is typically done when there is a concern for wound healing with only a primary suture line being intact or a concern for sudden increases in intra-abdominal pressure on abdominal incisions. Retention sutures are meant to increase/contribute to the tensile strength of the primary suture line and are placed laterally to the primary suture. Retention sutures are predominantly created with thicker nonabsorbable suture and are kept in place with a bolster, to prevent cutting into the skin when the incision is under stress, until the concern for improper wound healing has decreased, approximately 2–6 weeks postoperatively.

Table 5.2 Suture options for skin closure

Suture Options		
Absorbable	Braided	Vicryl
		Vicryl rapide
	Monofilament	Fast Absorbing Gut
		Chromic Gut
		Monocryl
Non-absorbable	Braided	Ethibond
		Silk
	Monofilament	Ethilon

5.5 Current Controversies/ Future Directions

Secure skin closure is an integral part of every surgical procedure and has routinely been performed with sutures, staples, and dermal adhesives. In recent years, dermal adhesive technology companies have made advances in their closure devices. One such device is a two-part skin closure system designed to approximate skin edges of an incision in place of or in addition to a traditional subcuticular stitch. Its components are a flexible, self-adhesive polyester mesh and a topical skin adhesive that is painted over the mesh. It keeps the traditional skin adhesive property of providing protection from organisms commonly responsible for surgical site infections (*S. aureus*, *S. epidermidis,* and *E. coli*). This new system also allows for a theoretical superior distribution of tension along the incision by creating individual points of tension and stress that are unavoidable with sutures and staples. There have yet to be any randomized controlled trials comparing this newer technology with traditional skin closure techniques.

Barbed suture wound closure devices eliminate the need to tie knots at skin closure without compromising the strength and security that traditional suture and traditional knot tying provide. The suture is designed to have multiple, unidirectional, circumferential barbs located along the entire length of the suture to grasp the tissue and distribute the tension across the wound. The main benefit that has been demonstrated between barbed sutures when compared to traditional suture has been the decreased OR time with barbed suture along with decreased suture utilization [8]. No cosmetic benefit was identified at 12 weeks between barbed suture and traditional suture.

Take-Home Points

- Tenets of incision and closure revolve around an understanding of anatomy, wound behavior, and healing.
- The major goal in choosing the optimal surgical incision is assuring adequate visualization.
- Three major goals of skin closure include minimizing wound-healing complications, achieving primary skin closure, and optimizing cosmesis.
- Take all necessary steps to prevent wound-healing complications.
- Primary closure of the skin requires healthy, well-vascularized tissue.
- Suture types can be broadly classified as absorbable versus nonabsorbable based on degradation properties. Choice depends on needs of the tissue in wound healing.

Editors' Corner

- Imaging studies should be routinely used to best plan the operative approach and decide on the most useful location and orientation of the incision.
- When planning a vertical midline incision, the surgical trainee should remember the basic anatomic characteristic of the linea alba: it is typically V shaped with its widest part in the epigastric area. Access at this location is typically safer.
- When planning a re-laparotomy, access should be sought a few centimeters proximal or distal to the previous incision to try and minimize the risk of bowel injury.
- Several of the incisions described in this chapter can be used as extraction sites after advanced laparoscopic procedures. While many surgeons favor low transverse incisions for such role (i.e., lap colon-rectal procedures), no final consensus has been reached on the ideal location for such incisions.

Suggested Readings

Roses RE, Morris JB. Incisions, closures, and management of the abdominal wound. In: Zinner MJ, Ashley SW, editors. Maingot's abdominal operations. 12th ed. Columbus: McGraw-Hill.

Skandalakis LJ, Skandalakis JE, Skandalakis PN. Surgical anatomy and technique: a pocket manual. 3rd ed. New York: Springer.

Fischer JF, Jones DB, Pomposelli FB, et al. Fischer's mastery of surgery. 6th ed. Philadelphia: Lippincott Williams & Wilkins.

Zollinger RM, Ellison EC. Zollinger's atlas of surgical operations. 10th ed. Columbus: McGraw-Hill.

Bland KI, Klimberg VS. Master techniques in surgery: breast surgery. 1st ed. Philadelphia: Lippincott Williams & Wilkins.

Oertli D, Udelsman R. Surgery of the thyroid and parathyroid glands. 2nd ed. Berlin: Springer.

References

1. Ly J, Mittal A, Windsor J. Systematic review and meta-analysis of cutting diathermy versus scalpel for skin incision. Br J Surg. 2012;99(5):613–20. https://doi.org/10.1002/bjs.8708.
2. Brown SR, Tiernan J. Transverse verses midline incisions for abdominal surgery. Cochrane Database Syst Rev. 2005. https://doi.org/10.1002/14651858.CD005199.pub2.
3. Seiler CM, Deckert A, Diener MK, et al. Midline versus transverse incision in major abdominal surgery: a randomized, double-blind equivalence trial (POVATI: ISRCTN60734227). Ann Surg. 2009;249(6):913–20.
4. Bland KI, Klimberg VS. Master techniques in surgery: breast surgery. 1st ed. Philadelphia: Lippincott Williams & Wilkins; 2011.
5. Zollinger RM, Ellison EC. Breast anatomy and incisions. In: Zollinger RM, Ellison EC, editors. Zollinger's atlas of surgical operations. 10th ed. Columbus: McGraw-Hill; 2016. http://accesssurgery.mhmedical.com.proxy.lib.ohio-state.edu/content.aspx?bookid=1755&sectionid=119131008. Accessed 12 Aug 2017.
6. NCCN clinical practice guidelines in oncology (NCCN guidelines): breast cancer. Version 2.2017. https://www.nccn.org/.
7. Joint Commission. The joint commission. 2017. https://www.jointcommission.org/.
8. Rubin JP, Capla JM, Dunn RM, Gusenoff J, Hansen J, Hunted J, Walgenbach K. A multicenter randomized controlled trial comparing absorbable barbed sutures versus conventional absorbable sutures for dermal closure in open surgical procedures. Aesthet Surg J. 2014;34(2):272–83.

6 Fundamentals of Retractors and Exposure

Michael B. Ujiki and H. Mason Hedberg

6.1 Introduction

Proper exposure is critical to maximizing safety and efficiency in the operating room. An operative field should be large enough to allow the operating surgeon and assistants to visualize critical anatomy and manipulate instruments comfortably and also no larger than necessary in order to minimize unnecessary trauma. There are many varieties of surgical retractors, and the ability to choose the right tool for the job can help meet the goal of keeping the view clear and the wound small.

Traditional stainless steel open surgical retractors were designed alongside the procedure they were intended to assist, with shapes that were carefully considered to meet a specific need. Effective, versatile designs have persisted to become common surgical instruments found in operating rooms worldwide. The evolution of material science, laparoscopic, and robotic procedures brought with them new instrumentation for retraction. Some minimally invasive retractors appear to be miniature versions of their open counterparts, while in some circumstances entirely new instrumentation has been developed to meet previously nonexistent needs.

The following chapter reviews technical considerations of surgical exposure, from patient positioning to economy of motion. A useful scalar paradigm for retraction is introduced: large-scale field exposure, effective recruitment of the operative assistant, and moment-by-moment use of the surgeon's nondominant hand. Additionally, types of surgical retractors available for open and laparoscopic surgery are described and categorized for convenient reference.

6.2 Exposure

6.2.1 Positioning and Gravity

Setting up the ideal operative field begins with patient positioning. Positioning must take into account the location of the surgeon and assistant with respect to the operative field, as well as the *fixed and universal surgical retractor—gravity*. Gravity can be especially useful for abdominal procedures given the mobility of some intra-abdominal organs. In general, once abdominal access has been obtained and initial exploration completed in a neutral position, the operating table should be adjusted for gravity retraction away from the operative field. This is

M. B. Ujiki (✉)
Department of Surgery, Grainger Center for Innovation and Simulation, NorthShore University HealthSystem, Evanston, IL, USA
e-mail: mujiki@northshore.org

H. Mason Hedberg
Department of Surgery, University of Chicago Medicine, Chicago, IL, USA
e-mail: herbert.hedberg@uchospitals.edu

F. Palazzo (ed.), *Fundamentals of General Surgery*, https://doi.org/10.1007/978-3-319-75656-1_6

accomplished by elevating the operative field with respect to the abdomen: appendectomy should be performed with the head down and right side up, cholecystectomy with the head and right side up [Editors' Note: *Move the target organ toward the surgeon*].

The utility of gravity differs between open and laparoscopic surgery. During open surgery, visualization is physically limited to an angle dependent upon the size of the incision and distance between the incision and the target organ. This restricts maneuverability of the table, and in some cases where gravity could be of assistance, packing and external retraction are utilized. Laparoscopic surgery brings the view to the operative field, so extreme table angles that would be inappropriate for open surgery can be advantageous. For example, steep reverse Trendelenburg is extremely useful for laparoscopic procedures in the upper abdomen.

6.2.2 Incision and Port Placement

Location of incision or laparoscopic ports is the second consideration when setting up the ideal operative field. The advantages of midline incisions for open surgery have been well described: blood supply to the abdominal wall is maintained, musculature is left intact for flaps such as TRAM, and access and closure can be performed relatively quickly [1]. A long midline laparotomy can access the entire abdomen, so incisions made initially small for local exploration can easily be extended when necessary. There are cases where incisions off the midline are appropriate, such as McBurney incision for appendectomy or right subcostal for cholecystectomy—patients may recover more quickly from a small incision directly overlying these structures than a larger midline laparotomy.

Up to half the operative complications that occur during laparoscopic surgery happen during initial port placement. The initial port may be placed after insufflation with a Veress needle, open with Hasson technique, or with an optical trocar. Each technique has advantages and disadvantages. For example, while direct optical entry poses a risk to intra-abdominal structures adhered to the abdominal wall, it has been shown to reduce iatrogenic injuries from initial trocar placement compared to Hasson technique in obese patients [2].

Once initial port placement is accomplished, additional ports can easily and safely be passed through the abdominal wall under visualization with the laparoscope and a cushion of pneumoperitoneum. A useful rule of thumb for laparoscopic port placement is triangulation, illustrated in Fig. 6.1. Working ports should be positioned such that when the instruments' tips are brought together at the operative target, there is a 45–75° angle between the instruments. This angular range allows the necessary ergonomics for most laparoscopic maneuvers. Usability of laparoscopic instruments is maximized when about half the length of the shaft is inside the abdomen. Regular adult instruments are 36 cm long, so working ports should be about 10–15 cm away from the location of the operative target as estimated on the skin (Fig. 6.2). Generally the best position for the camera to aid hand-eye coordination is behind and in between the working ports, although for some procedures ergonomics may be improved to have the camera to the outside of the two working ports. Additional assistant or retraction ports can be added laterally as needed [3].

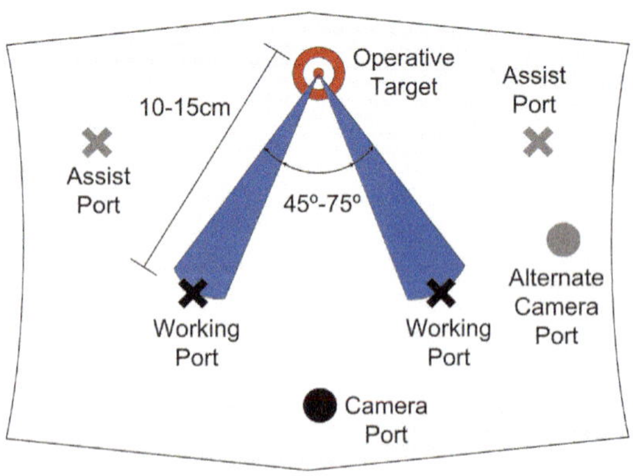

Fig. 6.1 Triangulation of working ports and assist port placement (top view)

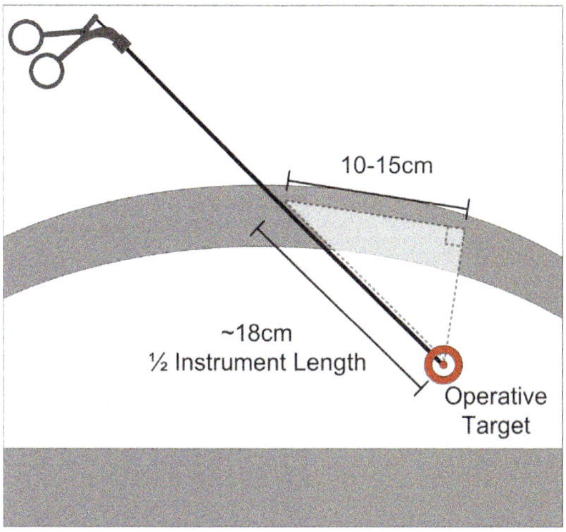

Fig. 6.2 Determining distance between working port and operative field

6.3 Retraction

It can be useful to consider three spaciotemporal levels of retraction during a surgical case in order to maintain ideal exposure at all times:

1. Large-scale field exposure
   On the largest scale is retraction that sets the stage for the entire operative field. This includes factors that are set and may remain unchanged for the duration of a case: patient positioning, gravity retraction, and self-retaining retractors. While these elements of exposure can be easy to "set and forget," it is important to consider adjusting them when visualization or ergonomics are compromised. It may be the case that various steps of a long operation benefit from subtle adjustments to gravity and self-retaining retractors. These adjustments can be worth the time when economy of motion subsequently improves.
2. Effective recruitment of the operative assistant
   The second level of retraction is that offered by the assistant; the assistant's hand is providing retraction at a smaller and more mobile scale than gravity or self-retaining retractors. It is the job of the surgeon to offer the correct instrument for the particular circumstance and to demonstrate appropriate positioning and tension. Over time, a good assistant will achieve synergy with the surgeon, anticipating the order of maneuvers and providing the correct exposure for each when needed.
3. Moment-by-moment use of the surgeon's nondominant hand
   The third level of retraction is the moment-by-moment adjustments made by the operating surgeon's nondominant hand. The only thing moving more than the surgeon's nondominant hand in the operative field is the surgeon's dominant hand. Motion-tracking studies of surgeons' instruments have demonstrated working-space volume, and path length of instrument tips can differentiate novice from expert surgeons [4]. The nondominant hand of novices tends to move more than the dominant hand, while the opposite is true of expert surgeons. Expert surgeons also operate in a volumetrically smaller space than novices. The shift in the use of the nondominant hand reflects improved economy of motion—making the appropriate exposure adjustments only when they are needed to improve performance of the dominant hand.

6.3.1 Retractors

Many types of surgical retractors have been developed over time. Many of the traditional retractors still in use today were developed alongside the procedures they are intended to assist, with specific shapes designed to provide exposure for a particular surgical maneuver. Both new materials and new procedures have continued the pursuit of designing the ideal tools to assist surgical exposure. This section will place various retractors into general categories and describe their distinguishing characteristics. See Tables 6.1, 6.2, and 6.4 for lists and brief descriptions of handheld, self-retaining, and laparoscopic retractors, respectively. Associated photographs are provided for specific examples. Tables 6.3 and 6.5 provide some retraction pearls for common open and laparoscopic procedures (Tables 6.4 and 6.5).

Table 6.1 Handheld retractors

Handheld		
Name	Description	Figure
Richardson retractor	Broad slightly saddled blade for body wall retraction	6.3a
Green retractor	An open-ended Richardson for visualization of retracted tissue	
Kocher retractor	Broad flat blade with inward bent tip	
Richardson-Eastman retractor	Double-ended Richardson	6.3b
Goelet retractor	Similar to but smaller than Richardson-Eastman	
US Army retractor	"Army-Navy" medium double ended with flat, narrow blades	6.3c
Mayo-Collins retractor	Like US Army with forked blades	
Mathieu retractor	One end like US Army, one end like Mayo-Collins	
Farabeuf retractor	Similar to but smaller than US Army with flat, solid handle	
Roux retractor	Farabeuf with saddle blades	
Parker retractor	Farabeuf with curved blades	
Parker-Mott retractor	Parker with one curved and one straight flat blade	
Little retractor	Small, curved blade for fine, superficial retraction	
Cushing vein retractor	Small, saddle blade for gentle retraction of vein or nerve	6.4a
Love nerve retractor	Thin, long handle with small curved blade	
Blair (Rollet) retractor	Small, fine rake for superficial retraction of wound edge	
Volkman retractor	Larger Blair—rake with blunt or sharp teeth	
Freeman facelift retractor	A rake with sharp, widely spaced prongs in a curvilinear pattern	
Ragnell retractor	Small, double ended with narrow, perpendicular spatulas	
Linde-Ragnell retractor	Ragnell with rough surface for increased friction	
Senn retractor	Small, one end like Ragnell, one end like Blair	6.4b
Davis retractor	Larger Ragnell	
Crile retractor	Similar to Davis or Ragnell with proportionally wider blades	
Jackson tracheal hook	Provides vertical elevation of the trachea for emergent airway	
Meyerding finger retractor	One end like a Ragnell or Blair, other end with a finger-loop	
Lahey retractor	Single-ended US Army or Ragnell with solid handle	
Langenbeck retractor	Similar to a Lahey with a thinner, deeper blade	
Skin hook	Small, pair of hooks for superficial retraction, raising skin flaps	6.4c
Deaver retractor	Broad, flat, and deep retractor with flat handle	6.5
Kelly retractor	Deaver-like blade with a formed handle	
Harrington retractor	"Sweetheart" heart-shaped end for deep, gentle retraction	6.6b
Davidson retractor	Broad, bent shape for scapula retraction	6.6a
Doyen retractor	Large, saddle blade for pelvic exposure	
Ribbon retractor	"Malleable" bendable strip for customizable use	6.7

Table 6.2 Self-retaining retractors

Self-retaining		
Name	Description	Figure
Weitlaner retractor	Opposing rakes with finger rings and ratchet-locking mechanism	6.8a
Gelpi retractor	Opposing spikes with finger rings and ratchet-locking mechanism	6.8b
Beckman retractor	A long Weitlaner with hinged ends	6.8c
Beckman-Weitlaner retractor	A Weitlaner with hinged ends	
Adson retractor	A long Weitlaner with ends at a fixed angle	
Beckman-Eaton retractor	A Beckman with broader rakes	
Bookwalter retractor system	Ring mounted to bed suspended over incision. Various retractors can be positioned to provide sustained, opposing tension	
Omni retractor system	Adjustable arms mounted to bed positioned around incision. Various retractors mount to arms to provide sustained tension	

Table 6.2 (continued)

Self-retaining		
Name	Description	Figure
Rultract Skyhook retractor system	Positions an adjustable arm vertically over the operative field to provide tension with retractors of various types and sizes	
Lone star retractor	Hooks with elastic tethers that can be stretched from a firm, circular scaffold to produce circumferential retraction	
Balfour retractor	A pair of deep, opposing retractors on rails to open a laparotomy, with a third retractor in between to apply perpendicular tension	6.9
Finochietto retractor	"Rib spreader" opposing blades with rack-and-pinion mechanism	
Wound protector	Set of plastic rings separated by a thin, flexible plastic cylinder	6.10

Table 6.3 Retraction pearls for common open procedures

Open procedures	Wrong	Right
Inguinal hernia	Using a metal retractor to retract cord structures	Using a soft retractor like a Penrose to prevent injuries
Cholecystectomy	Inadequate initial exposure leads to difficulty as the dissection proceeds deeper into the abdomen	A self-retaining retractor system can be helpful to achieve ideal exposure: right ribs elevated, Deaver or sweetheart to retract the liver, colon inferior, and stomach medial. Packs can be used to elevate segment IV and expose the porta hepatis
Laparotomy	"Set and forget" self-retaining retractor technique	Self-retaining retractor systems should be adjusted as the operation proceeds to provide ideal exposure in the operative area and relieve pressure on tissues when possible

Table 6.4 Laparoscopic retractors

Laparoscopic		
Name	Description	Figure
Hasson "S" retractor	Thin curved blades to aid open entry initial trocar placement	
Keith needle and suture	Can be passed across the abdominal wall to elevate structures	
Laparoscopic peanut	Simple shaft with cotton fabric tip	
Laparoscopic Deaver	Retractable curved blade for blunt dissection and retraction	
Fan retractor	End of shaft has spreadable blades to form broad surface	6.11
Nathanson retractor	Curved, rigid rod passed through abdominal wall, mounted to bed	
Articulating retractors	Rod with one to four joints that flex and lock. Can be inserted through port and mounted to bed for self-retained retraction	

Table 6.5 Retraction pearls for common laparoscopic procedures

Laparoscopic procedures	Wrong	Right
Inguinal hernia	Neglecting a full urinary bladder	Bladder should be emptied prior to surgery to avoid trocar injury and improve exposure
Cholecystectomy	Inadequate manipulation of gallbladder infundibulum	Infundibulum should be retracted toward the camera and laterally for best exposure of biliary anatomy
Exploration	Leaving the patient supine	Take advantage of gravity retraction to minimize unnecessary tissue manipulation

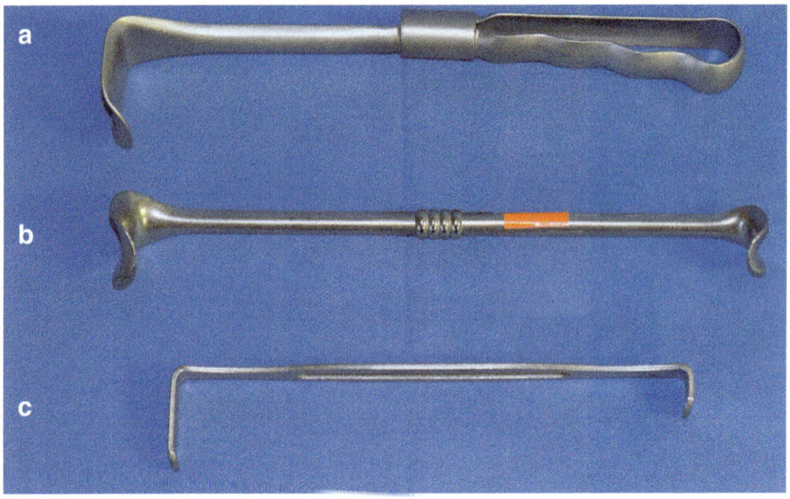

Fig. 6.3 Common handheld retractors. (**a**) Richardson, (**b**) Richardson-Eastman, (**c**) US Army

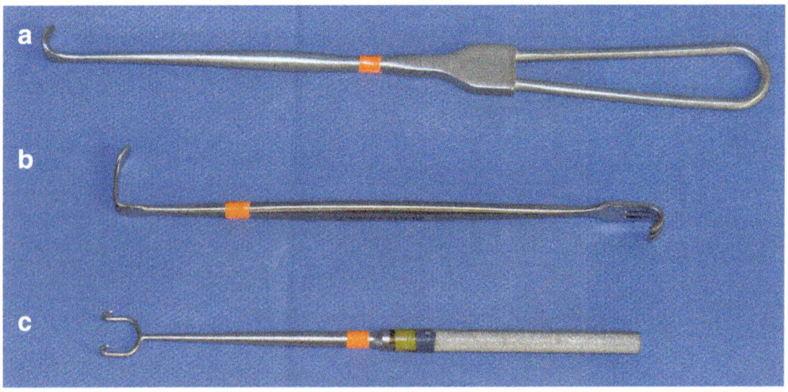

Fig. 6.4 Fine handheld retractors. (**a**) Cushing vein retractor, (**b**) Senn retractor, (**c**) skin hook

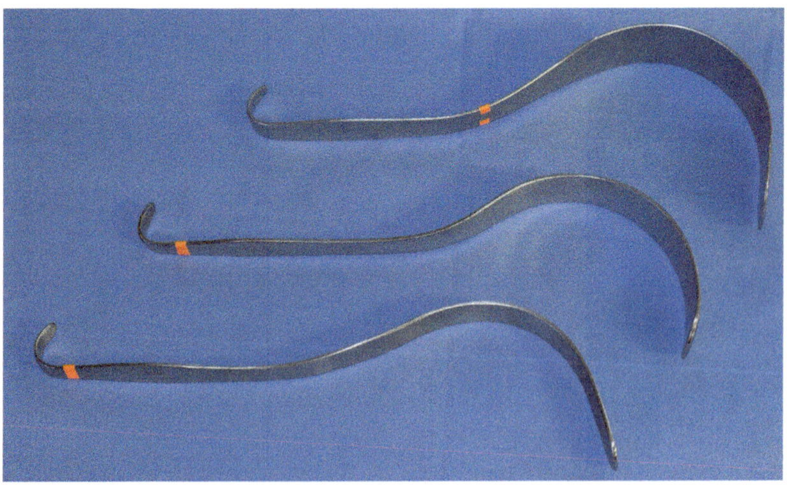

Fig. 6.5 Various Deaver retractors

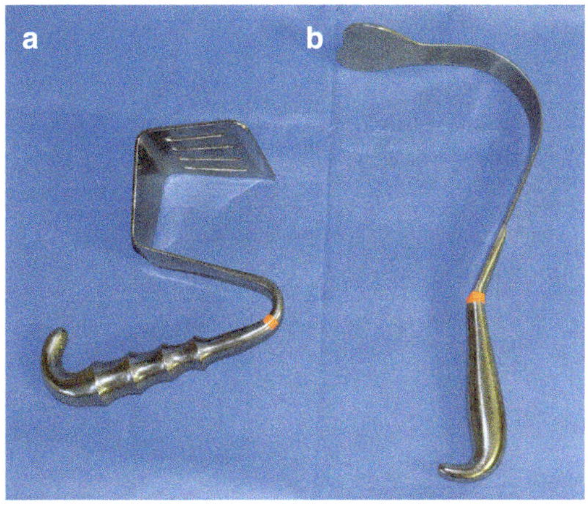

Fig. 6.6 (**a**) Davidson scapula retractor, (**b**) Harrington "sweetheart" retractor

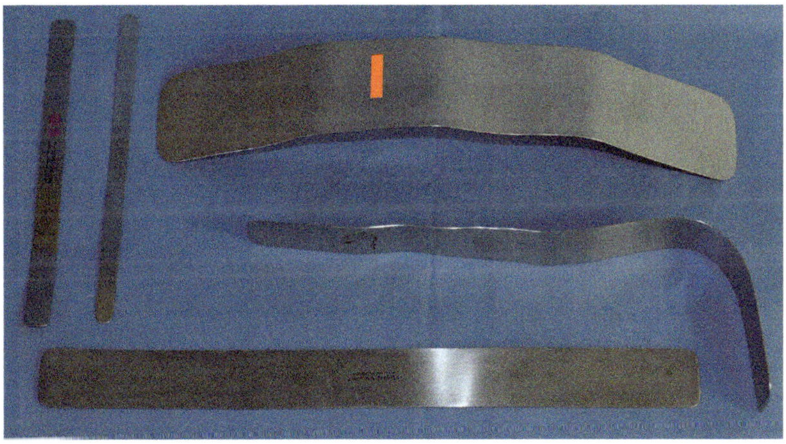

Fig. 6.7 Various malleable ribbon retractors

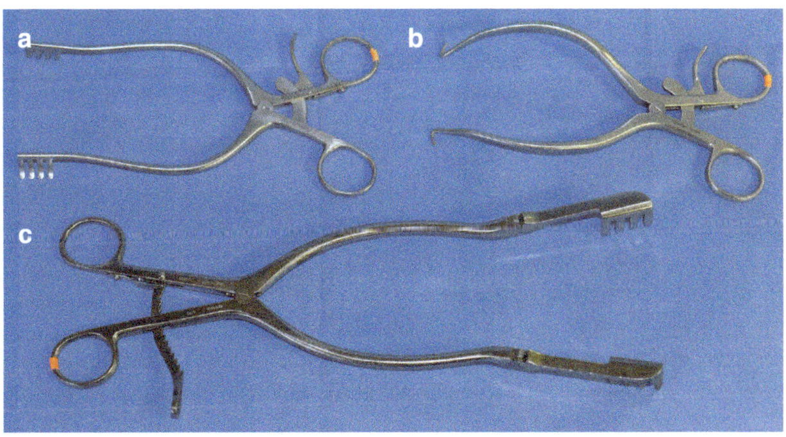

Fig. 6.8 (**a**) Weitlaner retractor, (**b**) Gelpi retractor, (**c**) Beckman retractor

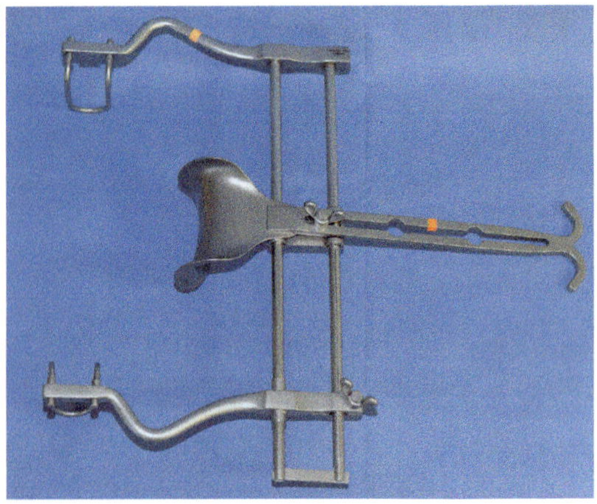

Fig. 6.9 Self-retaining Balfour retractor

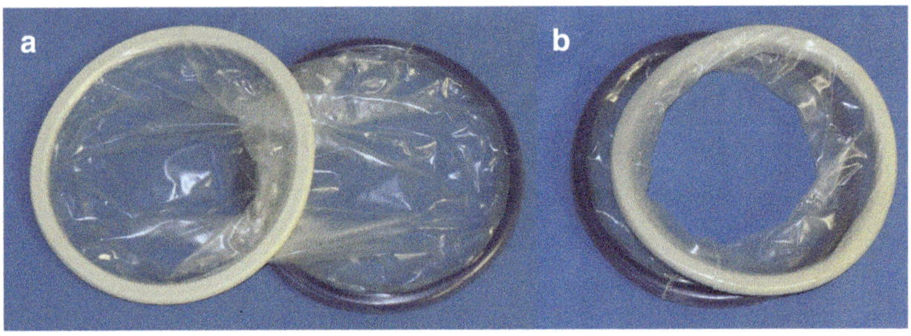

Fig. 6.10 Wound protector: This self-retaining retractor is a set of plastic rings separated by a thin, flexible plastic cylinder (**a**). One ring is placed through the incision, and the other is used to wrap and shorten the cylinder, which opens the incision and isolates wound edges (**b**)

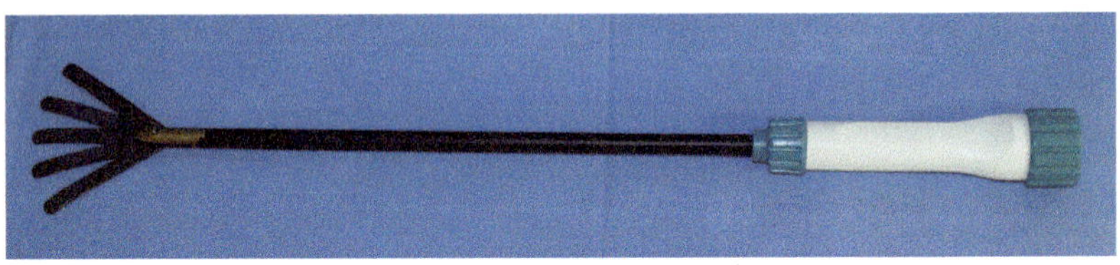

Fig. 6.11 Laparoscopic fan-style retractor

6.3.2 Handheld Retractors

Handheld retractors are meant to be mobile and easily repositionable. They are generally in the hands of the surgical assistant, who should change position in between maneuvers as appropriate to the procedure. All handheld retractors have two basic commonalities: the working end to manipulate tissue and the handle. They may be double ended, with two working ends and a handle in the middle, to allow rapid exchange between two types of working ends. Working ends come in two major varieties: blades or rakes.

Retractor blades are rectangular, positioned at a right angle to the handle. The intended use of bladed retractors determines the shape and height/width proportion of the blade. Blades come in three shapes: flat, curved, or saddled. Retractors with flat blades often come in two varieties, with or without a slightly inwardly bent distal tip that forms a lip to prevent retractor slippage. The US Army retractor (Fig. 6.3c) is a very common instrument that is manufactured both with and without a distal lip. Curved retractors conform to cylindrical structures for secure retraction. Saddle-shaped blades are similar to curved but have a second curve opposite and perpendicular to the first, like a hyperbolic paraboloid. This shape helps reduce tissue damage at the edges of the retractor. The Richardson (Fig. 6.3a) is a familiar retractor utilizing this shape. The flat portion of the Richardson's blade reflects its intended use against the abdominal wall, whereas the Cushing vein retractor (Fig. 6.4a) has no flat surface and is intended for gentle retraction of a cylindrical structure.

The second type of retractor working end is the rake. The individual prongs of rakes vary both in number and sharpness. For example, Fig. 6.4c is of a skin hook, which is a small retractor with two sharp prongs, intended to raise a thin, superficial layer to develop skin flaps. The hooks allow penetration and stable retraction of thin tissue without distorting or concealing the wound edge. The Senn retractor (Fig. 6.4b) features one end with multiple, thicker prongs, which results in less tissue penetration than the two hooks on the skin hook. The number, distribution, and sharpness of the rake determine the application it is best suited to.

6.3.3 Self-Retaining Retractors

Self-retaining retractors are appropriate for exposure that is expected to remain unchanged for long periods of time or when the hands available at the operating table are needed for more active tasks than retraction. They fall into two major categories: relatively small, self-contained instruments and large, table-mounted retraction systems.

In order to provide retraction without fixation to the operating table, self-contained instruments utilize opposing forces. One of the most familiar examples is the Weitlaner (Fig. 6.8a), which uses finger loops and a ratchet mechanism to direct two rakes away from each other. Two of these instruments placed perpendicularly to each other can provide excellent exposure through a small wound, such as with open inguinal hernia repair. Another example is the Lone Star, often used to retract the anus for transanal rectal surgery. The Lone Star is a circular plastic scaffold with slots to secure elastic bands that tether small hooks for tissue retraction. Opposing hooks are placed circumferentially, resulting in widening of the orifice and access to the rectum. Another notable self-contained retractor is commonly known as a wound protector (Fig. 6.10). This is a set of plastic rings connected by a cylindrical plastic sheet. One ring is passed through the wound, and the extracorporeal ring is turned around its circumference order to wrap and shorten the cylindrical sheet. As the sheet shortens, it applies pressure against the wound edges and forces them apart. This retractor isolates wound edges from the operative field, and has been shown to reduce risk of wound infection [5, 6].

Retraction systems are mounted to the operating table and can support multiple different retractors at once. Common examples are the Bookwalter and Omni systems. The Bookwalter involves mounting to the table a steel ring that surrounds the incision. Individual retractors are then secured to the ring. Similar to self-constrained retractors, the Bookwalter relies on opposing forces to keep the ring in centered; too much tension on one side or the other can skew the original fixation to the table. There are several different sizes of supporting rings to accommodate different sized surgical incisions. In contrast, the Omni system utilizes steel arms that can be positioned around the incision to support various retractors. This eliminates the need for different size components as with the Bookwalter rings. While both of these systems can be considered critical to long, open surgical cases, they also are bulky and can restrict access around the operating table.

Sustained pressure against tissues can result in ischemia and injury. Risk of injury is proportional to the quantity and duration of force applied and as such is more often associated with self-retaining retractors used during long cases. Clinically relevant retractor injury is rare when proper precaution is taken. Steel retractor blades of mounted retractor systems should be separated from tissue with moist laparotomy pads to provide padding and prevent tissue desiccation. Self-retaining retractors utilized in laparoscopic surgery carry the same risks, and ischemic injury due to laparoscopic liver retraction has been reported [7].

6.3.4 Laparoscopic Retraction

As with open surgery, various techniques and instrumentation for retraction have accompanied the development of laparoscopic procedures. Laparoscopic retractors can also be considered self-retaining or handheld. The simplest of the handheld laparoscopic retractors is the peanut, simply a shaft with a cotton tip. Some designs, such as one with spreading fanlike projections (Fig. 6.11), can increase surface area after passing through the trocar for more broad retraction. In the case of robotic surgery, a robotic assist arm can act as both a handheld and self-retaining retractor. The assist arm can be toggled and adjusted easily to change exposure and then left in place for as long as needed, providing an extremely versatile and easily adjustable retraction.

Anterior retraction of the left lobe of the liver is necessary for most laparoscopic procedures in the upper abdomen, and several approaches have been developed to serve this purpose. The Nathanson retractor is a curved steel rod that can be percutaneously introduced subxiphoid and rotated to retract the liver. A support mounted to the table holds the retractor in place. An alternate approach utilizes a trocar just inferior to the right lateral edge of the liver to introduce an articulating retractor, a rod that can be tightened into a polygonal shape. Articulating retractors may be exchanged through trocars as needed like any laparoscopic instrument or secured to the table for self-retaining retraction. A recent approach for liver retraction involves grasping the liver edge with a locking grasper, the end of which can be dropped from the device, leaving behind a magnet attached to the liver edge. This magnet can be directed to a larger magnet placed on the patient's skin to achieve incisionless, percutaneous liver retraction. Another simple but useful retraction technique in the upper abdomen is passing a Keith needle through the abdominal wall around the falciform. A gentle knot will keep the falciform suspended out of the way of the operative field.

Take-Home Points

Take-home points, to include a summary of the most important points (5–10 bullets):

- Perfecting exposure improves efficiency and safety.
- Spaciotemporal levels of retraction during a case:
  - Field exposure (positioning, gravity retraction)
  - Assistant retraction (appropriate instrumentation and guidance)
  - Surgeon's nondominant hand
- Know the correct retractor for the job at hand.
- Be mindful to avoid retractor injury during long cases.

Editors' Comments

- Learning to arrange the retractors for a specific procedure is a critical skill that any surgical trainee needs to concentrate on.
- While the surgeon should consider whether or not adequate exposure has been achieved, one should beware of how inefficient it is to frequently interrupt the procedure to adjust the retractors.
- "An accomplished surgeon practices economy of movements and economy of words," F.E. Rosato Sr., MD FACS.

Suggested Readings

Chassin's chapter on Incision, Exposure, Closure in open abdominal surgery: Scott-Conner CEH, editors. Chassin's operative strategy in general surgery. New York: Springer. p. 19–25.

Review and rationale for ergonomic laparoscopic port placement: Supe AN, Kulkarni GV, Supe PA. Ergonomics in laparoscopic surgery. J Minim Access Surg. 2010;6(2):31–6. https://doi.org/10.4103/0972-9941.65161.

References

1. Scott-Conner CEH, Chassin JL. Incision, exposure, closure. In: Scott-Conner CEH, editor. Chassin's operative strategy in general surgery. New York: Springer; 2014. p. 19–25.
2. Tinelli A, Malvasi A, Mynbaev OA, et al. Bladeless direct optical trocar insertion in laparoscopic procedures on the obese patient. JSLS. 2013;17(4):521–8. https://doi.org/10.4293/108680813X13693422519398.
3. Supe AN, Kulkarni GV, Supe PA. Ergonomics in laparoscopic surgery. J Minim Access Surg. 2010;6(2):31–6. https://doi.org/10.4103/0972-9941.65161.
4. D'Angelo A-LD, Rutherford DN, Ray RD, Laufer S, Mason A, Pugh CM. Working volume: validity evidence for a motion based metric of surgical efficiency. Am J Surg. 2016;211(2):445–50. https://doi.org/10.1016/j.amjsurg.2015.10.005.
5. Lee P, Waxman K, Taylor B, et al. Use of wound-protection system and postoperative wound-infection rates in open appendectomy. Arch Surg. 2009;144:872–5.
6. Sookhai S, Redmond HP, Deasy JM. Impervious wound-edge protector to reduce postoperative wound infection: a randomised, controlled trial. Lancet. 1999;353:1585.
7. Nozaki T, Kato T, Komiya A, Fuse H. Retraction-related acute liver failure after urological laparoscopic surgery. Curr Urol. 2013;7:199–203.

Fundamentals of Dissection

7

Neal S. McCall and Harish Lavu

7.1 Introduction

Surgery distinguishes itself from other fields of medicine by its emphasis on operator dependence. Studies suggest that surgical outcomes relate to not only *what* procedure is being performed but also *by the technical competency of the operating surgeon* [1–4]. Over a 5-year clinical time period, surgical trainees are expected to attain the skills to perform approximately 121 independent operations, despite the fact that on average, they will perform less than 15% of these procedures more than ten times during their residency [5–7]. And yet, research reveals that more than 60% of operative errors stem from improper surgical technique [8]. Human error—due to inadequate judgment, understanding, education, experience, or skill—thus remains among the most relevant factors in surgical morbidity and mortality outcomes [8–11]. This speaks to the importance of the fundamentals of surgical technique. There exists a great deal of literature about surgical dissection within the context of specific types of surgery and their respective considerations, yet few texts provide readers with an appreciation of the general and broad concepts as they relate to surgical dissection. This chapter explores fundamental surgical dissection techniques as well as more advanced instrumental techniques and their applications across many surgical fields.

N. S. McCall
Department of Surgery, Sidney Kimmel Medical College, Thomas Jefferson University, Philadelphia, PA, USA
e-mail: neal.mccall@jefferson.edu

H. Lavu (✉)
Jefferson Pancreas, Biliary and Related Cancer Center and the Department of Surgery, Thomas Jefferson University, Philadelphia, PA, USA

Sidney Kimmel Medical College, Thomas Jefferson University, Philadelphia, PA, USA
e-mail: Harish.lavu@jefferson.edu

7.2 General Concepts

7.2.1 Positioning

Conditions in the operative room should be designed to optimize the surgeon's visualization of the surgical field and allow for maximal exposure. Gravity should be used to a surgeon's advantage whenever possible. For example, many gynecologic procedures are facilitated by placing the patient in the Trendelenburg position, in which the patient's head is angled 15–30° toward the ground. This maneuver allows for easy mobilization of the small intestine away from the pelvis [12]. In contrast, the reverse Trendelenburg position (Fowler), placing the patient's feet 15–30° below the horizontal, can decrease engorgement of the jugular veins, facilitating safer dissection during head and neck surgery.

F. Palazzo (ed.), *Fundamentals of General Surgery*, https://doi.org/10.1007/978-3-319-75656-1_7

Positioning the patient in moderate Fowler position with the right side rotated down can also be helpful in the dissection of the left upper quadrant, allowing for greater exposure of the splenic flexure of the colon, tail of the pancreas, and spleen during operations involving this region of the body [13].

In the lithotomy position, the patient's hips are flexed to 80–90° and abducted 30–45° with feet placed in stirrups at the level of the knees. This provides the surgeon with maximal exposure of the perineum and rectum. A variant of this is the low lithotomy position, where the lower extremities are elevated to a lesser degree than full lithotomy. Care should be taken to avoid injuring the neuronal and vascular structures of the leg during this type of positioning. Notably, lithotomy position should be avoided for periods longer than 5 h to minimize the risk of fibular and femoral neuropathy and compartment syndrome [14, 15]. As any given operation progresses, especially if it necessitates work within multiple regions of the abdomen or body, it is important to reassess bed position periodically, ensuring that maximal exposure is always attained. For a further discussion of positioning and exposure, refer to Chaps. 4 and 6.

7.2.2 Lighting

The importance of adequate operative lighting during dissection cannot be understated. Before incision, luminaires should be equipped with a sterile handle and positioned with hinges at appropriate angles from one another to minimize mechanical interference during manipulation. On average, the overhead lights are readjusted every 7 to 8 min intraoperatively to ensure consistently optimal visualization of the field of dissection [16]. When possible, luminaires should be positioned such that the path of light is parallel to the surgeon's visual field of view, to prevent the development of eye fatigue from stray light. While standard surgical luminaires are adequate for most procedures, particularly deep or narrow surgical fields may necessitate the use of fiber-optic headlamps [17, 18]. The use of these devices has been shown to decrease complications associated with cardiovascular surgery by improving the surgeon's visualization of small surgical anastomoses [17]. Proper adjustment of the headlamp is vital; many surgeons find themselves readjusting their neck rather than their headlight intraoperatively. This can be avoided by focusing one's gaze on an object while maintaining the neck in a neutral position and adjusting the lamp using this gaze as a reference, prior to the commencement of the procedure.

7.2.3 Exposure and Planning

Incision planning should use standardized approaches so as to facilitate operative exposure, prevent injury to underlying structures, and optimize wound healing. For example, trocar placement in laparoscopic lower abdominal surgery should be carefully located so as to avoid injuring the inferior epigastric vessels. In open surgery, the length of the incision should be as small as possible while maintaining the surgeon's ability to have reasonable dexterity with their hands.

7.2.4 Imaging

Cross-sectional imaging has become an invaluable tool in preoperative planning for complex surgery. With special emphasis on vital structures at risk during a given operation (vascular, neuronal, ureters, etc.), this allows the surgeon at the time of the operation to dissect through difficult tissue planes with a mental 3D map of the relevant anatomical relationships. This becomes even more critical during laparoscopic or robotic operations, where tactile sensation is significantly diminished or completely absent. A careful review of imaging prior to surgery with a special emphasis on vital structures allows the surgeon to identify potentially uncommon but critical anatomic variants, such as a replaced right hepatic artery from the superior mesenteric artery during pancreaticoduodenectomy. This vessel can easily be injured during dissection along the lateral aspect of the common bile duct if the surgeon is unaware of its presence. Likewise, preoperative ultrasound has been shown in particularly inflamed cases of cholecystitis to predict the need for laparoscopic conversion to open surgery during cholecystectomy [19]. Cross-sectional imaging such as computed tomography (CT) and magnetic resonance imaging (MRI) can help to elucidate the relevant surgical anatomy and, in particular, define appropriate tissue dissection planes which allows for a more rapid as well as safe surgical technique [20]. The use of oral and intravenous contrast agents can further help to achieve diagnostic and therapeutic clarity.

7.3 Technical and Practical Considerations and Safety Precautions

The type of dissection technique used during a given operation is most often governed by the proximity of the dissection plane to vital surrounding structures. Sharp dissection during the incision is usually accomplished with a scalpel and is limited to incising the skin and upper dermis. Sharp dissection with Metzenbaum scissors is also commonly used to lyse intraabdominal adhesions and to carefully dissect inflamed tissue planes. Blunt dissection, on the other hand, often involves separating delicate (sometimes neurologic or vascular) structures along a more natural path with fingers or blunt instruments. It allows the surgeon to follow natural tissue planes rather than creating artificial ones.

7.3.1 Incision and Sharp Dissection

The scalpel fitted with a #11 or #15 blade [see Chap. 2 Appendix on instrumentation] should be held in the surgeon's dominant hand 3–4 cm from the tip of the blade, in the similar configuration as a pen is held with the index finger placed on the superior aspect. Alternatively, the scalpel fitted with a #10 blade may be held like the "bow of a violin" with the thumb on the medial aspect of the instrument and the four fingers supporting the lateral side [21]. The non-dominant hand (and eventually retractors) should be used on either side of the incision to apply adequate tension. The incision is begun with the tip of the scalpel but then should continue primarily with the belly of the blade (#10 blade) in a single sweeping motion. When multiple incisions are necessary, consider making the lower incision first to minimize blood obscuring the surgical field. Compression of the edges of the incision with fingertips and gauze can effectively control minor blood loss. The lower dermis and subcutaneous tissues are ideally divided with electrosurgery to limit bleeding (see "Instrumental Dissection").

Sharp scissor dissection is ideal when lysing intra-abdominal adhesions so as to avoid thermal/electric injury to surrounding structures and to prevent tearing of the serosal layer of the bowel. Severely inflamed tissues may also require sharp dissection to penetrate the hard or sometimes edematous tissue planes and to precisely stay on the appropriate track with the direction of the dissection.

7.3.2 Blunt Dissection

Splitting, a blunt dissection technique, generally involves inserting the closed, blunt tips of the scissors into tissues and then opening the scissors; this repeated rapid and gentle opening motion with the blunted ends facilitates the dissection [22]. *The splitting technique should be performed in a direction perpendicular to the strongest tissue, enabling dissection of the weaker connective fascia.* Alternatively, nearly closed scissors can be inserted into a previously defined plane and then advanced along a parallel path of weak connective tissue. Thicker, stronger fibrous tissue can be carefully dissected using the sharp aspect of the scissors. *Applying too much force during blunt dissection can result in unwanted injury to the tissues* [23]. For example, in the case of a dissection being carried out in the popliteal region, adipose tissue may obscure the peroneal nerve, and the use of blunt rather than sharp dissection can result in inadvertent injury [23, 24]. Thus, understanding the local tissue architecture and relevant anatomy is paramount to the choice of dissection technique.

Cautious manual tearing, otherwise known as *finger fracture*, is another technique to identify a plane of weakness in tissues. This is accomplished by first applying force between the index finger and thumb of the dominant hand on the tissue that one intends to separate. Care should be taken to avoid applying too much force during this maneuver, as it can result in the creation of false tissue planes. However, when used appropriately, the finger fracture technique can rapidly speed along a particular dissection.

Peeling is a technique used to liberate a flexible structure from adherent tissue by the use of friction generated by a blunt device [i.e., sponge, peanut, suction catheter tip]. The blunt device of choice is gently advanced in a repetitive fashion perpendicular to the area of adhesion to separate the tissue layers [editors' note: gentle additional rotating motion is critical to successfully applying this technique].

7.3.3 Instrumental Dissection

A number of instrumental dissection techniques are now available to the surgeon to facilitate safe surgery. For example, *water-jet dissection* is a form of blunt dissection which uses the high-pressure flow of water to separate tissues based on structure and resistance and has been employed in hepatic, renal, parotid, and orthopedic surgery. This technique is particularly effective in hepatic surgery, separating ductal structures and vessels from the overlying hepatic parenchyma. In at least one study, the implementation of water-jet dissection led to decreased operative transfusions, complications, and length of stay in hepatic surgery [25].

Hydrodissection is a technique that, though often confused with water-jet dissection, is unique in itself and does not require additional instrumentation. It involves the injection of saline under moderate pressure into the tissue planes using a common bulb syringe. This technique serves to increase the tissue volume, softens adhesions, expands the tissue plane, and can allow for transillumination [11, 26]. This is an extremely useful, yet underutilized, technique during a lysis of adhesion procedure. Dense, fibrous adhesions, when instilled with saline under moderate pressure from a bulb syringe, become soft and easier to dissect without injuring adherent viscera. Occasionally, an epinephrine solution may be preferred for vasoconstrictive hemostasis. This technique is frequently employed in many laparoscopic procedures as well as stress incontinence and pelvic organ prolapse procedures, where its use aids in the development of a plane underneath the pubocervical fascia for sling placement.

Following the initial skin incision, electrosurgery using the Bovie is often employed to dissect through subcutaneous tissues and to cauterize isolated small vessel bleeding. Caution should be used especially with monopolar electrosurgery, as it can cause adjacent tissue damage. When this is used to dissect through subcutaneous tissues and enter the abdominal cavity, it is crucial to protect underlying intraperitoneal structures, as shown in Fig. 7.1. Bipolar energy, though safer, is less effective at dissecting through larger amounts of tissue and is usually employed for cautery of small, focal, and delicate regions. Multiple Bovie® electrodessication systems, named after the father of modern electrosurgery, are available for a variety of surgical procedures. These are the most commonly utilized monopolar electrosurgical

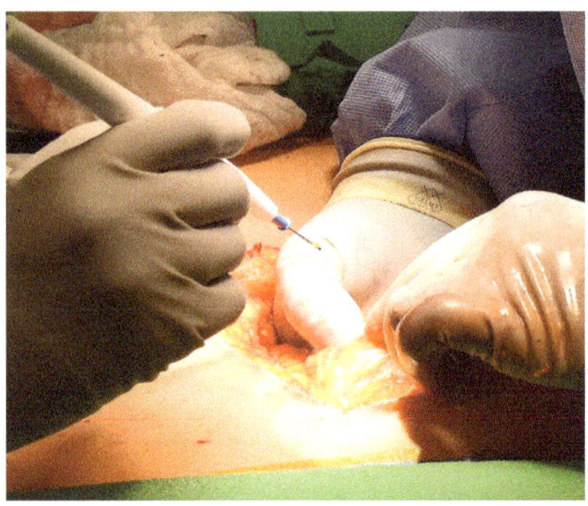

Fig. 7.1 Electrocautery dissection. In this photograph, the assistant surgeon is elevating tissue to be transected by electrocautery, so as to avoid injury to underlying intra-abdominal structures

instruments. The LigaSure® system is an example of a bipolar diathermy instrument that seals vessels clamped between its jaws up to seven millimeters in size, in 2–4 s of bursts of energy. It has been shown to reduce perioperative blood loss, procedure time, and length of stay in a variety of surgical settings [27, 28].

Surgeons may opt for ultrasound cutting and coagulation instruments, such as the Harmonic® system. These instruments convert mechanical force to heat by rupturing hydrogen atoms in the tissue. The main advantage of ultrasound dissection is a lower amount of thermal spread and adjacent tissue destruction compared to electrosurgical systems [29]. Modern versions of this system can now ligate vessels up to 7 mm in size [30].

Laser dissection and coagulation systems are yet another older alternative to electrosurgical systems. They can minimize adjacent tissue damage, providing the precise and controllable application of energy. Laser use is more common in ophthalmologic and cosmetic procedures, while its use has declined in gynecologic and general surgery procedures, primarily as a result of the development of electrosurgical systems [32]. These concepts are further and more in depth discussed in Chap. 9.

Despite the increasing importance of technology in the operating room, innovations alone cannot replace meticulous dissection and a fundamental understanding of anatomic landmarks [11]. In fact, when using advanced energy devices, it can be more difficult to follow natural tissue planes of dissection and easier to get off track, as these devices can create their own (potentially aberrant) planes of dissection.

7.3.4 Retraction

In terms of exposure, proper visualization of the surgical field would be impossible without adequate retraction [31]. As an example, during complex, open abdominal surgery, self-retaining retractors are often utilized. For example, the Bookwalter® and Omni-Tract® retraction systems provide a scaffolding on which multiple retractor blades can be attached to provide exposure to the surgical site. Intraoperative photographs of a Bookwalter retraction device are shown in Fig. 7.2a,b. An important consideration with these systems, as with all forms of retraction, however, is that the creation of very high tensile pressure on the tissues during retraction can result in damage and poor wound healing. For this reason, some newer retraction systems, such as the elastic LoneStar®, have replaced rigid metal with elastic, theoretically reducing the potential for tissue damage.

7.3.5 Traction and Counter-Traction

The principle of traction and counter-traction can dramatically improve the precision of surgical dissection. This technique increases the surgeon's visual field, by separating vital juxtaposed tissues

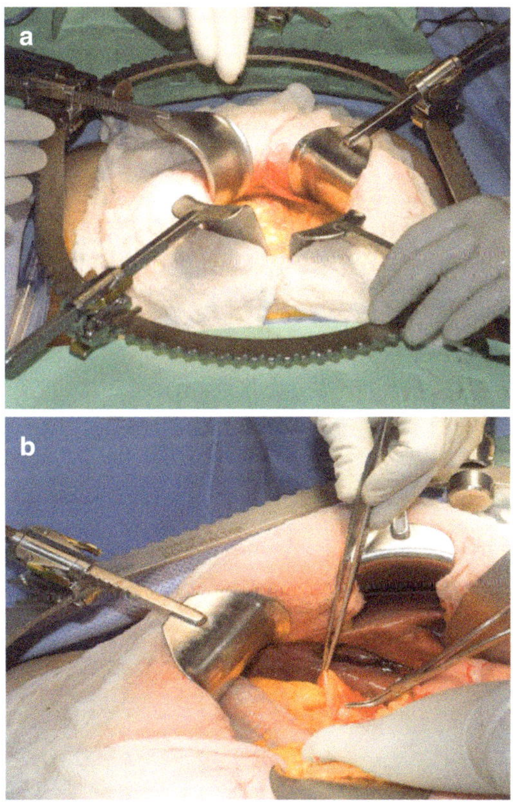

Fig. 7.2 Bookwalter® retraction system (**a**, **b**). A Bookwalter retraction system is shown before (**a**) and after (**b**) the abdomen is retracted, demonstrating improved deep and lateral abdominal exposure

and allowing for the identification of the appropriate tissue planes. As an example, the Kocher maneuver is an operative technique that allows the surgeon to mobilize the duodenum and pancreatic head out of the retroperitoneum. The peritoneal attachments of the duodenum are retracted laterally by the assistant surgeon, while the duodenum and pancreatic head are retracted medially by the surgeon, as shown in Fig. 7.3. This allows for the dissection to be carried out in an avascular plane.

During laparoscopic cholecystectomy, lateral traction is placed on the gallbladder at the level of Hartmann's pouch, which positions the cystic duct at a 90° angle to the common bile duct, minimizing the risk of inadvertent injury to the hepatic or common bile ducts [32] (Fig. 7.4a–d).

During mastectomy, the surgeon places traction on the underlying mammary tissue. Skin hooks are used by the assistant surgeon to create counter-traction to expose the appropriate plane of dissection. These hooks should be held perpendicular to the plane of dissection. Failure to do so may cause the flaps to be too thick, potentially allowing for cancerous breast tissue to remain adherent to the skin flap, whereas skin flaps that are made too thin can result in poor wound healing after surgery.

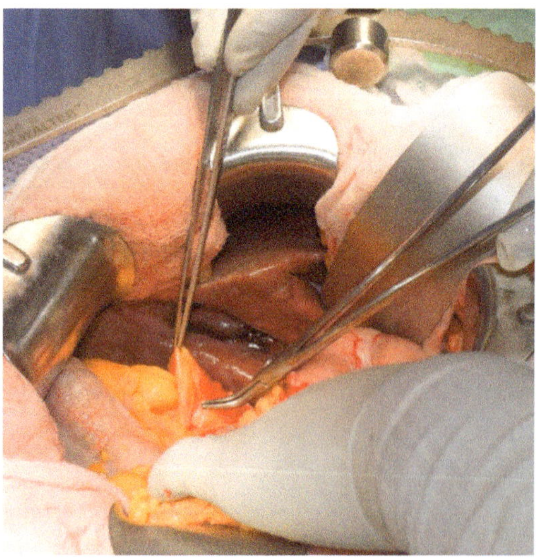

Fig. 7.3 The Kocher maneuver. A Kocher maneuver during pancreaticoduodenectomy is shown. The surgeon creates tension on the medial duodenal wall and pancreatic head, while the assistant creates counter-tension with the Debakey forceps on the retroperitoneal attachments to the duodenum. This allows for identification of the proper avascular tissue plane for dissection using the right angle

During open abdominal surgery for adhesive disease, hand retraction is used to create tension on the adhesion. This tension allows for a sharp dissection technique to be carried out using scissors. In situations where adequate tension is not able to be created, sharp dissection may be inappropriate or unsafe.

7.3.6 Tissue Planes

Proper identification of natural surgical planes, often avascular in nature, permits the safe isolation of anatomical structures and allows surgeons to avoid injury to vital structures. These planes are often convoluted, requiring a complex visuospatial and tactile acuity. Many examples abound and vary based upon a given operation. For example, the white lines of Toldt on the lateral borders of the ascending and descending colon are avascular reflections of posterior parietal peritoneum that are critical to properly identify during a hemicolectomy procedure or during exposure of the ureters. The performance of extraperitoneal hernia repair depends upon the ability to create a dissection plane within the preperitoneal space, which lies between the posterior rectus sheath and peritoneum. Another example is the plane between the pelvic parietal fascia and mesorectal fascia, referred to among colorectal surgeons as "the holy plane," which facilitates an oncologically sound en bloc resection of the mesorectum in patients with rectal cancer while sparing the sacral vessels and hypogastric nerves [33–36]. Improvement in the understanding of rectal anatomy led to the development of this technique and to substantially lower rectal cancer recurrence rates [36]. Pulmonary segmentectomy, a procedure minimizing the degree of parenchymal resection, depends entirely upon identification of the plane between the bronchopulmonary segments [34]. This plane can be accomplished by clamping the segmental bronchus and then gently inflating the

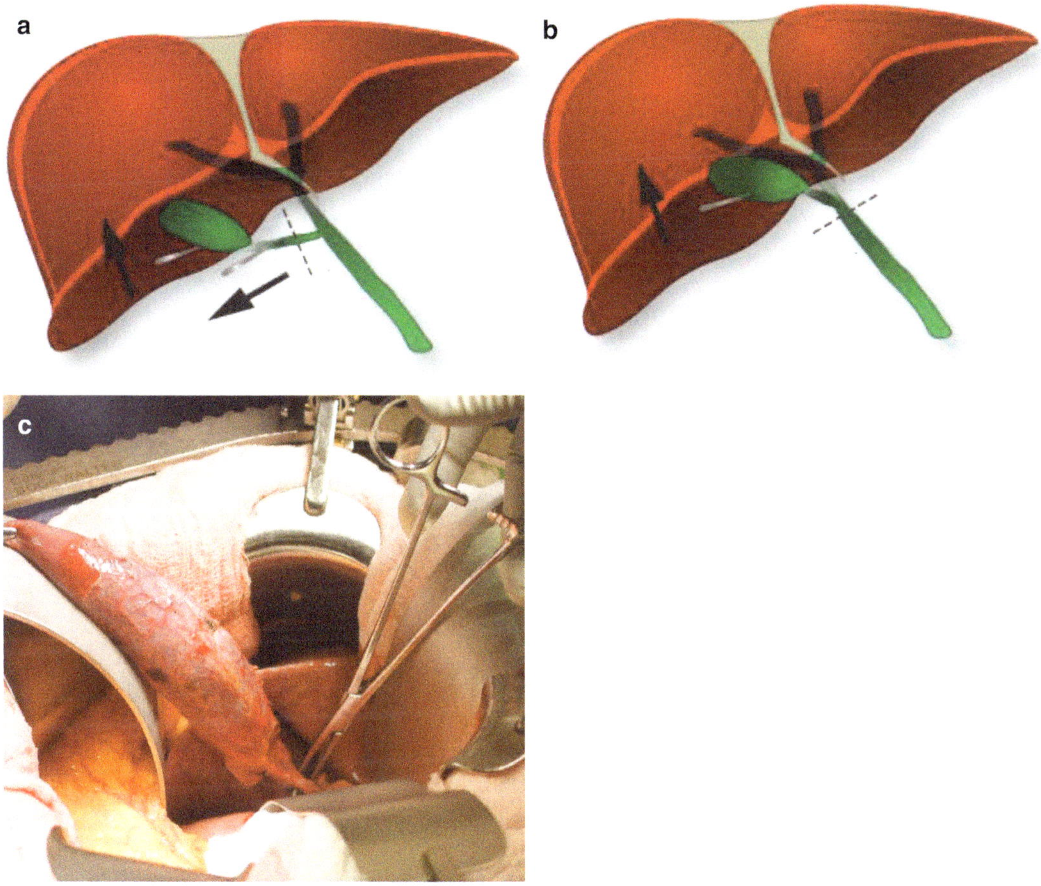

Fig. 7.4 Visualization of the triangle of Calot can prevent accidental transection of the common bile duct. (**a**) Lateral and cephalad traction has been applied to the gallbladder, allowing for safe transection of the cystic duct. (**b**) Inadequate lateral traction has been applied to the gallbladder resulting in the common bile duct being mistaken for the cystic duct. (**c**) Intraoperative photograph demonstrating the right angle clamp placed behind the cystic duct

lung. The intersegmental plane, defined by pulmonary veins and lymphatics, should lie at the junction of inflated and deflated tissue [33].

7.3.7 Inflamed Tissue

Dissection of acute or chronically inflamed tissue may require special consideration. Acutely inflamed tissue will often be more edematous and vascular than healthy tissue. Edema can distort the appearance and location of important anatomic landmarks, while the increased vascularity of inflamed tissues can obscure visualization of the dissection plane due to bleeding. Additionally, the presence of putrid or foul odors may signify infection or necrosis of tissue. In the setting of chronically inflamed tissue, fibrotic changes can also contribute to the distortion of normal anatomy. These changes may require use of sharp dissection in place of intended blunt dissection. Chronic inflammation may also predispose tissues to pathologic fistulous connections. The chronic inflammation of Crohn's disease predisposes the alimentary tract to fistulas, including anorectal, enterovesical, and enterocutaneous types [37]. Encountering abscesses or soft tissue infection should prompt adequate drainage and debridement. Regardless of the pathologic condition encountered, dissection should proceed in a direction from normal tissue toward inflamed tissue, identifying all normal landmarks before engaging altered ones. In complex, multistep operations, the order of the completed steps should be appropriately adjusted by the surgeon based upon the particular challenge a given case may pose. In such a case, the surgeon should complete the easiest, most straightforward steps prior to moving onto more difficult ones. This is important for two reasons. It keeps the operation moving forward in a timely fashion, and it also improves the visualization and mobilization of the tissues so that these are optimized prior to attempting to tackle the most difficult and potentially dangerous steps of the procedure.

7.3.8 Neoplasms

Surgical resection of a neoplasm requires several unique considerations with respect to dissection. Foremost, preoperative planning and review of imaging become paramount. Preoperative imaging is essential to confirm a given patient's candidacy for surgery, allow for the identification of anatomic abnormalities or variants, and give a sense of where the dissection must proceed to obtain negative surgical resection margins.

If the tumor is well-encapsulated and benign in nature, wide margins may not necessarily be indicated, and the surgeon can dissect closer to the margin of the capsule. However, it is important to consider that some malignant tumors may appear to be well-defined on imaging but in actuality demonstrate microscopic invasion of surrounding tissues. Some central nervous system tumors, most notably glioblastoma multiforme, may be impossible to delineate from healthy neuronal tissue. In this case, general anesthesia may be forgone for an awake craniotomy to ensure that surgical dissection does not result in a functional neurologic deficit [38]. It is important to be aware of the likely direction of spread of malignant tumors and the possibility of invasion or impingement of adjacent vital structures. For example, pancreatic adenocarcinoma frequently obstructs the bile and pancreatic ducts, resulting in biliary dilatation as well as pancreatic ductal dilation (termed "double-duct sign"). In locally advanced cases, pancreatic adenocarcinoma can involve the portal and superior mesenteric veins or superior mesenteric artery, which may preclude safe surgical resection.

As a general rule, resection of malignant tumors should proceed in a cautious fashion with the intent to remove the intact tumor as well as an appropriate margin of surrounding healthy tissue and the relevant lymph node basins for the tumor. Removal of large benign tumors, such as fibroids and posterior fossa masses, may be facilitated by debulking. This can be accomplished with radiofrequency, ultrasound, or electrosurgery as means to reduce the tumor volume [39].

7.4 Current Controversies and Future Directions

7.4.1 Cognitive Bias in Surgery

Research has demonstrated that cognitive biases play an important role in surgical errors, including wrong-patient, wrong-side, and wrong-procedure surgeries [40, 41]. One type of cognitive bias, confirmation bias, is defined as one's propensity to seek information to confirm rather than to challenge one's presumptions. Way et al. [42] retrospectively analyzed operative notes and videotapes of cholecystectomy cases complicated by common bile duct (CBD) injury. In some cases, the cystic duct was obscured by the infundibulum. Adequate cephalad and lateral traction of the gallbladder allows for what has been referred to as "the critical view of safety," as illustrated in Fig. 7.1a. However, inadequate lateral traction creates the illusion that the common bile duct is the cystic duct. Way et al. found that this illusion caused the inadvertent transection of the common bile duct, as shown in Fig. 7.1b–d. In these cases, the authors reasoned, the surgeon was betrayed by their subconscious brain's propensity to relate their visual field to that of the preconceived, mental image of the biliary tree.

While there exists evidence of the impact of nontechnical cognitive skills on surgeon performance, consensus on how to mitigate the impact of cognitive bias and nontechnical skill is lacking [40]. Moreover, unlike a surgeon's technical skills, a surgeon's ability to assess his or her own nontechnical skills is limited [43]. Research has suggested that simply requiring more operating experience is unlikely to be successful [42]. Way et al. assert that more liberalized use of technology, such as intraoperative cholangiography during cholecystectomy, could minimize the negative effects of surgeons' cognitive biases. Another alternative would be to implement systematic, process alterations [44]. During cholecystectomy, this could be the top-down approach to gallbladder dissection, which has been shown to be safer during open procedures [42]. However, alterations of operating room processes, such as those designed to confirm the correct patient and laterality, are still subject to a surgeon's cognitive biases [45]. Regardless, it remains imperative for future efforts to focus on both awareness of these biases and decreasing their associated risk.

Take-Home Points

- Surgeons should position patients in a manner to facilitate exposure and safety.
- Adequate lighting is imperative to accomplishing safe, effective dissection. Lighting in the operating room should be adjusted frequently throughout the procedure.
- Modern imaging techniques should be incorporated into a surgeon's preoperative planning and guide the operative approach.
- Sharp, blunt, and instrumental dissection should be chosen appropriately based on the given tissue planes.
- Dissection should always proceed in a direction from non-inflamed tissue toward inflamed or diseased tissue.
- Potentially malignant tissue should be dissected with the intent of en bloc resection along with the relevant lymph node basins.
- Surgeons should be aware of the impact of cognitive bias on their intraoperative decision-making.

Conflicts of Interest The authors have no conflicts of interest to declare.

Editors' Corner

- Blunt dissection: its basic concept can be summarized as finding the path of least resistance around/toward the target organ. Adequate balance between force to be used and traction applied is only learned with careful observation and practice with skilled mentors.
- Dissection during laparoscopic procedures presents special challenges for the surgeon as tactile feedback is lost and "finger fracture" techniques cannot be used. Splitting and peeling remain very useful resources for the surgeon and are commonly used by carefully employing advanced energy devices and dissectors like laparoscopic peanuts and laparoscopic suction cannulas. The presence of CO2 is a major aid during laparoscopic procedures as it will naturally tend to "open" up natural planes or not inflamed or fibrotic areas and guide the surgeon in identifying areas of easier dissection.

Suggested Readings

Kirk R. Basic surgical techniques. Edinburgh: Elsevier; 2010.

Karakousis CP. Principles of surgical dissection. J Surg Oncol. 1982;21:205–6.

Way LW, et al. Causes and prevention of laparoscopic bile duct injuries: analysis of 252 cases from a human factors and cognitive psychology perspective. Ann Surg. 2003;237:460–9.

References

1. AlJamal YN, Zendejas B, Gas BL, Ali SM, Heller SF, Kendrick ML, et al. Annual surgeon volume and patient outcomes following laparoscopic totally extraperitoneal inguinal hernia repairs. J Laparoendosc Adv Surg Tech A. 2016;26(2):92–8.
2. Al-Sahaf M, Lim E. The association between surgical volume, survival and quality of care. J Thorac Dis. 2015;7(Suppl 2):S152–5.
3. Amato L, Colais P, Davoli M, Ferroni E, Fusco D, Minozzi S, et al. [Volume and health outcomes: evidence from systematic reviews and from evaluation of Italian hospital data]. Epidemiol Prev. 2013;37(2-3 Suppl 2):1–100.
4. Sosa JA, Bowman HM, Gordon TA, Bass EB, Yeo CJ, Lillemoe KD, et al. Importance of hospital volume

in the overall management of pancreatic cancer. Ann Surg. 1998;228(3):429–38.
5. Bell RH, Biester TW, Tabuenca A, Rhodes RS, Cofer JB, Britt LD, et al. Operative experience of residents in US general surgery programs: a gap between expectation and experience. Ann Surg. 2009;249(5):719–24.
6. Khuri SF, Henderson WG, Daley J, Jonasson O, Jones RS, Campbell DA, et al. Successful implementation of the Department of Veterans Affairs' National Surgical Quality Improvement Program in the private sector: the patient safety in surgery study. Ann Surg. 2008;248(2):329–36.
7. Makary MA, Daniel M. Medical error-the third leading cause of death in the US. BMJ. 2016;353:i2139.
8. Fabri PJ, Zayas-Castro JL. Human error, not communication and systems, underlies surgical complications. Surgery. 2008;144(4):557–63; discussion 563.
9. Regenbogen SE, Greenberg CC, Studdert DM, Lipsitz SR, Zinner MJ, Gawande AA. Patterns of technical error among surgical malpractice claims: an analysis of strategies to prevent injury to surgical patients. Ann Surg. 2007;246(5):705–11.
10. Rogers SO, Gawande AA, Kwaan M, Puopolo AL, Yoon C, Brennan TA, et al. Analysis of surgical errors in closed malpractice claims at 4 liability insurers. Surgery. 2006;140(1):25–33.
11. Singh K, Ohri A. Anatomic landmarks: their usefulness in safe laparoscopic cholecystectomy. Surg Endosc. 2006;20(11):1754–8.
12. Buchwald H. Three helpful techniques for facilitating abdominal procedures, in particular for surgery in the obese. Am J Surg. 1998;175(1):63–4.
13. Poulin E, et al. Chap. 25: Splenectomy. In: ACS surgery: principles & practice. 6th ed. New York: WebMD; 2010.
14. Anema JG, Morey AF, McAninch JW, Mario LA, Wessells H. Complications related to the high lithotomy position during urethral reconstruction. J Urol. 2000;164(2):360–3.
15. Frezza EE. The lithotomy versus the supine position for laparoscopic advanced surgeries: a historical review. J Laparoendosc Adv Surg Tech A. 2005;15(2):140–4.
16. Knulst AJ, Mooijweer R, Jansen FW, Stassen LPS, Dankelman J. Indicating shortcomings in surgical lighting systems. Minim Invasive Ther Allied Technol. 2011;20(5):267–75.
17. Moriyama S, Kawasuji M. [Lighting and surgical exposure with head lamp and optical loupes]. Kyobu Geka. 2009;62(8 Suppl):633–7.
18. Browne D. A headlight for general surgery. Lancet. 1956;270(6909):191.
19. Tosun A, Hancerliogullari KO, Serifoglu I, Capan Y, Ozkaya E. Role of preoperative sonography in predicting conversion from laparoscopic cholecystectomy to open surgery. Eur J Radiol. 2015;84(3):346–9.
20. Jacobson FL. Chap. 3. Chest imaging: role of CT, PET/CT, and MRI. In: Sugarbaker DJ, Bueno R, Krasna MJ, Mentzer SJ, Zellos L, editors. Adult chest surgery. New York: McGraw-Hill; 2009.
21. Gross SD. In: Lee HC, editor. A system of surgery: pathological, diagnostic, therapeutic, and operative. 5th ed. Philadelphia: H.C. Lea; 1872.
22. Kirk R. Basic surgical techniques. Edinburgh: Elsevier; 2010.
23. Karakousis CP. Principles of surgical dissection. J Surg Oncol. 1982;21(4):205–6.
24. Karakousis CP. The technique of popliteal lymph node dissection. Surg Gynecol Obstet. 1980;151(3):420–3.
25. Vollmer CM, Dixon E, Sahajpal A, Cattral MS, Grant DR, Gallinger S, et al. Water-jet dissection for parenchymal division during hepatectomy. HPB (Oxford). 2006;8(5):377–85.
26. Naude GP, Morris E, Bongard FS. Laparoscopic cholecystectomy facilitated by hydrodissection. J Laparoendosc Adv Surg Tech A. 1998;8(4):215–8.
27. Araki Y, Noake T, Kanazawa M, Yamada K, Momosaki K, Nozoe Y, et al. Clipless hand-assisted laparoscopic total colectomy using Ligasure Atlas. Kurume Med J. 2004;51(2):105–8.
28. Targarona EM, Balague C, Marin J, Neto RB, Martinez C, Garriga J, et al. Energy sources for laparoscopic colectomy: a prospective randomized comparison of conventional electrosurgery, bipolar computer-controlled electrosurgery and ultrasonic dissection. Operative outcome and costs analysis. Surg Innov. 2005;12(4):339–44.
29. McCarus SD. Physiologic mechanism of the ultrasonically activated scalpel. J Am Assoc Gynecol Laparosc. 1996;3(4):601–8.
30. Bubenik LJ, Hosgood G, Vasanjee SC. Bursting tension of medium and large canine arteries sealed with ultrasonic energy or suture ligation. Vet Surg. 2005;34(3):289–93.
31. Steele PRC, Curran JF, Mountain RE. Current and future practices in surgical retraction. Surgeon. 2013;11(6):330–7.
32. Rossidis G. Chap. 1: Laparoscopic cholecystectomy. In: Operative techniques in surgery. 1st ed. Philadelphia: Lippincott Williams & Wilkins; 2015. p. 475–84.
33. Friedberg JS. Chap. 65. Segmentectomy. In: Sugarbaker DJ, Bueno R, Krasna MJ, Mentzer SJ, Zellos L, editors. Adult chest surgery. New York: McGraw-Hill; 2009.
34. Jones DR, Stiles BM, Denlinger CE, Antippa P, Daniel TM. Pulmonary segmentectomy: results and complications. Ann Thorac Surg. 2003;76(2):343–8; discussion 348.
35. Fell SC. Segmental resection. Chest Surg Clin N Am. 1995;5(2):205–21.
36. Abcarian H. Is the holy plane the last word? Dis Colon Rectum. 2016;59(2):160–1.
37. Su Y-R, Shih I-L, Tai H-C, Wei S-C, Lin B-R, Yu H-J, et al. Surgical management in enterovesical fistula in Crohn disease at a single medical center. Int Surg. 2014;99(2):120–5.
38. Brown T, Shah AH, Bregy A, Shah NH, Thambuswamy M, Barbarite E, et al. Awake craniotomy for brain

tumor resection: the rule rather than the exception? J Neurosurg Anesthesiol. 2013;25(3):240–7.
39. Brucker SY, Hahn M, Kraemer D, Taran FA, Isaacson KB, Krämer B. Laparoscopic radiofrequency volumetric thermal ablation of fibroids versus laparoscopic myomectomy. Int J Gynaecol Obstet. 2014;125(3):261–5.
40. Yule S, Flin R, Paterson-Brown S, Maran N. Non-technical skills for surgeons in the operating room: a review of the literature. Surgery. 2006;139(2):140–9.
41. Reason J. Safety in the operating theatre - part 2: human error and organisational failure. Qual Saf Health Care. 2005;14(1):56–60.
42. Way LW, Stewart L, Gantert W, Liu K, Lee CM, Whang K, et al. Causes and prevention of laparoscopic bile duct injuries: analysis of 252 cases from a human factors and cognitive psychology perspective. Ann Surg. 2003;237(4):460–9.
43. Arora S, Miskovic D, Hull L, Moorthy K, Aggarwal R, Johannsson H, et al. Self vs expert assessment of technical and non-technical skills in high fidelity simulation. Am J Surg. 2011;202(4):500–6.
44. Kaye AD, Fox CJ III, Urman RD. Operating room leadership and management. Cambridge: Cambridge University Press; 2012.
45. Thiels CA, Lal TM, Nienow JM, Pasupathy KS, Blocker RC, Aho JM, et al. Surgical never events and contributing human factors. Surgery. 2015;158(2):515–21.

Fundamentals of Surgical Hemostasis

8

Daniel J. Deziel

8.1 Fundamentals of Surgical Hemostasis

8.1.1 Introduction

Blood comes from blood vessels. Hence, the fundament of surgical hemostasis is control of blood vessels before, and after, they begin to spew their vital content. This essay will focus on principles for achieving mechanical hemostasis in the operating room. We will not invoke the coagulation cascade or recite a litany of intrinsic and acquired bleeding dyscrasias. Nor will we describe the physics of various energy sources or the safe use of the devices that dispense such hemostatic powers. These concepts are capably discussed in other chapters.

Surgeons accumulate a technical vocabulary for mechanical hemostasis at the operating table. We are taught by our mentors, we observe the traits of others, and we refine our techniques with experience. Modern textbooks give little heed to technical detail. The technical fundamentals presented in this chapter are evidence based only in experience. They are principles that are sculpted from a cumulative experience of 215 years of operating by seasoned surgeons. They are derived from a collective experience with an array of general abdominal, thoracic, oncologic, vascular, and transplant operations. They come from operative circumstances that are both routine and complex; many familiar, some scarcely believable; and most of them successful.

Many surgeons will have methods that are different from those discussed here. Surgeons must develop, from experience, the techniques that work best with their tools in their patients. There is no one way to assure hemostasis. However, there are ways that will be more effective, or less effective, and ways that will be defective. We present the ways that we teach at the table.

This chapter has a few disclaimers. The focus will be on the methods for handling blood vessels and for stopping blood loss during traditional open operations. Moreover, the focus will be on the use of traditional surgical instruments, rather than clips or staplers or energy devices. These latter accoutrements certainly have valuable applications, particularly during laparoscopic operations. However, every operating surgeon must have some familiarity with the traditional methods. These skills, for some patients, at some time, will become the ultimate life-sustaining measure. These necessary skills have also become less often learned and practiced by many current surgical trainees.

Adam Strickland, MD contributed all the pictures for this chapter

D. J. Deziel
Department of Surgery, Rush University Medical Center, Chicago, IL, USA
e-mail: daniel_j_deziel@rush.edu

F. Palazzo (ed.), *Fundamentals of General Surgery*, https://doi.org/10.1007/978-3-319-75656-1_8

For the most part, we intentionally avoid specification of the type of suture material used: permanent versus absorbable and braided versus monofilament. The surgeon must know the properties of each suture to determine its attributes and deficiencies. The surgeon must understand the function that a suture is intended to provide in a given situation. Informed by this, a surgeon will choose what works best with their own hands, in the environment at hand.

8.1.2 General Concepts

First, prevent bleeding. The prerequisite is to understand the anatomy; one must know what vessels one will find where. This means knowledge of "typical" anatomy as well as the natural variations that occur and, importantly, recognition of how the anatomy will be altered by pathologic conditions. The technical requisite is to establish proximal and distal control of blood vessels without inflicting trauma. This requires proper exposure and gentle handling of tissues during dissection.

Second, stop bleeding. Bleeding is to be controlled with alacrity and permanency and with adequate precision so as not to cause irreparable injury to vital vessels or to other structures. Management of active bleeding requires composure, exposure, and familiarity with techniques for handling disrupted vessels and diffusely bleeding surfaces and for inflow control.

8.1.3 Technical Considerations to Control Blood Vessels

Respect the integrity of the vessel. Dissect slowly, with minimal manipulation of the vessel itself. The idea is to move surrounding tissue away from the vessel while the vessel stays in place. Tissue can be teased, or pushed, or cut away. Tissue can be gently spread and divided with electrocautery. Adhesions around vessels are dealt with according to their consistency. Normal developmental adhesions can be moved bluntly. Stringy adhesions are cut with scissors. Dense adhesions are spread gradually with Adson-type clamps, if possible, and sharply divided in small increments. When cutting with a round-tipped scissors, the tip must go slightly past the tissue being divided. When there is little space, precise cutting is done with the tip of a more pointed scissors.

Respect the plane of the vessel wall. Tissue forceps with closed tips can be used to retract a vessel, gently going from side to side. DeBakey-type forceps are less likely to cause vascular damage compared to nonvascular forceps. Never squeeze an artery with any type of forceps. This may cause disruption of the vasa vasorum, subadventitial hematoma, intimal tears, and arterial dissection. The smaller the artery, the greater is the risk. While all arteries require careful dissection, there are some that tend to be particularly fragile and demand extra care; beware the internal iliac artery, the subclavian artery, and the pulmonary artery. If a vein must be maneuvered to facilitate dissection, it should be grasped bluntly across its near full diameter to avoid tearing.

When getting around the circumference of a vessel, use a blunt-tipped instrument like a Mixter clamp rather than a clamp that has jaws with more pointed tips. This is particularly important when dealing with frail vessels or when getting around veins that have walls that fold on themselves.

One needs to acquire the skill for feeling what is at the tip of the instrument. Put the tip of the instrument behind the vessel, spread, take the instrument out, and then place the instrument in again and spread again. Do not chew through the tissue by repeatedly opening and closing the jaws blindly while pushing the instrument behind the vessel. Under direct vision, see that the tip of the instrument comes around cleanly from behind the vessel and that it is not pushing a portion of the vessel wall ahead of it. Beware of branches on the backside of the vessel, particularly with veins, because the branching pattern is less constant.

Sometimes a loop is placed around a vessel to aid retraction. If used, the vessel must only be retracted gently because loops can cause damage. Do not retract a vessel with a double loop around it. Silicon loops slide on the vessel wall and may not retract as well as a fabric tape ("umbilical" or "core" tape). Fabric tape does not slide, but can injure the vessel, especially if dry.

Once identified and dissected, vessels can be controlled in several ways:

1. Sutures can be passed around the vessel and tied before the vessel is divided between the ties ("tying in continuity"). If the vessel is sturdy, it can be cut before the ties are cut. If the structure is tenuous, the suture should be cut before the vessel is cut so that the tie does not fall off (Fig. 8.1).
2. Two clamps can be placed on the vessel which is then divided between the clamps. Each clamped end of the vessel is then tied or suture ligated ("stick tied") (Fig. 8.2).
3. A suture can be passed around the vessel, and, while gently pulling up on the suture, one jaw of a clamp can be placed in the opening behind the vessel where the suture is. The clamp is moved down along the other side of the vessel and closed. The suture is tied. The vessel is divided, and the clamped end is either ligated or suture ligated (Fig. 8.3).
4. A vessel can be suture ligated in place before it is divided (Fig. 8.4).

The most appropriate of these techniques will depend upon the nature of the vessel, the length of vessel that is available, the amount of space

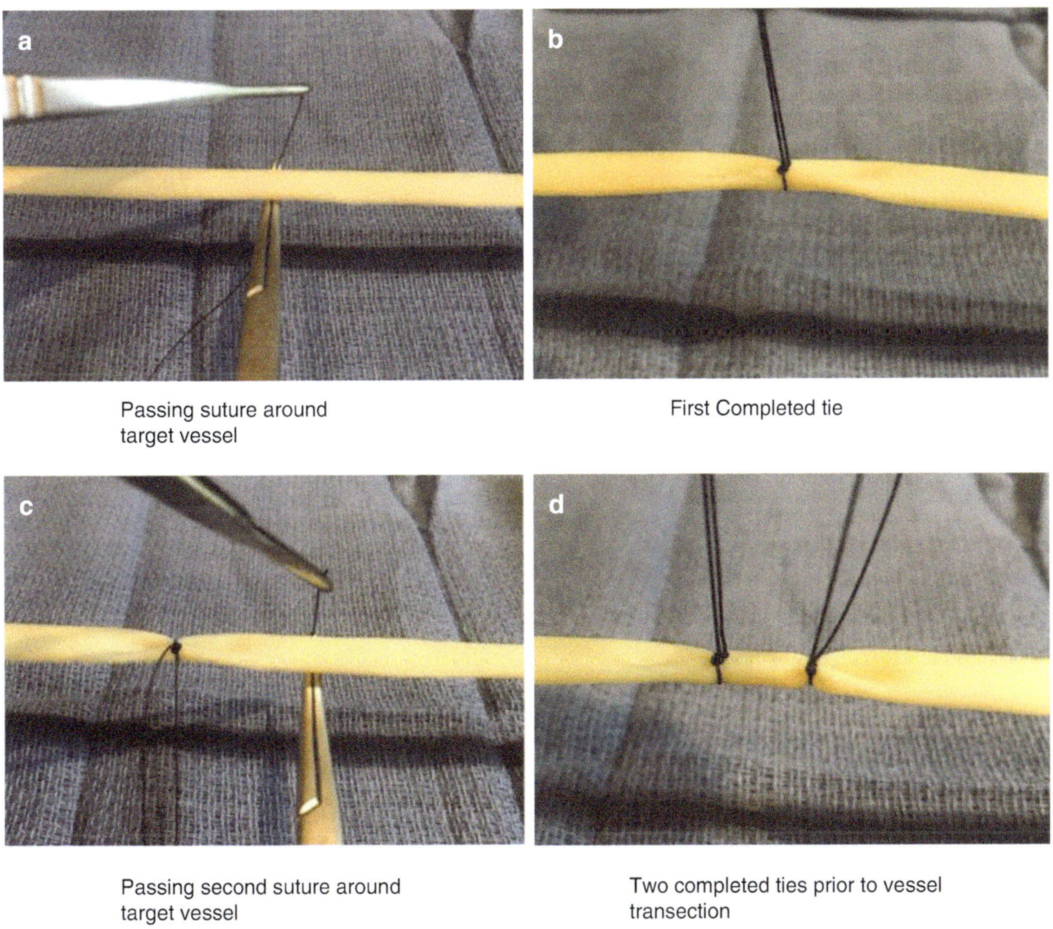

Fig. 8.1 (**a**–**d**) Depicts the steps of "tying in continuity." (**a**) Passing suture around target vessel. (**b**) First completed tie. (**c**) Passing second suture around target vessel. (**d**) Two completed ties prior to vessel transection

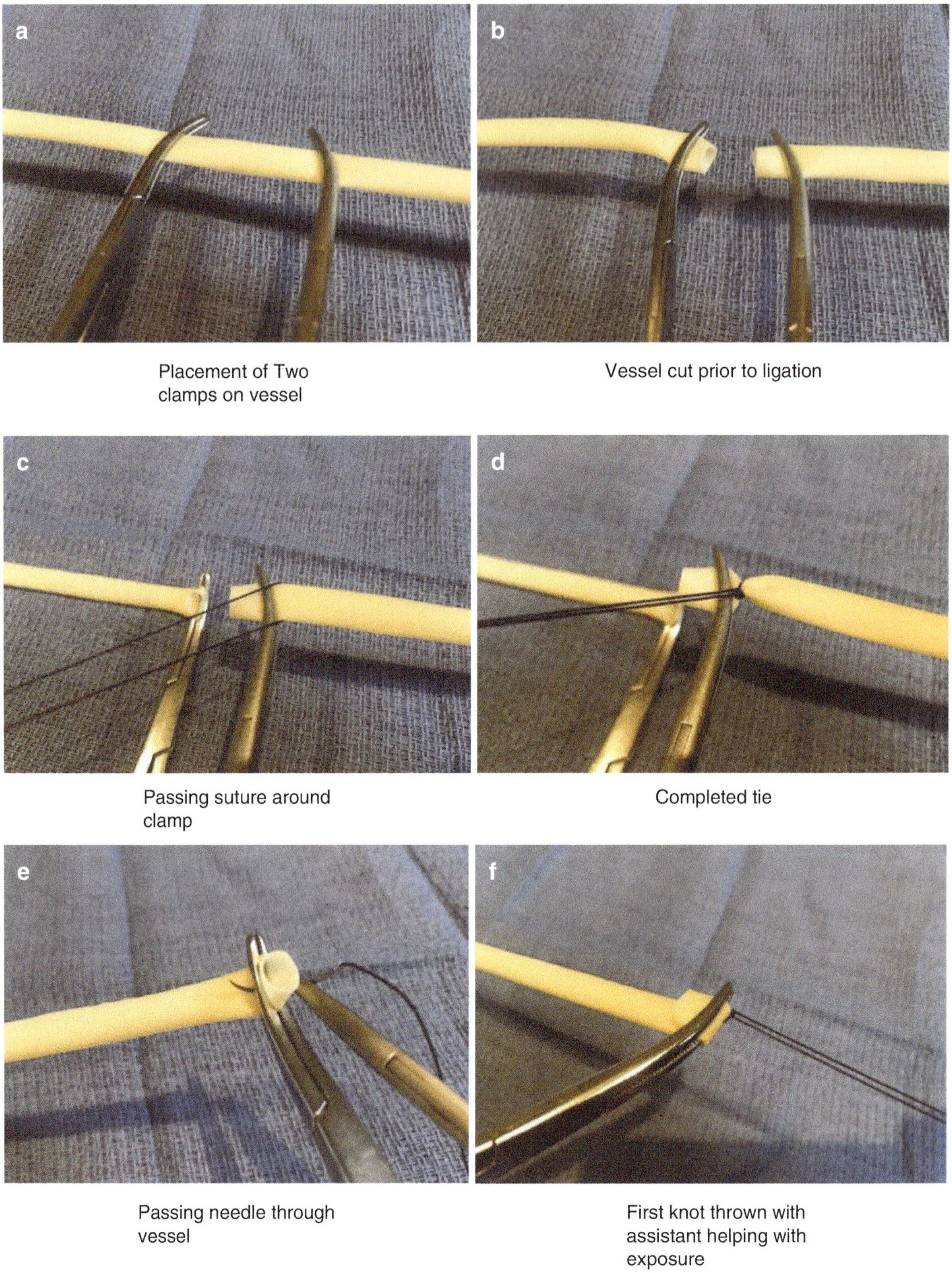

Fig. 8.2 Depict the steps of vascular control with division between clamps: (**a–d**) free hand tying, (**e–h**) suture ligature. (**a**) Placement of two clamps on vessel. (**b**) Vessel cut prior to ligation. (**c**) Passing suture around clamp. (**d**) Completed tie. (**e**) Passing needle through vessel. (**f**) First knot thrown with assistant helping with exposure. (**g**) Passing suture around clamp. (**h**) Completed suture ligation

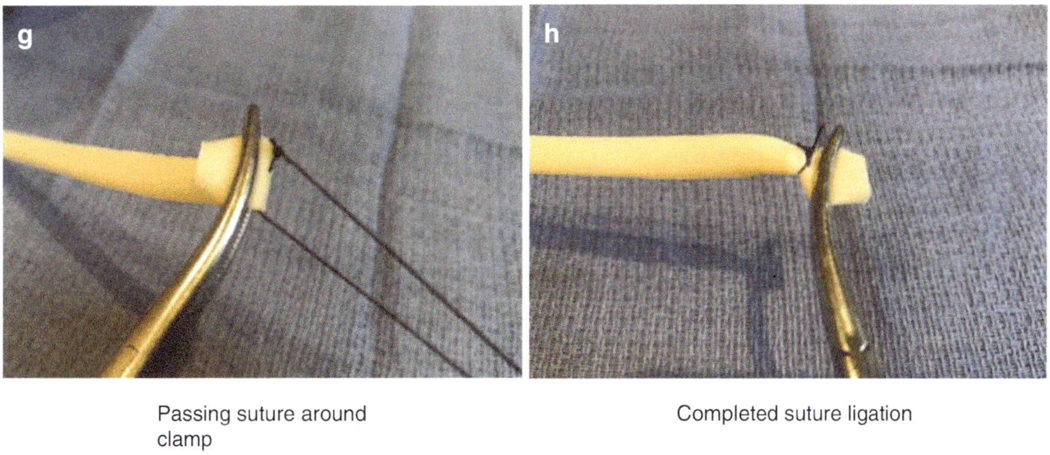

Fig. 8.2 (continued)

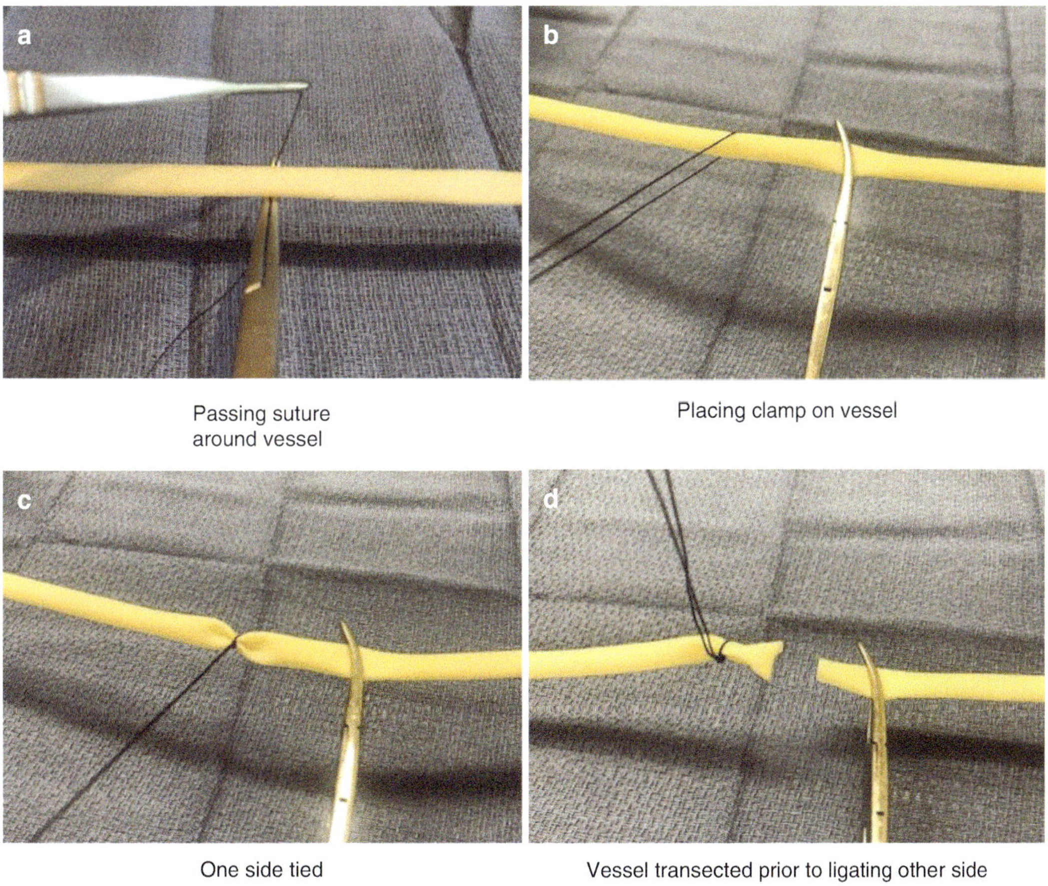

Fig. 8.3 Vascular control clamp-tie-divide-tie method (**a–d**). (**a**) Passing suture around vessel. (**b**) Placing clamp on vessel. (**c**) One side tied. (**d**) Vessel transected prior to ligating the other side

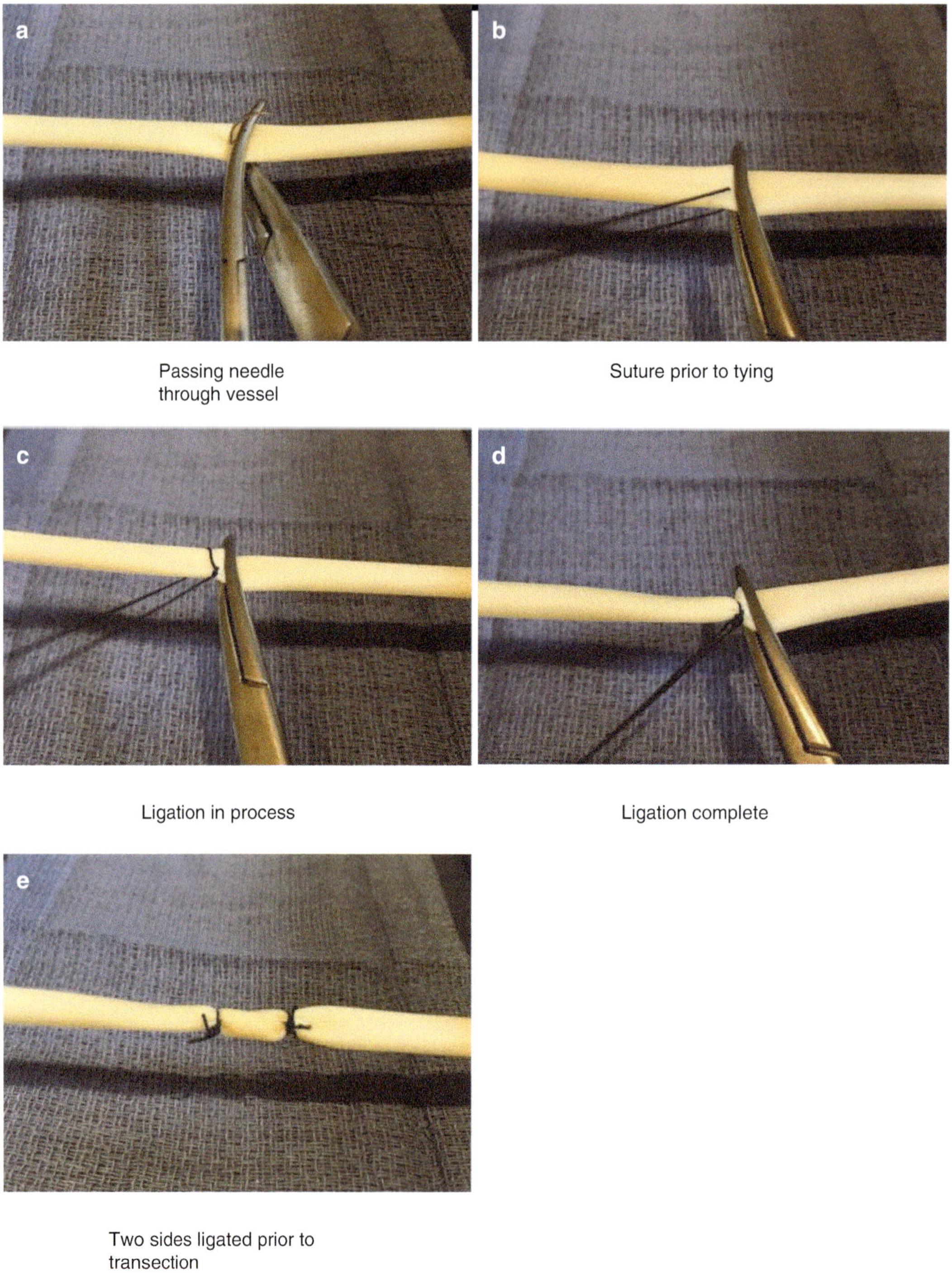

Fig. 8.4 Depicts technique to obtain vascular control with suture ligature (**a**–**e**). (**a**) Passing needle through vessel. (**b**) Suture prior to tying. (**c**) Suture passed around vessel after first throw. (**d**) Ligation complete. (**e**) Two sides ligated prior to transection

there is to work in, and to what extent the vessel will retract once divided. Tying, clamping, cutting, ligating, and suture ligating are the maneuvers necessary to perform these techniques; each has nuances.

When tying a suture down on a vessel in continuity, do not place the first throw too tightly because the suture can cut through the vessel; atherosclerotic vessels can crack and dissect. Use one-handed throws with the second throw in the same direction as the first and then cinch the suture down gently, but securely, and then place the squaring throw. *It is useful to first tie the side of the vessel that you are less worried about in order to feel how the vessel reacts to the suture. This tactile sense can guide safe management of the "business side."*

When clamping a vessel, close the clamp gently and slowly. Check the degree of pressure on the vessel with each increment of closure. The clamp needs only to occlude flow, usually only two or three steps up, more will cause injury.

When cutting a vessel, leave at least one to two millimeters outside of the tie or clamp. Close the scissors slowly. Only cut what you can see. A vessel that is to be anastomosed should be cut sharply with a blade.

When tying a vessel that has been clamped and divided, the index finger should be brought down on the suture in an orientation perpendicular to the shaft of the clamp and the suture tied at the tip of the clamp where there is space. Do not push the finger down parallel to the shaft or behind (under) the clamp where there is no space. Your hand must not push on the clamp or push down on the vessel. This will cause unwanted stretch and tension on the clamped tissue. When using a suture on a clamp as a passer, be certain that the suture is properly loaded at the tip of the jaws. Pass the suture around the shaft of the clamped vessel so that the knot will come down at the tip of the clamped vessel. Tie toward yourself and at the tip, not away from yourself or at the heel of the clamped vessel.

Named arteries, in general, should be doubly ligated on the source side with one tie being a suture ligature (stick tie). If there is any doubt, a stick tie will be the safest method to secure a vessel. Put the needle through the vessel near the center. Pass the suture around the heel and place a throw. Pass the heel of the needle around the tip of the clamp (deflect the tip with the shaft) and tie down under the tip side. The tie must come down below the site where the vessel was pierced by the needle. Do not pull up on the suture. With double ligation, the stick tie should be outside of the first tie or over it. An exception to suture ligation of arteries is when the artery will be anastomosed because the proximal vessel must not be damaged.

There is not always the luxury of having a well-exposed vessel with adequate space to clamp or to pass two ties. One example is division of the ascending lumbar vein off of the iliac vein during exposure for spine surgery. In this situation, the iliac side of the ascending lumbar vein can be stick tied in continuity. Put the needle through the vein, and then reverse the needle and pass the heel under the vessel and tie on top. The other side of the vein can be managed with a simple ligature or stick tie or clip. If there is no room, it can just be cut and pressure applied with a hemostatic agent such as gelfoam with thrombin.

A few tips for the management of specific vessels may be useful.

1. Mesenteric vessels

   Do not punch blindly through the mesentery with hemostats. Identify the vessels by dividing the peritoneum, and, with one hand behind the mesentery, pinch to feel the vessels and dissect the fat away with a clamp.

2. Hepatic veins

   Dissect initially until you are sure that you can get a vascular clamp on the caval side of the hepatic vein. If possible, during a liver resection, complete the division of the hepatic parenchyma before taking the hepatic vein(s). Place a vascular clamp such as a Satinsky or renal clamp on the hepatic vein with the tip of the clamp toward yourself. To create more room on the vein, place a blunt Mixter clamp around it, and gently strip the vein away from the cava toward the side coming out.

Cut the vein directly on the clamp that is coming out in order to leave as much vein outside of the clamp on the caval side as possible, at least 2 mm. The clamp on the specimen side can be oversewn and the suture tightened as the clamp is removed. If there is no adequate room, the specimen side of the vein can be ligated with an O suture. However, you then need to place a suture ligature over the silk to lock it; otherwise it will fall off.

The end of the divided vein on the caval side is oversewn with running suture (typically 4-0 or 5-0, single-armed prolene). The suture is placed on the vein outside of the clamp, away from the cava. Start at one end, place three throws after the first bite, and put a small clamp ("snap," "mosquito") on the end of the suture. Run the suture one direction, and then back, and then tie the suture with the vascular clamp still on the vein. When the clamp is removed, there may be bleeding, so be prepared to take additional bites. To do this, the needle of the running suture can be reloaded in the needle holder. Alternatively, a fresh needle with new suture can be loaded to provide more length. The snapped end of the suture can be used to pull up on the vessel so that it does not retract if additional suturing is necessary.

3. Portal vein

   During tumor resection, control the portal vein and its branches as well away from the tumor site as possible. Some prefer to pass loops around the vessel for proximal and distal control. When the portal vein is divided during hepatic resection, there may not be sufficient room to oversew the remaining end outside of the vascular clamp as described for the hepatic vein. In this circumstance, a running suture can be placed under the clamp by two methods. The jaws of the clamp can be sewn over and over with the suture and the clamp gently removed as the suture is tightened. Alternatively, the suture can be run back and forth under the clamp and tied prior to removing the clamp. With either method, it is advisable to have another needle with suture loaded and ready in case it is needed.

8.1.4 Technical Considerations to Stop Bleeding

There are useful principles for achieving hemostasis when bleeding occurs. These include management of injured vessels by suture techniques and methods for control of diffuse bleeding from raw surgical surfaces and maneuvers for emergent occlusion of major arterial inflow.

8.1.4.1 Pressure and Suture

When unexpected bleeding occurs, the first maneuver, always, is to apply direct pressure. This can be with a finger, a blunt instrument, a sponge, a laparotomy pad, or other tissue. Temporary proximal and distal tamponade of large veins, such as the inferior vena cava or portal vein, can be obtained with sponges on ring forceps ("stick sponge"). Bleeding often occurs when operating in a hole, so do not dig a deeper hole. Do not try to grasp for vessels that cannot be seen, or blindly place clamps or clips or sutures. Simply apply pressure, suction the blood to clear the field, and assess the magnitude of the situation. You will need exposure. If there is major bleeding, you will need help. Call for another surgeon early. Alert the anesthesia and nursing teams to ready the resources that may be required.

Assess whether the bleeding is from a vital or a non-vital vessel. A non-vital vessel can be readily dealt with; a vital vessel must be repaired without compromising flow.

When the end of a bleeding vessel is visible, compress it from the side with a forceps; do not try to grab the end. Put a right-angled clamp on the vessel and either tie or stick tie it, depending upon its size and on how well it is exposed. If you cannot see the true substance of the vessel, stick tie it. When bleeding is from the side of a vessel, a "figure of 8" stitch can be placed over it, or a suture can be placed on either side. Sometimes, two right-angled clamps can be placed, one from each side so the tips touch or overlap slightly, and the clamps can be oversewn. When the vessel is not well seen, your finger or a blunt forceps can focally tamponade the bleeding and you can suture under it. If there is a lateral injury to a vital vessel, such as the portal vein or superior mesenteric vein, carefully place a small vascular clamp so as not to occlude the vessel. If the defect is limited, a primary repair may suffice. If there is any risk for stenosis, a vein patch is used.

Blind suturing is to be avoided but, on occasion, may be unavoidable. Some circumstances where it may be required include bleeding from the cut surface of the liver or from a difficult retroperitoneum or pelvis, particularly during redo operations. It is more applicable for control of bleeding that is primarily venous.

When it must be resorted to, use large needles (an MH needle works for liver), and take mass suture bites. Avoid blind suturing near critical structures. A rare exception might be in a crashing, hypotensive patient if tamponade or inflow control cannot be achieved. In this desperate scenario, rapid suturing, including even what you do not want to suture, may prevent the immediate demise of the patient.

8.1.4.2 Diffuse Bleeding

There are several methods for managing diffusely bleeding surfaces. Application of local hemostatic materials and pressure is often effective. We have long had success with gelfoam soaked in thrombin as the topical hemostatic preparation. Gelfoam is derived from denatured animal skin gelatin and alone has no intrinsic hemostatic action. However, it serves as an efficient and absorbable carrier for thrombin. Laparotomy pads work better than sponges for pressure on top of the gelfoam/thrombin because the interstices of the lap pad are smaller. The argon beam coagulator is useful for superficial bleeding over a broad area.

Gauze packing can successfully tamponade bleeding from difficult surfaces, especially when the patient is coagulopathic. Examples include bleeding from liver injury and from the retroperitoneum in cases of necrotizing pancreatitis or retroperitoneal hematoma and pelvic bleeding from the presacral plexus. If available, large sheets of gelfoam can be placed first. Pack the bleeding site tightly with unfurled rolls of Kerlix gauze. The rolls are 13 ft long. Usually, two or three rolls are needed. The end of each roll is brought out separately through a lateral counter-incision or through a portion of the primary incision. When packing, you will need to keep track of the rolls in the sequence that they were placed so that the most superficial roll can later be removed first and the deepest roll last. A simple way to mark them is to tie one knot on the roll to come out first, two on the second, and so on.

The rolls are usually removed at the bedside beginning within about 24 h. They can be dampened with dilute hydrogen peroxide that is allowed to soak in. Then, slowly, start to pull out the first and most superficial roll. Stop if fresh blood and clots emanate. A burgundy color is good. Only one roll is removed at a time, but they should all be out by about the second postoperative day. When the last roll is out, a brief sigh of relief is permitted.

8.1.4.3 Inflow Control

There are ways to stem rapid abdominopelvic hemorrhage by temporarily occluding aortic inflow. Supraceliac control can be obtained in the abdomen at the level of the diaphragm. The aorta is located above the stomach to the right of the esophagus. Go through the gastrohepatic ligament and feel for the aorta deep between the diaphragmatic crura overlying the spine. Try to see it, if possible; the muscle of the diaphragm can be cut. Compress the aorta firmly with your hand or fist or with a stick sponge. Take a long vascular clamp and, with the jaws closed, put the tip on the spine. Move the clamp to your right (the left side of the patient) until just past the spine, and open the jaws to spread the tissue. Close, lift the clamp up slightly, open the jaws, put it back down, and clamp the vessel.

When the aorta cannot be clamped on the abdomen, keep it manually compressed while you or an assistant quickly opens the left chest. Do an anterior thoracotomy in the left 6th or 7th interspace. Lift the lung. The aorta is under the esophagus (which is to be avoided). Manually feel for the aorta which can be tactilely identified as a rubbery structure even when it is essentially non-pulsatile. Open the pleura, and finger dissect to get your thumb and finger around the vessel and clamp it.

On occasion, if there is no other good access, it may be possible to establish supradiaphragmatic occlusion of the aorta by a retrograde approach. Expose the infrarenal aorta and make a small transverse aortotomy. If you have the luxury, advance a 30 cm^3 aortic occlusion balloon. If desperate, take a large clamped Foley[1] catheter, push it up the vessel above the diaphragm, and inflate the balloon. There will still be some collateral bleeding, but this maneuver may afford enough time to continue.

Rapid control of inflow to the iliac artery may be necessary. A particular example is with trocar injury during an attempted laparoscopic operation. Make a midline incision and compress the aorta against the spine at the pelvic inlet.

Unrelenting pelvic hemorrhage during operations for trauma or resection or large malignancies can be slowed by ligation of both internal iliac arteries at their origin.

The Pringle[2] maneuver will temporarily control liver bleeding from hepatic arterial and portal venous sources [1]. Encircle the hepatoduodenal ligament by getting the index finger of your left hand into the foramen of Winslow behind the hepatoduodenal structures with your thumb on top. Divide adhesions if present, and open the lesser sac so that your thumb and fingertips touch.

The hepatoduodenal ligament can be occluded with a vascular clamp or a Rumel[3] tourniquet. Position an angled PV clamp through the finger opening from your right with the handle on the left side of the patient. Alternatively, pass an umbilical tape through the opening with either a clamp or two fingers. Wider tape is preferred so it does not cut through the tissue when tightened. Cut a length of red rubber catheter as a Rumel tourniquet. The diameter of the catheter should be large enough to allow the end of the catheter to fold around the tissue when tightened. While holding the tape in the left hand, advance the catheter down over the umbilical tape. This is done with a clamp in the right hand held perpendicular to the catheter. The thumb of the right hand pushes the clamp down against the end of the catheter to advance it over the tape. Do not pull up on the tape; there should not be movement of the tissue upward. When the catheter has cinched the tissue adequately, close the clamp on the tape at the top of the end of the catheter. Clamp the tape only; do not clamp on the catheter.

Take-Home Points

- Know the anatomy.
- Proximal and distal control.
- Respect the integrity of blood vessels when dissecting, clamping, and ligating.
- Control bleeding by direct pressure first.
- Control serious bleeding with composure, exposure, and assistance.

Legion of Honor

The author wishes to recognize the following master surgeons whose shared lifetime of operative experience contributed to the principles distilled in this chapter:

Alexander Doolas MD
Marshall D. Goldin MD
Martin Hertl MD, PhD
Keith W. Millikan MD

[1]Frederic Eugene Basil Foley (1891–1966), American urologist

[2]James Hogarth Pringle (1863–1941), Australian born Glasgow surgeon

[3]William Ray Rumel (1911–1977), American cardiothoracic surgeon

Reference

1. Pringle JH. Notes on the arrest of hepatic hemorrhage due to trauma. Ann Surg. 1908;48:541–9.

9 Fundamentals of Energy Utilization in the Operating Room

Amin Madani and Carmen L. Mueller

9.1 Introduction

Energy devices are ubiquitously used for almost all operations. These include traditional electrosurgical monopolar devices to more advanced bipolar sealing devices and ultrasonic dissectors. Despite their utility to achieve hemostasis, dissect tissue planes, and ablate lesions, the operator should bear in mind their potential to cause intraoperative injuries and should take the necessary steps to mitigate the risks of iatrogenic injury. Energy devices in minimally invasive surgery can be especially hazardous due to the fact that a significant portion of the instruments are located outside the field of view and can lead to unexpected energy diversion. Other injuries include operating room fires and interference with implantable devices, such as pacemakers and cardiac defibrillators.

Adverse events related to energy devices are a significant public safety issue. In the case of electrosurgery, injuries are estimated to occur at an incidence of approximately 40,000/year [1] or approximately 1–2 per 1000 operations during laparoscopy [2]. As many as one-fifth of the surgeons have reported personally experiencing a stray electrosurgical burn injury during laparoscopy, while half of the surgeons know of a colleague who has experienced a similar event [3]. In addition, hundreds of millions of dollars are spent annually for medical-legal claims related to inadvertent electrosurgical burn injuries [4, 5].

This chapter summarizes the most common energy devices, potential injuries that can occur from their utilization, and steps that can be taken to mitigate their risk.

9.2 Electrosurgery

Electrosurgery is the most common form of energy (i.e., "Bovie"), which is radiofrequency (RF) alternating current that is applied across tissues. The rapid oscillation of polarities across the cells and tissues causes a resultant elevation in intracellular temperatures from the frictional forces of rapidly moving ions. This leads to various effects on the tissues, including vaporization, desiccation, and protein coagulation. Contrary to its commonly used misnomer "cautery," electrosurgery does not actually apply passive transfer of heat to tissues and instead produces currents that have the potential to be diverted to other conductors and subsequently cause electrosurgical burn injuries.

All electrosurgery is bipolar by nature, meaning that two electrodes are attached to the patient to create a closed-loop circuit, without grounding the patient (also a common misconception) (Fig. 9.1). Nevertheless, the position and function

A. Madani · C. L. Mueller (✉)
Department of Surgery, McGill University, Montreal, QC, Canada
e-mail: carmen.mueller@mcgill.ca

F. Palazzo (ed.), *Fundamentals of General Surgery*, https://doi.org/10.1007/978-3-319-75656-1_9

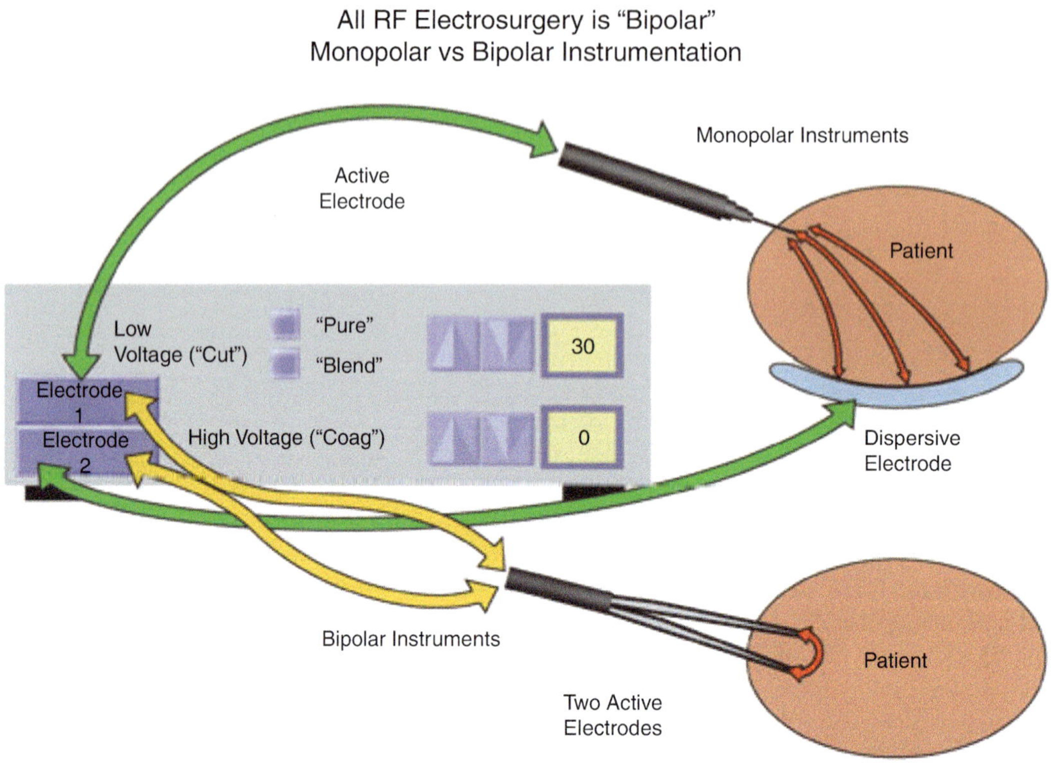

Fig. 9.1 Schematic of energy circuit differences between monopolar and bipolar electrosurgical devices

of the electrodes can vary, allowing the surgeon to use a monopolar or bipolar system. In a *monopolar* setup, the surgeon utilizes one electrode ("active electrode") in the surgical field as a handheld device, whereas the second electrode is attached to the patient outside the field of view as a large pad that disperses the current on a large surface area ("dispersive electrode"). These electrodes are then connected to the electrosurgical unit (ESU)—the large generator that delivers RF energy at defined levels of power, current, and/or voltage. In a *bipolar* setup on the other hand, both electrodes are active electrodes, which are included within the instrument itself without the need for a dispersive electrode—making it a very useful tool for achieving hemostasis of tissue that is grasped between both electrodes. In addition, many bipolar devices have advanced configurations, such as the ability to measure the tissue impedance between the jaws of the two active electrodes to ensure optimal hemostasis, as well as cutting blades to divide desiccated tissue. These tools are ideal when dissecting through highly vascularized tissues, such as omentum or mesentery.

In most settings, the ESU is set at a specific power (e.g., "30 coag," "30 cut"), delivering preset energy through the circuit per unit time, irrespective of whether "cut," "coag," or "blend" functions are used to activate the device. While the device is activated and energy is being delivered, these different buttons modulate the current in different ways, whereby the end result is that there is significantly greater voltage (and therefore thermal effect) with the "coag" mode compared to the "cut" mode (Fig. 9.2). A common misconception is that "cut" mode is used for "cutting" and that "coag" mode is used for tissues desiccation, whereas in fact "coag" is used most commonly for tissue dissection. In fact, both modalities vaporize tissues that come into contact with the active electrode tip. The difference however is the resultant collateral thermal spread, which is substantially more when the "coag"

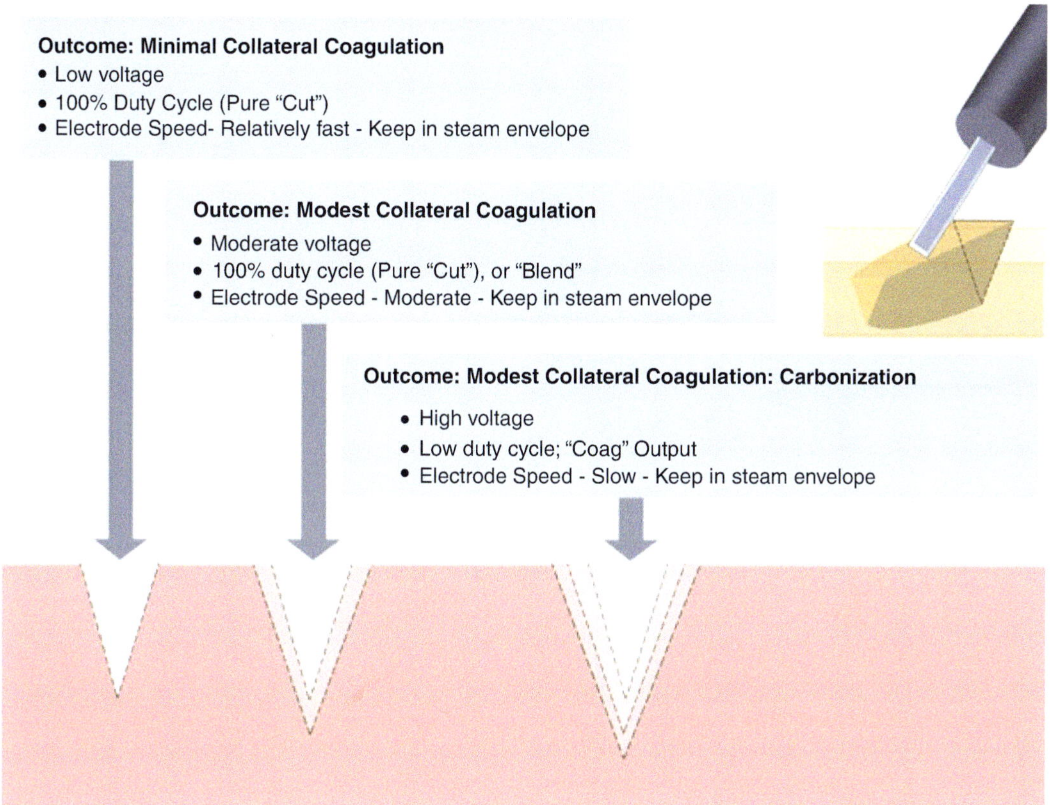

Fig. 9.2 Schematic of tissue injury created using different electrosurgical monopolar device settings

mode, or a higher power on the ESU (e.g., "coag 60" as opposed to "coag 30"), is used. Whereas in some cases the collateral thermal spread is beneficial in order to avoid small bleeding vessels, in other circumstances, it may be safer to use a lower power setting or the "cut" function when dissecting in the vicinity of a critical structure such as the common bile duct, phrenic nerve, or ureter. It is also advisable to avoid using high-energy settings on the skin, minimize desiccation of the skin edges, and optimize wound healing.

9.3 Adverse Events

Electrosurgical injuries can be categorized based on their mechanism: current diversion injuries, active electrode injuries, and dispersive electrode injuries [6].

Current diversion injuries are extremely dangerous during minimally invasive surgery, mostly due to their unfamiliarity by surgeons. Since the bulk of the instrument is located outside the field of view on a monitor, these instruments often come into contact with other structures without the knowledge of the operator (Fig. 9.3). It is not uncommon to assume that as long as the metal tip of a fully insulated instrument is clearly seen on a monitor without being activated near any critical structures, those inadvertent injuries will not occur. This assumption is wrong. Stray current can travel anywhere along the shaft of the instrument, regardless of whether the insulation is fully intact or not. In fact, most current diversion injuries are not initially recognized and lead to delayed patient manifestations, such as diffuse peritonitis and intra-abdominal sepsis in a postoperative patient with a bowel injury [7–9].

Insulation failure is a very common source of injury during minimally invasive surgery [3, 10, 11], such that insulated instruments may possess a break in insulation somewhere along their shaft

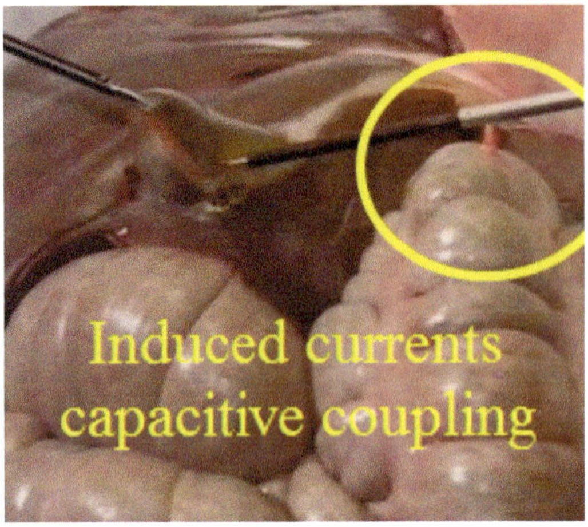

Fig. 9.3 Induced currents capacitive coupling

Table 9.1 Recommendations for decreasing the risk of electrosurgical injuries, as adopted from the Society of American Gastrointestinal and Endoscopic Surgeons' Fundamental Use of Surgical Energy™ curriculum (http://www.fuseprogram.org) [6]

• Use the lowest power setting necessary for the intended tissue effect
• Use the current with the lowest voltage possible for the intended tissue effect (i.e., "cut" as opposed to "coag")
• Use active electrode monitoring systems for inspecting insulation on electrosurgical instruments
• Avoid activation of electrosurgical devices in open air
• Use brief (2–3 s) intermittent activations
• Activate the instrument only when the active electrode is entirely in the field of view
• Use either all metal or all plastic cannulas
• Clear the electrode tip of built-up eschar (increases the risk of current arcing)
• Avoid bundling cords and various instruments together
• Place unused electrosurgical devices in an insulated holster

causing possible current diversion. It is important to recognize that defective insulation tends to be invisible to the naked eye or with careful inspection. Moreover, smaller insulation defects lead to smaller areas of contact with tissues and therefore greater concentration of current and resultant thermal effect. Current standards recommend routine screening for insulation failure using specialized active electrode monitoring systems [12].

Capacitive coupling and antenna coupling are phenomena whereby active electrodes, once activated, transmit and receive electromagnetic waves to other adjacent conductors (virtue of the fact that they conduct alternating current), without direct contact through nonconductive media (such as air or by touching fully insulated instruments). These can be anything from surrounding wires, the laparoscope, other instruments in the surgical field, and even electrocardiogram monitoring wires. The consequence is that the adjacent conductor, which was previously not electrically active, induces the electromagnetic wave into a current—a current that can now travel to other unexpected sites and cause potential injuries outside the field of view [13–15]. Various steps can be taken to decrease the risk of current diversion (Table 9.1). *It is imperative to emphasize the importance of avoiding open-air activation of electrosurgical devices, such that the active electrode is activated without actually making contact with the target tissue.* Should the situation occur where current is diverted, by activating the device in such a manner, all current will be diverted in this alternative pathway as opposed to its intended circuit. *For example, activating the hook in midfield during laparoscopic cholecystectomy may divert the current to the nearby duodenum or common bile duct, rather than to the tissue intended to be dissected.* In contrast, if contact is made with the target tissue, the current will prefer the intended trajectory as it is the path of least resistance, and the current and resultant thermal effect through the alternative pathway is minimized and often negligible. Furthermore, it is advised to avoid bundling wires to other conductors such as the laparoscope camera cord or towel clamps and to use the lowest energy (lowest power and voltage) necessary to obtain the intended tissue effects [6].

Finally, current diversion can occur through direct coupling, a mechanism through which one conductor makes direct contact (or arcs current) with another conductor. In some instances, this is done intentionally, such as when a bleeding vessel is grasped between the jaws of forceps and the active electrode is activated while making contact with the forceps, causing vessel sealing. Nonetheless, this can also occur inadvertently if the instrument is activated while making contact with another conductor (such as the laparoscope or another non-insulated metal instrument) that is in contact with non-target tissues.

Other forms of injuries occur in relation to the active electrode, such as with collateral thermal spread with higher-voltage settings (e.g., "coag" mode instead of "cut" mode or "coag 40" instead of "coag 25") or direct injury from residual heat at the tip of the instruments, even after a period of activation. This form of injury is much more common in laparoscopy and especially more concerning with the use of advanced bipolar and ultrasonic devices, whose tips can reach temperatures well above the threshold necessary to cause cell death. Furthermore, injuries can occur in relation to the dispersive electrode, whose function is to act as the return electrode to the ESU. Given that it transmits the same current as that which travels through the active electrode, it is important that the pad sticks very well over a large surface area to keep the current density at a minimum and avoid burn injuries at that site.

9.4 Ultrasonic Energy Devices

Ultrasonic devices convert electrical energy to mechanical energy allowing the instrument tip to vibrate at extremely high frequencies. As the energy is applied to the tissues between the jaws of the instrument, this leads to a frictional force that causes vaporization, desiccation, and protein coagulation. There are various factors that determine the type of tissues effect. The most important is the frequency of blade excursion, with a higher frequency (often denoted as "MAX") leading to more efficient cutting but less hemostasis and lower frequency ("MIN") causing more hemostasis but less efficient cutting. Other factors include the degree of compression of the tissues between the jaws, with greater compression improving cutting but decreasing hemostasis, as well as the tension on the tissues (such as from lifting to provide more efficient cutting).

One of the reasons why ultrasonic devices have proven very versatile is the fact that the lower blade (oscillating blade) can also be used in a manner similar to a scalpel for tissues that are under sufficient tension. Their advantage over electrosurgery also includes the lack of current passing through the patient, eliminating the risk of electrosurgical burns and electromagnetic interference with other devices, such as pacemakers. Nonetheless, ultrasonic devices are notorious for causing very high temperatures at the tip of the instrument. This can be problematic during minimally invasive surgery where there is a lack of tactile feedback. The operator should be cognizant of this and avoid using the tip of the instrument as a grasper (such as to move bowel in the peritoneal cavity) as this can lead to delayed injuries with dire consequences.

9.5 Argon Beam Plasma Coagulator (APC)

The APC is a form of monopolar energy device that uses the current to ionize argon gas and to arc current from the active electrode tip to the target tissues without making actual contact with the tissues. This requires high-voltage energy and leads to superficial desiccation of tissue with minimal penetration by "spraying" current on the target—a process called fulguration. Fulguration can also be achieved with traditional monopolar electrosurgery using high-voltage settings and is particularly useful for bleeding raw surfaces, such as on the liver and spleen. APC can also be used during endoscopic procedures for controlling superficial mucosal lesions [16]. Risks include excessive buildup of argon gas in the peritoneal cavity, gas embolism, and abdominal compartment syndrome. The lowest effective flow rate should be maintained, and if this form of energy is used during laparoscopic surgery, *it is advisable to consistently maintain one port open.*

9.6 Energy-Related Emergencies

9.6.1 Operating Room Fires and Explosions

Hundreds of operating room fires occur every year in the USA alone, and while these are relatively rare and mostly minor, approximately 5% are associated with disfiguring injuries or death [17]. The surgical team should be properly trained in fire prevention strategies and be familiar with institutional protocols to deal with such unexpected events (Table 9.2).

Three factors are required for a fire to occur. First, there needs to be a source of heat or ignition (spark). In the operating room, the most common source is electrosurgery. Other sources include laser, the fiber-optic light cable, or the light source during laparoscopy. During laparoscopic procedures, the surgical team should be careful not to place the light source in contact with the drapes, as even a few seconds is sufficient time for it to set fire to the drapes. Instead, the light source should be placed on "standby" before the start of the case and subsequently turned off before disconnecting it from the laparoscope at the end of the case. The second element for a fire is the need for a fuel source, examples of which include the drapes or alcohol-based prepping agents. It is important not to apply the surgical drapes until flammable liquids have fully dried and any pooling of prep fluid is removed. Lastly, there needs to be an oxidizer (e.g., oxygen or nitrous oxide). Approximately 50% of fires tend to occur in "oxygen-enriched zones" near the head, neck, and upper chest [17]. The team can minimize the risk of fires by keeping oxygen concentrations below 30% whenever possible and limiting the use of open-source oxygen (such as nasal prongs and oxygen masks, as opposed to supraglottic airways or endotracheal intubation), which can lead to oxygen tenting under the drapes. Lastly, gastrointestinal surgeons and endoscopists should be aware that bowel content contains various explosive compounds, such as hydrogen-air mixtures and methane. Mannitol can lead to the production of methane gas and is therefore contraindicated as a bowel preparation [18, 19].

Table 9.2 Strategies for decreasing the risk of operating room fires, as adopted from the Society of American Gastrointestinal and Endoscopic Surgeons' Fundamental Use of Surgical Energy™ curriculum (http://www.fuseprogram.org) [6]

• Minimize the use of open oxygen (e.g., face masks, nasal cannula)
• Minimize oxygen concentration and beware of oxygen enrichment under the drapes
• Do not apply drapes until flammable prepping fluid has fully dried
• Remove spilled and pooled prepping agents
• Connect the fiber-optic light cable before activating the light source
• Turn off the light source before disconnecting the light cable
• Seal the surgical site tightly from oxygen source tenting under the drapes
• Use the lowest possible power and voltage for the intended tissue effect using energy devices

9.6.2 Managing Operating Room Fires

Responding to a fire in the operating room requires a coordinated effort by all members of the operating team, including surgeons, anesthesiologists, and nurses [20]. First, flow of oxygen should be immediately stopped, followed by disconnection of the breathing circuit. While this is occurring at the head of the bed, another team member should immediately remove all burning material off the patient (including the endotracheal tube in the case of an airway fire). Subsequently, the fire should be extinguished using either the fire extinguisher or saline from the nurse's table. Finally, as a team member activates the fire alarm and notifies the appropriate authorities, the patient should have their breathing restored (may require re-intubation) using room air and their injuries managed.

9.7 Special Considerations

9.7.1 The Use of Energy in Patients with Implantable Devices

Energy devices can also cause electromagnetic interference (EMI) with implantable electronic devices in patients, most commonly with cardiac implantable electronic devices (CIED), such as pacemakers, ventricular assist devices, and defibrillators. While interference can also occur with other devices, including various nerve and spinal cord stimulators, infusion pumps, cochlea implants, and many others, CIEDs are particularly problematic due to the millions of patients who are currently treated with a CIED and the potential cardiovascular effects that can result from interference. Potential effects of EMI include inappropriate triggering, reprogramming or inhibition of the pacemaker or defibrillator, unintended asynchronous pacing, and generation of electrical current in the wires, causing arrhythmias or thermal tissue injury [21].

The most common source of EMI is from RF electrosurgery—specifically monopolar devices, including those used in open surgery, minimally invasive surgery, endoscopic procedures, radiofrequency ablation procedures, and electrocardiographic monitors. *Of note, ultrasonic devices generate mechanical energy as opposed to electromagnetic energy and are therefore safer in patients with CIEDs. Also, bipolar instruments cause significantly less interference and are also recommended over monopolar devices.*

Because the mechanism of action of EMI with CIEDs is similar to that which occurs with current diversion injuries (i.e., antenna coupling and capacitive coupling), similar recommendations are advised for surgeons wishing to minimize the risk of interference. These include using the lowest-energy settings necessary to get the intended tissue effects (e.g., using lower power settings and low-voltage current such as "cut" whenever possible) and ensuring that the active electrode cord does not cross the chest wall in the vicinity of the implanted device. Furthermore, during setup of the patient, the team should make sure that the intended current vector through the patient (path from the active electrode to the dispersive electrode) does not cross the CIED system to cause interference. *This can be achieved by keeping the dispersive electrode as close as possible to the surgical site where the active electrode is activated and as far away as possible from the CIED* [22]. In fact, animal studies suggest that increasing the distance between the active electrode (energy source) and CIED decreases EMI in a dose-response fashion up to 10 cm [22]. Also, whenever possible, monopolar laparoscopic instruments ought to be substituted in favor of either an ultrasonic dissector or advanced bipolar instrument—especially if the dissection is above the umbilicus and the patient is pacemaker dependent.

In most instances, the patient will present preoperatively, in which case surgeons should ensure that the appropriate consultation with an anesthesiologist and/or cardiologist takes place. Often, the pacemaker needs to be reprogrammed to an asynchronous mode to avoid unintended inhibition of its function when EMI is mistaken as cardiac activity, among patients who are pacing dependent and when the surgical site is in the vicinity of the mediastinum. However, reprogramming should usually be avoided in patients who are prone to ventricular tachyarrhythmia. Also, rate-adaptive functions and anti-tachyarrhythmia functions in patients with defibrillators may need to be suspended to avoid being triggered in the presence of EMI. In such cases, the entire surgical team should be aware of these alterations on the day of the operation, with temporary pacing equipment and defibrillators immediately available, in the event that the patient requires resuscitation.

Rarely, it may be neither feasible nor practical to obtain preoperative consultation for patients with CIEDs who require emergency surgery. In addition to the aforementioned precautions, a magnet can also be placed overtop the CIED on the patient's chest to shield it against any EMI. For pacemakers, this may result in asynchronous pacing, whereas for defibrillators, it can often temporarily disable the anti-tachyarrhythmia functions. *While removal of the magnet normally restores the CIED back to its original function, this may not always be the case, and permanent damage may ensue. A cardiology consultation should be sought postoperatively.*

Conclusion

Surgical energy devices are extremely useful for a broad range of applications in the operating room. To date, various forms of energy exist in a number of different configurations. Yet, despite their proven usefulness, they remain a source of iatrogenic injury. It is imperative that operators acquaint themselves with the appropriate utilization of each device, the many pitfalls that can occur, and steps to take to use such devices safely and effectively.

Take-Home Points

- Electrosurgical energy devices vary in the type of energy used and the manner in which that energy is delivered to the tissues to create a desired effect.
- Knowledge of the differences between electrosurgical devices allows the operator to select the best tool for the desired application.
- Each type of device can cause undesirable effects (adverse events) and the operator must familiarize themselves with the possible adverse outcomes associated with each device to be used.

Suggested Readings

Feldman LS, Fuchshuber P, Jones DB. The SAGES manual on the fundamental use of surgical energy (FUSE). New York: Springer; 2012.

References

1. Lee J. Update on electrosurgery. Outpatient Surg. 2002;2:44–53.
2. Nduka CC, Super PA, Monson JR, Darzi AW. Cause and prevention of electrosurgical injuries in laparoscopy. J Am Coll Surg. 1994;179:161–70.
3. Tucker RD. Laparoscopic electrosurgical injuries: survey results and their implications. Surg Laparosc Endosc. 1995;5:311–7.
4. Perantinides PG, Tsarouhas AP, Katzman VS. The medicolegal risks of thermal injury during laparoscopic monopolar electrosurgery. J Healthc Risk Manag. 1998;18:47–55.
5. Chandler JG, Voyles CR, Floore TL, Bartholomew LA. Litigious consequences of open and laparoscopic biliary surgical mishaps. J Gastrointest Surg. 1997;1:138–45. discussion 145
6. Feldman L, Fuchshuber P, Jones DB, editors. The SAGES manual on the fundamental use of surgical energy (FUSE). New York: Springer; 2012.
7. Sankaranarayanan G, Resapu RR, Jones DB, Schwaitzberg S, De S. Common uses and cited complications of energy in surgery. Surg Endosc. 2013;27:3056–72.
8. Agarwal BB, Gupta M, Agarwal S, Mahajan K. Anatomical footprint for safe laparoscopic cholecystectomy without using any energy source: a modified technique. Surg Endosc. 2007;21:2154–8.
9. Polychronidis A, Tsaroucha AK, Karayiannakis AJ, Perente S, Efstathiou E, Simopoulos C. Delayed perforation of the large bowel due to thermal injury during laparoscopic cholecystectomy. J Int Med Res. 2005;33:360–3.
10. Montero PN, Robinson TN, Weaver JS, Stiegmann GV. Insulation failure in laparoscopic instruments. Surg Endosc. 2010;24:462–5.
11. Tixier F, Garcon M, Rochefort F, Corvaisier S. Insulation failure in electrosurgery instrumentation: a prospective evaluation. Surg Endosc. 2016;30:4995–5001.
12. Vancaillie TG. Active electrode monitoring. How to prevent unintentional thermal injury associated with monopolar electrosurgery at laparoscopy. Surg Endosc. 1998;12:1009–12.
13. Jones EL, Robinson TN, McHenry JR, Dunn CL, Montero PN, Govekar HR, Stiegmann GV. Radiofrequency energy antenna coupling to common laparoscopic instruments: practical implications. Surg Endosc. 2012;26:3053–7.
14. Robinson TN, Barnes KS, Govekar HR, Stiegmann GV, Dunn CL, McGreevy FT. Antenna coupling--a novel mechanism of radiofrequency electrosurgery complication: practical implications. Ann Surg. 2012;256:213–8.
15. Townsend NT, Jones EL, Paniccia A, Vandervelde J, McHenry JR, Robinson TN. Antenna coupling explains unintended thermal injury caused by common operating room monitoring devices. Surg Laparosc Endosc Percutan Tech. 2015;25:111–3.
16. Postgate A, Saunders B, Tjandra J, Vargo J. Argon plasma coagulation in chronic radiation proctitis. Endoscopy. 2007;39:361–5.
17. ECRI Institute. Health devices: top 10 health technology hazards for 2011. 2010.
18. Avgerinos A, Kalantzis N, Rekoumis G, Pallikaris G, Arapakis G, Kanaghinis T. Bowel preparation and the risk of explosion during colonoscopic polypectomy. Gut. 1984;25:361–4.
19. Keighley MR, Taylor EW, Hares MM, Arabi Y, Youngs D, Bentley S, Burdon DW. Influence of oral mannitol bowel preparation on colonic microflora and the risk of explosion during endoscopic diathermy. Br J Surg. 1981;68:554–6.
20. Brunt LM. Fundamentals of electrosurgery part II: thermal injury mechanisms and prevention. In: Feldman LS, Fuchshuber P, Jones DB, editors. The SAGES manual on the fundamental use of surgical energy (FUSE). New York: Springer; 2012. p. 61–79.
21. Jones S, Rozner M. Integration of energy systems with other medical devices. In: Feldman LS, Fuchshuber P, Jones DB, editors. The SAGES manual on the fundamental use of surgical energy (FUSE). New York: Springer; 2012. p. 181–94.
22. Robinson TN, Varosy PD, Guillaume G, Dunning JE, Townsend NT, Jones EL, Paniccia A, Stiegmann GV, Weyer C, Rozner MA. Effect of radiofrequency energy emitted from monopolar "Bovie" instruments on cardiac implantable electronic devices. J Am Coll Surg. 2014;219:399–406.

10 Fundamentals of Stapling Devices

Christina Souther and Kenric Murayama

10.1 History of Stapling

The design of the first surgical stapler with resemblance to our current devices is credited to Humer Hultl in 1908 [1–4]. Prior to Hultl's stapler, which applied four parallel lines of wire hooks [3, 4], Henroz had anastomosed dog bowel with metal rings in 1826, and John Murphy created the Murphy button in 1892 which again used rings to join structures [2]. Hultl's device, however, was similar to the staplers we use today. Hultl's reason for pursuing the development of a mechanical device for anastomosis was to control spillage of bowel contents in an effort to decrease infection; he intended to create a device that would make operations cleaner, faster, and easier to perform [2]. To produce the first surgical stapler, Hultl enlisted the assistance of Peter Fischer who created the product which Hultl had envisioned. His first device, although innovative, was noted to be heavy and difficult to use by its operators [2]. The stapler was also difficult to clean between uses. Major improvements were made in the 1920s by Aladar Petz, who used silver clips rather than thin steel wires [3, 4]. His "Petz clamp" was notably easier to maneuver especially during the application and removal of the device and was lighter than Hultl's version [2–4]. This stapler also fired parallel staple lines similar to Hultl's product.

In the 1930s, replaceable cartridges were developed by H. Friedrich so that multiple loads of staples could be fired in succession without preparing an entirely separate device [1]. The simultaneous application of staples and division of the stapled viscera was pioneered in the Soviet Union during the 1950s through the 1970s [2]. The Russian staplers also featured a staggered rather than a parallel staple line configuration which was found to increase hemostasis. Mark Ravitch is credited with bringing staplers to widespread use in the United States and also optimizing the devices by allowing customization based on tissue type and size [2]. He created multiple different cartridges which could be loaded onto the same stapler base allowing for immediate customization for variable tissues during a surgery. These cartridges differed both in staple size and length of staple line creating the ability to tailor the stapler to each specific tissue type and length of tissue involved. He also developed the circular stapler allowing for end-to-end stapled anastomosis creation [1, 5]. Leon Hirsch, who formed the United States Surgical Corporation in the 1960s, contributed to the streamlining of surgical stapler function by optimizing the structure of the stapler and creating disposable cartridges for easy and efficient loading of the staples [6].

C. Souther · K. Murayama (✉)
Department of Surgery, John A Burns School of Medicine, University of Hawaii at Manoa, Honolulu, HI, USA
e-mail: kenricm@hawaii.edu

F. Palazzo (ed.), *Fundamentals of General Surgery*, https://doi.org/10.1007/978-3-319-75656-1_10

10.2 Mechanics of Stapling

The majority of surgical staplers in use today form staples in a "B" shape when fired against the anvil [7]. The "B" shape of the staple was designed to hold tissue securely but to allow small vessels to pass through the staples allowing for adequate perfusion [8]. The stapling device first compresses the tissue to be stapled causing elongation of the tissue. Allowing time for full compression and elongation of the tissue is important for adequate staple line formation but compression for an extended period of time can lead to tissue damage [1, 7, 9]. These considerations are important especially when using the staplers that complete their compression when they are first closed. Other models do not fully compress the tissue until they are fired so the compression time cannot be altered as easily. Longer duration of compression prior to firing the stapler has been associated with fewer anastomotic leaks and more adequate hemostasis of the staple line [7]. However, adequate compression does not only depend on duration; it is also affected by patient characteristics such as overall systemic health, including nutritional status and vascular supply. The tissue makeup is also important for adequate stapling. The ratio of liquid to solid components of the tissue and the elasticity of the tissue play important roles as well [7]. Tissue with higher liquid content requires longer compression time to reduce the fluid at the site of stapling and allow the tissue to elongate evenly. The longer compression time also allows the staple to form a tighter "B" shape which has been associated with decreased bleeding at the staple line [10, 11]. Short tight staples are also thought to decrease the chance of forming a stricture at the site [7]; however prolonged compression may increase the risk of local ischemia. *In choosing a staple cartridge for a particular operation, the thickness of the tissue must be considered* (Table 10.1). Creating a staple that is too tall can lead to gaps between the staple and tissue ultimately resulting in anastomotic leaks or bleeding at the staple line [7, 10, 11]. However, a staple which is too short can lead to anastomotic leaks as well, due to excessive compression of the tissue leading to ischemia and subsequent breakdown of the anastomosis [7]. Another key feature of creating a robust stapled anastomosis is the lack of force placed on the staple line during creation [7, 8]. Sheer forces and torque can lead to tearing of tissue or misalignment of the staples leading to both immediate injury requiring immediate revision and also subtle damage that is not recognized until the postoperative period during which complications arise. Easy firing of the stapler is important to avoid placing additional force or tension on the staple line during its creation.

In open cases, to avoid applying additional force to the tissues, the anvil can be inserted first followed by the cartridge instead of attempting to align both ends simultaneously. Holding the stapler steady with one hand or having an assistant stabilize the tissues that will be approximated can help to avoid tearing. The other hand should be used to fire the stapler slowly and smoothly, avoiding jarring movements especially when reaching the end of the staple line. To open the stapler, the trigger must be pulled back, and the tissue must remain stabilized during this step so

Table 10.1 Staple height and tissue applications for common laparoscopic staplers

Tissue	Covidien		Covidien tri-staple	Ethicon		Stomach	Small bowel	Large bowel	Rectum
Thin-mesentery	Gray	2 mm	Gray	White	2.6 mm				
Thin-vascular	White	2.6 mm	Gold				X		
Medium	Blue	3.5 mm	Gold/Purple	Blue	3.6 mm	X	X	X	X
Medium-thick	Gold	3.8 mm	Purple	Gold	3.8 mm	X		X	X
Thick	Green	4.8 mm		Green	4.1 mm	X			X
Extra-thick			Black	Black	4.2 mm	X			

that inordinate force is not placed on the newly created staple line.

In laparoscopic cases, the staplers can be manipulated in multiple directions by articulation. Articulating the stapler prior to placing it in contact with tissues is ideal to avoid grasping the tissue with the stapler as it is adjusted. The laparoscopic staplers have a narrow end which acts as the anvil; this narrow end should be inserted through any window in the tissue (e.g., between an appendix and mesoappendix), and the larger side should be applied externally to avoid forcing the larger side of the stapler through a small opening.

10.3 Current Devices

Surgical staplers used today are largely disposable and have become much easier to operate. Most of the devices have both an open and a laparoscopic counterpart. Linear staplers are available with multiple types of handles and cartridge configurations, allowing for tension-free application in various settings. The linear staplers include both models which apply staple lines and divide the tissue between the staple lines during the firing (GIA staplers) and also models which apply a staple line without any severing of tissue (TA staplers) [8]. These staplers require the operator to divide the tissue sharply after firing the stapler. Both of these linear staplers are available in endomechanical versions as well for use in laparoscopy and thoracoscopy. A modification of the linear stapler is a curved staple load fired in the same way with a blade between the staple lines, allowing for control and division of tissues in difficult to reach areas, such as the rectum. The curve allows the stapler to be applied to a structure deep in the pelvis or in another narrow area without placing torque on the stapler and thus decreasing the risk for shear of the tissues [7].

Circular staplers have been developed mainly for the creation of end-to-end anastomoses. The circular staplers allow firing of staple lines circumferentially and also excise a ring of tissue allowing connection of the two lumens. Circular staplers are generally used near an end of the GI tract as the stapler itself must be inserted through the tubular viscera and aligned with a prepositioned anvil in the other end of the planned anastomosis but can also be inserted via an enterotomy. The introduction of circular staplers allowed for stapled anastomoses in areas where tissues are difficult to mobilize, making distal rectal stapled anastomoses possible and much more facile [7].

10.4 Applications of Surgical Staplers

The widespread use of surgical staplers over the last half century has led to adaptation of the technology for use in multiple organ systems and various modes of operation. The original staplers were created for use in gastrointestinal surgery, and much of the data regarding technical aspects of staple size choice and outcomes have been derived from the field of bariatric surgery [7, 10, 11]. Staplers are used frequently in bariatric surgery: linear staplers for division of the stomach in sleeve gastrectomy and jejunojejunal anastomoses in gastric bypass and circular staplers for gastrojejunal anastomoses in gastric bypass. Shorter staple heights are associated with lower postoperative bleeding rates when circular staplers are used for the gastrojejunal anastomosis [10, 11]. Special attention must be paid to the size of the staples used on the stomach due to the varying thickness of the stomach in different anatomic regions in contrast to the colon which tends to be more uniform in thickness. Longer staples are generally used in the distal stomach as the distal stomach tends to be thicker [7]. Long staple lines, although sometimes necessary, can cause additional complications, especially leaks [12, 13]. In addition, a higher number of intersections of staple lines are associated with a higher risk of leak [13]. This situation typically occurs when creating a stapled anastomosis between two segments of bowel which already have stapled ends. This increased risk can be mitigated by inverting one staple line into another [13].

Throughout the gastrointestinal tract, linear staplers can be used to divide the small bowel or colon without spillage of contents, and curved staplers with long handles can be used to reach deep into the pelvis to divide the distal sigmoid colon or rectum without placing tension on the colon or torque on the device. Circular staplers are used frequently for distal sigmoid or rectal anastomoses. Ideally a single staple load is used to divide bowel as the use of multiple linear staplers for the same anastomosis can result in higher rate of anastomotic leak [7], making the curved stapler that can traverse the rectum in one application safer.

Esophagectomies and the subsequent anastomoses can be performed using both linear and circular staplers. Emergent situations such as bleeding esophageal varices can be managed with stapling devices as well by obtaining hemostasis using staplers to divide the esophagus and control the bleeding, followed by reanastomosis using additional staplers after the enlarged veins have been controlled [14].

Division of the pancreas can be simplified with the use of a stapler, and this method is commonly used for sealing the remaining portion of the pancreas after distal pancreatectomy [15]. Appropriate choice of staple height [15] and adequate compression duration [7, 16] are important for the prevention of pancreatic fistula in these cases. The thickness of the pancreas has been found to independently predict formation of a pancreatic fistula after stapled distal pancreatectomy making the decision to use the stapler and the choice of cartridge significant [17].

Linear staplers can be used in open and laparoscopic hepatic resections both for the division of the liver parenchyma itself and also for vascular control for the segment undergoing removal [18, 19]. As in other organ systems, the thickness of the liver can affect the success of staple line. In vitro studies have suggested that the liver measuring more than 10 mm in thickness can have other important factors influencing risk of staple line failure including stiffness which does not seem to play a role in the liver which is not as thick [18]. Staplers have also been used to divide enlarged cystic ducts in biliary operations during which a clip cannot fit entirely across the duct [20].

Pulmonary surgery has benefited from the use of staplers in lung resections [5, 7]. However, the air distribution in the lungs can make the thickness of the tissue more variable than in other organs. Since additional air is located in the periphery of the lung, the compression time and pressure required during application of the stapler are lower than those required in more central portions of the lung which contain bronchial tissue and more blood to displace prior to firing the stapler [7]. Baseline pulmonary health must be considered when stapling lung parenchyma as the thickness can be affected by malignancies, fibrosis, and chemical damage, while bronchopleural fistulae are more likely in emphysematous lung parenchyma [7]. Overall, the stapling of lungs leads to better aerostasis than hand-sewn pulmonary resections [7]. Methods including folding over the edges of bronchi prior to anastomosis to decrease tension placed at the center of the staple line have been employed to improve the success rate of pulmonary stapling [21].

10.5 Current Controversies

Given that leaks or bleeding are dreaded complications of endomechanical devices, the staple lines can be reinforced by the use of several "buttressing" materials which can be absorbable or permanent. Many surgeons advocate for their use, but the need for reinforcement, as well as the method providing the most benefit, is widely debated. Some authors report no benefit in reinforcing staple lines [22]. In several studies, decreased leak rates and lower rates of bleeding have been seen after oversewing the staple line [23–26]. Some advocate using bovine tissue buttresses rather than simply suture reinforcements to the staple line [23–25]. There is some concern for stenosis which can occur when additional sutures are placed, so care should be taken when reinforcing staple lines to avoid decreasing the patency of the anastomosis [26].

10.6 Summary

The first surgical stapler designed by Hultl initially designed to control spillage of bowel contents and improve asepsis paved the way for the modern devices which make many operations easier to accomplish and increase their efficiency. Many organs can be divided and anastomosed using stapling devices, and a variety of modifications have been made to suit tissues of different character and size. Surgeons must pay close attention to mechanical aspects of staple application, including each patient's baseline health, comorbidities, and tissue composition, to fully obtain the benefits of these devices and avoid complications by using the tailored stapling products available for each clinical situation.

Take-Home Messages

- Tissue depth and composition must be taken into consideration when choosing staple size.
- It is important to avoid torque on the tissues when firing staplers.
- Surgeons should become familiar with stapling devices and their possible complications despite the relative ease of operating they provide.

References

1. Baker RS, Foote J, Kemmeter P, Brady R, Vroegop T, Serveld M. The science of stapling and leaks. Obes Surg. 2004;14:1290–8.
2. Klimczak A, Miroslawska-Kempinska B, Mik M, Dziki A. Evolution of the mechanical suture. Pol Przegl Chir. 2013;85:44–6.
3. Olah A. Aladar Petz, the inventor of the modern surgical staplers. Surgery. 2008;143:146–7.
4. Robiscek F, Konstantinov I. Humer Hultl: the father of the surgical stapler. J Med Biogr. 2001;9:16–9.
5. Steichen FM, Ravitch MM. Mechanical sutures in surgery. Br J Surg. 1973;60:191–7.
6. Kleinfield NR. U.S. Surgical's checkered history. New York Times. May 13, 1984.
7. Chekan E, Whelan RL. Surgical stapling device-tissue interactions: what surgeons need to know to improve patient outcomes. Med Devices. 2014;7:305–18.
8. Ravitch MM, Steichen FM. Technics of staple suturing in the gastrointestinal tract. Ann Surg. 1972;175:815–35.
9. Nakayama S, Hasegawa S, Hida K, Kawada K, Sakai Y. Obtaining secure stapling of a double stapling anastomosis. J Surg Res. 2015;193:652–7.
10. Nguyen NT, Dakin G, Needleman B, Pomp A, Mikami D, Provost DA, Scott DJ, Jones DB, Gallagher S, Gagner M, Murr M. Effect of staple height on gastrojejunostomy during laparoscopic gastric bypass: a multicenter prospective randomized trial. Surg Obes Relat Dis. 2010;6:477–84.
11. Sakran N, Assalia A, Sternberg A, Kluger Y, Troitsa A, Brauner E, Van Cauwenberge S, De Visschere M, Dillemans B. Smaller staple height for circular stapled gastrojejunostomy in laparoscopic gastric bypass: early results in 1,074 morbidly obese patients. Obes Surg. 2010;21:238–43.
12. Ito M, Sugito M, Kobayashi A, Nishizawa Y, Tsunoda Y, Saito N. Relationship between multiple numbers of stapler firings during rectal division and anastomotic leakage after laparoscopic rectal resection. Int J Color Dis. 2008;23:703–7.
13. Lee S, Ahn B, Lee S. The relationship between the number of intersections of staple lines and anastomotic leakage after the use of a double stapling technique in laparoscopic colorectal surgery. Surg Laparosc Endosc Percutan Tech. 2017;27:273–81.
14. Steichen FM, Ravitch MM. Mechanical sutures in esophageal surgery. Ann Surg. 1980;191:373–81.
15. Kim H, Jang J, Son D, Lee S, Han Y, Shin YC, Kim JR, Kwon W, Kim S. Optimal stapler cartridge selection according to the thickness of the pancreas in distal pancreatectomy. Medicine. 2016;95(35):e4441.
16. Nakamura M, Ueda J, Kohno H, Aly MYF, Takahata S, Shimizu S, Tanaka M. Prolonged peri-firing compression with a linear stapler prevents pancreatic fistula in laparoscopic distal pancreatectomy. Surg Endosc. 2011;25:867–71.
17. Okano K, Oshima M, Kakinoki K, Yamamoto N, Akamoto S, Yachida S, Hagiike M, Kamada H, Masaki T, Suzuki Y. Pancreatic thickness as a predictive factor for postoperative pancreatic fistula after distal pancreatectomy using an endopath stapler. Surg Today. 2013;43:141–7.
18. Tsukane M, Kobayashi Y, Otsuka Y, Maeda T, Yamazaki N, Watanabe H, Ando T, Kaneko H, Fujie MG. Effect of the thickness and nonlinear elasticity of tissue on the success of surgical stapling for laparoscopic liver resection. Conf Proc IEEE Eng Med Biol Soc. 2014;2014:353–6.
19. Yao D, Wu S. Application of stapling devices in liver surgery: current status and future prospects. World J Gastroenterol. 2016;22:7091–8.
20. Odabasi M, Muftuoglu MAT, Ozkan E, Eris C, Yildiz MK, Gunay E, Abuoglu HH, Tekesin K, Akbulut S. Use of stapling devices for safe cholecystectomy in acute cholecystitis. Int Surg. 2014;99:571–6.

21. Aoki T, Ozeki Y, Watanabe M, Tanaka S. Cartilage folding method for main bronchial stapling. Ann Thorac Surg. 1998;65:1800–1.
22. Timucin A, Aras O, Karip B, Memisoglu K. Staple line reinforcement methods in laparoscopic sleeve gastrectomy: comparison of burst pressures and leaks. JSLS. 2015;19:e2015.00040.
23. Al HGN, Haddad J. Preventing staple-line leak in sleeve gastrectomy: reinforcement with bovine pericardium vs. oversewing. Obes Surg. 2013;23:1915–21.
24. Mery CM, Shafi BM, Binyamin G, Morton JM, Gertner M. Profiling surgical staplers: effect of staple height, buttress, and overlap on staple line failure. Surg Obes Relat Dis. 2008;4:416–22.
25. Shikora SA, Mahoney CB. Clinical benefit of gastric staple line reinforcement (SLR) in gastrointestinal surgery: a meta-analysis. Obes Surg. 2015;25:1133–41.
26. Taha O, Abdelaal M, Talaat M, Abozeid M. A randomized comparison between staple-line oversewing versus no reinforcement during laparoscopic vertical sleeve gastrectomy. Obes Surg. 2017;28(1):218–25.

11 Fundamentals of Drain Management

Guillaume S. Chevrollier, Francis E. Rosato, and Ernest L. Rosato

11.1 Introduction

11.1.1 General Concepts

The types, indications, and placement of drains are often confusing to the surgical trainee. In general, surgical drains are placed to evacuate an unwanted collection of fluid, blood, or air. Intraoperatively, drains are placed to drain infected areas and potential spaces at risk for fluid accumulation and secondary infection. As a general rule, drains should never be placed with the goal to drain blood, as hemostasis should be achieved by the completion of any case. Drains are also commonly utilized to decompress hollow organs such as the stomach and bladder during the perioperative recovery period when paralytic ileus or close monitoring needs are common. Specialized drains placed in the GI tract can serve to decompress segments of bowel, preventing anastomotic dehiscence. Additionally, they can help control potential areas of fistula formation from the liver, biliary tree, and pancreas. Specialized genitourinary drains, such as the percutaneous nephrostomy tube and the suprapubic catheter, have been developed to decompress the obstructed kidneys and bladder, respectively. When widespread soilage and peritoneal contamination from a perforated viscus occur, specialized drains are indicated through which irrigation and drainage can be obtained. Recently, the use of intraoperatively placed drains has been associated with higher rates of postoperative deep space infection and fistula formation, calling into question their use in routine surgical procedures.

Although evidence is relatively lacking outside of plastic and breast surgery, some surgeons advocate for the use of continued antibiotic prophylaxis for the duration of certain postsurgical drains [1].

11.1.2 History of the Surgical Drain

The origins of the surgical drain can be traced as far back as 400 BC, specifically to Hippocrates, who first reported the use of cloth and small tubes to drain infected spaces. For centuries, passive drainage with makeshift tools persisted, using such materials as animal bones, catgut, horsehair, cloth, glass, and metal tubing. Passive drainage remained the only form of operative drainage until the end of the nineteenth century, when William Halstead

G. S. Chevrollier · F. E. Rosato · E. L. Rosato (✉)
Department of Surgery, Sidney Kimmel Medical College, Thomas Jefferson University, Philadelphia, PA, USA
e-mail: Ernest.Rosato@jefferson.edu

F. Palazzo (ed.), *Fundamentals of General Surgery*, https://doi.org/10.1007/978-3-319-75656-1_11

popularized the radical mastectomy. By raising skin flaps during the mastectomy, a large potential space was created, which inevitably filled with fluid and often required re-operative drainage. It wasn't until 1947, when a general surgeon named David Murphey applied suction to a perforated drain, that a successful post-mastectomy drainage device became available. Although Murphey's system allowed only for intermittent suction, rapid improvements and modifications over the next decade would allow for the application of continuous suction to the surgical drain. Over the ensuing years, various modifications have allowed the modern surgeon to overcome such basic barriers as drain clogging and collapse, leading to the vast number of surgical drains and drainage systems available today [2].

11.1.3 Drain Sizes

Drains are typically described in terms of their size either on the French scale or the gauge system.

11.1.3.1 The French Scale

Surgical catheters are generally sized using the French (Fr.) scale, which is a direct measure of the catheter's outer diameter. By definition, the size in French is equal to three times the catheter's external diameter in millimeters (mm), as demonstrated by the equation below:

$$\text{Fr.} = 3 \times d, \text{where } d = \text{outer diameter in mm}$$

For example, a 3 Fr. catheter has an outer diameter of one millimeter, a 6 Fr. catheter has an external diameter of 2 mm, and so on. Practically speaking, the French size is a close approximation of the catheter's outer circumference in millimeters, where a 10 Fr. catheter has an outer circumference of approximately 10 mm and a 20 Fr. catheter has an outer circumference of approximately 20 mm. It is important to note again that the French size is reflective of a catheter's OUTER circumference, and because the intraluminal diameter depends mainly on wall thickness, the French size is not reflective of intraluminal size or flow rate [3].

Table 11.1 The French scale and gauge system

French scale		Gauge scale	
French size	Outer diameter (mm)	Needle gauge	Outer diameter (mm)
3	1	32	0.24
4	1.33	30	0.31
5	1.67	28	0.36
6	2	27	0.41
7	2.33	26	0.46
8	2.67	24	0.56
9	3	23	0.64
10	3.33	22	0.71
11	3.67	21	0.81
12	4	20	0.90
13	4.33	19	1.07
14	4.67	18	1.27
15	5	17	1.47
16	5.33	16	1.65
18	6	15	1.83
20	6.67	14	2.11
24	8	13	2.41
28	9.33	12	2.77
30	10	11	3.05
32	10.67	10	3.40

11.1.3.2 The Gauge System

The other commonly used scale is the gauge system, which also measures the outer diameter of a needle, catheter, or drain, and is generally reserved for describing the size of hypodermic needles. This scale was initially developed for wire manufacturing and is mathematically much less intuitive than the French scale. On the French scale, a rising value corresponds to a larger catheter or tube size. By contrast, the gauge system has an inverse relationship between gauge and size, where a higher gauge corresponds to a smaller catheter size (Table 11.1) [3, 4].

11.2 Technical Considerations: Drain Types

There are four common classes of drains: open drains, closed drains, closed drains with suction, and sump drains—with and without irrigation.

11.2.1 Open Drains

Open drains are the oldest and simplest type of surgical drain. These drains are placed into a collection or open wound and drain either across a pressure gradient or with the assistance of capillary force to the outside environment, where the drained fluids usually collect in an absorbent-type dressing. The presence of the drain also prevents skin closure or wound healing over the deep tissue space, allowing for healing by secondary intention and prevention of abscess formation or recurrence. Since the system is open to the environment, this type of drainage system is not sterile and is by definition considered contaminated. Examples of common open drains include wound wicks, gauze wound packing, Penrose drains, and setons. These drains are commonly used in heavily contaminated surgical cases to prevent or treat a closed space infection.

11.2.2 Closed Drains

Closed drainage systems utilize a perforated drainage catheter, which is connected to a drainage receptacle via a closed tubing system. The entire system is isolated from the external environment and is better protected from external bacterial contamination. The drained fluids move from the higher pressure (intra-abdominal) or tissue space to the lower pressure (external environment). Drainage is often facilitated by movement, cough or strain, which create a pressure gradient to direct flow externally. These drains are utilized by surgeons and interventional radiologists for the drainage of postoperative fluid collections and for viscus decompression. Some examples of closed drains are discussed below.

11.2.2.1 The Pigtail Catheter

The most common interventional radiology (IR) drain is the pigtail catheter, which must be inserted percutaneously under direct radiologic supervision. Specifically, the pigtail catheter is placed using the Seldinger technique over a wire to guide the drain to its desired location. Once the drain is in correct position, the guidewire is removed, allowing the distal end of the catheter to coil onto itself and form a locking tip, or "pigtail," that allows it to remain inside a collection (Fig. 11.1).

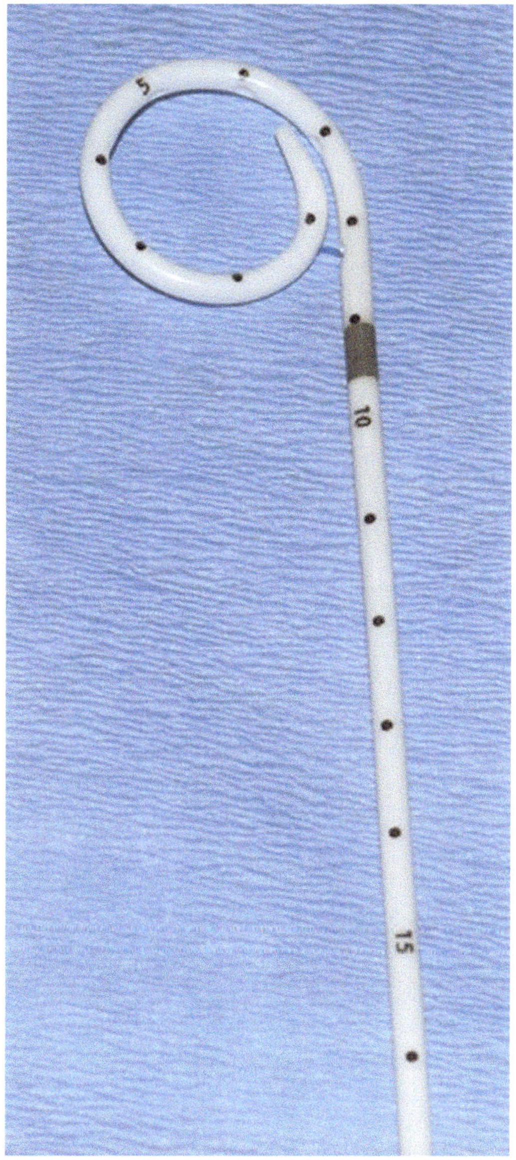

Fig. 11.1 Pigtail catheter with coiling, locking tip

11.2.2.2 Hollow Viscus Drains

Surgeons may also utilize closed drainage systems intraoperatively to decompress a hollow viscus which may have a tenuous suture closure and high risk of postoperative leak into the

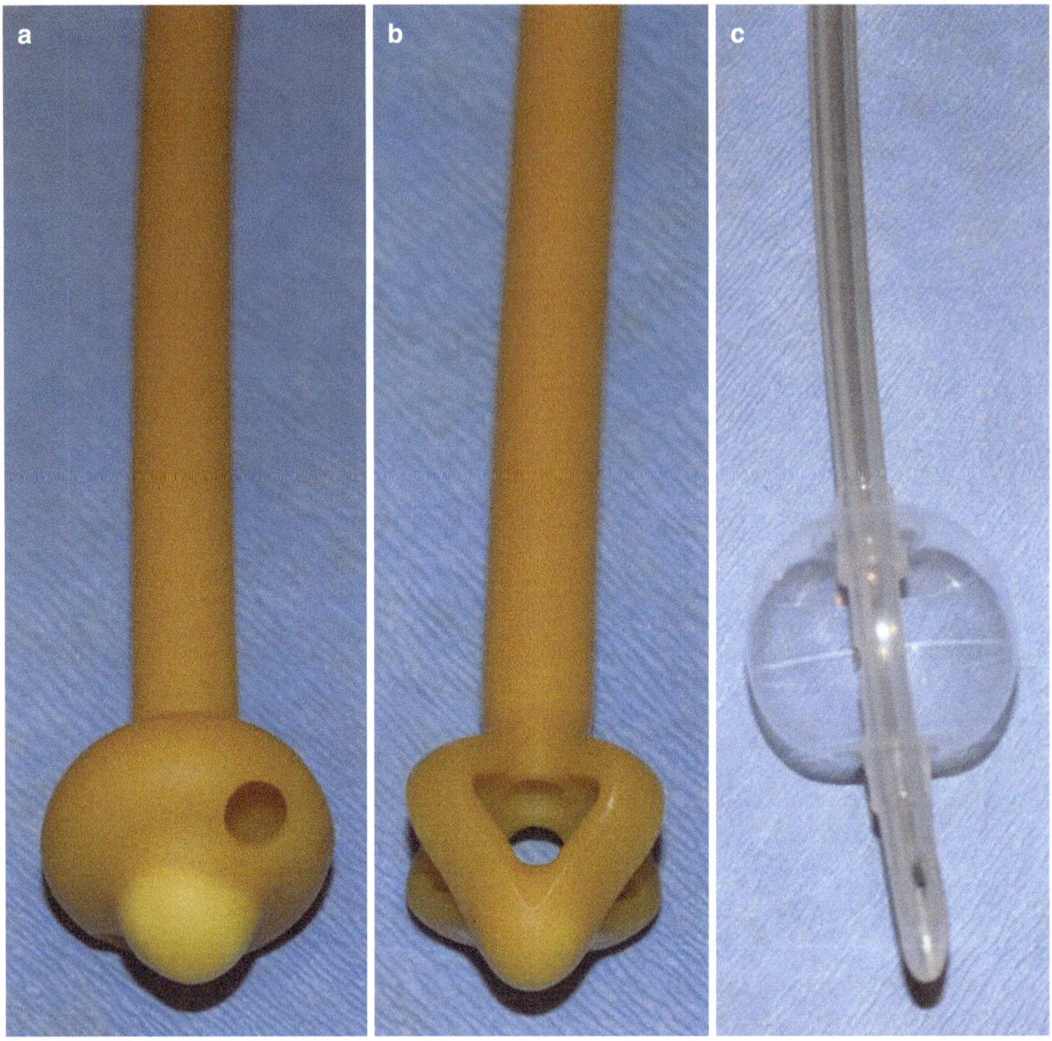

Fig. 11.2 Hollow viscus drains with different retention mechanisms. (**a**) Mushroom catheter. (**b**) Malecot catheter. (**c**) Foley catheter with balloon tip

peritoneal cavity. These types of tubes are often used to decompress the biliary tree (T-tubes), gallbladder (mushroom catheter or Malecot catheter) (Fig. 11.2a, b), stomach (gastrostomy tube or G-tube) (Fig. 11.3), duodenal stump (duodenostomy tube or D-tube), and genitourinary tract (Foley catheter, suprapubic catheter, and percutaneous nephrostomy tube) (Fig. 11.2c). These drains have flanges, extensions, or balloons which help with drainage and retention within the lumen (Fig. 11.2). They are usually constructed from soft rubber or silicone and therefore collapse and fail to drain if strong suction is applied. Prolonged use can lead to a permanent fistula from the hollow viscus to the skin, which may require surgical closure.

11.2.2.3 Gastric Tubes

Special consideration should be given to the gastrostomy tube (G-tube), a very common yet often mismanaged drain. Although G-tubes can be placed for palliative decompression, they are more often used for long-term enteral feeding access. G-tubes allow for both decompression of the stomach by opening it to a drainage bag and "venting" and for feeding by injecting tube feeds

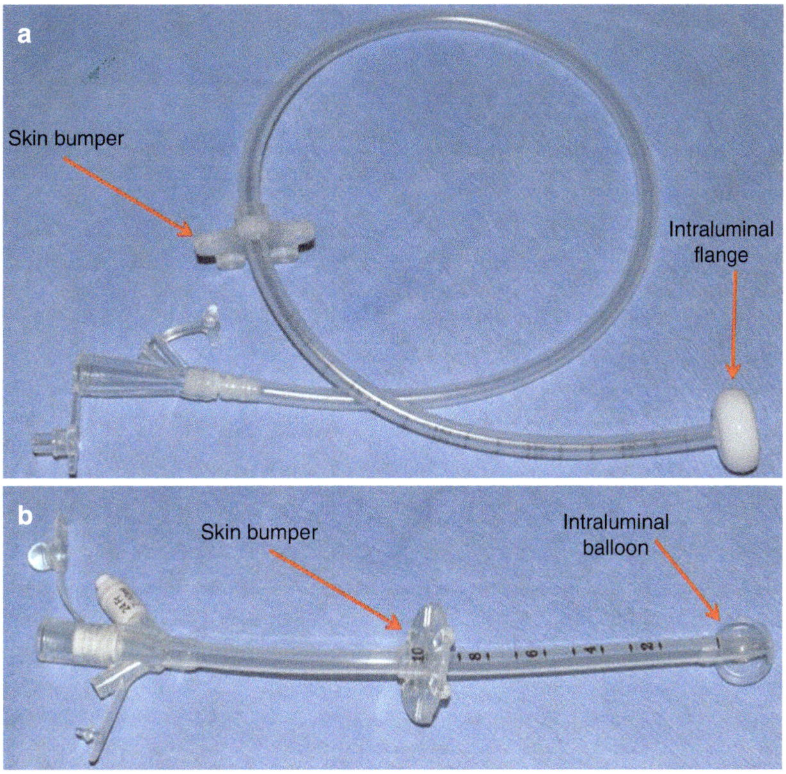

Fig. 11.3 Gastric tubes. (**a**) Percutaneous endoscopic gastrostomy (PEG) tube. (**b**) MIC G® tube (Halyard Health, Inc., Alpharetta, GA)

directly into the stomach. G-tubes mainly come in one of two forms: the percutaneous endoscopic gastrostomy (PEG) tube or the MIC G® tube (Halyard Health, Inc., Alpharetta, GA), the main difference being the presence of a flange or a balloon at the intracorporeal extremity of the catheter (Fig. 11.3).

11.2.2.4 The PEG and the MIC G-tubes

With endoscopic assistance, the PEG tube is advanced down the esophagus and into the stomach. Under direct endoscopic visualization, the tube is externalized by pulling it through the gastric wall, abdominal wall, and overlying skin. A plastic flange at the proximal end of the tube is used to pull the gastric wall up to the abdominal wall and locked in place with a bumper applied to the skin surface (Fig. 11.3a). Within approximately 14–21 days, the tract epithelializes and the stomach scars to the abdominal wall, making bedside tube removal or exchange generally safe thereafter. Once deemed appropriate for removal, the surgeon simply pulls on the tube with enough force to dislodge the gastric flange through the tract and out through the skin. Once the PEG is removed or dislodged, it cannot be replaced into the tract, as the proximal flange cannot fit back into the tract. If replacement is desired and as long as the tract is well established, a MIC G-tube can be reinserted. This tube is designed like a Foley catheter with a balloon at the tip. This design allows the introduction of the catheter from the skin, bypassing the need for endoscopy. Subsequent inflation of the balloon secures the tube within the gastric lumen (Fig. 11.3b). As is the case with Foley catheters, it is important to remember that the balloon should only be filled with water and never with saline. Over time, saline will precipitate to form salt crystals that can perforate the balloon or clog the lumen of the side port, preventing deflation of the balloon.

11.2.2.5 Troubleshooting the G-tube

Two very common issues arising in patients with G-tubes are dislodgment and obstruction. If the tube falls out of its tract after the 14–21-day mark, a Foley catheter may be placed safely in the tract to prevent it from closing or narrowing until a new tube can be placed. For elderly or malnourished patients, it can take up to 4–6 weeks for the tract to mature. Once replaced, correct position can be confirmed with simple auscultation of air injected into the stomach. Although often unnecessary, placement can also be confirmed at the bedside by injecting contrast into the G-tube and obtaining an abdominal X-ray. Visualization of the gastric rugae confirms adequate placement.

Another common problem encountered is occlusion of the G-tube, often from administration of improperly crushed or dissolved medications or precipitation of tube feeds. Generally, this can be resolved by applying gentle positive pressure with warm water into the obstructed lumen. If this fails, instilling a 50:50 mixtures of orange juice and soda and allowing it to percolate within the tube for 30 minutes often breaks up the occlusion. Pancrelipase solution has also been reported as an effective clog-busting agent. Finally, if this fails, a specially designed de-clogging brush can be used; however, this is associated with a risk of damage to the tube and even to bowel if improperly used. The same unclogging principles can be applied to the more temporary Dobhoff tubes, which are thin, single lumen catheters that are strictly used for feeding. Dobhoffs travel from the nose to either the stomach (nasogastric) or to the duodenum (nasoduodenal) if post-pyloric feeding is desired.

11.2.2.6 T-tubes

Another noteworthy tube with which the surgical trainee must gain familiarity is the T-tube (Fig. 11.4), which is most commonly used as a platform for biliary tree reconstruction and biliary anastomoses, as well as for decompression of biliary strictures and blockages. A T-tube is designed in the shape of the letter T, with the longer end of the tube (the base of the T) extending from the biliary tree to the external environment. The two shorter ends (top of the T) lie within the biliary tree at the site of anastomosis or repair. When removal is appropriate, a T-tube cholangiogram can be performed to ensure that

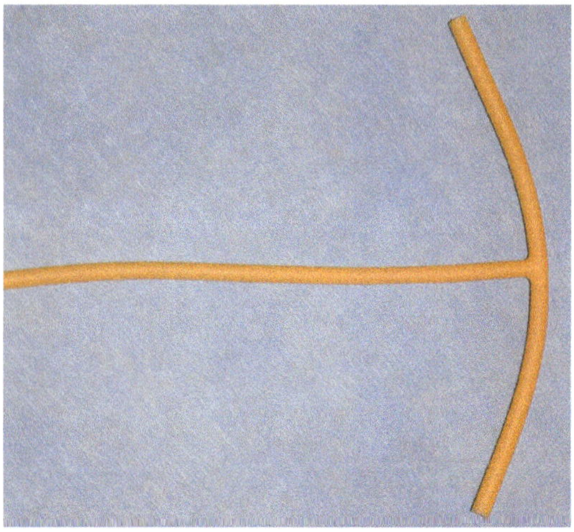

Fig. 11.4 T-tube

there is no intra-abdominal extravasation of contrast, confirming an intact and well-healed biliary tree. A number of modifications can be made to the T-tube intraoperatively to facilitate placement, optimize flow within the tube, minimize trauma to the biliary tree, and avoid a post-removal bile leak. The first option is to incise the T-tube along the length of its intraluminal portion (Fig. 11.5b). A second option is to cut a "gutter" along this same intraluminal portion of the T-tube (Fig. 11.5d). Others prefer to create a "notch" in the segment of the drain that sits directly across from the draining lumen at the top of the T (Fig. 11.5e). These modifications allow the T-tube to fold on itself more easily with traction, facilitating removal. With all of these modifications, the intraluminal ends can also be beveled to facilitate insertion (Fig. 11.5c).

11.2.3 Closed Suction Drains

Closed suction drains are among the most commonly used drains in the surgeon's armamentarium. These are classically utilized to drain potential spaces left after an extirpative procedure or infected spaces and abscesses. They also play a role in the management of high-risk anastomoses, where a controlled fistula may be preferable to returning to the OR for revision or where there are limited revision options

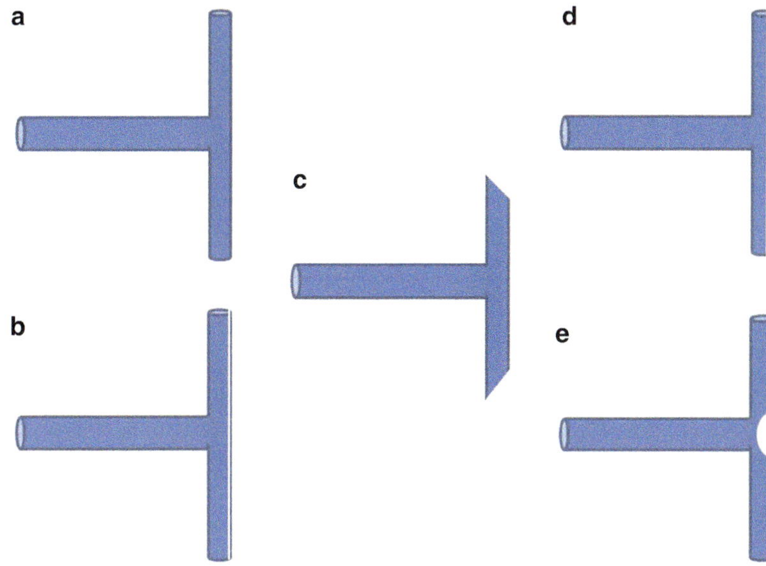

Fig. 11.5 T-tube modifications. (**a**) Unaltered T-tube. (**b**) Incision made along intraluminal length. (**c**) Beveled ends of intraluminal portion. (**d**) "Gutter" creation along length of intraluminal portion. (**e**) "Notch" creation in middle of intraluminal portion

(pancreaticojejunostomy or esophagojejunostomy). Common drain styles include the Jackson-Pratt (JP) and Blake drainage systems. These drains have channels or holes that facilitate drainage into the tube along their length. These are connected to a low-pressure suction bulb which maintains constant negative pressure, enhancing the flow of fluids to the external receptacle (Fig. 11.6).

11.2.3.1 Proper Use of the Closed Suction Drain

When placing these drains, care must be taken to ensure that all side-holes and channels are contained within the tissues. If this is not ensured, external air will enter into the bulb from the drain's externalized holes or channels, and the drain will be unable to maintain suction. *Closed suction drains should never be connected to direct wall suction or unregulated vacuum.* This has been reported to cause direct suction injury to surrounding organs and vasculature, sometimes with fatal consequences. The negative pressure and closed system minimize bacterial migration into the drained space.

Controversy exists over whether these drains may promote anastomotic leak and fistula formation if they are placed in proximity to a fresh intestinal anastomosis. Further, there is currently no evidence of any benefit derived from routine drainage of bowel anastomoses [5]. *Drains should therefore not be used for routine anastomotic drainage.*

Finally, closed suction drains are not indicated to drain actively bleeding spaces. Relying on these drains to control and monitor bleeding and hematoma formation is a mistake which can lead to delayed recognition of significant hemorrhage, hemorrhagic shock, and serious morbidity. The prudent surgeon should achieve meticulous hemostasis by the completion of the surgical procedure.

11.2.4 Sump Drains

Sump drains are designed with an additional channel in the tubing which enables air to be drawn into the drained space and prevents collapse of the tissues around the catheter. These drains require constant suction to draw fluids out of the desired space and into the suction canister. The inflowing air travels through a separate channel in the tube and prevents a vacuum seal from forming around the drain while allowing the dependent fluid to travel into the drainage holes and out through the tubing. This "sump" design enables continued evacuation of a space or organ

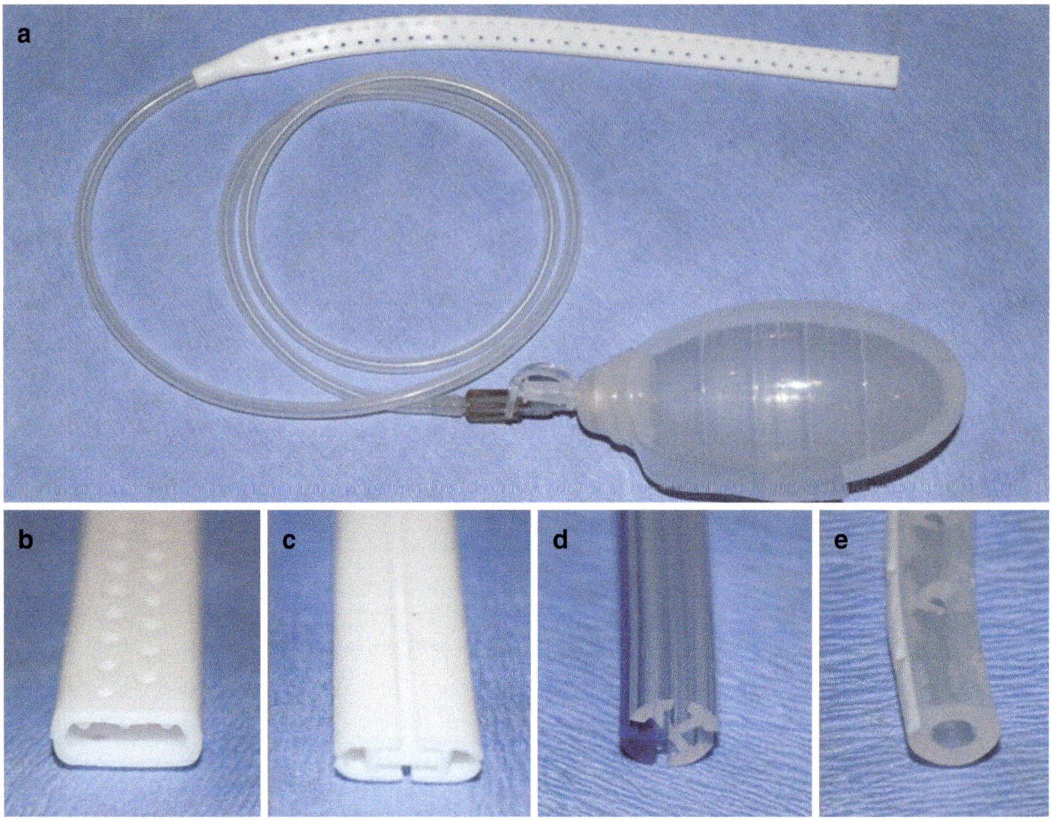

Fig. 11.6 Closed suction drains. (**a**) Jackson-Pratt® (JP) (Cardinal Health, Waukegan, IL) drain with attached tubing and suction bulb. (**b**) Flat Jackson-Pratt® (JP) drain. (**c**) Flat BLAKE® (Ethicon US, LLC., Cincinnati, OH) drain. (**d**) Round BLAKE® hubless drain. (**e**) Round perforated drain

over time and minimizes suction trauma from continuous vacuum pressure against a mucosal lining. Common examples are nasogastric (NG) decompression tubes (Salem Sump) and triple-channel Davol drains (containing suction, sump, and irrigation channels) for evacuation of debris-laden abscesses, as well as some long intestinal decompression tubes (Fig. 11.7).

11.2.4.1 Ensuring Proper Function

The key to successful decompression with this style of drain is to maintain a clear air inflow channel, which enables constant sump drainage of the space. This is usually confirmed by listening for the "whistling" of air through the inflow port. If the port is blocked, it can be cleared by a quick blast of air through the port with a bulb syringe or slip-tip syringe. A one-way filter is often placed over the air intake port to filter the entering air to prevent fluid from backing up into the air port and breaking the sump effect. It is imperative that the filter be placed in the correct orientation to allow unobstructed airflow.

11.2.4.2 The Nasogastric (NG) Tube and its Proper Placement

NG tube placement is one of the most commonly performed bedside procedures by the early surgical trainee and, although very common, can have devastating consequences if improperly placed. The first step in placement is to approximate the appropriate length of tubing by measuring the distance from the tip of the patient's nose, around the back of the ear, and to the xiphoid process. In an awake patient, the tube is lubricated with water-soluble lubricant. The patient is asked to tilt their head back allowing the tube to be gently advanced until the first level of resistance is felt, when the tip of the

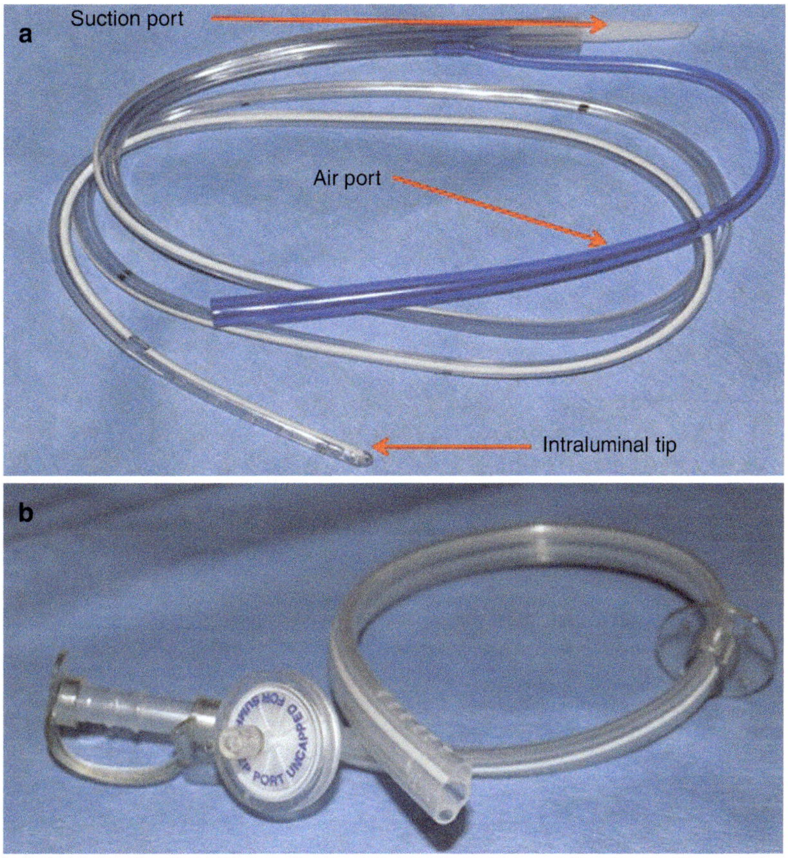

Fig. 11.7 Salem Sump drains. (**a**) Nasogastric (NG) tube. (**b**) Triple-channel Davol drain

tube is abutting the back wall of the oropharynx. At this point, the patient may gag, and it is important to give the patient the time necessary to adjust to the presence of the tube in this location. When ready, the patient is instructed to bring their chin to their chest, allowing for widening of the esophageal opening and narrowing of the airway to avoid endotracheal placement. The tube is then gently advanced in a slightly downward direction to avoid the cribriform plate, while the patient is instructed to swallow water through a straw, allowing for gentle passage of the tube down the esophagus and across the gastroesophageal (GE) junction. Placement can be confirmed by auscultation of air being injected into the stomach. A good indicator that the tube is not in the airway is to ask the patient to phonate. If phonation is possible, the NG tube is unlikely to be positioned through the vocal cords. Once proper position is confirmed, the tube is secured to the nose with tape or can be bridled in place in patients at risk of premature self-removal.

Prior to insertion, it is important to ask the patient if they have had nasopharyngeal surgery in the past, as this may be a contraindication to blind NG tube placement and may require otolaryngology consultation for placement under direct visualization. In these patients, blind advancement of the tube could result in penetration of the cribriform plate and intracranial NG tube placement with devastating neurological consequences.

11.2.4.3 The Triple-Channel Sump Drain

Triple-channel Davol drains (Fig. 11.7b) are utilized for decompression of debris-laden cavities and abscesses which are likely to clog the average closed suction drainage system. They employ a sump design which prevents the development of a vacuum seal and offer a third port through which continuous irrigation can be delivered to break up solid particles in the cavity and facilitate their evacuation. These drains are often employed

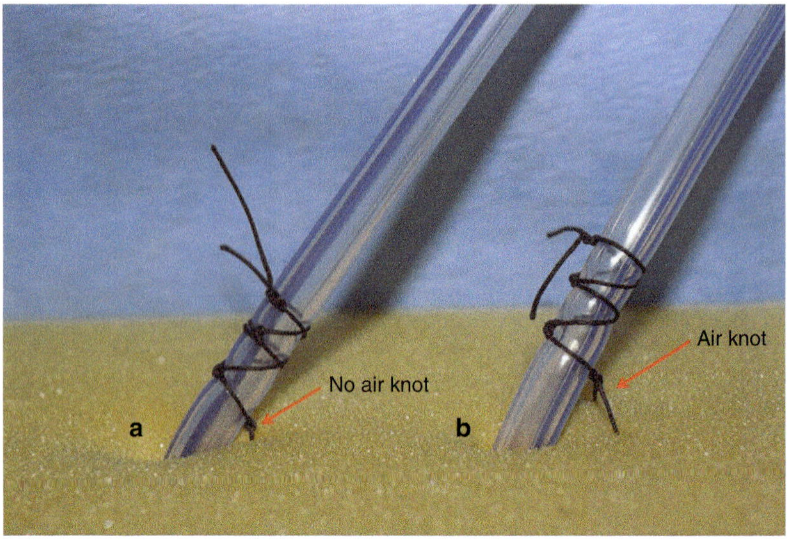

Fig. 11.8 Securing of the surgical drain with 360° wraps. (**a**) Initial suture tied down to the skin to approximate the skin at drain site. (**b**) Initial suture tied as air knot to facilitate removal and decrease patient discomfort

for drainage of infected necrotic tissues especially following debridement of infected pancreatic necroses as an alternative to open abdominal packing.

11.3 General Drain Care

11.3.1 Securing the Surgical Drain

As a general rule, any surgical drain should be sutured in place to prevent accidental removal with patient repositioning or ambulation. Nonabsorbable suture is generally recommended. Monofilament suture is commonly preferred, offering a potentially lower risk of infection compared to braided suture, which can allow for bacterial trapping and growth within its braids.

If using the initial stitch to concomitantly close the drain incision, we recommend a single interrupted stitch across the incision, adjacent to the drain. When the incision is about the size of the drain, a single interrupted stitch is placed to the side of the incision and tied into an air knot so as to decrease pain at the site and make it easier to remove when discontinuing the drain. After placement and tying of the initial skin stitch, both sides of the suture are passed circumferentially around the drain, and a surgeon's knot is laid down onto the drain. The ends are then passed around the drain 360° and tied again as a surgeon's knot. With each knot laid onto the drain itself, one should observe an indentation into the drain material, ensuring that the suture is tight enough to hold the drain securely in place, yet not so tight as to occlude the lumen of the drain. This 360-degree wrap can be repeated as many times as desired. The anchoring stitch should be positioned in such a way as to direct the drain inferiorly and laterally, making it more comfortable for the patient and avoiding the potential for any kinking of the tube postoperatively (Fig. 11.8).

11.3.2 "Cracking Back" the Surgical Drain

At times, it may be appropriate to slowly remove a drain over a period of days (usually 1–2 cm/day) so that the drained cavity can slowly close down over time. This technique theoretically reduces the risk of fluid re-accumulation in a potential space and allows the tract to close down gradually from the inside out with application of negative pressure. To do this, the suture is cut between the skin knot and the first drain knot, and the remaining suture encircling the drain is removed, leaving the drain unsecured with an adjacent skin stitch still in place. The drain can now be pulled back a desired length. Next, a new piece of suture is passed within the loop of the original skin suture. This new piece of suture is then secured to the tube as described above in 360-degree fashion. Intuitively, this process is made easier if at the time of initial drain placement, it is secured with an air knot.

11.3.3 "Milking" the Surgical Drain

To ensure proper function of bulb-suction drains, these should be "milked" every 4–6 h to prevent stasis within the drain, which could lead to eventual clot formation or accumulation of debris. To do this, the drain is pinched with one hand just above skin level, while the contralateral hand secures the drain at skin level to avoid transmitting any pull to the skin sutures. The pinched fingers are then slid together down the length of the drain, milking any fluid or particles out of the drain and into the bulb. To facilitate this process, liquid soap or alcohol swabs can be placed between the fingers to reduce friction on the drain. Proper drain care is critical to maintaining adequate function and ensuring that the indwelling drain does not become a nonfunctioning "dead" tube.

11.3.4 Removing the Surgical Drain

11.3.4.1 When to Remove the Surgical Drain

The timing of drain removal remains debatable. The classic teaching is to remove a drain once it drains less than 25–30 cm^3 over a 24-h period; however, this remains very much up to the operating surgeon and is highly dependent on the clinical scenario.

11.3.4.2 Drain Removal Technique

Once it is determined appropriate to remove the surgical drain, a number of key precautionary measures should be taken to avoid any damage to the tissues surrounding the drain and provide a relatively comfortable experience for the surgical patient. First, the securing suture is cut, remembering to cut only one side and to pull the suture out of the skin from the opposite side. Intuitively, cutting both sides of the suture flush at the skin place the patient at risk of having retained suture that can be difficult to remove. Second, prior to removal, the drain must be taken off suction so as to reduce the amount of stress applied to the surrounding tissues. Third, the patient must be instructed or distracted to "relax" the musculature through which or around which the drain may be traveling. This relaxation can be accomplished by distracting the patient or with deep breathing. Last, the rate of pull on the tube should be kept slow and constant. If excessive resistance is felt, one should stop pulling on the drain and confirm that the patient is as relaxed as feasible. Sometimes, turning the drain 360° back and forth can also overcome any "catch" of the drain. Of utmost importance, one should remember never to readvance a drain into its tract once it has been pulled out, as any portion of exposed drain is considered contaminated and should never be reinserted into its sterile tract. Finally, upon removal, the tip of the drain should be checked for integrity. When placing a drain with side-holes, if trimming a drain to size, it is advisable to cut the drain between two side-holes, as the side-holes themselves constitute the area of a drain that is most prone to fracture. Ensuring that the side-holes are intact at time of removal reassures the surgeon that no part of the drain has fractured. If there remains any concern that a part of the drain may have fractured during removal, a plain film should be obtained to confirm absence of a retained foreign body.

11.4 Complications of the Surgical Drain

11.4.1 Managing the Fractured Drain and the Nonremovable Drain

If drain fracture is confirmed radiologically at time of removal, the indwelling portion must be retrieved. This can be accomplished with IR consultation and attempted access through the existing tract. If this fails, return to the operating room is mandatory for removal of foreign body. Rarely, at the time of removal, one may find that the resistance is simply too strong to overcome safely. If this happens, inadvertent drain suturing at time of placement or excessive fascial tightness around the drain must be suspected. One should never attempt to overcome significant resistance by simply overpowering the tube, as this can lead to significant visceral and tissue damage. These two scenarios are often undiscernible, and both require IR consultation for attempted removal under direct visualization. If this fails, return to the operating room for controlled retrieval should be performed.

11.4.2 Fistula Formation

At times, the surgical drain may start putting out enteric contents when a fistula from either large or small bowel has formed. Depending on the patient's clinical condition and on the output, this may be managed conservatively but typically requires a complete work-up to rule out intra-abdominal abscesses/collections. Once the output decreases to the desired daily amount, the drain can be slowly "cracked back" as described above, allowing the tract to slowly close from the inside out.

11.4.3 Bleeding at the Site

Bleeding from the site of the drain is another commonly encountered problem for the surgical trainee, especially in the coagulopathic or anticoagulated patient. When bleeding is detected, gentle pressure should first be applied in an attempt to achieve hemostasis. If hemostasis is not achieved with continued pressure, gentle traction can be placed on the tube in an attempt to identify the source of bleeding within the tract. If a bleeding vessel is clearly identifiable, bedside cautery may be used after application of local anesthetic, making sure to avoid burning the skin or the drain itself. A simple figure-of-8 stitch may also be applied to control the bleeding vessel. If diffuse ooze is encountered or a bleeding vessel is not identified, hemostatic agents similar to those used in the operating room can be applied. Lastly, a purse-string suture can be used to circumferentially appose the bleeding tract to the drain itself. Coagulation parameters should be checked for any reversible causes. In the anticoagulated patient, it may be appropriate to hold anticoagulation and potentially even reverse it if deemed appropriate. However, the risks of thrombosis must be weighed against the risks of persistent bleeding, and this decision is highly individualized to the patient.

11.4.4 Accidental Drain Removal

In addition to ensuring proper drain positioning and securing at time of placement, additional steps can be taken to avoid accidental drain removal. The cognitively altered patient is at particularly high risk of premature drain removal. When dealing with a delirious patient, it is prudent to use such adjuncts as an abdominal binder to cover the drain site and direct the drain out of the patient's reach. If there is clinical concern that the patient may cause harm to his or herself, then protective mitts and/or restraints may be appropriate. Unfortunately, not all accidental removals will be prevented, and if this occurs, the site should first be dressed with an absorptive dressing. The patient can either be observed clinically or plans should be made for immediate replacement by interventional radiology depending on the clinical situation.

11.5 Special Considerations: Tube Thoracostomy and Negative-Pressure Wound Therapy (NPWT)

11.5.1 Chest Tubes and Pleural Space Drainage

11.5.1.1 Chest Tube Basics

Drainage of the pleural space is required for evacuation of air, blood, and fluid collections in the thoracic cavity which may cause infection, lung trapping, lung compression, or respiratory compromise with hemodynamic instability from

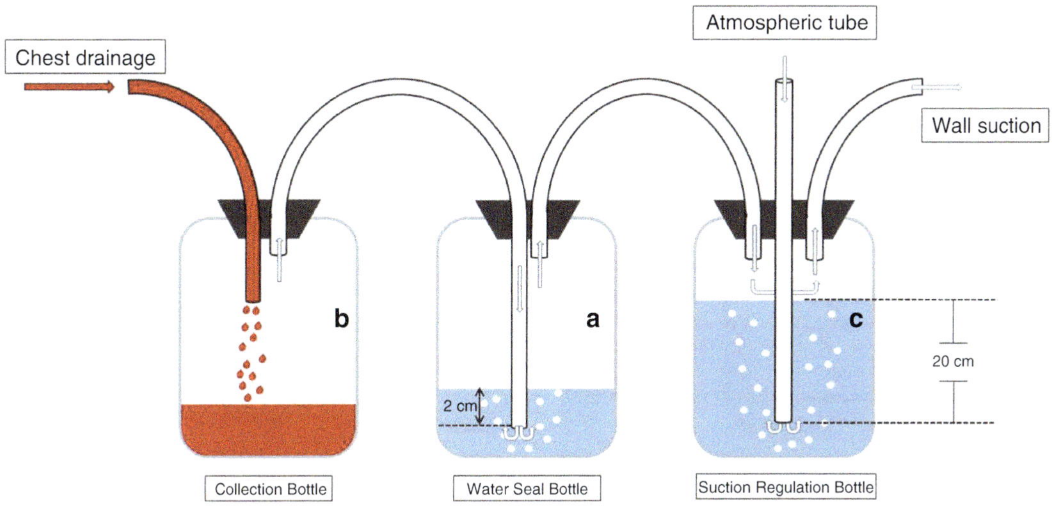

Fig. 11.9 Original three-bottle system for chest tube drainage. (**a**) The "water seal" bottle acts as a one-way valve to allow evacuation of intrapleural contents. The tube in this bottle is conventionally kept 2 cm below water. (**b**) The "collection bottle" allows evacuation and accumulation of fluid while keeping the underwater seal level constant in "water seal" bottle. (**c**) The "suction regulation" bottle allows for increased negative pressure to be applied safely to the pleural cavity and is conventionally maintained with 20 cm of H_2O

pressure buildup. Increased intrathoracic pressure results in mediastinal shift, leading to decreased cardiac blood return and ultimately cardiogenic shock. This tension pneumothorax physiology is most commonly the result of a traumatic or iatrogenic injury to the lung parenchyma resulting in one-way passage of air into the pleural space and subsequent increase in intrapleural pressure. The tension pneumothorax requires immediate decompression. As a temporizing measure in the unstable patient, needle decompression can be performed by inserting a 14-gauge angiocatheter in the second intercostal space in the midclavicular line until chest tube thoracostomy materials become available. Regardless of the indication for placement, once properly positioned, the chest tube requires a drainage system that will maintain negative intrathoracic pressure and enable drainage and collection of the intrapleural fluids and air.

11.5.1.2 The Original Three-Bottle System

The original design for a chest tube drainage system was comprised of a three-bottle system (Fig. 11.9). The first bottle is the "water seal" bottle, which acts as a one-way valve to allow evacuation of intrapleural contents. An increase in intrathoracic pressure with either expiration or coughing forces intrapleural fluid and air into the chamber. Because of surface tension and the gravitational pull onto the column of water, reentry into the pleural cavity is prevented. In this first bottle, the distance between the end of the tube and the surface of the water is critical. The deeper the end of the tube sits below water, the greater the resistance to flow into the bottle. Therefore, the tube is conventionally kept at a level approximately 2 cm below water. With accumulation of fluid, relying only on this single chamber system would result in incomplete decompression of the pleural space as the resistance created by the rise in fluid would eventually cause the pressure in the bottle to equilibrate with the intrathoracic pressure, preventing any further flow of intrathoracic contents into the bottle.

The addition of a second bottle or "collection bottle" overcomes this challenge by allowing for the evacuation and accumulation of fluid while keeping the underwater seal level at a constant

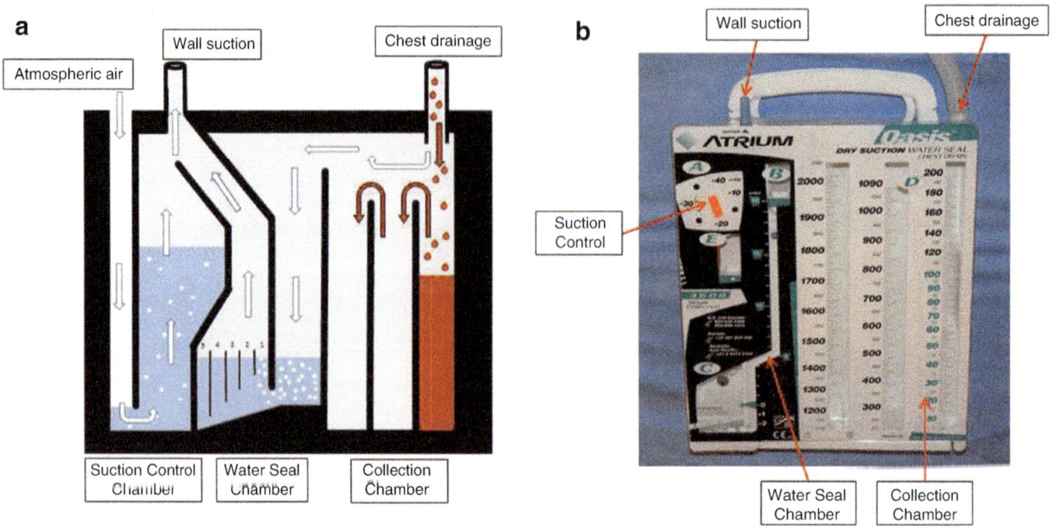

Fig. 11.10 (**a**) Schematic representation of the three-bottle system integrated into a single unit. (**b**) Oasis™ dry suction water seal chest drain (Atrium Medical Corporation, Hudson, NH)

2 cm in the first bottle. This prevents an increase in resistance to flow from the pleural space with evacuation of the chest cavity.

A third "suction regulation" chamber is introduced into the system to allow for increased negative pressure to be applied safely to the pleural cavity. In this chamber, an atmospheric tube is required, running from the external environment into a predetermined height of water within the third bottle. The height of water in this chamber (typically 20 cm) determines the pressure that will be applied across the system into the pleural cavity. When external suction is applied to the third chamber, air is drawn from the external environment into the atmospheric tube, and bubbling will occur once the pressure in the canister reaches −20 cm H_2O or the pressure equals to the height of the water column in cm. As wall suction is increased, a constant amount of negative pressure within the system is maintained by the increased entry of environmental air into the chamber, as manifested by increased amounts of bubbling within the chamber. The atmospheric air entering the third chamber is immediately evacuated via the vacuum tube into the wall suction device. The now-constant level of negative pressure (−20 cm H_2O) is transmitted to the other two chambers and to the intrathoracic space, speeding up the evacuation of the pleural cavity and thereby accelerating or maintaining lung expansion. It is important to understand that as long wall suction exceeds −20 cm H_2O, this conventional −20 cm H_2O of pressure is maintained across the entire system irrespective of the amount of negative pressure generated by wall suction.

11.5.1.3 Today's Chest Tube and Developing Technologies

Although today's collection systems are much more compact, the three-bottled design remains as a three-chambered device integrated into a single unit (Fig. 11.10a), such as the Oasis™ dry suction water seal chest drain (Atrium Medical Corporation, Hudson, NH) (Fig. 11.10b). Recently, new medical devices such as the Thopaz® digital chest drainage system (Medela LLC—Healthcare, McHenry, IL) have been developed to accomplish the same physiology using digital technology and built-in suction control.

11.5.1.4 Chest Tube Insertion

Although the insertion technique is beyond the scope of this chapter, it is important to recognize that insertion can be performed using either the open or closed technique. In the closed technique, a trocar is used to blindly insert the tube into the pleural space. This technique is fraught with

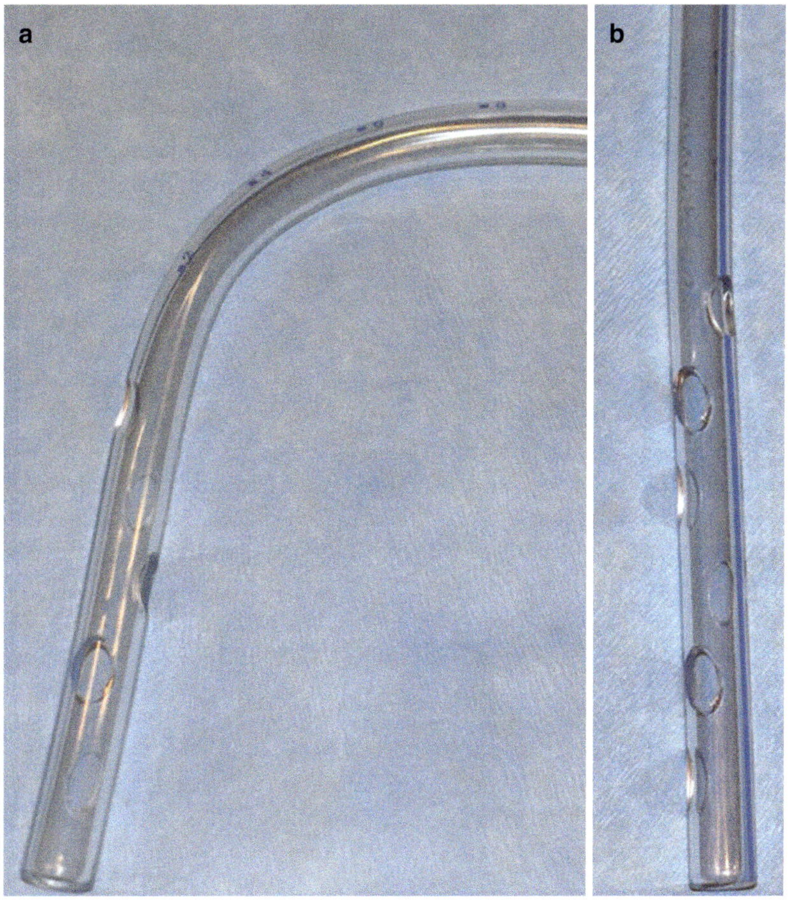

Fig. 11.11 Different chest tube shapes. (**a**) Curved chest tube. (**b**) Straight chest tube

dangers and strongly discouraged, as it places the patient at high risk of lung injury and damage to the great vessels from poorly controlled trocar insertion, which can have devastating consequences. Instead, the open technique is a much safer and precise method of chest tube insertion. Depending on the indication for placement, chest tube location may vary. Traditionally recommended landmarks to safely place a chest tube identify an area between the anterior and midaxillary lines in the fourth or fifth intercostal space.

11.5.1.5 Choosing the Appropriate Chest Tube and Location

As a general principle, larger chest tubes should be placed for the evacuation of hemothoraces and empyemas, as smaller tubes are easily clogged by clots or debris. Smaller tubes can be used for evacuation of simple fluid and air. Generally, chest tubes placed for fluid should be positioned posteriorly and in a basilar location, as fluid will fall to dependent portions of the pleural cavity. Chest tubes placed for air should be positioned anteriorly and apically as air rises anteriorly in the supine patient and apically when upright. These are designed in either straight or curved form to allow for easier positioning based on desired location (Fig. 11.11).

11.5.1.6 Applying Suction to the Chest Tube

The appropriate use and level of suction applied to chest tubes remain heavily debated. Proponents of suction argue that suction should allow the injured lung to re-expand and stay approximated to the chest wall, thereby speeding up healing of the inured lung. However, those who oppose the prolonged use of suction argue that negative pressure causes damage to the lung parenchyma and prevents or slows the resolution of air leaks by maintaining airflow through the injured distal airway. There is currently no consensus on how long and when to apply suction to the chest tube, and this aspect of management remains very much dependent on the surgeon.

11.5.1.7 Special Precautions

Special consideration should be directed to chest tube placement in patients with large hemothoraces and large pleural effusions.

11.5.1.8 The Large Pleural Effusion

One of the potential complications of chest tube placement in patients with large pleural effusions generally present for 3 days or more is the development of re-expansion pulmonary edema, which can lead to severe respiratory compromise. This results from rapid re-expansion of a collapsed lung and is thought to arise secondary to increased alveolar permeability that results from overly rapid lung re-expansion. This complication can be avoided at the time of chest tube placement by briefly clamping the chest tube after drainage of 1.5 L of fluid to allow the lung time to adjust. Intermittent re-clamping should be performed for every 1.5 L drained.

11.5.1.9 The Massive Hemothorax

When evacuating a large hemothorax, the volume of blood evacuated should be carefully monitored. In certain specific instances, life-threatening hemorrhage is likely, and surgical exploration is therefore warranted to identify and repair the source of bleeding. The indications for operative exploration are:

- Evacuation of 1500 mL of blood at time of initial placement
- Chest tube output of 150–250 mL/h for 2–4 h
- Persistent need for blood transfusions to maintain hemodynamic stability [6]

11.5.1.10 Chest Tube Removal

The timing of chest tube removal remains very much up to surgeon and institutional preference, as there is no clear evidence for optimal timing of chest tube removal. When placed for fluid evacuation, the decision is usually based on the daily amount of fluid drainage. When placed for air evacuation, the surgeon can test for resolution of lung injury by testing for an "air leak." In doing so, the awake patient is asked to cough to generate a brisk rise in intrathoracic pressure. If air bubbles are observed in the water seal chamber, air is still evacuating the pleural space, and thus, the lung has not yet healed. Removal of the chest tube in the setting of an air leak would lead to a pneumothorax. In the intubated patient, the same process can be observed during inspiration, when positive pressure is applied to the airways.

When removal of the chest tube is deemed appropriate, the tube should be pulled in early expiration. This is the phase of respiration when the lungs fill the chest cavity and there is no negative intrathoracic pressure to draw air into the pleural space, reducing the risk of a post-removal pneumothorax. An occlusive dressing is typically applied until the tract is closed and air can no longer enter the pleural space from the skin (usually 24–48 h).

11.5.2 Negative-Pressure Wound Therapy (NPWT)

11.5.2.1 NPWT Basics

Negative-pressure wound therapy (NPWT) and vacuum-assisted closure (VAC) therapy are becoming increasingly common adjuncts in the treatment of both acute and chronic wounds. Traditionally, the system is designed using a vacuum pump, which applies negative pressure to a porous material (sponge, gauze, foam, etc.) placed directly within a wound (Fig. 11.12). This system serves to contract the wound, reduce edema, remove fluid and infectious material, and promote tissue regeneration by promoting blood flow and fibroblast migration, accelerating granulation tissue formation [7, 8]. Although not all wounds have been shown to benefit from the use of the wound VAC, recent evidence has shown significant benefit in the treatment of vascular surgery patients, as well as in the treatment of burn wounds, skin grafts, and diabetic foot ulcers [9–11].

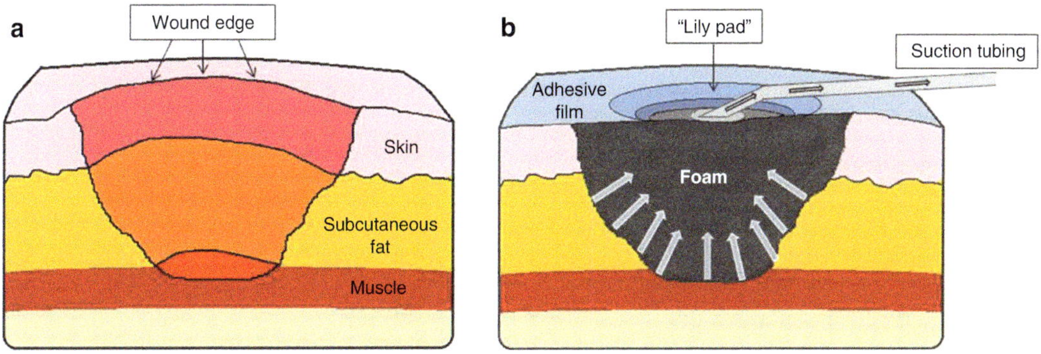

Fig. 11.12 (**a**) Unprotected wound. (**b**) Wound containing indwelling sponge with overlying film and "lily pad" connected to V.A.C.® (KCI—An Acelity Company, San Antonio, TX) therapy canister

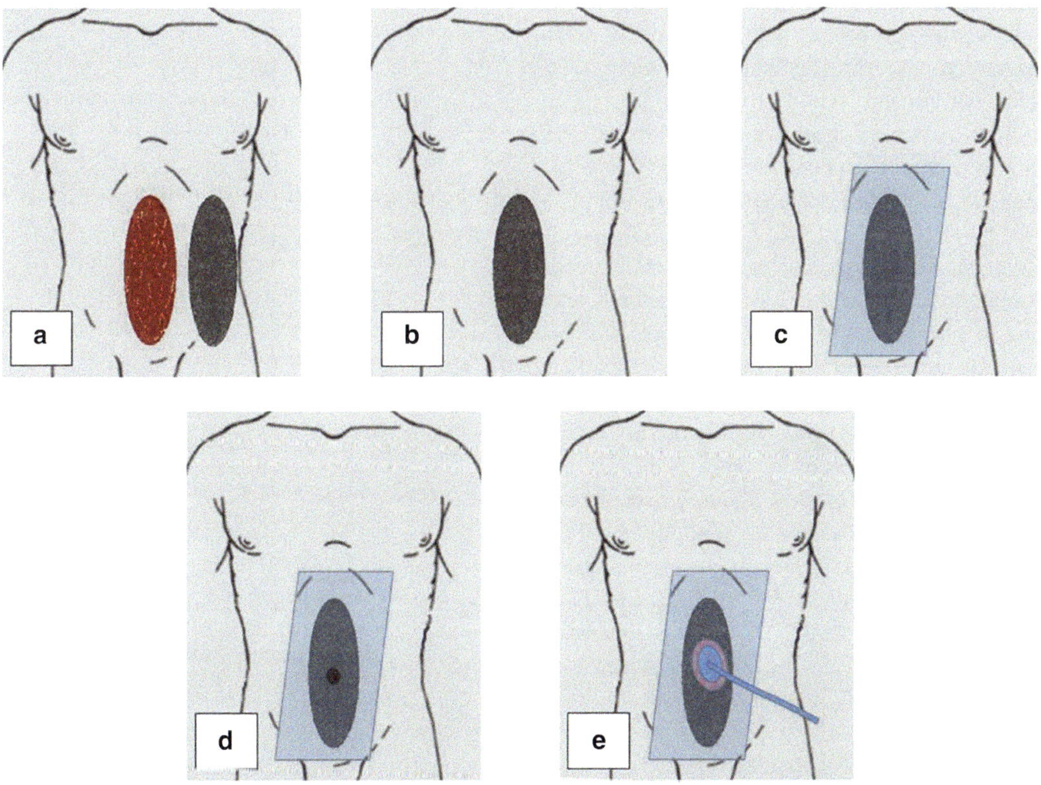

Fig. 11.13 Wound V.A.C.® application. (**a**) Sponge cut to appropriate size. (**b**) Sponge placed into wound. (**c**) Adhesive film applied over sponge and surrounding the skin, forming an occlusive dressing. (**d**) Dime-sized defect created in the film directly overlying the foam. (**e**) "Lily pad" applied over defect and connected to V.A.C.® machine

11.5.2.2 Applying the Wound VAC

In applying the wound VAC (Fig. 11.13), a piece of foam is cut to a size that is slightly smaller than the wound itself and laid within the wound bed. An occlusive film is then applied to cover the entire wound. A small dime-sized defect is created in the film directly overlying the foam, and the tubing is connected to this defect via an occlusive "lily pad" adapter. The tubing is then hooked to the vacuum device, and negative pressure is applied to the desired level of suction ranging from −25 to −200 mmHg. Generally, this dressing is changed every 2–3 days. Theoretically, with each dressing change, the wound bed heals and shrinks in size as it is gradually replaced by granulation tissue. The VAC is continued until the wound can either be left unprotected or skin grafted depending on size and depth.

11.5.2.3 Precautionary Measures for Applying the Wound VAC

With the traditional VAC, care must be taken to ensure that the surface of the indwelling sponge only comes into contact with subepidermal tissue, as any contact directly onto the epidermis has potential to cause skin necrosis with the application of suction. In general, the typical foam dressing should not be applied directly onto the nerves, blood vessels, or viscera (with the exception of open abdomen VACs—see Chap. 20) [7]. Ideally, only one single piece of sponge is laid into the wound to minimize the risk of inadvertently leaving sponge within the wound. If multiple pieces of sponge are required, they should be counted and documented with each VAC change. Finally, care should be taken to avoid placing the lily pad on weight-bearing areas of the body, as this can lead to pressure ulcers. In such instances, as in the care of sacral decubitus ulcers, for example, creation of a "skin bridge" is generally recommended to extend a foam bridge away from the wound. Foam is placed onto the healthy skin that is covered by occlusive dressing, and the lily pad is placed at the end of this "bridge" on a non-weight-bearing area.

11.5.2.4 Other Applications

There are many variations in the design and applications of the original wound VAC. A number of different types of foams exist, with differences in composition, porosity, and antimicrobial properties. These developments have enabled the application of negative-pressure wound therapy to extend far beyond nonhealing or large postoperative wounds. The incisional VAC allows for atraumatic foam to be applied directly onto incisions. Recent data suggest that incisional VACs can decrease the rate of wound infections in certain high-risk wounds [8]. Another new development is the open abdomen (OA) VAC to provide temporary abdominal wall closure. This type of abdominal wall closure is discussed in further detail in Chap. 20.

Take-Home Points

- The surgical trainee must become familiar with the various types, indications, and appropriate placement of surgical drains.
- The French scale is generally used to measure catheters and tubes and has a direct relationship to drain size, while the gauge system is generally used to measure hypodermic needles and has an inverse relationship to size.
- The four common classes of drains are open drains, closed drains, closed drains with suction, and sump drains with and without irrigation.
- Chest tube thoracostomy is an essential skill that must be familiar to all surgical trainees, and understanding how chest tube drainage works is critical to proper management of the chest tube.
- Negative-pressure wound therapy is a rapidly advancing technology that is quickly expanding in terms of its application; however, despite its many theoretical advantages over standard wound therapy, more prospective studies are needed to truly elucidate its benefits in various patient populations.
- When postoperative bleeding is suspected on clinical grounds, remember that drain output can be very unreliable as drains can clot and fail to evacuate accumulated blood.

Suggested Reading

Meyerson JM. A brief history of two common surgical drains. Ann Plast Surg. 2016;77(1):4–5.

Urbach DR, Kennedy ED, Cohen MM. Colon and rectal anastomoses do not require routine drainage: a systematic review and meta-analysis. Ann Surg. 1999;229(2):174.

Mowery NT, et al. Practice management guidelines for management of hemothorax and occult pneumothorax. J Trauma Acute Care Surg. 2011;70(2):510–8.

Dumville JC, et al. Negative pressure wound therapy for treating surgical wounds healing by secondary intention. Cochrane Database Syst Rev. 2015;6:CD011278.

References

1. Edwards BL, et al. Use of prophylactic postoperative antibiotics during surgical drain presence following mastectomy. Ann Surg Oncol. 2014;21(10):3249–55.
2. Meyerson JM. A brief history of two common surgical drains. Ann Plast Surg. 2016;77(1):4–5.
3. Iserson KV. J.-F.-B. Charriere: the man behind the "French" gauge. J Emerg Med. 1987;5(6):545–8.
4. Ahn W, Bahk J-H, Lim Y-J. The "gauge" system for the medical use. Anesth Analg. 2002;95(4):1125.
5. Urbach DR, Kennedy ED, Cohen MM. Colon and rectal anastomoses do not require routine drainage: a systematic review and meta-analysis. Ann Surg. 1999;229(2):174.
6. Mowery NT, et al. Practice management guidelines for management of hemothorax and occult pneumothorax. J Trauma Acute Care Surg. 2011;70(2):510–8.
7. Dumville JC, et al. Negative pressure wound therapy for treating surgical wounds healing by secondary intention. Cochrane Database Syst Rev. 2015;6:CD011278.
8. Acelity. KCI. An Acelity company negative pressure wound therapy technology. 2017. http://www.acelity.com/products/tech/vac. Accessed 22 June 2017.
9. Acosta S, Björck M, Wanhainen A. Negative-pressure wound therapy for prevention and treatment of surgical-site infections after vascular surgery. Br J Surg. 2016;104(2):e75–84.
10. Kantak NA, Mistry R, Halvorson EG. A review of negative-pressure wound therapy in the management of burn wounds. Burns. 2016;42(8):1623–33.
11. Hasan MY, Teo R, Nather A. Negative-pressure wound therapy for management of diabetic foot wounds: a review of the mechanism of action, clinical applications, and recent developments. Diabetic Foot Ankle. 2015;6(1):27618.

Fundamentals of Flexible Endoscopy for General Surgeons

12

Robert D. Fanelli

12.1 Introduction

Modern flexible endoscopes are marvels of medical science. Thin, highly flexible tubular devices illuminated with powerful light sources, with channels for irrigation, suction, and lens clearance, which permit tissue sampling, injection of substances, and the introduction of adjunctive devices like clips and stents, have dramatically altered the landscape of surgical practice since their widespread introduction. The introduction of new, less invasive procedures, those done endoscopically instead of surgically, changed surgical practice forever. From the time that Ponsky introduced percutaneous endoscopic gastrostomy (PEG) [1], McCune described endoscopic retrograde cholangiopancreatography (ERCP) [2], Sugawa used a flexible endoscope to accurately identify the source of upper GI bleeding during laparotomy [3], and Youmans Jr. used a flexible endoscope to treat upper GI bleeding [4], surgeons without endoscopic skills suddenly became ill prepared for the future of general surgery.

Once a set of tools improved the diagnostic yield and target localization for lesions like intestinal tract cancers and sites of GI bleeding, there has been a continual explosion in endoscopic practice since the advent of therapeutic endoscopy, and endoscopy has emerged as a mainstay of clinical practice. During the 1970s and 1980s, while many general surgeons focused on traditional surgical developments and their busy operative practices, others continued the quest for increasingly less invasive methods for the diagnosis and treatment of common problems, as demonstrated in Table 12.1. GI bleeding, intestinal polyps, and common bile duct stones became the targets of these advancements, among other things, and before long surgeons found that endoscopic methods of treatment had changed the

Table 12.1 The history of endoscopy is an important part of our rich surgical heritage

Which were developed by surgeons? All of these major endoscopic innovations were:	
Colonoscopy	Turell
Endoscopic control of hemorrhage	Gaisford, Sugawa
Polypectomy	Shinya, Wolf
Endoscopic retrograde cholangiopancreatography (ERCP)	McCune, Shorb
Variceal band ligation	Steigman
Percutaneous endoscopic gastrostomy (PEG)	Ponsky, Gauderer
Biliary stenting	Sohendra

R. D. Fanelli
Department of Surgery, The Guthrie Clinic, Sayre, PA, USA

The Geisinger Commonwealth School of Medicine, Scranton, PA, USA

Albany Medical College, Albany, NY, USA

F. Palazzo (ed.), *Fundamentals of General Surgery*, https://doi.org/10.1007/978-3-319-75656-1_12

landscape of surgical practice. Continued development in the field of flexible endoscopy has pushed boundaries of treatment beyond the operating room, and other specialists have claimed this tool and the set of procedures developed around it as their own, in an attempt to exclude surgeons from practicing this art for the benefit of their patients. The flexible GI endoscope, however, owes its development to surgery and remains well entrenched in our discipline.

12.2 General Concepts

It isn't possible to provide anything but an introduction to a broad field like surgical endoscopy, which includes numerous primary and adjunctive procedures, through a chapter in a textbook. Whole texts have been devoted to each of the flexible endoscopy procedures commonly employed in practice, and the reader interested in more than the fundamental viewpoints presented herein is advised to seek additional information from the recommended reading list, below, and other sources. Acquisition of endoscopic skills requires direct clinical exposure, an immersion experience, and use of a validated tool to assess competence after training has been conferred by an expert endoscopist [5]. This is the role of the Flexible Endoscopy Curriculum developed by the American Board of Surgery, Inc. (ABS), to guide the acquisition of skills in this set of techniques central to the past, present, and future of surgery. Assessment requires the measurement of accomplishment against a validated yardstick, and surgeons are fortunate to have access to assessment through the Fundamentals of Endoscopic Surgery program and testing modules, produced by the Society of American Gastrointestinal and Endoscopic Surgeons (SAGES), the first such program ever created for the objective assessment of endoscopy skills regardless of specialty [6]. This program removes economic bias from assessment and credentialing determinations and promotes a patient-first approach by ensuring that standards of training and achievement are met [7].

The inclusion of flexible GI endoscopy within surgical practice improves the performance and outcomes of gastrointestinal surgery. At its very basic level, the endoscope is a tool that, when used to provide inspection at the conclusion of an operation involving GI tract reconstruction or anastomosis, confirms for patients and surgeons that the intended goals of surgery have been safely accomplished. At the very least, all surgeons who operate on the GI tract should have great facility with the use of endoscopes to leak test anastomoses, inspect mucosal surfaces for ischemia, and gauge the appropriateness of reconstructive procedures, like Nissen fundoplication, or the completeness of dissections important to optimal outcomes, like during esophageal myotomy for achalasia. Intraoperative endoscopy has become a critically important part of GI surgery [8]. Without robust experience with these basic endoscopic approaches, surgeons will not be positioned to move forward with progressive therapies, like peroral endoscopic myotomy (POEM), peroral pyloromyotomy (POP), or endoscopic mucosal resection (EMR), for example, or other procedures that rely on the flexible endoscopy platform.

Rural surgeons have long found that surgical endoscopy is an important part of their practices as they often provide patients with screening, diagnostic, and therapeutic services that otherwise would not be available in their communities. A 2005 publication revealed that rural surgeons were observed to have performed more endoscopic procedures than operative procedures, important to their communities and practices, and that these skills in flexible GI endoscopy are an essential component to general surgery practice in rural regions of the United States [9]. The results of this same publication, summarized in Table 12.2, demonstrated also that while rural surgeons performed more endoscopy than their urban colleagues, the number of flexible GI endoscopy procedures performed by urban surgeons was substantial as well and concluded that endoscopy remains an important tool for surgical patient care in all situations. Regardless of practice setting, surgeons are encouraged to maintain their endoscopy skills and incorporate these skills into practice for the benefit of their patients and communities.

Table 12.2 Comparison of cases reported by urban and rural general surgeons applying for ABS recertification

	Rural	Urban	*p* Value
General	211	305	<0.0001
Endoscopy	220	77	<0.0001
Gynecology	18	5	<0.0001
Obstetrics	6	1	0.0003
Laparoscopic	94	119	0.016
	$n = 421$	$n = 114$	

Adapted from Heneghan et al. [9]

At the time of this writing, great uncertainty exists about future policies that will be central to the American healthcare system. Regardless of which plan emerges as the framework that will guide how we care for patients in this country going forward, putting flexible GI endoscopes in the hands of surgeons makes sense economically. Evaluations of the healthcare labor force suggest that combining the capabilities of specialists, and tearing down traditional silos of care, may be more efficient and may improve the quality and expedience of care [10]. Surgeons who combine their extensive knowledge and experience in the treatment of conditions and symptoms like gastroesophageal reflux disease, gastrointestinal hemorrhage, GI malignancy, and dysphagia and abdominal pain, as some examples, are likely to provide a more economically efficient approach to the care of these patients when involved early, as they have the broadest array of diagnostic and therapeutic capability available to be deployed for the benefit of the patient. By eliminating delays and costly but not always additive consultations with other specialists, the surgeon is able to swiftly assemble an evaluation that benefits the patient in a cost-efficient manner.

While there is no question that incorporating flexible GI endoscopy into surgical practice serves the needs of our patients today, it will be an increasingly important set of skills for future generations of surgeons. Numerous surgical procedures that already have been replaced by endoscopic approaches are listed in Table 12.3. The flexible endoscope has emerged as an exciting platform upon which future minimally invasive surgical procedures will be based. Consider the positive impact of effective colonoscopic screening and endoscopic ablation for patients with Barrett esophagus, for example, and the use of EMR or endoscopic submucosal dissection (ESD) for those with early rectal or esophageal cancer. Traditional surgical approaches will continue to be less commonly necessary, and less invasive therapies based on the flexible GI endoscopy platform will emerge as new standards in our approach to many patients. Surgeons who do not develop and maintain their skills in surgical endoscopy will miss the opportunity to participate in the next epoch of our specialty.

Table 12.3 Surgical procedures already replaced by endoscopic approaches (partial list)

Esophagus	Foreign body removal
	Stricture management
	Palliation of malignancy
	Variceal hemorrhage management
	Achalasia
	GERD (early)
	Barrett esophagus
Stomach	Hemorrhage management
	Pyloric obstruction
	Gastroparesis
	Foreign body management
	Enteral feeding access
	Obesity (early)
Pancreaticobiliary	Management of choledocholithiasis
	Biliary stricture management
	Periampullary neoplasm (benign)
	Complicated pancreatitis, walled-off pancreatic necrosis
	Pseudocyst drainage
Colon	Polypectomy
	Intestinal hemorrhage
	Colonic stricture
	Acute colonic obstruction
	Management of hemorrhoid disease

Another important example an evolution that surgeons must participate in is the burgeoning field of bariatric endoscopy. While there are few at present who would argue that any of the currently available endoscopic therapies for obesity compare with the effectiveness of gastric bypass and sleeve gastrectomy, new technical developments, combinations of pharmacologic and endoscopic approaches, and therapeutic improvements will develop, and there is great likelihood that an endoscopic treatment model will emerge that serves the needs of many patients well [11]. In order for surgeons to remain relevant to their patients in all areas of our specialty, we must embrace the flexible endoscopy platform and apply its principles liberally in preparation for a future that incorporates these techniques in ways we might not even imagine presently.

12.3 Practical Considerations

Unless a surgeon in training sets out to master flexible GI endoscopy, and pursues specialized training opportunities, it is unlikely that she is going to acquire the skills necessary to offer full spectrum diagnostic and therapeutic endoscopy to her community of patients. However, the incorporation of flexible GI endoscopy into surgical practice should not be seen as an all or none proposition. It is completely reasonable that a foregut surgeon or bariatric surgeon will develop expertise in upper endoscopy, as the minimum, and offer those services to patients to address preoperative, intraoperative, and postoperative concerns and forego the dedicated additional training that would be required to add ERCP to their practice. Similarly, a colorectal surgeon would be expected to develop and maintain expertise in colonoscopy as a minimum, although given the significant plasticity seen in specialty practices, maintaining skills in upper GI endoscopy may be warranted [12]. Although I support the notion that surgical endoscopists develop a broad range of skills and recognized expertise in as many endoscopic procedures as possible, we all tailor our skill sets to the needs of our communities, to our clinical interests, and to the particular circumstances of our careers. Surgeons are encouraged to begin broadly and acquire the wide-ranging set of endoscopic skills that will support them in offering patients an optimal choice of procedures and superb clinical outcomes, but if that is not possible, or not feasible given one's area of subspecialization, then maintaining expertise in the endoscopic procedures central to their field of practice is what will serve patients best.

There is no question that the best time for surgeons to learn to perform flexible GI endoscopy procedures is within the structured learning environment of their residency and fellowship training. This is why SAGES and the ABS have taken such measures as developing FEC and FES programs that seek to increase the endoscopic competence of our surgical workforce going forward in order to maximally benefit patients. Surgeons who did not learn endoscopy during their training must make special efforts to attain this knowledge and skill and gain clinical experience. The pursuit of fellowship opportunities is available to surgeons able to take time away from their practice, and individualized programs of instruction and assessment are possible as well but vary from locale to locale. Mentorship is a hallmark of the surgical community, and surgeons interested in further training and ongoing education aimed at achieving mastery of new skills are advised to seek out mentorship arrangements that will work best in their individual environments.

12.4 Specific Procedures

Although it would be an impossible task to discuss in detail each of the basic and advanced endoscopic techniques that are incorporated into a full spectrum surgical endoscopy practice that might include expertise in EGD, enteroscopy, ERCP, EUS, and colonoscopy and their adjuncts as its mainstays, for most surgeons, the fundamental procedures that will be employed are EGD and colonoscopy. These will be detailed below.

12.4.1 Esophagogastroduodenoscopy (EGD)

EGD provides for detailed inspection of the mucosal surfaces of the esophagus, stomach, and early duodenum. This study is indicated for the evaluation of symptoms that persist despite conservative treatment, alarm symptoms such as dysphagia and odynophagia, and surveillance of treated malignancy or premalignant conditions or in lieu of radiographic or other evaluation where the therapeutic advantage of endoscopy adds value [13].

Consent for EGD is based on a discussion of the potential risks associated with the procedures, the potential benefits to be gained, and the alternatives for investigation or treatment that might be used instead. Patients are selected according to local standards of the unit where EGD will be performed, but general health and airway assessments are important to the appropriate selection and treatment of patients. Nasal oxygen, complete cardiac, oximetry, and, increasingly, capnographic monitoring are utilized, and intravenous access is established for the administration of both fluids and sedative agents and rescue medications when needed.

Equipment is selected and tested prior to any endoscopic procedure, and in particular, the planned procedure is central to these selections. Each endoscope has at least one working channel through which endoscopic tools are deployed, and it is important that the endoscopist ensures that the selected endoscope will accept the tools necessary for the planned procedure (Fig. 12.1). Once the equipment has been selected and tested, an appropriate pre-procedure safety check completed, and the patient sedated either by the endoscopist or an anesthesiologist, the procedure may begin.

The endoscope is advanced under direct vision at all times, and carbon dioxide insufflation, preferred over room air insufflation because of its more rapid absorption that results in improved patient comfort, is used to distend the lumen of the organ being inspected in order to provide the best view possible and aid in complete inspection of the mucosal surfaces. As the endoscope is advanced over the base of the tongue, it is passed into the proximal esophagus and directed into the center of the lumen as it is advanced distally (Fig. 12.2). Mucosal surfaces are inspected along the way, noting pathology and securing samples for biopsy as needed. The endoscope is then advanced into the stomach and advanced toward the pylorus. Novice endoscopists often struggle with advancement into the distal stomach, but this can be accomplished more easily if the endoscopist rotates themselves slightly toward their right to face toward the head of the patient, so that the endoscope advances along the greater curvature of the stomach. This maneuver aligns the scope with the pylorus, and after inspection, the pylorus then is intubated to examine the duodenum.

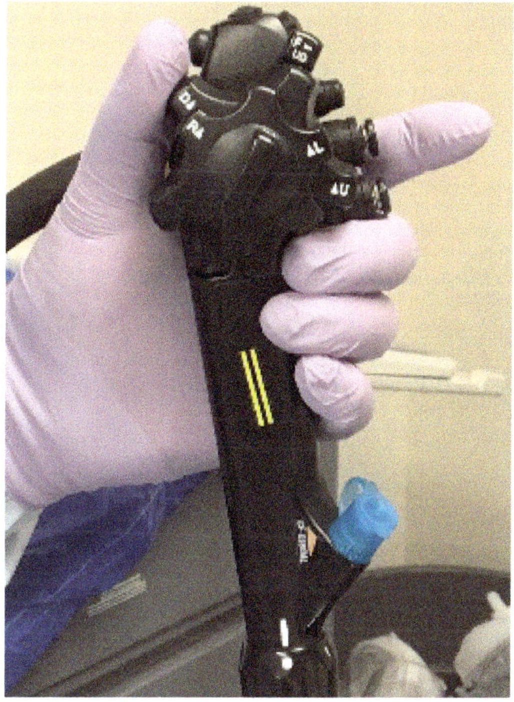

Fig. 12.1 The head of the endoscope is held in the left hand, index finger poised to insufflate, suction, or cleanse the lens. Proper balance is important to ergonomic function

Throughout most of an upper endoscopy, torque on the shaft of the endoscope is effective in exposing mucosal surfaces to the left and right of center, for inspection. As the endoscope is advanced through the duodenal bulb, the directional wheels of the endoscope become more important. As the endoscope advances toward the second portion of the duodenum, the endoscopist once again takes an oblique step forward with the left foot, rotates her body toward her right, and rotates the large directional wheel counterclockwise and the small directional wheel clockwise, delivering the tip of the endoscope into the

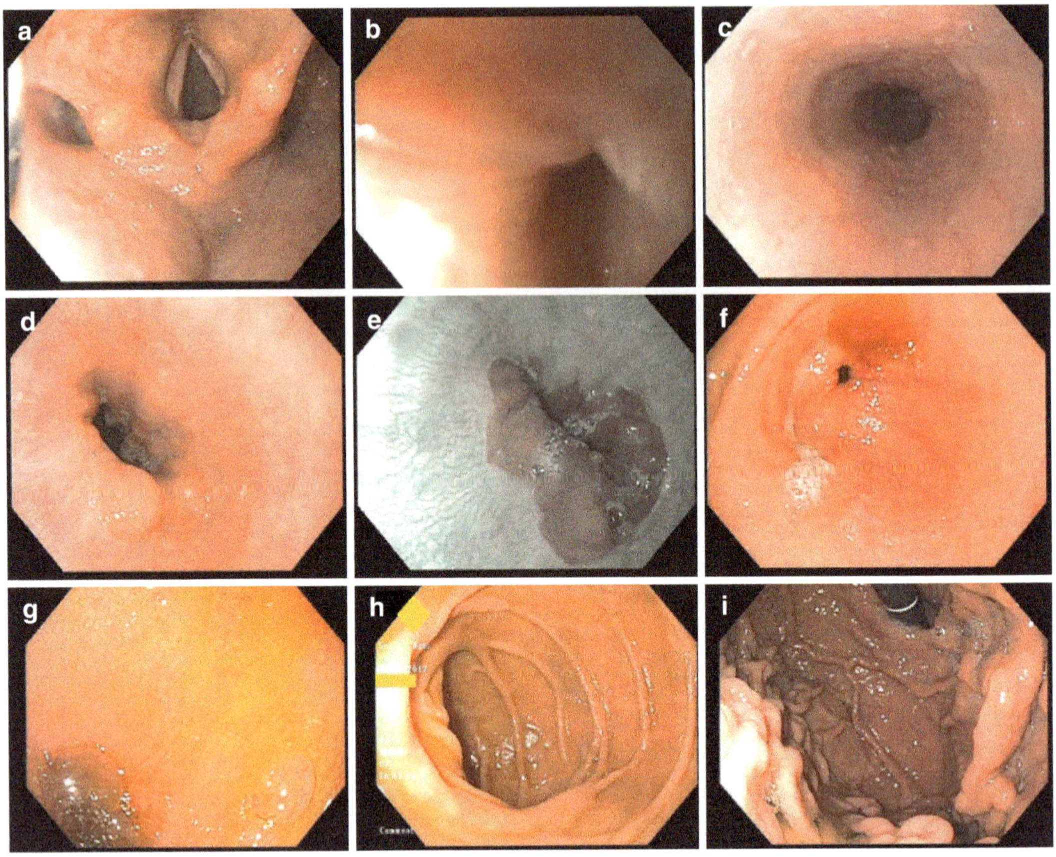

Fig. 12.2 (**a**) The vocal cords are seen superior to the esophageal introitus (red arrow), where the endoscope will be introduced. (**b**) The esophageal introitus yields to gentle insertion and insufflation as the gastroscope is advanced. (**c**) The body of the esophagus is inspected and observed, noting mucosal abnormalities, altered peristalsis, and other abnormalities. Note that the gastroscope remains centered in the lumen. (**d**) The esophagogastric junction is inspected for erosions, metaplasia, gaping, and other abnormalities using white light. (**e**) The esophagogastric junction is inspected for metaplasia and other abnormalities using narrow bandwidth illumination. (**f**) After advancement along the greater curvature, the pylorus is inspected from the antrum. (**g**) The duodenal bulb is evaluated after gentle advancement of the gastroscope through the pylorus. (**h**) The descending duodenum is inspected after advancement of the gastroscope. Note the biliary ampulla on the medial wall (red arrow). (**i**) Retroflexed view of the esophagogastric junction demonstrates the gastroscope entering the stomach in the region of the hiatus. Note the small hiatus hernia (red arrow)

descending duodenum. This is the deepest extent of insertion in the average procedure, and the careful observation of mucosal surfaces continues during slow withdrawal of the endoscope, and samples for biopsy are obtained as needed using a biopsy forceps designed for the endoscope in use. Care should be taken to inspect for pathology, obtain tissue samples that will be helpful in diagnosis, and observe all important anatomic structures, like the major papilla, seen more easily on the medial duodenal wall if the shaft of the endoscope is slightly rotated clockwise during withdrawal. Great care should be taken to avoid taking biopsies from the medial wall in order to avoid inadvertent biopsy of the major or minor papillae.

The endoscopist should develop a systematic approach to mucosal inspection, so that there is great consistency in the quality of examination. Once the duodenal inspection has been completed, retroflexion is accomplished by rotating the large directional wheel counterclockwise while laying the head of the endoscope over toward the left and withdrawing the endoscope shaft back toward the hiatus. This position permits inspection for and measurement of a hiatus hernia, and careful inspection will most often permit delineation between sliding and paraesophageal hernias.

Once anteflexed, the now forward facing endoscope is used to decompress the stomach of excess insufflation, and the esophagogastric junction is inspected once again. Narrow bandwidth illumination, present in high-definition endoscopes, shifts the spectrum of light emitted and is useful in identifying mucosal changes associated with Barrett esophagus. The esophagus is thoroughly inspected, and as the endoscope is withdrawn, once the pharynx is cleared, the suction button on the endoscope should be kept depressed until some fluid is suctioned through the channel and the gastroscope safely laid on a back table for reprocessing. This simple maneuver keeps fluids from dripping on the patient and staff, and onto the shoes of the endoscopist, while the endoscope is transitioned from bedside to back table.

Photo documentation is an important part of each endoscopic procedure, and it is generally accepted that capturing images of (1) the esophagogastric junction using white light and narrow bandwidth illumination, if available, (2) the retroflexed view of the gastric cardia and hiatus, (3) the forward view facing the pylorus, and (4) the duodenal bulb and (5) descending duodenum are a reasonable standard to achieve in most, if not all, upper endoscopy procedures.

12.4.2 Colonoscopy

Colonoscopy provides for detailed inspection of the mucosal surfaces of the colon, and as often as technically feasible, the terminal ileum. This study is indicated for the evaluation of symptoms that persist despite conservative treatment, alarm symptoms such as bleeding, and surveillance of treated malignancy or premalignant conditions and, most commonly, for screening for polyps and colorectal cancer where the combined diagnostic and therapeutic capabilities of colonoscopy hold advantage over other screening methods.

One measure necessary to perform colonoscopy that is not required for EGD is bowel preparation. Although there are numerous commercial bowel preparations available, they can be sorted into two general categories; high-volume lavage preparations and split-dose preparations. The latter are generally better tolerated and are more effective in cleansing the colon, but the former are less expensive and more likely to have lower patient copay levels. It is recommended that surgeons performing colonoscopy emphasize to patients the critical importance of a complete bowel preparation. Without adequate preparation in advance of colonoscopy, achieving near complete mucosal inspection will not be possible, and the risk of a missed lesion is increased.

Consent for colonoscopy is based on a discussion of the potential risks associated with the procedure and its adjunctive measures, the potential benefits to be gained, and the alternatives for investigation or treatment that might be used instead. Patients are selected according to local standards of the unit where colonoscopy will be performed, but general health and airway assessments are important to the appropriate selection and treatment of patients. Nasal oxygen, complete cardiac, oximetry, and, increasingly, capnographic monitoring are utilized, and intravenous access is established for the administration of both fluids and sedative agents and rescue medications when needed.

Equipment is selected and tested prior to any endoscopic procedure, and in particular, the planned procedure is central to these selections. Each colonoscope has one working channel through which endoscopic tools are deployed, and it is important that the endoscopist ensure that the selected colonoscope will accept the tools necessary for the planned procedure, and that the tools that might be needed are of a length sufficient to match that required for use through a colonoscope. Once the equipment has been selected and tested, an appropriate pre-procedure safety check completed and all monitoring devices have been attached and baseline measurements recorded, the patient then is asked to

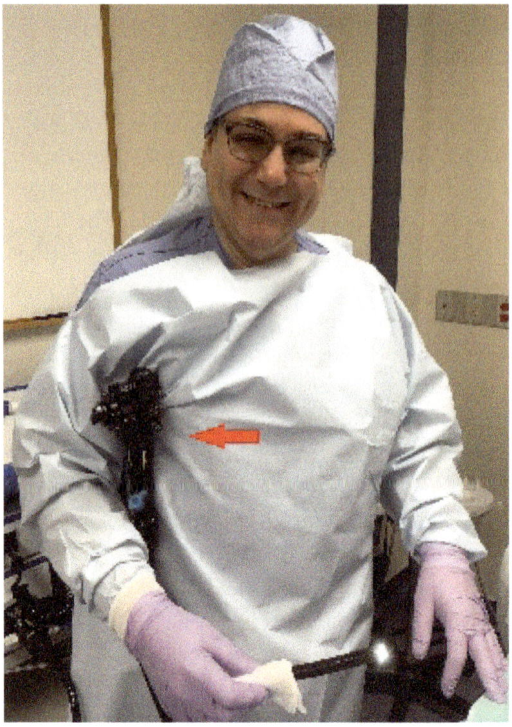

Fig. 12.3 The head of the colonoscope is held between the upper right arm and chest wall (red arrow), the tip in the double-gloved right hand, and the colonoscope shaft and electronic umbilicus are gently looped without twists in preparation for the introduction of the colonoscope

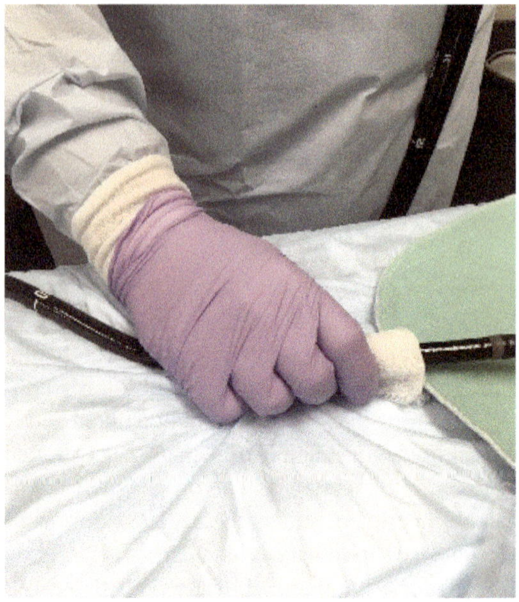

Fig. 12.4 The right hand glove is kept clean by using a fresh gauze pad for manipulation of the shaft of the colonoscope. Contaminating the directional wheels, snares and biopsy forceps, and air and suction buttons with lubricant adds unnecessary difficulty to colonoscopy

lie in the left lateral decubitus position, and the patient is sedated either by the endoscopist or an anesthesiologist.

Water-soluble lubricant then is dabbed onto the anus using a gauze pad, administered by the endoscopist using the right hand. One glove is worn on the left hand and two are worn on the right hand (Fig. 12.3). As the head of the colonoscope is held between the right upper arm and lateral chest with its shaft forming a gentle U-shaped loop beside the surgeon, the endoscopist uses the left hand to elevate the right buttock of the patient and uses the right hand, holding the tip of the colonoscope, to first perform a digital rectal examination and then to introduce the colonoscope into the rectum. The outer right glove then is removed and discarded, and the head of the colonoscope held in the left hand while the right hand, grasping the colonoscope using a gauze pad, is used to advance and withdrawal the colonoscope (Fig. 12.4). Great care should be taken to maintain as clean the operational head and control wheels of the colonoscope; contamination with fluids or lubricant makes handling the colonoscope significantly more challenging throughout the remainder of the procedure. The colonoscope is advanced under direct vision at all times, and carbon dioxide insufflation, preferred over room air insufflation because of its more rapid absorption that results in improved patient comfort, is used to distend the lumen of the colon in order to provide the best view possible and aid in as complete an inspection of mucosal surfaces as is possible.

The colonoscope is advanced throughout the colon under direct vision, inspecting the mucosal surfaces both during insertion and withdrawal. Several anatomic regions in the colon can prove challenging during insertion, particularly the often-tortuous sigmoid colon, the splenic flexure, and the hepatic flexure, but loop reduction, limited insufflation, external support, and other nuances learned over time will permit complete intubation and inspection in the overwhelming majority of patients. Once the cecum has been reached, it is usually identified by the confluence of the three teniae coli in the cecal pit, leading to the appendiceal orifice seen at the base of the cecum. The ileocecal valve will be seen as a more pronounced fold than the others, often fatty in appearance with a slightly more yellow coloration, and often, the orifice into the ileum can be seen. Gently maneuvering the colonoscope toward this lumen, and insufflating while advancing slightly, will permit intubation of the terminal ileum in a majority of patients (Fig. 12.5).

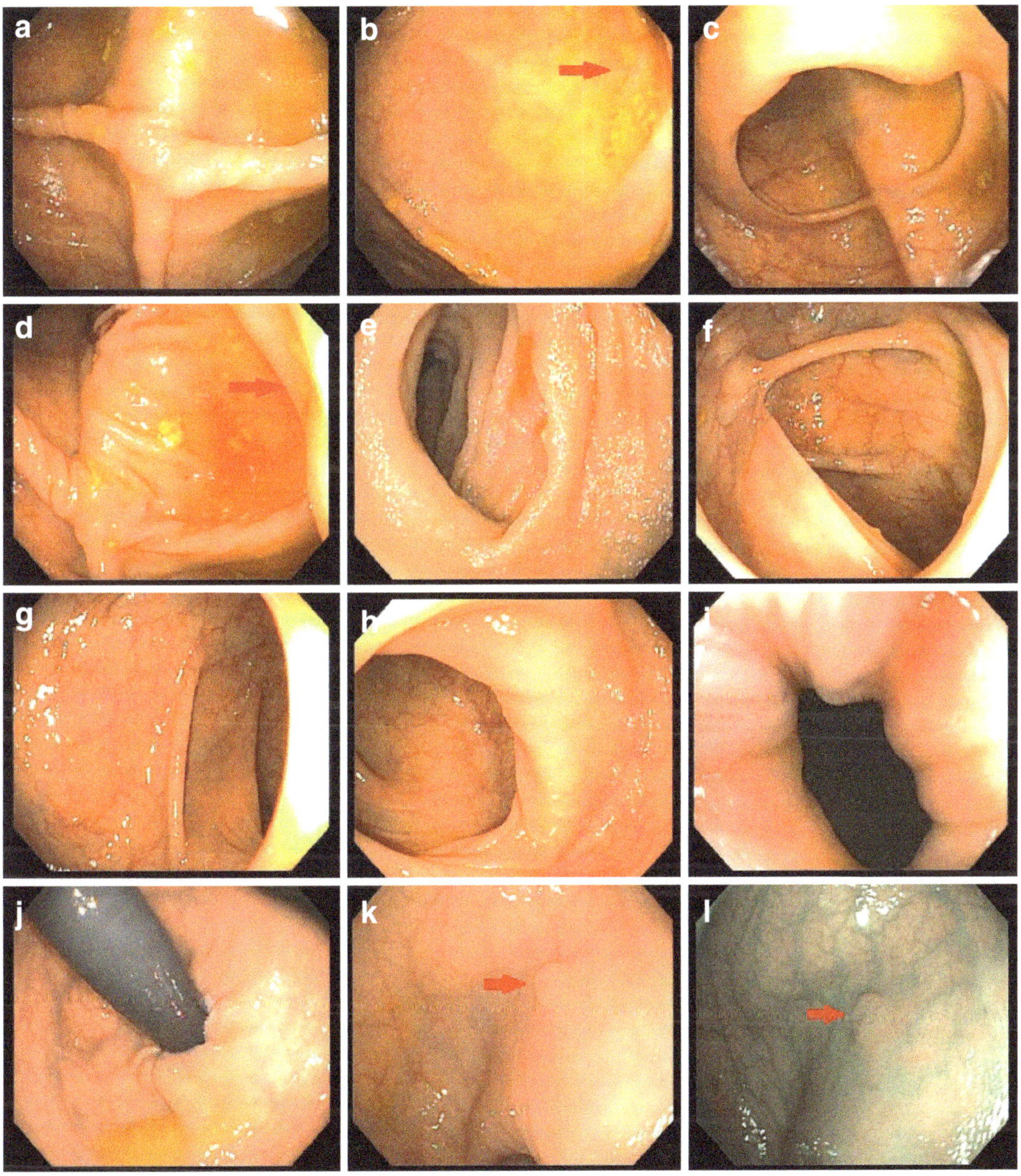

Fig. 12.5 (**a**) Cecal intubation is recognized by the confluence of the teniae coli, (**b**) the appendiceal orifice, and (**c**) the ileocecal valve. (**d**) The dimpled surface of the ileocecal valve (red arrow) permits entry into (**e**) the terminal ileum with just the right amount of tip deflection, insufflation, and colonoscope advancement. The (**f**) hepatic flexure and (**g**) splenic flexure are recognizable landmarks in most patients, and (**h**) the sigmoid colon has noticeably thicker folds than the more proximal colon. (**i**) Visual inspection of the anal canal supplements digital rectal examination performed at the outset, and (**j**) retroflexion within the rectal vault completes the distal examination. (**k**) Visualization of a small polyp (red arrow) is enhanced using (**l**) narrow bandwidth illumination for confirmation

The colon is carefully inspected again during withdrawal, taking care to visualize each mucosal surface as thoroughly as possible. Biopsies should be taken when indicated, using appropriately configured biopsy forceps, and polyps should be removed using standard polypectomy techniques. The decision to perform hot or cold polypectomy is based on patient factors, polyp size and morphology, endoscopist experience, and anatomic location. Traditionally, therapeutic maneuvers and specimen acquisition have been performed during withdrawal, but polypectomy, biopsy, and tissue sampling may be done safely during insertion of the colonoscope as well [14]. Tissue removed using any of these techniques routinely is sent for histopathologic analysis, although there has been recent enthusiasm for discarding obviously benign tissues, to reduce costs [15]. After the entirety of the colonic mucosa has been inspected as precisely as possible, the colonoscope is withdrawn to the level of the dentate line, inspecting circumferentially, and the colonoscope retroflexed within the rectum by rotating the large directional wheel counterclockwise while slowly and gently advancing the colonoscope into the mid-rectum. Often, rotating the colonoscope by its shaft will assist in this maneuver. Once anteflexed again, the suction button on the endoscope should be depressed to decompress the colon and rectum and should be kept depressed until some fluid is suctioned through the channel and the colonoscope safely laid on a back table for reprocessing. This simple maneuver keeps fluids from dripping on the patient and staff, and onto the shoes of the endoscopist, while the colonoscope is transitioned from bedside to back table.

Photo documentation is an important part of each colonoscopy, and it is generally accepted that capturing images of (1) the cecal pit, (2) ileocecal valve, (3) terminal ileum, (4) and retroflexed view of the rectum serve as a minimum suggested standard. To this, photos of all pathology encountered are highly advised, and some endoscopists early in their experience will include photos of the splenic and hepatic flexures, transverse colon, and other anatomic features as well.

Take-Home Message

Flexible GI endoscopy is an important set of skills for the general surgeon. Mastery, as in all forms of procedural intervention, requires training, assessment, current practice and experience, and continuing education. The surgeon planning to incorporate endoscopy into clinical practice in a meaningful way should strive for excellence in all aspects of patient care related to this undertaking and should determine which particular endoscopic procedures are essential to their current and future patient service. Specifically, surgical endoscopists must master the principles of patient selection, pre-procedure evaluation, and sedation and should familiarize themselves with the many useful evidence-based guidelines that inform these processes [13]. Surgical endoscopists should strive for excellence in the performance of those endoscopic procedures germane to their patient populations and should master adjunctive therapeutic measures and procedures, recognition of pathology, and management of lesions encountered. The management of complications, arrangement of appropriate follow up based on findings and pathology, and expertise in the recovery needs of patients undergoing endoscopic procedures all are central to expertise in this field. Whether choosing to offer basic endoscopy services, like EGD and colonoscopy, or advanced procedures that include enteroscopy, ERCP, and EUS, surgical endoscopists should approach the acquisition and maintenance of skills in flexible GI endoscopy the same way they would approach any set of procedures central to their practice.

Recommended Reading

Zetka JR Jr. Surgeons and the scope. Ithaca: ILR Press; 2003.

Marks JM, Dunkin BJ. Principles of flexible endoscopy for surgeons. New York: Springer; 2013.
Ponsky JL. Atlas of surgical endoscopy. St. Louis: Mosby Year Book; 1992.

References

1. Gauderer MW, Ponsky JL, Izant RJ Jr. Gastrostomy without laparotomy: a percutaneous endoscopic technique. J Pediatr Surg. 1980;15(6):872–5.
2. McCune WS, Shorb PE, Moscovitz H. Endoscopic cannulation of the ampulla of vater: a preliminary report. Ann Surg. 1968;167(5):752–6.
3. Lucas CE, Sugawa C. Diagnostic endoscopy during laparotomy for acute hemorrhage from the upper part of the gastrointestinal tract. Surg Gynecol Obstet. 1972;135(2):285–6.
4. Dudley HA, St John DB, Yeomans ND. Early endoscopy in haematemesis and melaena. Br Med J. 1973;2(5869):772–3.
5. Poulose BK, Vassiliou MC, Dunkin BJ, Mellinger JD, Fanelli RD, Martinez JM, et al. Fundamentals of endoscopic surgery cognitive examination: development and validity evidence. Surg Endosc. 2014;28(2):631–8.
6. Hazey JW, Marks JM, Mellinger JD, Trus TL, Chand B, Delaney CP, et al. Why fundamentals of endoscopic surgery (FES)? Surg Endosc. 2014;28(3):701–3.
7. Pearl J, Fellinger E, Dunkin B, Pauli E, Trus T, Marks J, et al. Guidelines for privileging and credentialing physicians in gastrointestinal endoscopy. Surg Endosc. 2016;30(8):3184–90.
8. Fanelli RD. Intraoperative endoscopy: an important adjunct to gastrointestinal surgery. Tech Gastrointest Endosc. 2013;15(4):184–90.
9. Heneghan SJ, Bordley JT, Dietz PA, Gold MS, Jenkins PL, Zuckerman RJ. Comparison of urban and rural general surgeons: motivations for practice location, practice patterns, and education requirements. J Am Coll Surg. 2005;201(5):732–6.
10. Kocher R, Sahni NR. Rethinking health care labor. N Engl J Med. 2011;365(15):1370–2.
11. Fanelli RD, Andrew BD. Is endoluminal bariatric therapy a new paradigm of treatment for obesity? Clin Gastroenterol Hepatol. 2016;14(4):507–15.
12. Fleming CA, Khan Z, Andrews EJ, Fulton GJ, Redmond HP, Corrigan MA. "Is general surgery still relevant to the subspecialised trainee?" a 10 year comparison of general versus specialty surgical practice. World J Surg. 2015;39(2):297–302.
13. Committee ASoP, Early DS, Ben-Menachem T, Decker GA, Evans JA, Fanelli RD, et al. Appropriate use of GI endoscopy. Gastrointest Endosc. 2012;75(6):1127–31.
14. Sanaka MR, Parsi MA, Burke CA, Barnes D, Church J, Rizk M, et al. Adenoma detection at colonoscopy by polypectomy in withdrawal only versus both insertion and withdrawal: a randomized controlled trial. Surg Endosc. 2015;29(3):692–9.
15. Rees CJ, Rajasekhar PT, Wilson A, Close H, Rutter MD, Saunders BP, et al. Narrow band imaging optical diagnosis of small colorectal polyps in routine clinical practice: the detect inspect characterise resect and DISCARD 2 (DISCARD 2) study. Gut. 2017;66(5):887–95.

13 Fundamentals of Prosthetic Materials for the Abdominal Wall

Udai S. Sibia, Adam S. Weltz, H. Reza Zahiri, and Igor Belyansky

13.1 Introduction

The earliest hernias were repaired by primary closure of the defect with catgut, silk, or metal wire [1]. Without the use of mesh, primary defect closure alone was demonstrated to be associated with higher rates of hernia repair failure [2, 3]. Benjamin Pease, a surgeon and innovator, first sought to incorporate prosthetic materials in hernia repair when he filed a patent titled "Nonmetallic Mesh Surgical Insert for Hernia Repair." Several years later, Usher would be the first to describe the use of this patented material (polypropylene mesh) for hernia repair [4]. The use of polypropylene mesh was furthered by Lichtenstein for inguinal hernias [5]. Contemporary surgical practice enjoys the luxury of choosing from a vast pool of mesh products, which have consistently been shown to reduce recurrence rates compared to primary closure alone [6–8]. While experts and studies have attempted to define the ideal mesh and its characteristics, data supports proper mesh and patient selection for optimal outcomes post-hernia repair.

Mesh products are broadly categorized into synthetic permanent, synthetic bioabsorbable, and biologic types. Mesh characteristics such as chemical composition, pore size (i.e., microporous or macroporous), filament structure (i.e., monofilament or multifilament), and biodegradability influence the intensity of the foreign body reaction elicited by the mesh material and are important characteristics to consider when selecting a prosthetic material for your patients. The following sections will help define important features of various mesh products available today and the parameters to consider when selecting them.

13.2 General Concepts

The principles of functional tissue engineering are the foundation to manufacture hernia mesh [9]. Mesh is either "knitted" or "woven." Knitted meshes are continuous filaments looped around another [10]. Woven mesh contains a series of parallel strands alternatively passed over and under another series of parallel strands to be positioned perpendicularly to each other. Synthetic meshes, except expanded polytetrafluoroethylene (ePTFE), are usually knitted and more porous and flexible than woven meshes [11].

Mesh weight and pore size are key aspects of mesh design. The weight of the mesh depends on the weight and amount of material used (weight/unit area) [12]. Mesh can be lightweight (typically 33 g/cm^2), medium

U. S. Sibia · A. S. Weltz · H. R. Zahiri
I. Belyansky (✉)
Department of Surgery, Anne Arundel Medical Center, Annapolis, MD, USA
e-mail: ibelyansky@aahs.org

F. Palazzo (ed.), *Fundamentals of General Surgery*, https://doi.org/10.1007/978-3-319-75656-1_13

weight (~60 g/cm^2), or heavy weight (~100 g/cm^2). Small pore sizes impede soft tissue ingrowth and normal healing granulomatous reactions which can lead to encapsulation of the entire mesh leading to stiffness and reduced flexibility. Access to antimicrobial agents and host immune cells to bacteria is also impeded with small pore-sized mesh [13, 14]. For that reason, microporous synthetic meshes such as ePTFE are difficult to salvage from infection and frequently require explantation [15–17]. Larger pore sizes (>75 μm) allow infiltration by macrophages, fibroblasts, blood vessels, and collagen [12].

All meshes trigger an immune response after implantation [18]. Although an acute inflammatory response is an important step in the wound healing process [19], chronic inflammation can lead to mesh-related complications of erosion, migration, and contracture [20–23]. Filament structure and chemical composition of mesh can influence the intensity of the foreign body reaction. Monofilament polyester mesh elicits a reduced foreign body reaction compared to multifilament polyester mesh or monofilament polypropylene mesh in a rodent model [24]. The biocompatibility of mesh is important to its design and is measured by the quantity of macrophages and granulocytes, granuloma size, vascularization, collagen deposition, and mesh migration [25].

13.3 Mesh Types

13.3.1 Synthetic Permanent Mesh

The use of synthetic permanent mesh is standard practice to repair most hernia defects. Polymeric materials commonly used to manufacture permanent mesh include polyester, polypropylene (PP), ePTFE, and more recently polyvinylidene fluoride (PVDF). The benefits of synthetic mesh are well described. Monofilament mesh elicits a reduced inflammatory and foreign body reaction and offers better bacterial clearance when compared to multifilament mesh [24, 26–30]. Lightweight macroporous mesh is thought to have greater tissue integration and lower long-term rates of chronic pain as opposed to heavyweight mesh [31–33]. Notably, monofilament lightweight mesh has a high incidence of mechanical failure in open incisional hernia repairs [34]. The next sections will describe individual characteristics of the different types of synthetic mesh.

13.3.1.1 Polyester

Polyester mesh is synthesized using alcohol and carboxylic acid [35]. It is biocompatible, hydrophilic, strong, durable, and resistant to most chemicals. Studies have demonstrated higher rates of tissue regeneration compared to PP mesh [36, 37]. Polyethylene terephthalate (PET) is a semi-aromatic copolymer that was an early polyester mesh used in the repair of inguinal and abdominal hernias [38]. However, some have found that PET mesh may be prone to hydrolytic degradation reducing its mechanical strength over time [39].

Mesh infection is a dreaded complication of prosthetic hernia repair. Some synthetic meshes such as Parietex (PCO) composite mesh™ (Medtronic, USA) have multifilament structural properties designed to promote tissue ingrowth. In the setting of an infection, multifilament polyester meshes are very difficult to salvage and often result in chronic wound infections requiring complete surgical resection of infected mesh [40, 41].

Monofilament lightweight polyester mesh such as Parietex TCM (Medtronic, USA) has been reported to have a higher incidence of mechanical failure in open incisional hernia repair [34]. Newer constructs such as Versatex™ (Medtronic, USA) and Symbotex™ (Medtronic, USA) are monofilament, macroporous, medium-weight meshes that offer improved textile strength, mesh integration, and favorable tissue ingrowth [42]. ProGrip™ (Medtronic, USA) meshes are self-fixating meshes which may result in decreased postoperative pain associated with traditional tack fixation. They are composed of a textile PET and microgrip polylactic acid material. Self-fixating mesh is particularly useful during inguinal hernia repair which carries a risk for nerve and vascular injury due to tack fixation.

13.3.1.2 Polypropylene

Polypropylene mesh is the most commonly implanted synthetic surgical mesh, with more than one million implanted annually worldwide [43]. The mesh offers high chemical resistance, good mechanical stability, and durable strength at a low cost [44]. It is inert, hydrophobic, biocompatible, and resistant to biological degradation [45].

The choice of mesh for clean-contaminated/contaminated ventral hernia repair remains debatable. Recent studies have shown that macroporous, medium-weight meshes may be used safely in the retromuscular space with significantly lower wound morbidity and more durable outcomes versus a similar cohort of biologic repairs in clean-contaminated ventral hernia repairs [46]. This is likely secondary to improved bacterial clearance and faster integration of macroporous synthetics.

13.3.1.3 Expanded Polytetrafluoroethylene (ePTFE)

Polytetrafluoroethylene is a synthetic fluoropolymer produced by free radical polymerization of tetrafluoroethylene [35]. It is highly hydrophobic and does not degrade in the abdominal wall. Studies have shown mesh fragmentation, fracture lines, and detachments in the presence of bacterial contamination [17].

13.3.1.4 Polyvinylidene Fluoride (PVDF)

Polyvinylidene fluoride is produced by the polymerization of vinylidene difluoride [35]. It is highly inert and thermoplastic and exists in four different crystalline phases, exhibiting different physiochemical and mechanical properties [47]. The mesh is durable and more resistant to hydrolysis or degradation than PET [48]. PVDF retains 92.5% of its strength after 9 years of implantation [49].

13.3.2 Synthetic Bioabsorbable Mesh

Bioabsorbable mesh products are single- or double-layered monofilament polymers that gradually degrade over time [35]. These mesh products have been promoted to be used in contaminated fields to address hernia defects [50], although there is a paucity of literature regarding long-term outcomes when used for this indication. Once implanted, the mesh provides the structural framework for the remodeling of the abdominal wall by host tissues, which restores its support. Depending on the specific mesh, they are fully resorbed within 2–36 months [51]. Accurate long-term recurrence rates with absorbable mesh remain to be determined, although they are likely higher when compared to synthetic mesh [52].

There are several synthetic bioabsorbable mesh products available on the market. Gore Bio-A (WL Gore and Associates, USA) mesh is comprised of polyglycolic acid and trimethylene carbonate and has been shown to be efficacious in terms of long-term recurrence and quality of life for contaminated ventral hernia repairs [53]. It may be an alternative to biologic and synthetic permanent meshes in these complex repairs. Phasix™ (Bard Davol Inc., USA) and TIGR® Matrix (Novus Scientific, USA) are newer products that degrade over several months [54–58]. Phasix™ is a monofilament mesh, while TIGR® Matrix is a multifilament copolymer of glycolide, lactide, and trimethylene carbonate. In vivo studies have shown that the extent of adherent bacteria corresponds to the estimated filament surface area [40]. The increased surface area of multifilament meshes may therefore promote the persistence of bacteria resulting in chronic infections.

13.3.3 Biologic Mesh

Biologic mesh products are generally harvested from allogenic (i.e., human) or xenographic (i.e., bovine, porcine, and equine) collagen sources and are comprised of a variety of tissues (i.e., dermis, pericardium, and small intestine submucosa) [35, 51]. The species and types of tissue define the structural and compositional properties of the biologic mesh. The mode of processing (i.e., cross-linking process) determines the mechanical properties of mesh, with cross-linked mesh being stronger than non-cross-linked mesh. A variety of biologic mesh products with

Table 13.1 Properties of biologic mesh

Trade name	Manufacturer	Species	Tissue type	Intentionally cross-linked	Sterilization method
AlloDerm, X-Thick	LifeCell Corp., Branchburg, NJ	Human	Dermis	No	Not terminally sterilized
AlloMax	C.R. Bard/ Davol, Inc., Warwick, RI	Human	Dermis	No	Low-dose gamma
CollaMend	C.R. Bard/ Davol, Inc., Warwick, RI	Porcine	Dermis	Yes 1-ethyl-(3-dimethylaminopropyl)-carbodiimide (EDC) hydrochloride	Ethylene oxide
CollaMend FM	C.R. Bard/ Davol, Inc., Warwick, RI	Porcine	Dermis (fenestrated)	Yes (EDC)	Ethylene oxide
FlexHD	Ethicon, Inc., Somerville, NJ	Human	Dermis	No	Decontamination with ethanol and peracetic acid (not terminally sterilized)
Fortive	RTI Biologics, Inc., Alachua, FL	Porcine	Dermis	No	RTI's Tutoplast® Tissue Sterilization Process with low-dose gamma irradiation
GraftJacket	Wright Medical Technology, Inc., Arlington, TN	Human	Dermis	No	Not terminally sterilized
OrthADAPT	Synovis Orthopedic and Woundcare, Irvine, CA	Equine	Pericardium	Yes (proprietary)	Proprietary
PeriGuard	Synovis Surgical Innovations, St. Paul, MN	Bovine	Pericardium	Yes (glutaraldehyde)	Ethanol and propylene oxide
Permacol	Covidien, Norwalk, CT	Porcine	Dermis	Yes (hexamethylene diisocyanate)	Gamma irradiation
Strattice-firm	LifeCell Corp., Branchburg, NJ	Porcine	Dermis	No	E-beam
SurgiMend	TEI Biosciences, Inc., Boston, MA	Bovine (fetal)	Dermis	No	Ethylene oxide
Surgisis, Biodesign	Cook Medical, Bloomington, IN	Porcine	Small intestine submucosa	No	Ethylene oxide
Veritas	Synovis Surgical Innovations, St. Paul, MN	Bovine	Pericardium	No	E-beam
XenMatrix	C.R. Bard/ Davol, Inc., Warwick, RI	Porcine	Dermis	No	E-beam

different characteristics are available for hernia repairs (Table 13.1).

Decellularization is the process of removing cells and cellular debris from the harvested tissues [51]. Biologic mesh undergoes a decellularization process to prevent a host's immune response against the implanted mesh. Residual donor cellular debris can lead to an inflammatory response in the recipient causing fibrosis. Depending on the species and tissue, there are many ways of processing biologic mesh. These include acidic or basic solutions, chelating agents [59, 60], detergents [61–63], enzymes [64, 65], hypertonic or hypotonic solutions [66, 67], solvents [61, 62, 68], and toxins [69].

Mesh degradation is prevented by cross-linking of acellular scaffolds to increase material stability in vivo [70]. Cross-linking is achieved with chemicals. These include carbodiimides [71–74], glutaraldehyde [75–77], and hexamethylene diisocyanate [75]. The harvested collagen matrix in turn facilitates cellular repopulation and neovascularization of the implanted field to form granulation tissue and subsequent epithelialization. This process may be further enhanced through the addition of growth factors to the matrix. Autologous tissue grafts such as fascia lata and dura mater may also be used in certain cases for abdominal wall defects when contamination or risk of infection is high [78–80].

Allogenic mesh has higher recurrence rates than xenographic mesh [81]. Porcine dermal collagen mesh has been reported to have lower rates of seroma formation, decreased morbidity, lower failure rates, and longer time to failure in contaminated or infected fields when compared to allogenic dermal or porcine intestinal collagen-based mesh [82, 83]. Heavily cross-linked porcine dermal mesh offers a heightened foreign body reaction and an early inflammatory response [84, 85]. Lighter cross-linked porcine mesh has fewer adhesions and complications [86]. Cost is a major barrier to the widespread use of biologic mesh [87]. Furthermore, literature is inconclusive on the advantages of biologic mesh over synthetic mesh in the contaminated field [88–90].

13.4 Special Considerations: Prevention of Infectious Complications

Literature reports infection rates for abdominal wall hernia repairs from 0.5 to 30% [80, 91], with onset of infection up to 39 months after implantation [92, 93]. The most common contaminating organism is *Staphylococcus aureus* [94]. Other contaminating organisms include *Staphylococcus epidermidis*, *Escherichia coli*, anaerobes/*Enterococcus*, *Pseudomonas*, *Proteus*, and *Klebsiella*. Many factors including patient comorbidities, history of wound complications, operative urgency, operative complexity, technical approach, and mesh selection influence mesh infection rates [94–97]. Mesh type and construct may also impact rates of infection post-surgery. Overall, PP mesh has been associated with infection rates of 2.0–4.2% [98, 99] compared to 0.5–9.2% for ePTFE used in open hernia repairs [100–102].

13.4.1 Preventative Measures

Prevention is the best strategy to avoid bacterial contamination of the prosthesis during the initial implantation [97]. Below is a list of technical considerations to minimize the risk of mesh infection:

- Maintaining meticulous surgical technique
- Minimizing dissection and tissue undermining with selective use of closed suction drains to eliminate large dead spaces
- Minimizing mesh handling
- Minimizing contact between mesh and surrounding operative environment including the skin
- Donning new gloves when handling mesh for implantation
- Careful assessment of the wound to ensure good vascularization and absence of necrotic debris

13.4.2 Antibiotic Prophylaxis

In vitro studies indicate that biofilm formed by common bacteria such as *S. aureus* and *E. coli* plays a critical role in antimicrobial defense mechanism. Some studies have indicated a possible reduction of deep infections after inguinal hernia repair with application of a single dose of cefamandole applied directly to the wound or gentamicin placed on the mesh in vivo or in vitro [103–105]. Others have indicated that biofilms may be reduced with the use of diclofenac and ibuprofen, which may reduce infectious complications [106]. These studies have helped to form the foundation for antibiotic prophylaxis and antibiotic-coated mesh products.

However, antibiotic prophylaxis in elective hernia repair remains a debated topic. The 2009 European Hernia Society guidelines recommend avoiding the use of prophylaxis in low-risk patients but consider it in patients at a high risk (>4–5%) of surgical site infections [107]. Nevertheless, a review of 85,033 patients in the Herniamed Registry revealed that antibiotic prophylaxis significantly reduced the risk for postoperative infectious complications [108]. As expected, this benefit was less pronounced in laparoscopic procedures which utilize much smaller wounds. Current practice largely mandates at least one dose of prophylactic antibiotics 1 h prior to incision [109].

13.4.3 Other Strategies to Counter Mesh Infection

In vitro studies have shown that antibiotic-coated mesh products are effective at reducing the risk for postoperative SSIs [110–117]. Gentamicin-coated PVDF mesh is effective against all strains except gentamicin-resistant *Escherichia coli* [110–113]. Vancomycin-coated polyester and PP meshes are effective against *Staphylococcus aureus* and *Staphylococcus epidermidis* [114–118]. PP-coated ofloxacin or ofloxacin-rifampin mesh has limited cytotoxicity and effectively combats gram-positive and gram-negative organisms [115, 119]. One must always be cautious with the use of antibiotics to prevent the emergence of new antibacterial-resistant strains.

13.4.4 Novel Strategies to Counter Mesh Infection

Hydrophobic anti-adhesive substances such as polyvinylpyrrolidone, polyethylene glycol, polyethylene oxide, and polydimethylsiloxane substantially reduce the number and strength of microorganisms adhering to prosthetic surfaces [113, 120, 121]. Polydimethylsiloxane is also known to prevent adhesions when placed in direct contact with visceral loops.

The use of non-antibiotic agents with antimicrobial properties has recently gained attention because it minimizes the emergence of resistant strains [122]. For example, natural peptides are currently being used on catheters for their antimicrobial activity, which may also benefit prosthetic hernia repair [123]. Lysostaphin is a bacterial endopeptidase which when coated onto PP meshes contaminated in vitro or to collagen biomeshes in a contaminated subcutaneous implant model has shown antimicrobial properties against *Staphylococcus* [124–126]. Biopolymers are effective at preventing the formation of methicillin-resistant *Staphylococcus aureus* (MRSA) biofilms [127]. Allicin is a natural compound that inhibits the growth of *Staphylococcus epidermidis* [128]. An antiseptic triclosan, often applied onto PP mesh, has been shown to reduce the incidence of SSIs [129–132].

Recently, the use of thin porous PP mesh, implanted in the retromuscular space, has been described to be a safe alternative to biologic meshes in contaminated wounds [46]. This allows permanent repair of the hernia defect without incurring higher mesh infection rates.

13.4.5 Mesh Explantation

Mesh explantation is commonly indicated with resistant mesh infection [133]. Several studies have correlated mesh explantation with the use of ePTFE mesh, onlay position, and enterotomy during surgery and postoperative surgical site infections [94, 134]. Conservative treatments such as antimicrobial agents and drainage of fluid collections may allow salvation of the mesh repair when polyester and PP mesh is used in the repair but rarely for infected ePTFE mesh [1, 135].

13.5 Technical Considerations

13.5.1 Technical Approach

The field of abdominal wall reconstruction for complex hernias has historically employed open techniques to restore the abdominal wall anatomy [136–138]. Open approaches, while efficacious when performed properly, have been associated with higher perioperative morbidity and longer length of hospital stays [139–143]. Recently, the revolution of minimally invasive surgery (MIS) has extended to encompass the field of abdominal wall reconstruction. Although MIS approaches are technically more demanding, they have been shown to reduce wound morbidity, expedite return of bowel function, and decrease hospital length of stay. Furthermore, MIS repairs may substantially decrease overall hospital costs [144, 145]. These findings have in turn fueled new interest in adopting minimally invasive techniques using laparoscopic and robotic platforms to address hernias, increasing 40% since 2009 [146].

13.5.2 Mesh Selection

The selection of mesh for clean-contaminated or contaminated fields during ventral hernia repair remains debatable. The advantage of biologic mesh in contaminated operative fields is that it may reduce the need for additional procedures aimed at mesh explantation. The disadvantage of biologic mesh is that it predisposes patients for latent hernia recurrences. Recent studies have challenged these data contingent on an important technical point [46, 147]. In clean-contaminated cases, the use of medium-weight macroporous synthetic mesh offers the advantage of a more durable repair with improved bacterial clearance and faster integration into the abdominal wall when positioned in the retrorectus or preperitoneal spaces [46]. While the technical and financial significance of these findings may be tremendous [148], it is important to note that development of retromuscular or preperitoneal space is more time-consuming and technically challenging. Prospective multicenter trials are needed to confirm the reproducibility and lower morbidity associated with these techniques when performed in clean-contaminated fields.

13.5.3 Mesh Implantation

Mesh may be implanted as onlay, inlay, retrorectus sublay, or underlay relative to the defect (Fig. 13.1). Inlay mesh is secured to the defect fascial edges. This technique, although com-

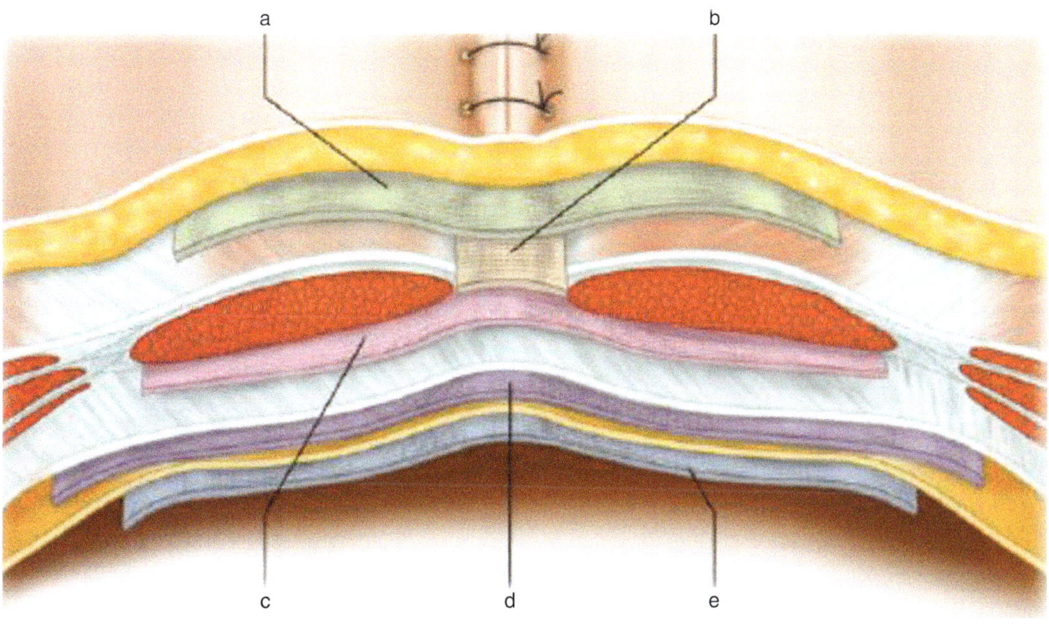

Fig. 13.1 Diagram of ventral hernia and mesh positioning (**a**) onlay mesh, (**b**) inlay mesh, (**c**) retrorectus sublay mesh, (**d**) underlay preperitoneal, (**e**) underlay intraperitoneal © Novitsky YW. Hernia Surgery. Cham: Springer; 2016

monly used in the past, may be falling out of favor due to high recurrence rates [136, 149].

Underlay techniques secure the mesh either to the peritoneum intraperitoneally or, more recently, to the posterior rectus sheath preperitoneally. The intraperitoneal underlay technique allowed direct contact between mesh and visceral contents of the abdomen leaving the repair prone to adhesions, mesh erosion, fistulas, and bowel obstruction [150]. The retrorectus repair, popularized by Rives and Stoppa, countered this problem by placing the mesh between the rectus abdominis muscle and its fascia [151–153]. A 2013 systematic review of 62 articles of ventral hernia repairs concluded that the hernia recurrence rates were the lowest for retrorectus (5%) and underlay (7.5%) mesh placements when compared to onlay (17%) or interposition (17%) placements [154].

The increasing utilization of minimally invasive techniques along with recent data supporting primary closure of the abdominal wall defect to enhance mesh incorporation has led to modifications of the traditional sublay placement of mesh. One of the most significant developments in this realm has been laparoscopic transversus abdominis release to reconstruct the linea alba [151, 155, 156]. Additionally, the MIS approach with mesh implantation into the retrorectus or preperitoneal spaces have allowed for superior repair of more complex defects with reduced morbidity for patients. Therefore, the retrorectus and the more recently described preperitoneal mesh placement are likely the safest options for hernia repair, as long as the surgeon is trained and is facile with these techniques.

13.5.4 Mesh Fixation

Mesh fixation techniques are many and can range from transfascial sutures to adhesive agents. While transfascial fixation has been deemed a more stable approach to secure mesh, the use of fibrin sealant or other biologic glues in place of transfascial sutures has been reported as an alternative, with support from studies that suggest reduced incidence of chronic postoperative pain (>3 months), impacting up to 27% of patients [157–168]. The pathophysiology of chronic pain associated with transfascial sutures is thought to stem from entrapment of neurovascular fibers running in between internal oblique and transversus abdominis muscles [160–165]. Patients with transfascial suture mesh fixation may be 12 times more likely to report pain at the 6-month follow-up when compared to those with fibrin glue mesh fixation [165].

While some studies have correlated the use of glue fixation with increased seroma rates [166], recent studies have contradicted those findings [164, 165, 167]. Hernia recurrence rates continue to be one of the most important outcome measures in quality in hernia care. In retromuscular repairs, it has been reported that the use of fibrin glue does not increase the rate of hernia recurrence when compared to transfascial fixation [165]. The recurrence rate for fibrin glue fixation of mesh in the retromuscular position at a median follow-up of 1 year is 2.5% [166]. It remains to be seen whether recurrence rates increase at longer follow-ups. The key to the use of glue fixation in retromuscular or preperitoneal spaces is adequate dissection to develop an adequate space for wide mesh placement. There is yet no long-term data regarding complete elimination of fixation in combination with retromuscular dissection.

Macroporous synthetic meshes rapidly integrate into the retromuscular space [168, 169]. Once integrated, mesh implant serves to provide the needed shear forces to off-load the tension on the defect closure, and the use of transfascial fixation may be less important. Heavyweight and biologic meshes take longer to integrate than macroporous meshes [168, 169]; therefore, many still recommend the use of transfascial or more permanent fixation methods with heavyweight and biologic meshes.

Inconsistent with current cost containment efforts, the immediate costs associated with use of adhesive fixatives may be as high as $1000 per case [165]. It remains to be determined if the costs incurred with use of fixatives

Take-Home Points

- Mesh reinforcement is seen by most as the standard of care in most hernia repairs for its ability to decrease hernia recurrence rates.
- There is no one ideal mesh product for every clinical situation.
- Hernia repair and choice of prosthetic materials must be tailored to specific patient factors.
- Minimizing wound-related complications may decrease recurrence rates.

will be offset by lowered recurrence rates or other benefits such as reduced treatments for chronic pain.

Suggested Readings

Novitsky YW. Hernia surgery. Cham: Springer; 2016.

Todros S, Pavan PG, Natali AN. Synthetic surgical meshes used in abdominal wall surgery: Part I-materials and structural conformation. J Biomed Mater Res B Appl Biomater. 2017;105(3):689.

References

1. Wood J. Lectures on hernia and its radical cure. Br Med J. 1885;1:1279–83.
2. Thomas A, Rogers A. Edoardo Bassini and the wound that inspires. World J Surg. 2004;28(110): 1060–2.
3. George CD, Ellis H. The results of incisional hernia repair: a twelve year review. Ann R Coll Surg Engl. 1986;68(4):185–7.
4. Usher FC, Ochsner J, Tuttle LLD Jr. Use of Marlex mesh in the repair of incisional hernias. Am Surg. 1958;24:969.
5. Lichtenstein IL, Shulman AG, Amid PK, et al. The tension free hernioplasty. Am J Surg. 1989;157:188–93.
6. Scott NW, McCormack K, Graham P, et al. Open mesh versus non-mesh for repair of femoral and inguinal hernia. Cochrane Database Syst Rev. 2002;4:CD002197.
7. EU Hernia Trialists Collaboration. Repair of groin hernia with synthetic mesh: meta-analysis of randomized controlled trials. Ann Surg. 2002;235:322–32.
8. EU Hernia Trialists Collaboration. Mesh compared with non-mesh methods of open groin hernia repair: systematic review of randomized controlled trials. Br J Surg. 2000;87:854–9.
9. Butler DL, Goldstein SA, Guilak F. Functional tissue engineering: the role of biomechanics. J Biomech Eng. 2000;122:570–5.
10. Rastegarpour A, Cheung M, Vardhan M, Ibrahim MM, Butler CE, Levinson H. Surgical mesh for ventral incisional hernia repairs: understanding mesh design. Plast Surg. 2016;24(1):41.
11. Cobb WS, Peindl RM, Zerey M, Carbonell AM, Heniford BT. Mesh terminology 101. Hernia. 2009;13:1–6.
12. Bilsel Y, Abci I. The search for ideal hernia repair; mesh materials and types. Int J Surg. 2012;10(6):317–21.
13. Martakos P, Karwoski T. Healing characteristics of hybrid and conventional polytetrafluoroethylene vascular grafts. ASAIO J. 1995;41:M735–41.
14. Klinge U, Klosterhalfen B. Modified classification of surgical meshes for hernia repair based on the analyses of 1,000 explanted meshes. Hernia. 2012;16: 251–8.
15. Collage RD, Rosengart MR. Abdominal wall infections with in situ mesh. Surg Infect. 2010;11:311–8.
16. Sanchez VM, Abi-Haidar YE, Itani KM. Mesh infection in ventral incisional hernia repair: Incidence, contributing factors, and treatment. Surg Infect. 2011;12:205–10.
17. Bellon JM, Contreras LA, Bujan J. Ultrastructural alterations of polytetrafluoroethylene prostheses implanted in abdominal wall provoked by infection: Clinical and experimental study. World J Surg. 2000;24:528–31.
18. Klosterhalfen B, Klinge U, Rosch R, Junge K. Long-term inertness of meshes. In: Schumpelick V, Nyhus L, editors. Meshes: benefits and risks. Berlin: Springer; 2004. p. 170–8.
19. Enoch S, Leaper DJ. Basic science of wound healing. Surgery. 2005;23:37–42.
20. Brown CN, Finch JG. Which mesh for hernia repair? Ann R Coll Surg Engl. 2010;92:272–8.
21. Junge K, Klinge U, Rosch R, et al. Functional and morphologic properties of a modified mesh for inguinal hernia repair. World J Surg. 2002;26:1472–80.
22. Welty G, Kinge U, Klosterhalfen B, et al. Functional impairment and complaints following incisional hernia repair with different polypropylene meshes. Hernia. 2001;5:142–7.
23. Klinge U, Junge K, Stumpf M, et al. Functional and morphological evaluation of a low-weight, monofilament polypropylene mesh for hernia repair. J Biomed Mater Res. 2002;63:129–36.
24. Nguyen PT, Asarias JR, Pierce LM. Influence of a new monofilament polyester mesh on inflammation and matrix remodeling. J Investig Surg. 2012;25(5):330.

25. Brandt CJ, Kammer D, Fiebeler A, Klinge U. Beneficial effects of hydrocortisone or spironolactone coating on foreign body response to mesh biomaterial in a mouse model. J Biomed Mater Res A. 2011;99:335–43.
26. Asarias JR, et al. Influence of mesh materials on the expression of mediators involved in wound healing. J Investig Surg. 2011;24(2):87–98.
27. Sanders D, Lambie J, Bond P, Moate R, Steer JA. An in vitro study assessing the effect of mesh morphology and suture fixation on bacterial adherence. Hernia. 2013;17(6):779–89.
28. Blatnik JA, et al. In vivo analysis of the morphologic characteristics of synthetic mesh to resist MRSA adherence. J Gastrointest Surg. 2012;16(11):2139–44.
29. Bryan N, et al. In vitro activation of human leukocytes in response to contact with synthetic hernia meshes. Clin Biochem. 2012;45(9):672–6.
30. Orenstein SB, et al. Comparative analysis of histopathologic effects of synthetic meshes based on material, weight, and pore size in mice. J Surg Res. 2012;176(2):423–9.
31. Schmidbauer S, et al. Heavy-weight versus low-weight polypropylene meshes for open sublay mesh repair of incisional hernia. Eur J Med Res. 2005;10(6):247–53.
32. Cobb WS, et al. Textile analysis of heavy weight, midweight, and light weight polypropylene mesh in a porcine ventral hernia model. J Surg Res. 2006;136(1):1–7.
33. Cobb WS, Kercher KW, Heniford BT. The argument for lightweight polypropylene mesh in hernia repair. Surg Innov. 2005;12(1):63–9.
34. Petro CC, Nahabet EH, Criss CN, Orenstein SB, von Recum HA, Novitsky YW, et al. Central failures of lightweight monofilament polyester mesh causing hernia recurrence: a cautionary note. Hernia. 2015;19(1):155–9.
35. Todros S, Pavan PG, Natali AN. Synthetic surgical meshes used in abdominal wall surgery: Part I-materials and structural conformation. J Biomed Mater Res B Appl Biomater. 2017;105(3):689.
36. Gonzalez R, Fugate K, McClusky D, Ritter EM, Lederman A, Dillehay D, Smith CD, Ramshaw BJ. Relationship between tissue ingrowth and mesh contraction. World J Surg. 2005;29:1038–43.
37. Burger JW, Halm JA, Wijsmuller AR, ten Raa S, Jeekel J. Evaluation of new prosthetic meshes for ventral hernia repair. Surg Endosc. 2006;20:1320–5.
38. Wolstenholme JT. Use of commercial Dacron fabric in the repair of inguinal hernias and abdominal wall defects. Arch Surg. 1956;73:1004–8.
39. Maarek JM, Guidoin R, Aubin M, Prud'homme RE. Molecular weight characterization of virgin and explanted polyester arterial prostheses. J Biomed Mater Res. 1984;18:881–94.
40. Klinge U, Junge K, Spellerberg B, Piroth C, Klosterhalfen B, Schumpelick V. Do multifilament alloplastic meshes increase the infection rate? Analysis of the polymeric surface, the bacteria adherence, and the in vivo consequences in a rat model. J Biomed Mater Res. 2002;63(6):765.
41. Hanna M, Dissanaike S. Mesh ingrowth with concomitant bacterial infection resulting in inability to explant: a failure of mesh salvage. Hernia. 2015;19(2):339.
42. Medtronic. Hernia repair. http://www.medtronic.com/covidien/products/hernia-repair/. Accessed 11 May 2017.
43. Cobb WS, Kercher KW, Heniford BT. Laparoscopic repair of incisional hernias. Surg Clin North Am. 2005;85:91–103.
44. Robinson TN, Clarke JH, Schoen J, Walsh MD. Major mesh related complications following hernia repair. Surg Endosc. 2005;19:1556–60.
45. Read RC. Milestones in the history of hernia surgery: prosthetic repair. Hernia. 2004;8:8–14.
46. Majumder A, Winder JS, Wen Y, Pauli EM, Belyansky I, Novitsky YW. Comparative analysis of biologic versus synthetic mesh outcomes in contaminated hernia repairs. Surgery. 2016;160(4):828.
47. Laroche G, Marois Y, Guidoin R, King MW, Martin L, How T, Douville Y. Polyvinylidene fluoride (PVDF) as a biomaterial: From polymeric raw material to monofilament vascular suture. J Biomed Mater Res. 1995;29:1525–36.
48. Klinge U, Klosterhalfen B, Ottinger AP, Junge K, Schumpelick V. PVDF as a new polymer for the construction of surgical meshes. Biomaterials. 2002;23:3487–93.
49. Laroche G, Marois Y, Schwarz E, Guidoin R, King MW, Paris E, Douville Y. Polyvinylidene fluoride monofilament sutures: can they be used safely for long-term anastomoses in the thoracic aorta? Artif Organs. 1995;19:1190–9.
50. Dayton MT, Buchele BA, Shirazi SS, Hunt LB. Use of an absorbable mesh to repair contaminated abdominal-wall defects. Arch Surg. 1986;121:954–60.
51. Novitsky YW. Hernia surgery. Cham: Springer; 2016.
52. Engelsman AF, van der Mei HC, Ploeg RJ, Busscher HJ. The phenomenon of infection with abdominal wall reconstruction. Biomaterials. 2007;28:2314–27.
53. Rosen MJ, Bauer JJ, Harmaty M, et al. Multicenter, prospective, longitudinal study of the recurrence, surgical site infection, and quality of life after contaminated ventral hernia repair using biosynthetic absorbable mesh: the COBRA study. Ann Surg. 2017;265(1):205–11.
54. Deeken CR, Matthews BD. Characterization of the mechanical strength, resorption properties, and histologic characteristics of a fully absorbable material (poly-4-hydroxybutyrate-PHASIX mesh) in a porcine model of hernia repair. ISRN Surg. 2013;2013:238067.
55. Martin DP, Badhwar A, Shah DV, et al. Characterization of poly-4-hydroxybutyrate mesh for hernia repair applications. J Surg Res. 2013;184:766–73.

56. Hjort H, Mathisen T, Alves A, Clermont G, Boutrand JP. Three year results from a preclinical implantation study of a long-term resorbable surgical mesh with time-dependent mechanical characteristics. Hernia. 2012;16:191–7.
57. Peeters E, van Barneveld KW, Schreinemacher MH, et al. One-year outcome of biological and synthetic bioabsorbable meshes for augmentation of large abdominal wall defects in a rabbit model. J Surg Res. 2013;180:274–83.
58. Ruiz-Jasbon F, Norrby J, Ivarsson ML, Bjorck S. Inguinal hernia repair using a synthetic long-term resorbable mesh: results from a 3-year prospective safety and performance study. Hernia. 2014;18:723–30.
59. Zhang AY, Bates SJ, Morrow E, Pham H, Pham B, Chang J. Tissue-engineered intrasynovial tendons: optimization of acellularization and seeding. J Rehabil Res Dev. 2009;46:489–98.
60. Rieder E, Kasimir MT, Silberhumer G, Seebacher G, Wolner E, Simon P, et al. Decellularization protocols of porcine heart valves differ importantly in efficiency of cell removal and susceptibility of the matrix to recellularization with human vascular cells. J Thorac Cardiovasc Surg. 2004;127:399–405.
61. Cartmell JS, Dunn MG. Effect of chemical treatments on tendon cellularity and mechanical properties. J Biomed Mater Res. 2000;49:134–40.
62. Woods T, Gratzer PF. Effectiveness of three extraction techniques in the development of a decellularized bone-anterior cruciate ligament-bone graft. Biomaterials. 2005;26:7339–49.
63. Deeken CR, White AK, Bachman SL, Ramshaw BJ, Cleveland DS, Loy TS, et al. Method of preparing a decellularized porcine tendon using tributyl phosphate. J Biomed Mater Res B Appl Biomater. 2011;96:199–206.
64. Meyer SR, Chiu B, Churchill TA, Zhu L, Lakey JR, Ross DB. Comparison of aortic valve allograft decellularization techniques in the rat. J Biomed Mater Res Part A. 2006;79:254–62.
65. Lynch AP, Ahearne M. Strategies for developing decellularized corneal scaffolds. Exp Eye Res. 2013;108:42–7.
66. Gillies AR, Smith LR, Lieber RL, Varghese S. Method for decellularizing skeletal muscle without detergents or proteolytic enzymes. Tissue Eng Part C Methods. 2011;17:383–9.
67. Gratzer PF, Harrison RD, Woods T. Matrix alteration and not residual sodium dodecyl sulfate cytotoxicity affects the cellular repopulation of a decellularized matrix. Tissue Eng. 2006;12:2975–83.
68. Horowitz B, Bonomo R, Prince AM, Chin SN, Brotman B, Shulman RW. Solvent/detergent-treated plasma: a virus-inactivated substitute for fresh frozen plasma. Blood. 1992;79:826–31.
69. Badylak SF. Decellularized allogeneic and xenogeneic tissue as a bioscaffold for regenerative medicine: factors that influence the host response. Ann Biomed Eng. 2014;42:1517–27.
70. Scales JT. Tissue reactions to synthetic materials. Proc R Soc Med. 1953;46:647–52.
71. Damink LHHO, Dijkstra PJ, vanLuyn MJA, vanWachem PB, Nieuwenhuis P, Feijen J. Cross-linking of dermal sheep collagen using a water-soluble carbodiimide. Biomaterials. 1996;17:765–73.
72. Abraham GA, Murray J, Billiar K, Sullivan SJ. Evaluation of the porcine intestinal collagen layer as a biomaterial. J Biomed Mater Res. 2000;51:442–52.
73. Billiar K, Murray J, Laude D, Abraham G, Bachrach N. Effects of carbodiimide crosslinking conditions on the physical properties of laminated intestinal submucosa. J Biomed Mater Res. 2001;56:101–8.
74. Olde Damink LH, Dijkstra PJ, van Luyn MJ, van Wachem PB, Nieuwenhuis P, Feijen J. vitro degradation of dermal sheep collagen cross-linked using a water-soluble carbodiimide. Biomaterials. 1996;17:679–84.
75. Khor E. Methods for the treatment of collagenous tissues for bioprostheses. Biomaterials. 1997;18:95–105.
76. Courtman DW, Errett BF, Wilson GJ. The role of crosslinking in modification of the immune response elicited against xenogenic vascular acellular matrices. J Biomed Mater Res. 2001;55:576–86.
77. HardinYoung J, Carr RM, Downing GJ, Condon KD, Termin PL. Modification of native collagen reduces antigenicity but preserves cell compatibility. Biotechnol Bioeng. 1996;49:675–82.
78. Tiengo C, Giatsidis G, Azzena B. Fascialata allografts as biological mesh in abdominal wall repair: preliminary outcomes from a retrospective case series. Plast Reconstr Surg. 2013;132:631E–9E.
79. Miyamoto Y, Watanabe M, Ishimoto T, Baba Y, Iwagami S, Sakamoto Y, Yoshida N, Masuguchi S, Ihn H, Baba H. Fascialata on lay patch for repairing infected incisional hernias. Surg Today. 2015;45:121–4.
80. Kama NA, Coskun T, Yavuz H, Doganay M, Reis E, Akat AZ. Autologous skin graft, human dura mater and polypropylene mesh for the repair of ventral abdominal hernias: an experimental study. Eur J Surg. 1999;165:1080–5.
81. Beale EW, Hoxworth RE, Livingston EH, Trussler AP. The role of biologic mesh in abdominal wall reconstruction: a systematic review of the current literature. Am J Surg. 2012;204:510–7.
82. Slater NJ, van der Kolk M, Hendriks T, van Goor H, Bleichrodt RP. Biologic grafts for ventral hernia repair: a systematic review. Am J Surg. 2013;205:220–30.
83. Smart NJ, Marshall M, Daniels IR. Biological meshes: a review of their use in abdominal wall hernia repairs. Surgeon. 2012;10:159–71.
84. Novitsky YW, Rosen MJ. The biology of biologics: basic science and clinical concepts. Plast Reconstr Surg. 2012;130:9S–17S.
85. Clemens MW, Selber JC, Liu J, et al. Bovine versus porcine acellular dermal matrix for complex

abdominal wall reconstruction. Plast Reconstr Surg. 2013;131:71–9.
86. Butler CE, Burns NK, Campbell KT, Mathur AB, Jaffari MV, Rios CN. Comparison of cross-linked and non-cross-linked porcine acellular dermal matrices for ventral hernia repair. J Am Coll Surg. 2010;211:368–76.
87. Peppas G, Gkegkes ID, Makris MC, Falagas ME. Biological mesh in hernia repair, abdominal wall defects, and reconstruction and treatment of pelvic organ prolapse: a review of the clinical evidence. Am Surg. 2010;76:1290–9.
88. Bellows CF, Smith A, Malsbury J, Helton WS. Repair of incisional hernias with biological prosthesis: a systematic review of current evidence. Am J Surg. 2013;205:85–101.
89. Ditzel M, Deerenberg EB, Grotenhuis N, et al. Biologic meshes are not superior to synthetic meshes in ventral hernia repair: an experimental study with long-term follow-up evaluation. Surg Endosc. 2013;27:3654–62.
90. Hiles M, Record Ritchie RD, Altizer AM. Are biologic grafts effective for hernia repair? A systematic review of the literature. Surg Innov. 2009;16:26–37.
91. Falagas ME, Kasiakou SK. Mesh-related infections after hernia repair surgery. Clin Microbiol Infect. 2005;11:3–8.
92. Coda A, Botto-Micca F, Botto-Micca F. Reoperations for chronic infections following prosthetic hernia repair. Hernia. 1998;2:163–7.
93. Leber GE, Garb JL, Alexander AI, et al. Long-term complications associated with prosthetic repair of incisional hernias. Arch Surg. 1998;133:378–82.
94. Bueno-Lledó J, Torregrosa-Gallud A, Sala-Hernandez A, Carbonell-Tatay F, Pastor PG, Diana SB, et al. Predictors of mesh infection and explantation after abdominal wall hernia repair. Am J Surg. 2017;213(1):50.
95. Bueno J, Sosa Y, Gomez I, et al. Infeccion de la protesis en la reparacion herniaria. Nuestra experiencia en 5 anos. Cir Esp. 2009;85:158–63.
96. Petersen S, Henke G, Freitag M, et al. Deep prosthesis infection in incisional hernia repair: predictive factors and clinical outcome. Eur J Surg. 2001;167:453–7.
97. Mann D, Prout J, Havranek E, et al. Late-onset deep prosthetic infection following mesh repair of inguinal hernia. Am J Surg. 1998;176:12–4.
98. Dunne JR, Malone DL, Tracy JK, et al. Abdominal wall hernias: risk factors for infection and resource utilization. J Surg Res. 2003;111:78–84.
99. Neumayer L, Giobbie-Hurder A, Jonasson O, et al. Open mesh versus laparoscopic mesh repair of inguinal hernia. N Engl J Med. 2004;350:1819–27.
100. Gonzalez AU, De la Portilla F, Albarran GC. Large incisional hernia repair using intraperitoneal placement of ePTFE. Am J Surg. 1999;177:291–3.
101. LeBlanc KA. Laparoscopic incisional and ventral hernia repair: how to avoid and handle complications. Hernia. 2004;8:323–31. 24
102. Berger D, Bientzle M, Muller A. Postoperative complications after laparoscopic incisional hernia repair. Surg Endosc. 2002;16:1720–3.
103. Lazorthes F, Chiotasso P, Massip P, et al. Local antibiotic prophylaxis in inguinal hernia repair. Surg Gynecol Obstet. 1992;175:569–70.
104. Musella M, Guido A, Musella S. Collagen tampons as aminoglycoside carriers to reduce postoperative infection rate in prosthetic repair of groin hernias. Eur J Surg. 2001;167(2):130.
105. Wiegering A, Sinha B, Spor L, et al. Gentamicin for prevention of intraoperative mesh contamination: demonstration of high bactericide effect (in vitro) and low systemic bioavailability (in vivo). Hernia. 2014;18:691–700.
106. Reslinski A, Dabrowiecki S, Gowacka K. The impact of diclofenac and ibuprofen on biofilm formation on the surface of polypropylene mesh. Hernia. 2015;19:179–85.
107. Simons MP, Aufenacker T, Bay-Nielsen M, et al. European Hernia Society guidelines on the treatment of inguinal hernia in adult patients. Hernia. 2009;13:343–403.
108. Köckerling F, Bittner R, Jacob D, Schug-Pass C, Laurenz C, Adolf D, et al. Do we need antibiotic prophylaxis in endoscopic inguinal hernia repair? Results of the Herniamed Registry. Surg Endosc. 2015;29(12):3741.
109. The Centers for Medicare and Medicaid Services. Surgical care improvement project. https://innovation.cms.gov/Files/x/ACE-Quality-Measures.pdf. Accessed 13 Aug 2017.
110. Junge K, Rosch R, Klinge U, et al. Gentamicin supplementation of polyvinylidenfluoride mesh materials for infection prophylaxis. Biomaterials. 2005;26:787–93.
111. Klink CD, Binnebosel M, Lambertz A, et al. In vitro and in vivo characteristics of gentamicin-supplemented poly-vinylidenfluoride mesh materials. J Biomed Mater Res A. 2012;100:1195–202.
112. Junge K, Klinge U, Rosch R, et al. Improved collagen type I/III ratio at the interface of gentamicin-supplemented polyvinylidenfluoride mesh materials. Langenbeck's Arch Surg. 2007;392:465–71.
113. Binnebosel M, von Trotha KT, Ricken C, et al. Gentamicin supplemented polyvinylidenfluoride mesh materials enhance tissue integration due to a transcriptionally reduced MMP-2 protein expression. BMC Surg. 2012;12:1.
114. Fernandez-Gutierrez M, Olivares E, Pascual G, et al. Low-density polypropylene meshes coated with resorbable and biocompatible hydrophilic polymers as controlled release agents of antibiotics. Acta Biomater. 2013;9:6006–18.
115. Guillaume O, Garric X, Lavigne JP, et al. Multilayer, degradable coating as a carrier for the sustained release of antibiotics: preparation and antimicrobial efficacy in vitro. J Control Release. 2012;162:492–501.
116. Letouzey V, Lavigne JP, Garric X, et al. Is degradable antibiotic coating for synthetic meshes provide

protection against experimental animal infection after fascia repair? J Biomed Mater Res B Appl Biomater. 2012;100:471–9.
117. Laurent T, Kacem I, Blanchemain N, et al. Cyclodextrin and maltodextrin finishing of a polypropylene abdominal wall implant for the prolonged delivery of ciprofloxacin. Acta Biomater. 2011;7:3141–9.
118. Harth KC, Rosen MJ, Thatiparti TR, et al. Antibiotic releasing mesh coating to reduce prosthetic sepsis: an in vivo study. J Surg Res. 2010;163:337–43.
119. Guillaume O, Lavigne JP, Lefranc O, et al. New antibiotic eluting mesh used for soft tissue reinforcement. Acta Biomater. 2011;7:3390–7.
120. Saldarriaga Fernandez IC, Mei HC, Metzger S, et al. In vitro and in vivo comparisons of staphylococcal biofilm formation on a cross-linked poly(ethylene glycol)-based polymer coating. Acta Biomater. 2010;6:1119–24.
121. Legeay G, Poncin-Epaillard F, Arciola CR. New surfaces with hydrophilic/hydrophobic characteristics in relation to (no)bioadhesion. Int J Artif Organs. 2006;29:453–61.
122. Yurko Y, McDeavitt K, Kumar RS, et al. Antibacterial mesh: a novel technique involving naturally occurring cellular proteins. Surg Innov. 2012;19:20–6.
123. von Eiff C, Jansen B, Kohnen W, Becker K. Infections associated with medical devices: pathogenesis, management and prophylaxis. Drugs. 2005;65:179–214.
124. Belyansky I, Tsirline VB, Montero PN, et al. Lysostaphin coated mesh prevents staphylococcal infection and significantly improves survival in a contaminated surgical field. Am Surg. 2011;77:1025–31.
125. Belyansky I, Tsirline VB, Martin TR, et al. The addition of lysostaphin dramatically improves survival, protects porcine biomesh from infection, and improves graft tensile shear strength. J Surg Res. 2011;171:409–15.
126. Satishkumar R, Sankar S, Yurko Y, et al. Evaluation of the antimicrobial activity of lysostaphin-coated hernia repair meshes. Antimicrob Agents Chemother. 2011;55:4379–85.
127. Dinjaski N, Fernandez-Gutierrez M, Selvam S, et al. PHACOS, a functionalized bacterial polyester with bactericidal activity against methicillin-resistant Staphylococcus aureus. Biomaterials. 2014;35:14–24.
128. Zhai H, Pan J, Pang E, Bai B. Lavage with allicin in combination with vancomycin inhibits biofilm formation by Staphylococcus epidermidis in a rabbit model of prosthetic joint infection. PLoS One. 2014;9:e102760.
129. Edmiston CE, Seabrook GR, Goheen MP, et al. Bacterial adherence to surgical sutures: can antibacterial-coated sutures reduce the risk of microbial contamination? J Am Coll Surg. 2006;203:481–9.
130. Rasic Z, Schwarz D, Adam VN, et al. Efficacy of antimicrobial triclosan-coated polyglactin 910 (Vicryl_ Plus) suture for closure of the abdominal wall after colorectal surgery. Coll Antropol. 2011;35:439–43.
131. Hoshino S, Yoshida Y, Tanimura S, et al. A study of the efficacy of antibacterial sutures for surgical site infection: a retrospective controlled trial. Int Surg. 2013;98:129–32.
132. Cxakmak A, Cirpanli Y, Bilensoy E, et al. Antibacterial activity of triclosan chitosan coated graft on hernia graft infection model. Int J Pharm. 2009;381:214–9.
133. Trunzo JA, Ponsky JL, Jin J, et al. A novel approach for salvaging infected prosthetic mesh after ventral hernia repair. Hernia. 2009;13:545–9.
134. Hawn M, Gray S, Snyder C, et al. Predictors of mesh explantation after incisional hernia repair. Am J Surg. 2011;202:28–33.
135. Brown RH, Subramanian A, Hwang CS, et al. Comparison of infectious complications with synthetic mesh in ventral hernia repair. Am J Surg. 2013;205:182–7.
136. Breuing K, Butler CE, Ferzoco S, et al. Incisional ventral hernias: review of the literature and recommendations regarding the grading and technique of repair. Surgery. 2010;148:544–58.
137. Novitsky YW, Elliott HL, Orenstein SB, et al. Transversus abdominis muscle release: a novel approach to posterior component separation during complex abdominal wall reconstruction. Am J Surg. 2012;204:709–16.
138. Mason RJ, Moazzez A, Sohn HJ, et al. Laparoscopic versus open anterior abdominal wall hernia repair: 30-day morbidity and mortality using the ACS-NSQIP database. Ann Surg. 2011;254(4):641–52.
139. Heniford BT, Park A, Ramshaw BJ, et al. Laparoscopic repair of ventral hernias: nine years' experience with 850 consecutive hernias. Ann Surg. 2003;238:391–9.
140. Itani KM, Hur K, Kim LT, et al. Comparison of laparoscopic and open repair with mesh for the treatment of ventral incisional hernia: a randomized trial. Arch Surg. 2010;145:322–8.
141. Sauerland S, Walgenbach M, Habermalz B, et al. Laparoscopic versus open surgical techniques for ventral or incisional hernia repair. Cochrane Database Syst Rev. 2011;3:CD007781.
142. Salvilla SA, Thusu S, Panesar SS. Analyzing the benefits of laparoscopic hernia repair compared to open repair: a meta-analysis of observational studies. J Minim Access Surg. 2012;8:111–7.
143. Zhang Y, Zhou H, Chai Y, et al. Laparoscopic versus open incisional and ventral hernia repair: a systematic review and meta-analysis. World J Surg. 2014;38:2233–40.
144. Weltz AS, Turcotte JT, Sibia US, Zakharov E, Wu N, Turner TR, Zahiri HR, Belyansky I. The trend toward minimally invasive complex abdominal wall reconstruction: is it worth it? Surg Endosc. 2017. https://doi.org/10.1007/s00464-017-5850-0.
145. Martin-del-Campo LA, Weltz AS, Belyansky I, Novitsky YW. Comparative analysis of perioperative outcomes of robotic versus open transversus abdominis release. Surg Endosc. 2016;32(2):840–5.

146. Savitch SL, Shah PC. Closing the gap between the laparoscopic and open approaches to abdominal wall hernia repair: a trend and outcomes analysis of the ACS-NSQIP database. Surg Endosc. 2016;30(3):3267–78.
147. Chamieh J, Tan WH, Ramirez R, Nohra E, Apakama C, Symons W. Synthetic versus biologic mesh in single-stage repair of complex abdominal wall defects in a contaminated field. Surg Infect. 2017;18(2):112–8.
148. Reynolds D, Davenport DL, Korosec RL, Roth JS. Financial implications of ventral hernia repair: a hospital cost analysis. J Gastrointest Surg. 2013;17(1):159–66.
149. Hawn MT, Snyder CW, Graham LA, Gray SH, Finan KR, Vick CC. Long-term follow-up of technical outcomes for incisional hernia repair. J Am Coll Surg. 2010;210(5):648–55.
150. de Vries Reilingh TS, van Geldere D, Langenhorst B, de Jong D, van der Wilt GJ, van Goor H, Bleichrodt RP. Repair of large midline incisional hernias with polypropylene mesh: comparison of three operative techniques. Hernia. 2004;8(1):56–9.
151. Rives J, Lardennois B, Pire JC, Hibon J. Large incisional hernias. The importance of flail abdomen and of subsequent respiratory disorders. Chirurgie. 1973;99(8):547–63.
152. Belyansky I, Zahiri HR, Park A. Laparoscopic transversus abdominis release, a novel minimally invasive approach to complex abdominal wall reconstruction. Surg Innov. 2016;23(2):134.
153. Stoppa RE. The treatment of complicated groin and incisional hernias. World J Surg. 1989;13(5):545–54.
154. Albino FP, Patel KM, Nahabedian MY, Sosin M, Attinger CE, Bhanot P. Does mesh location matter in abdominal wall reconstruction? A systematic review of the literature and a summary of recommendations. Plast Reconstr Surg. 2013;132(5):1295–304.
155. Cheesborough JE, Dumanian GA. Simultaneous prosthetic mesh abdominal wall reconstruction with abdominoplasty for ventral hernia and severe rectus diastasis repairs. Plast Reconstr Surg. 2015;135:268–76.
156. Novitsky YW, Fayezizadeh M, Orenstein SB. Outcomes of posterior component separation with transversus abdominis muscle release and synthetic mesh sublay reinforcement. Ann Surg. 2016;264:226–32.
157. Hirsch H, Nagatomo K, Gefen J, et al. Mesh fixation with fibrin sealant in totally extraperitoneal hernia repair. J Laparoendosc Adv Surg Tech A. 2016;27(3):259–63.
158. Berney CR, Descallar J. Review of 1000 fibrin glue mesh fixation during endoscopic totally extraperitoneal (TEP) inguinal hernia repair. Surg Endosc. 2016;30(10):4544–52.
159. Kukleta JF, Freytag C, Weber M. Efficiency and safety of mesh fixation in laparoscopic inguinal hernia repair using *n*-butyl cyanoacrylate: long-term biocompatibility in over 1300 mesh fixations. Hernia. 2012;16(2):153–62.
160. Iqbal CW, Pham TH, Joseph A, et al. Long-term outcome of 254 complex incisional hernia repairs using the modified Rives-Stoppa technique. World J Surg. 2007;31:2398–404.
161. Hanna EM, Byrd JF, Moskowitz M, et al. Outcomes of a prospective multi-center trial of a second-generation composite mesh for open ventral hernia repair. Hernia. 2014;18(1):81–9.
162. Vermeulen J, Alwayn I, Stassen LP. Prolonged abdominal wall pain caused by transfascial sutures used in the laparoscopic repair of incisional hernia. Surg Endosc. 2003;17(9):1497.
163. LeBlanc KA. Laparoscopic incisional hernia repair: are transfascial sutures necessary? A review of the literature. Surg Endosc. 2007;21(4):508–13.
164. Brill JB, Turner PL. Long-term outcomes with transfascial sutures versus tacks in laparoscopic ventral hernia repair: a review. Am Surg. 2011;77(4):458–65.
165. Weltz AS, Sibia US, Zahiri HR, Schoeneborn A, Park A, Belyansky I. Operative outcomes after open abdominal wall reconstruction with retromuscular mesh fixation using fibrin glue versus transfascial sutures. Am Surg. 2017;83(9):937–42.
166. Azoury SC, Rodriquez-Unda Nm Soares KC, et al. The effect of TISSEEL fibrin sealant on seroma formation following complex abdominal wall hernia repair: a single institutional review and derived cost analysis. Hernia. 2015;19(6):935–42.
167. Canziani M, Frattini F, Cavalli M, et al. Sutureless mesh fibrin glue incisional hernia repair. Hernia. 2009;13(6):625.
168. Köhler G, Koch OO, Antoniou SA, et al. Prevention of subcutaneous seroma formation in open ventral hernia repair using a new low-thrombin fibrin sealant. World J Surg. 2014;38(11):2797.
169. Sadava EE, Krpata DM, Gao Y, et al. Wound healing process and mediators: implications for modulations for hernia repair and mesh integration. J Biomed Mater Res A. 2014;102(1):295–302.

Fundamentals of Basic Laparoscopic Setup

14

Marc Rafols, Navid Ajabshir, and Kfir Ben-David

14.1 Introduction

Laparoscopic surgery has rapidly expanded during the last few decades but has been around for more than a century. Earliest reports of endoscopy of natural orifices date back to 936–1013 A.D. in medieval Spain where an Arabian by the name of Albukasim was performing primitive esophagoscopies to remove foreign bodies and possibly early cystoscopy. During the early 1800s, Philipp Bozzini is credited with creating one of the first endoscopic devices used to examine the urethra, female bladder, rectum, ear, mouth, and nasal cavity. Reports also indicated that Bozzini's device may have been used to examine the peritoneum of corpses via minilaparotomies. Throughout the 1800s many physicians and scientist have been accredited with the development of more sophisticated endoscopies including Desormeaux, Nitze, and Kussmaul. But it was George Kelling, in 1901, that was the first to use a laparoscope to examine the peritoneal cavity as a procedure he labeled celioscopy. It was not until the 1930s that laparoscopy was used for interventional procedures such as lysis of adhesions and diagnostic biopsy. Laparoscopy laid latent until the 1970s when gynecologists began using it routinely. After the advent of fiber optics, once the video computer chip allowed for projections and magnification of images on a monitor, laparoscopic surgery expanded exponentially. The first laparoscopic cholecystectomy was performed by French physician Mouret in 1987. Technological advances in instrumentation and laparoscopic devices continue to grow in all fields of surgery [1, 2].

14.2 General Concepts

14.2.1 Preoperative Evaluation and Patient Selection Criteria

When deciding whether laparoscopic surgery is the best option for the patient, the surgeon must take a thorough medical history. Pertinent questions include any prior abdominal, pelvic surgery, radiation exposure, radioactive implants, joint prosthesis, or arthritis that may limit patient positioning, significant pulmonary, or cardiac conditions that might be affected by pneumoperitoneum or anesthesia, any deep vein thrombosis (DVT) or coagulation disorders, and any previous complications/reaction to anesthesia in previous surgeries. One must also inquire about medication history, particularly chronic steroid use, as this may interfere with healing and may require stress doses during the perioperative period. Cardiac or pulmonary medications should be continued at the time of surgery.

M. Rafols · N. Ajabshir · K. Ben-David (✉)
Mount Sinai Medical Center, Comprehensive Cancer Center, Miami Beach, FL, USA
e-mail: kfir.bendavid@msmc.com

F. Palazzo (ed.), *Fundamentals of General Surgery*, https://doi.org/10.1007/978-3-319-75656-1_14

Physical exam should be performed prior to any surgery. Attention to prior incisions, hernias, masses, location of tenderness, presence of peritonitis, and rectal or vaginal exams when necessary are imperative for accurate diagnosis. A routine cardiac and pulmonary workup should include a chest X-ray and electrocardiogram with a cardiologist clearance when required. The American Society of Anesthesiologists (ASA) classification is important for laparoscopic surgery as patients that fall into ASA classes 4 and 5 may not be candidates for a laparoscopic approach as they may not be able to tolerate the physiologic changes that accompany pneumoperitoneum [3].

During the preoperative discussion, the surgeon must review the risks and benefits of undergoing laparoscopic surgery. Special attention must be given to the expected postoperative course, the associated complications, the possibility of having to convert to open surgery, and the anticipated recovery time. Informed consent must include the possibility of conversion to open or any other anticipated procedures that may possibly be performed during the surgery.

The patient's body habitus is also important to preoperative planning. Obese patients can have a very thick abdominal wall and may require longer trocars and special considerations when creating pneumoperitoneum safely. In thin patient, the close proximity of the aorta and inferior vena cava (IVC) to the abdominal wall poses a risk of injury when entering the abdomen. Techniques for avoiding injury to the aortoiliac vasculature are direct visualization with open Hasson approach, using an optical trocar, placing Veress needle at Palmer's point, and elevating the abdominal wall; all of these will be further elaborated later in the chapter.

Laparoscopic surgery is not amenable to every patient. Absolute contraindications for laparoscopic surgery include inability to tolerate laparotomy, hypovolemic shock, or inability for the facility to provide appropriate postoperative care. Relative contraindications include inability to tolerate general anesthesia, long-standing peritonitis which increases risk of bowel injury during trocar insertion, large incarcerated ventral or inguinal hernias, large abdominal/pelvic masses that may limit working space, or severe cardiopulmonary disease [4].

Coinciding abdominal findings require extra precautions and may even preclude one from being able to undergo laparoscopic surgery. Previous hernia repairs may pose a particular problem as trocar insertion may cause injury to any bowel that is adherent to the mesh or trauma to the mesh itself. Patients with distended bowel are also at risk for intestinal injury, and attempts for nasogastric decompression should precede operative intervention. Care must also be taken when entering the abdomen in patients with history of peritonitis or pelvic inflammatory disease which both increase the risk of adhesions and inadvertent enterotomy. The presence of any abdominal aortic aneurysms must be noted prior to inserting trocars as inadvertent damage will be devastating. Hepatosplenomegaly could also potentially lead to massive hemorrhage if either organ is accidentally damaged during trocar insertion. Cirrhotic patients generally have an increased risk of coagulopathy intraoperatively, and the appropriate blood products should be readily available in the operating room if bleeding is expected. Also patients with ascites may need special attention to fluid and colloid replacement. Ascites leaking out of port sites postoperatively can result in delayed healing and increased risk of infection. Efforts to medically control ascites prior to surgery should be made, if possible.

14.2.2 Operating Room Setup

Basic room setup is reflected in Fig. 14.1. Typically, a tower console will house the insufflator, energy source, and camera interface with its light source (Figs. 14.2 and 14.3). Aligning these in a single area allows for consolidation of the necessary connections as a single track from the operative field to the console. With up to seven or more connections, disorganization and entanglement can lead to difficult maneuvering of instruments, will frustrate the surgeon and operating room staff, and ultimately compromise the surgery and safety of the patient.

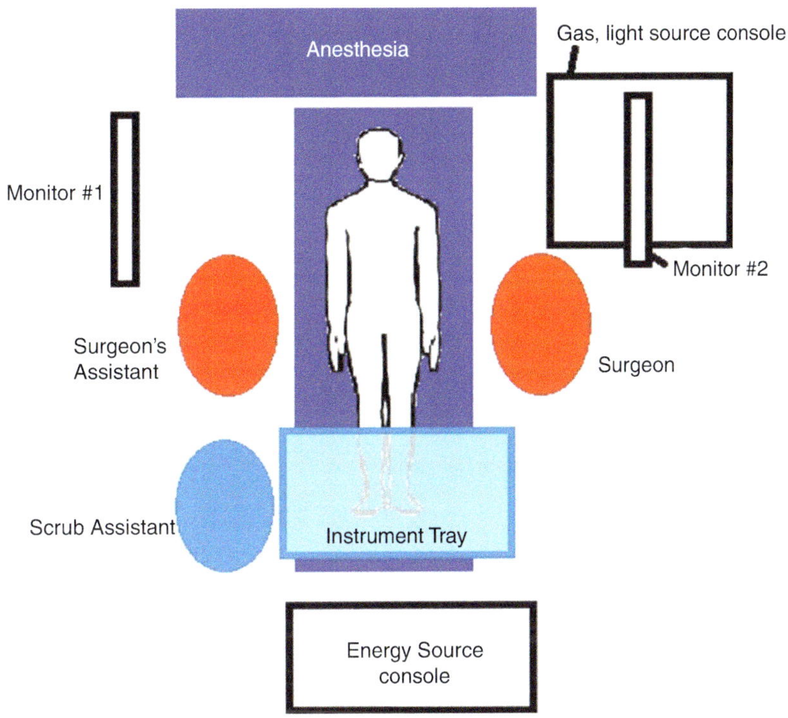

Fig. 14.1 Basic operating room lay out

Video monitors should be positioned across from the operating surgeon and ideally, multiple screens can be strategically positioned so that all participants, including the anesthesia team, surgical assistants, and circulating nurse, may view and be aware of how the surgery is progressing. Room lighting should be actively adjusted based on the stage of the procedure. Initially, overhead and surgical lights should be on, as would occur in any typical open surgical approach. Once intra-abdominal access is established, overhead lights should be dimmed and surgical lights shut off. The darkened room will contrast against a brightly lit screen and will allow for best and safest visualization of the operative field. At the conclusion of surgery, room lights and surgical lights are turned on again to facilitate closure of the abdominal wall layers.

14.2.3 Patient Positioning

Patient positioning often depends on the operative field needed. Most laparoscopic surgeries require the patient to be in the supine position. Some procedures may require temporary maneuvering of the bed in the Trendelenburg or reverse Trendelenburg positioning. This allows gravity to assist in mobilizing intra-abdominal contents to facilitate visualization. If working on the esophagus or left liver, patient positioning may need to be in lithotomy position, with legs in stir-ups and the surgeon positioned in-between the legs. For a retroperitoneal approach, such as nephrectomy or retroperitoneal aortic surgery, the best exposure is achieved by placing the patient in the lateral decubitus position and then flexing the table at the waist to spread the lateral plane as well as the intercostal space for thoracoscopic access.

14.2.4 Surgeon Positioning

The surgeon is positioned opposite the surgical field and across from the video monitor. He or she should have an uncompromised vantage point to safely accomplish the goals of the operation. Often, assistants will be asked to hold the camera or retract tissue. With limited space, a great deal of flexibility and dexterity is necessary to do this effectively.

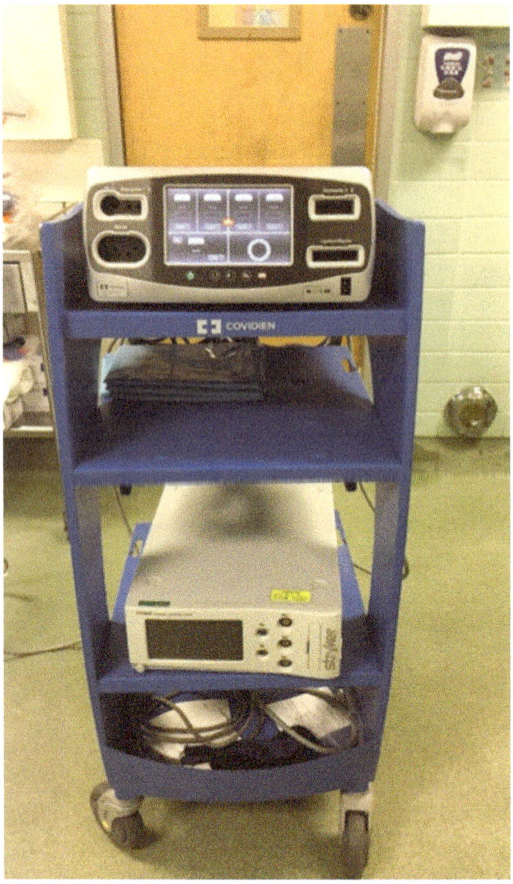

Fig. 14.2 Energy source console

14.2.5 Instruments

There exist a wide variety of instruments used in laparoscopic surgery, and the list grows daily, also due to the growth of hybrid procedures which may require combining laparoscopic techniques with ultrasonography, endoscopy, or fluoroscopy. It is important to have a number of these instruments and modalities readily available, including instruments for a potentially open approach. Nowadays, most instruments used in traditional, open surgery are available for use in laparoscopic surgery with the necessary size and length modifications that allow for functionality, despite entry via 5–12 mm ports. Unfortunately, many of these are limited in their degrees of freedom [wrist-like motion] forcing the laparoscopic surgeon to adjust his or her technique. This limiting factor and subsequent learning curve forced upon the surgeon is one reason for the delay in widespread adoption of minimally invasive laparoscopic surgery when it was first being performed. Fortunately, increases in volume have proportionally increased new medical devices such as knot pusher, Bovie hook, Endo Catch bag, and Endo Stitch™. Figure 14.4a–i depicts the basic essential equipment to perform laparoscopic surgery.

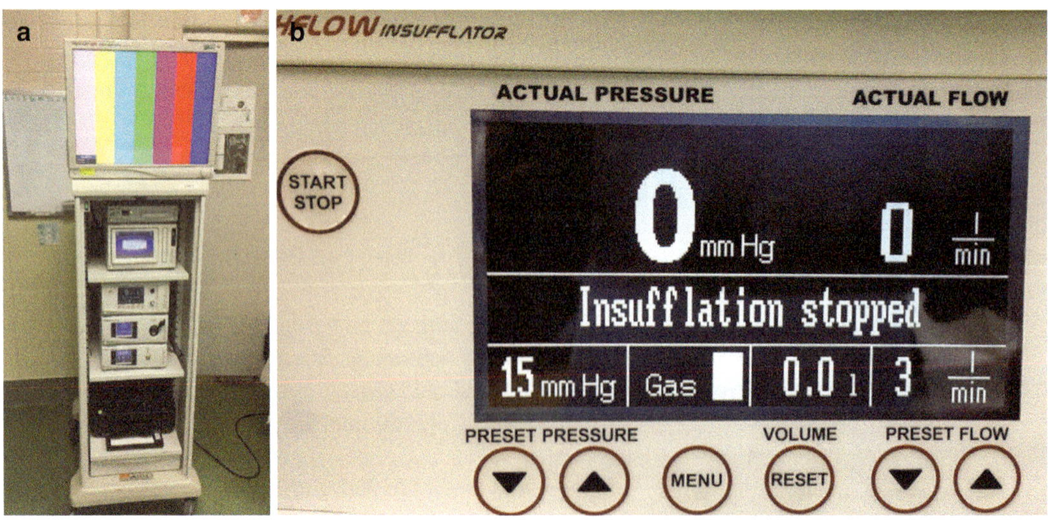

Fig. 14.3 (**a**) Video monitor console with gas, light, and camera source. (**b**) Insufflator monitor

14.2.6 Establishing Pneumoperitoneum

In order for appropriate visualization and maneuvering to take place within the abdomen, creating a surgical field with adequate separation of tissues is required. This is primarily done by insufflating the workspace cavity with a gaseous substance. Mechanical lift devices do exist; however, due to their bulk, inferior exposure, and increased postoperative pain, they may prove to be more of a nuisance. Several options exist for establishing pneumoperitoneum such as Air, N_2O, helium, neon, argon, and CO_2. The latter has been the most studied and used. It is important to consider both the gas-specific and pressure-specific effects of each option, especially since these substances may absorb into the patient's circulatory system to different extents and subsequently induce dangerous physiologic

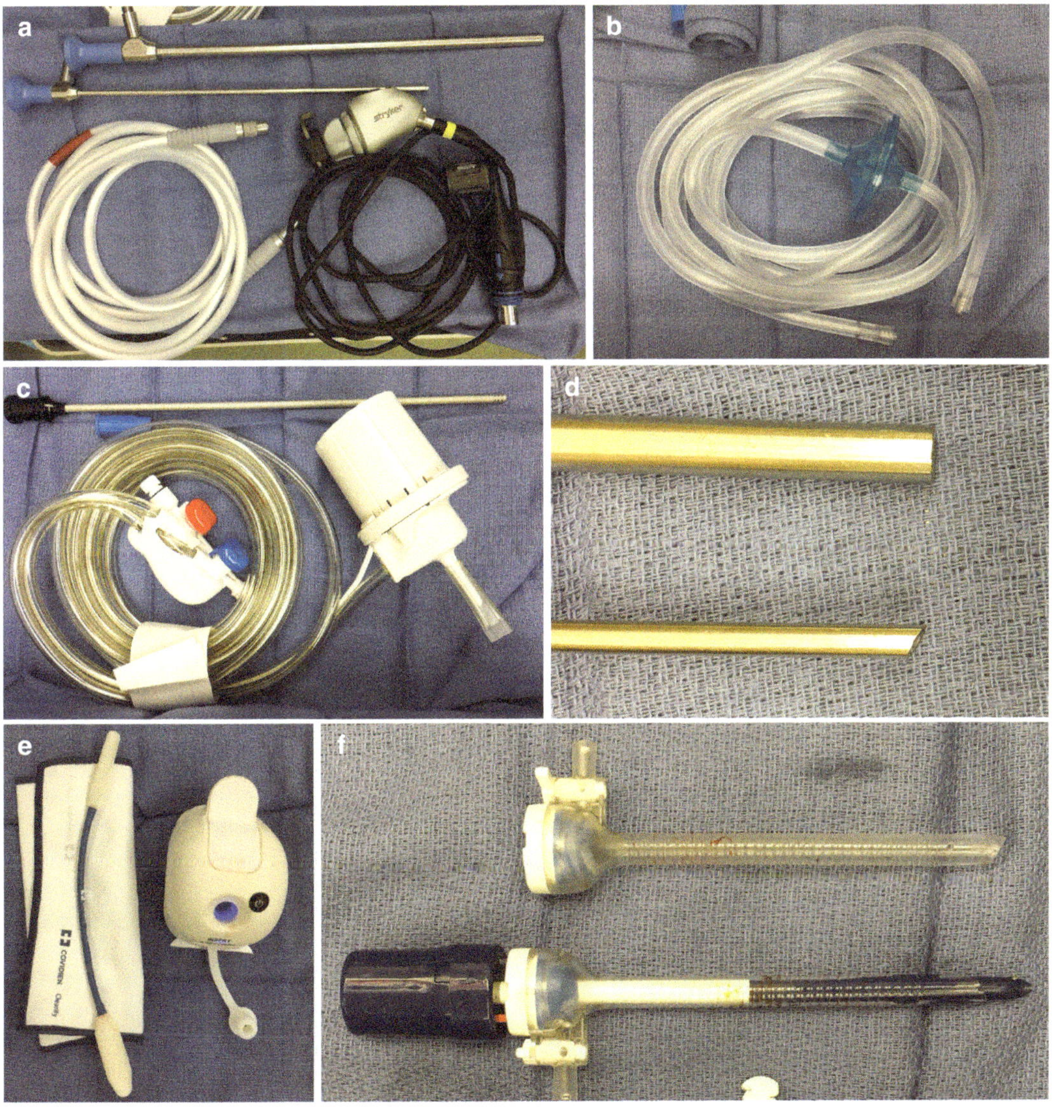

Fig. 14.4 Assorted basic equipment. (**a**) Laparoscopes (top), light source (left), and camera (right). (**b**) Insufflation tubing. (**c**) Suction irrigator. (**d**) 0 (top) and 30 (bottom) degree laparoscope. (**e**) Scope warmer. (**f**) Trocar. (**g**) Grasping instruments. (**h**) Scissors. (**i**) Maryland

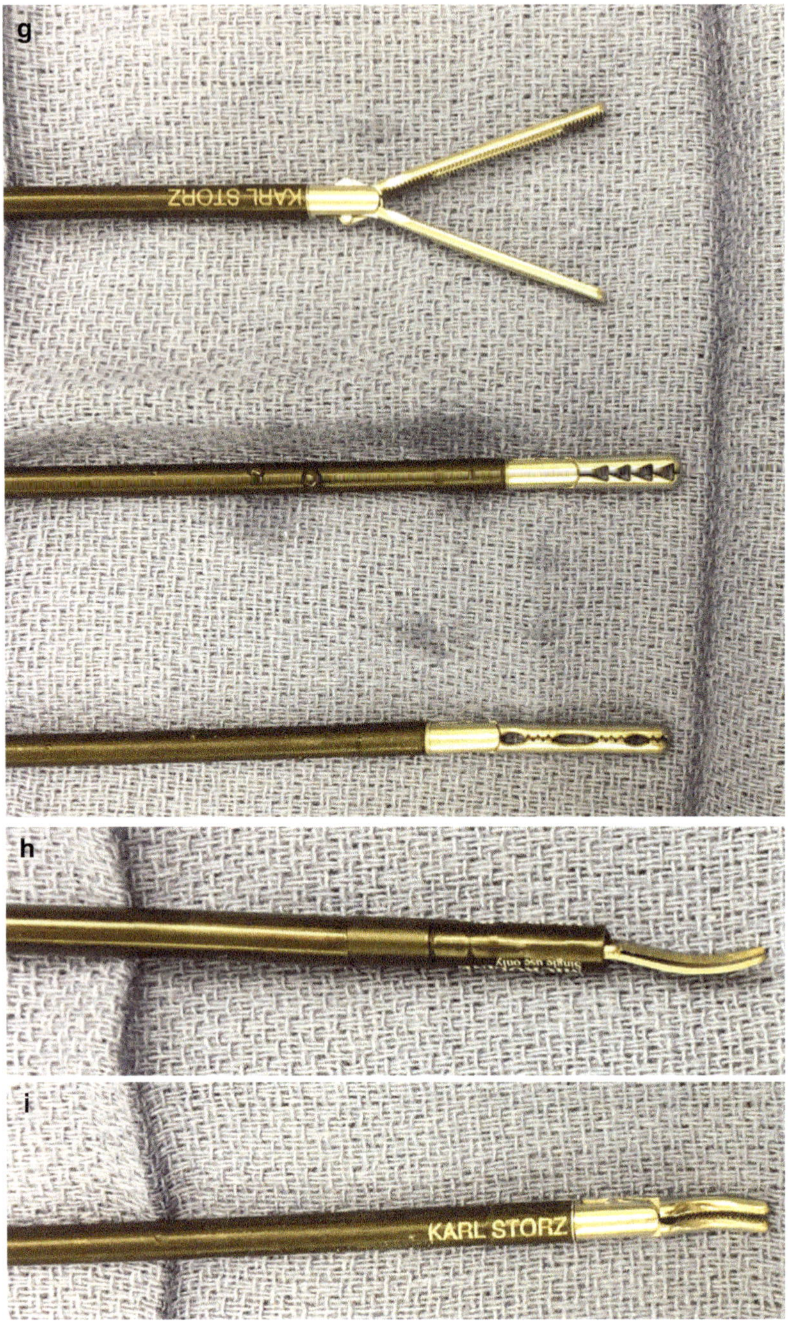

Fig. 14.4 (continued)

responses. Those with poor absorption such as the inert gasses have an increased risk for gas embolus. With CO_2 on the other hand, diffusion into the patient's tissue can result in hypercarbia and ensuing acidosis, increased afterload, even myocardial stress [5]. The physiologic changes associated with CO_2 pneumoperitoneum will be discussed later in this chapter.

When deciding upon where to initially gain entry, it is important to consider what may be found underneath the skin. The surgeon's first choice is at the umbilicus. The umbilical stalk naturally converges the tissue planes, and an approach here will minimize the depth of tissue layers traversed. Alternatively, in patients with previous surgical scarring especially at the midline, access via Palmer's point (3 cm below the left costal margin, midclavicular line) may provide safe entry in avoiding potentially adhered loops of bowel.

14.2.6.1 Veress Needle

In the virgin abdomen, one method of gaining entry to the abdomen is with the use of a Veress needle (Fig. 14.5). This spring-loaded needle is designed to retract its pointed end upon interface with resistance. Thus, when the surgeon "pops" through the abdominal wall fascia and then the peritoneum, it is understood that there now exists direct access from the environment to the peritoneal space. Anterior retraction or lifting of the

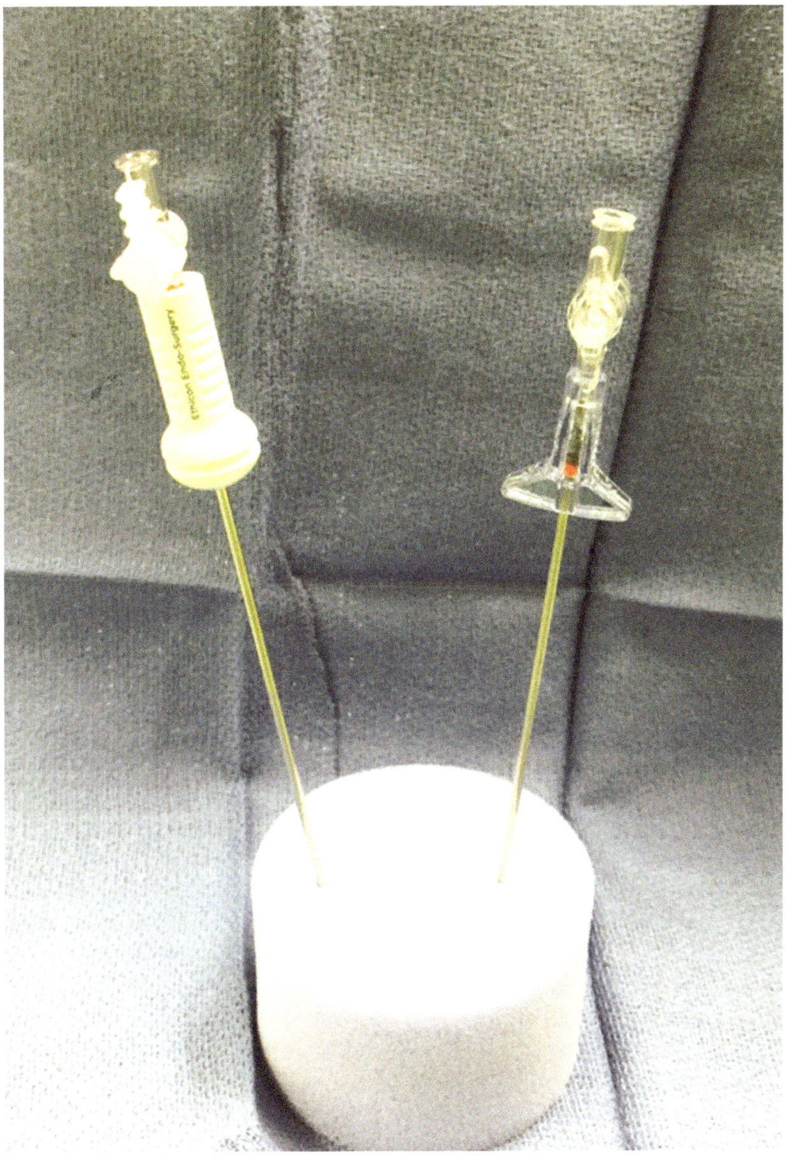

Fig. 14.5 Veress needle

abdominal wall layers, such as with two penetrating towel clamps, away from the viscera can facilitate safe entry. The gaseous substance of choice can flow via the needle's shaft and insufflation of the abdomen begins. With pressure feedback monitoring on the insufflation console, low (<5 mmHg) starting pressure ensures the needle's tip is outside of abdominal wall layers. Further, the surgeon may instill normal saline and note the ease with which it enters the abdomen. Infiltrating with normal saline and noting clear fluid return on aspiration confirm the needle tip rests outside loops of bowel.

Once the abdomen is appropriately inflated to 15 mmHg, standard trocars, e.g., 5 or 10 mm in diameter, may be introduced with a now minimized possibility of organ injury. Trocar tips are generally aimed away from the sacral promontory and the great vessels. Often, the initial trocar placement is performed under direct laparoscopic visualization through an optic trocar. Once this is placed, the remaining trocars are placed under direct visualization as they are inserted through the abdominal incisions.

14.2.6.2 Hasson Technique

When a patient has had multiple previous abdominal surgeries, it is advisable to gain entry via a more direct route in the event adhesions from previous surgeries have developed and fixed loops of bowel or other organs are against the peritoneal surface. The initial incision is then made adjacent to or within the umbilicus. Dissection is carried down through Camper's and Scarpa's fascia into the paucity of abdominal wall musculature at midline which allows entry into the peritoneal cavity. Securing the fascia on either side of the incision can be achieved with two clamps or stay sutures allowing for elevation away from intra-abdominal organs and a safe incision through the fascia and peritoneum. Now, a blunted trocar (Fig. 14.6) may be advanced into the abdomen. Replacing the clamps with suture that can be wrapped around the trocar for added security is the final step prior to passing the trocar tip into the abdominal cavity. If preferred, a clean finger swipe can add reassurance prior to trocar entry.

14.2.6.3 Optical Trocar

A hybrid of the aforementioned approaches is peritoneal cavity access with a direct optical see-through trocar. Here, the 0° laparoscope is placed within the transparent 5 mm trocar, and the surgeon is able to visualize the abdominal wall layers as the trocar rotates and separates the fascia and muscle fibers. Guided entry is performed following small skin incision made wide enough to accommodate the trocar. Then, a twisting motion with controlled entry is performed with visualization of each abdominal wall layer with the end point here being visualization beyond the peritoneal lining and within the abdominal cavity. This technique may be combined with Veress pneumoperitoneum prior to entry, though insufflation may also begin after trocar entry.

14.2.7 Troubleshooting Common Problems

There exist a number of common hiccups that can easily derail the progress of a surgery. Many of these will resolve with a quick fix; however,

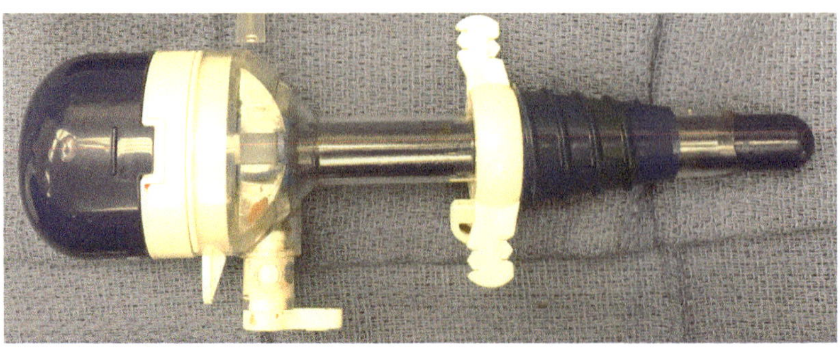

Fig. 14.6 Blunted trocar for Hasson technique

the procedure may be severely hampered without knowledge of such remedies. For instance, when establishing and maintaining pneumoperitoneum, high-pressure readings could signal insufflation of an incorrect tissue plane, i.e., within the abdominal wall and hollow viscus. It is best to begin insufflating the abdomen with a low-flow setting (e.g., 3 L/min). If the monitor reads an unexpectedly high pressure, insufflation should be immediately stopped, and the trocar should be repositioned followed by careful exploration of all underlying organs. Once in the correct tissue plane, insufflation can be expedited with a "high flow" rate (e.g., 40 L/min). For reference, a typical insufflator monitor is depicted in Fig. 14.3b.

Further, when initially viewing via a laparoscope, the temperature difference between the room and the abdomen will produce fogging of the lens until these equalize. To prevent this, a scope warmer (Fig. 14.4e) can be employed to adjust the temperature of the lens and defogging solution can be applied to the scope's tip. To expedite having a clear view once inside the abdomen, a gentle and brief wiping of the camera against the liver, peritoneum, or omentum is safe. Other reasons why there may be a subpar image include if the camera is out of focus or the light adjustment was not previously white balanced.

14.2.8 Physiologic Effects of Pneumoperitoneum

The most common gas used for pneumoperitoneum is carbon dioxide (CO_2) because it is relatively cheap and widely available, suppresses combustion, is rapidly absorbed into the peritoneum, and is easily eliminated from the body. Nonetheless CO_2 pneumoperitoneum has a physiologic effect on the human body. These effects can be divided into chemical gas-specific or mechanical pressure-specific effects. During the procedure monitoring of cardiac rhythm, oxygen saturation, end-tidal CO_2, heart rate, blood pressure, and urine output is critical to safe laparoscopic surgery.

14.2.8.1 Gas-Specific Effects

CO_2 is readily absorbed into the circulatory system and carried to the alveoli. The diffusion coefficient of CO_2 is 20 times greater than that of oxygen making it very soluble in the blood. The lungs eliminate CO_2 during expiration by increasing minute ventilation which is the primary mechanism of eliminating CO_2. Also, the bone can buffer up to 12 L of CO_2. Normally these mechanisms prevent hypercarbia and respiratory acidosis. However, when the limits of the body's buffers are overwhelmed, there will be an increased arterial P CO_2 and an abrupt increase in end-tidal CO_2. This will eventually lead to a decrease in the serum pH. These changes can be seen in patients with severe cardiopulmonary disease in the first 15–20 min of pneumoperitoneum, after which a steady state will be achieved. These physiologic changes may also be seen during long cases. In these circumstances, the anesthesiologist may require the patient to come off pneumoperitoneum and hyperventilate the lungs. Off-loading CO_2 may be achieved by an increase respiratory rate or tidal volume, keeping in mind that a respiratory rate greater than 20 breaths per minute may cause worsening of hypercapnia secondary to poor oxygen exchange. If the tidal volume is increased too much, barotrauma or excessive movement of the surgical field may result. Severe respiratory acidosis is uncommon if patient has normal pulmonary function, but it could lead to tachycardia as well as an increase in systemic vascular resistance and blood pressure, thus leading higher myocardial oxygen demand and risk for cardiac ischemia. Changes in cerebrovascular autoregulation can also be seen with high serum CO_2 levels [3, 4].

14.2.8.2 Pressure-Specific Effects

Pneumoperitoneum can also increase intra-abdominal (IA) pressures and can affect the cardiovascular, pulmonary, and renal organ systems [5]. Increased IA can decrease renal blood flow, glomerular filtration rate, and urine output. Frequently there is an observed intraoperative oliguria secondary to decreased renal venous flow [6]. This is immediately reversible when pneumoperitoneum is completed at the end of the case. Pneumoperitoneum can also indirectly increase renin and antidiuretic hormone levels leading to sodium retention and free water absorption. On the other hand, this effect can take up to 1 h to reverse.

Elevated IA pressure affects the cardiovascular system in many ways. One of the benefits of laparoscopic surgery is that insensible fluid loss is much less when compared to open abdominal surgery. Nonetheless, during laparoscopic surgery intravenous fluids are required for fluid shifting occurs with lower extremity venous pooling, third spacing, as well as blood loss. In hypovolemic patients, excessive IA pressure may compress the inferior vena cava and reduce blood return to the heart and thus preload and cardiac output. This, combined with reverse Trendelenburg positioning, promotes venous stasis and venous thrombosis. It is important to prevent venous thrombosis on a patient to patient basis. This includes sequential compression devices (SCD) and chemical prophylaxis including agents like heparin or low molecular weight heparin. For quick procedures >60–90 min, excessive deep vein thrombosis (DVT) prophylaxis is not warranted since the risk of DVT is significantly low [4].

Increased IA pressure on a paralyzed diaphragm is transferred to thoracic cavity. This increases the filling pressure in both the right and left atrium. This can be avoided by maintaining the IA pressure <20 mmHg [7]. Increased intrathoracic pressure may also increase the peak inspiratory pressure, making barotrauma more likely. However, even in patients with chronic obstructive pulmonary disease, ruptured blebs resulting in pneumothorax are rare after laparoscopic surgery.

14.2.9 Trocar Positioning

Trocar placement is paramount to a seamless operation. When not thoughtfully planned ahead of time, the surgery may be wrought with frustration at the expense of patient safety. Several cardinal guidelines exist that the surgeon should bear in mind. First, trocars should be placed with appropriate distance from each other. This creates space and allows for efficient movement within the abdomen. Trocars placed within 3 cm of each other are not only redundant but facilitate collision of instruments within the abdomen. Ideally, there should be at least 10 cm between the surgeon's right and left hands.

Although the camera can technically be placed in any of the ports that accommodate its size, one port should intentionally be designated as the camera port. A commonly used analogy is that of the baseball diamond, where first and third base are the surgeon's right and left hands, respectively, second base is the target organ, and this leaves home plate to be the designated camera port (Fig. 14.7).

Prior to making any incision, the surgeon must be mindful of several additional factors which may not result in a perfect diamond, though would be ultimately be more beneficial for the patient. For example, incisions within previous scars or hidden within natural creases and folds make for a better cosmetic outcome for the patient with the avoidance of a new, visible scar. Further, prodding the outside surface of the abdomen while visualizing the indentation made from within can assist in avoiding placement of a trocar within potentially dangerous territory, such as within an area of dense adhesion that may contain viscera. Figures 14.8 and 14.9 demonstrate typical trocar placement for laparoscopic appendectomy and cholecystectomy, respectively.

14.3 Alternative Approaches

14.3.1 Single-Incision Laparoscopic Surgery (SILS)

SILS has recently entered into the limelight of general surgery. The concept of SILS has been around for some time. As early as the 1970s, Dr. Raimund Wittmoser, the "father" of modern thoracoscopic surgery of the autonomic nervous system, used a single-intercostal incision through which he inserted a multifunctional port which contained all the instruments and optics. Since

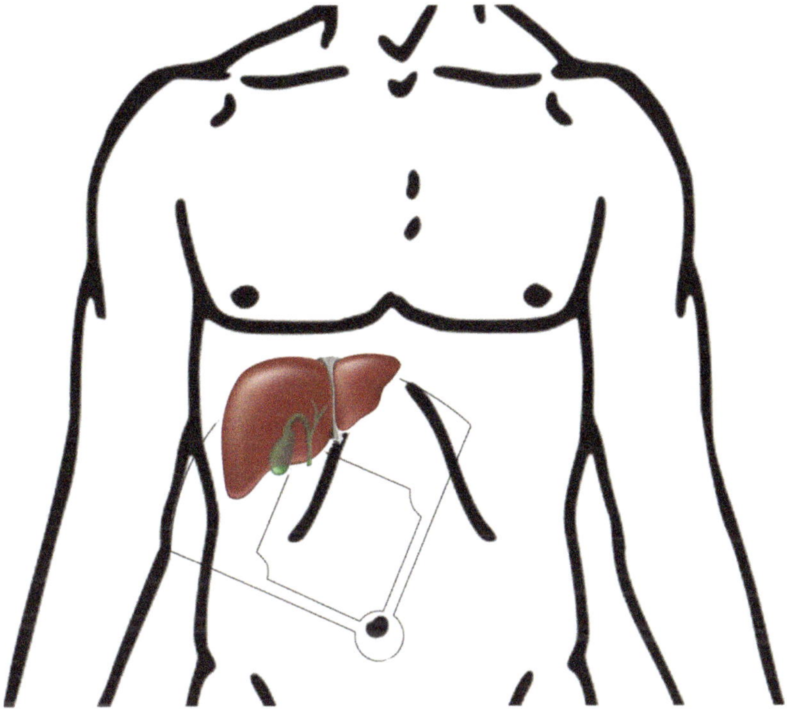

Fig. 14.7 "Baseball diamond" analogy for trocar placement for, as an example, laparoscopic cholecystectomy

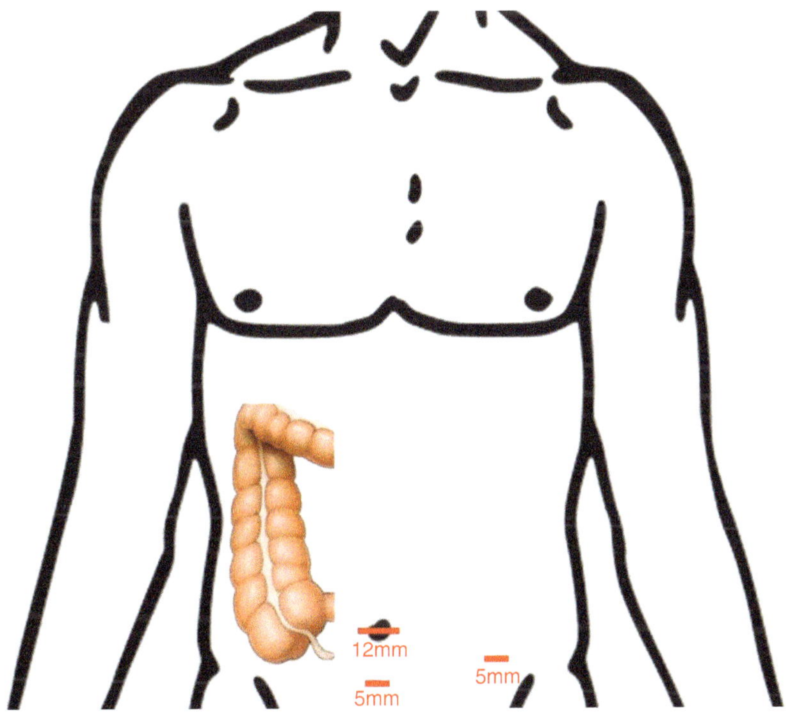

Fig. 14.8 Typical trocar placement for laparoscopic appendectomy

there have been multiple published articles establishing its resourcefulness as a standard of laparoscopic surgery, many surgeons have attempted various surgical procedures using this technique. The foundation of SILS is the use of a single trocar site where multiple laparoscopic instruments

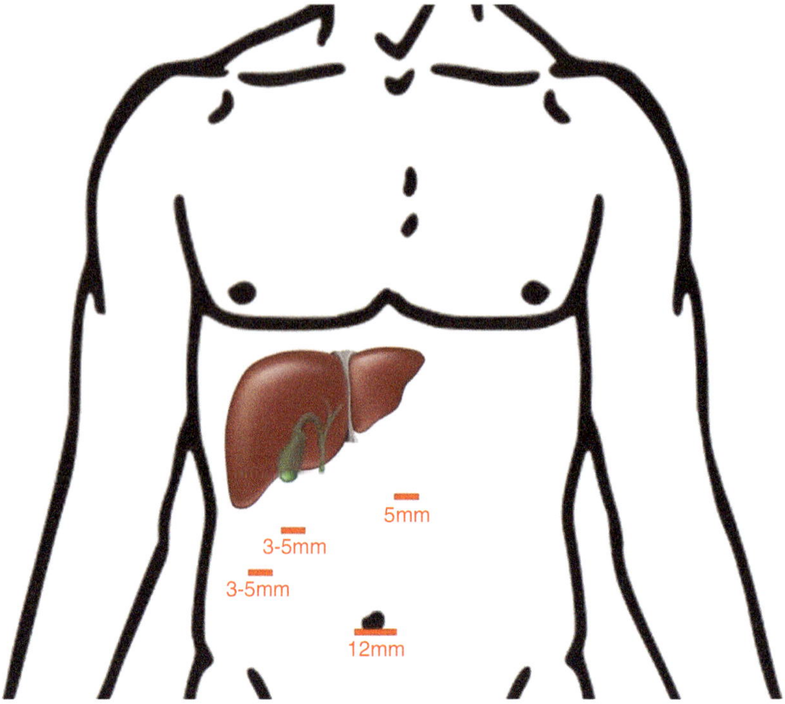

Fig. 14.9 Typical trocar placement for laparoscopic cholecystectomy

are manipulated via a multiport system. Placement of the trocar at the umbilicus allows for minimal visible scar and thus theoretically more aesthetically appealing than traditional laparoscopic surgical scars. However, many surgeons have questioned its practicality for routine use over traditional laparoscopic surgery. The ideal patient for SILS is one with lower body mass index (BMI), early disease, and no previous abdominal surgery.

SILS appendectomy has been described in many pediatric cases, but as the patient size and weight increase, as does the difficulty of the procedure and conversion rates. Adult SILS appendectomy was reviewed in a large meta-analysis of randomized control studies. The result was longer operating time and higher rate of conversion. There were no differences between the two groups in visual analogue pain scores, doses of analgesics, overall complication rates, wound infection, or cosmesis.

One of the most commonly performed SILS surgeries is the single-incision laparoscopic cholecystectomy. Comparable results have been reported for SILS versus traditional four-port cholecystectomy. Rivas et al. reported operating times of 50 min always attaining a critical view using a two-port and three-port SILS technique under experienced hands [8]. Acute cholecystitis is a factor associated with a lower success rate 59.9 vs 93.0% and longer operative time of 78 vs 70 min. A BMI >30 was also associated with longer operative times [9]. A recent meta-analysis pooling ten randomized control studies evaluated SILC vs laparoscopic cholecystectomy and found that although there were improved postoperative pain and cosmesis scores, there was a significant increase in major complications (CBD injury, requirement for reexploration, and large vessel injury) with a relative risk of 3.0 as well as an increase in minor complications. Operation times were significantly longer in the SILC group with a mean difference added time of 23 min. No difference was noted in requirement for conversion to open or addition of extra port sites were noted [10].

14.3.2 Extracavitary MIS

Extracavitary laparoscopic surgery is a technique that uses balloon attached to a laparoscopic camera to develop a space in the extraperitoneal or extrafascial plane and then use low-pressure insufflation to maintain it open. Extracavitary laparoscopic surgery uses the same instrumentation as traditional laparoscopic surgery. Not entering the peritoneum will avoid the risk of adhesion formation. Also, insufflation of extraperitoneal space is associated with less physiologic disturbances than pneumoperitoneum. Yet, CO_2 may produce extensive subcutaneous emphysema if high pressures are used during insufflation. Direct absorption of CO_2 into the subcutaneous space may lead to metabolic acidosis.

Gaining access to the extracavitary space may be performed by two different techniques, via balloon dissection or subcutaneous laparoscopic/endoscopic devices. Balloon dissection is the most commonly employed technique for good for extraperitoneal hernia repair and the retroperitoneal approach used for adrenalectomy, lumbar discectomy, necrotic pancreatectomy, and occasionally for para-aortic lymph node dissection.

Totally extraperitoneal hernia repair is the most frequent extraperitoneal MIS performed. An infraumbilical incision is made contralateral to the hernia site. The anterior rectus sheath is incised transversely, and the rectus muscle sin retracted laterally to allow a 10 mm blunt trocar. Either a blunt dissection (Fig. 14.10a) or by balloon dissector (Fig. 14.10b) is then used to develop the preperitoneal space under direct visualization. Once this potential space has been created, the extraperitoneal space is insufflated to 10 mm hg to avoid excessive subcutaneous emphysema. This results in a surgical field/working space that is reduced, but it avoids the complications associated with intraperitoneal laparoscopic surgery like adhesions and trocar site hernias and reduces risk of intestinal damage and post-op ileus.

14.3.3 Hand-Assisted Laparoscopic Surgery (HALS)

At times, the goals of surgery are unable to be fully met while exclusively employing the laparoscopic approach. This is especially true when the operation necessitates the use of tactile feedback such as in feeling for tumor. Several systems (Fig. 14.11: GelPort™, Applied Medical) exist that allow the surgeon inserts his or her hand through a large, airtight port which maintains pneumoperitoneum. This, of course, necessitates a larger abdominal wall incision upwards of 7 8 cm. Proponents of HALS argue it may assists with the learning curve of laparoscopy, retraction, blunt finger dissection, allows for rapid control to bleeding vessels, and can be used

a b

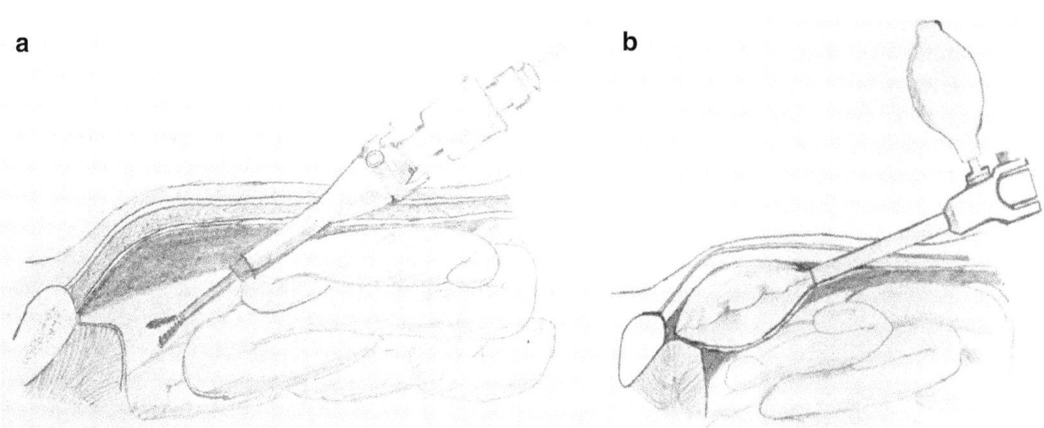

Fig. 14.10 (**a**) TEP direct access with blunt dissection. (**b**) Balloon-assisted dissection

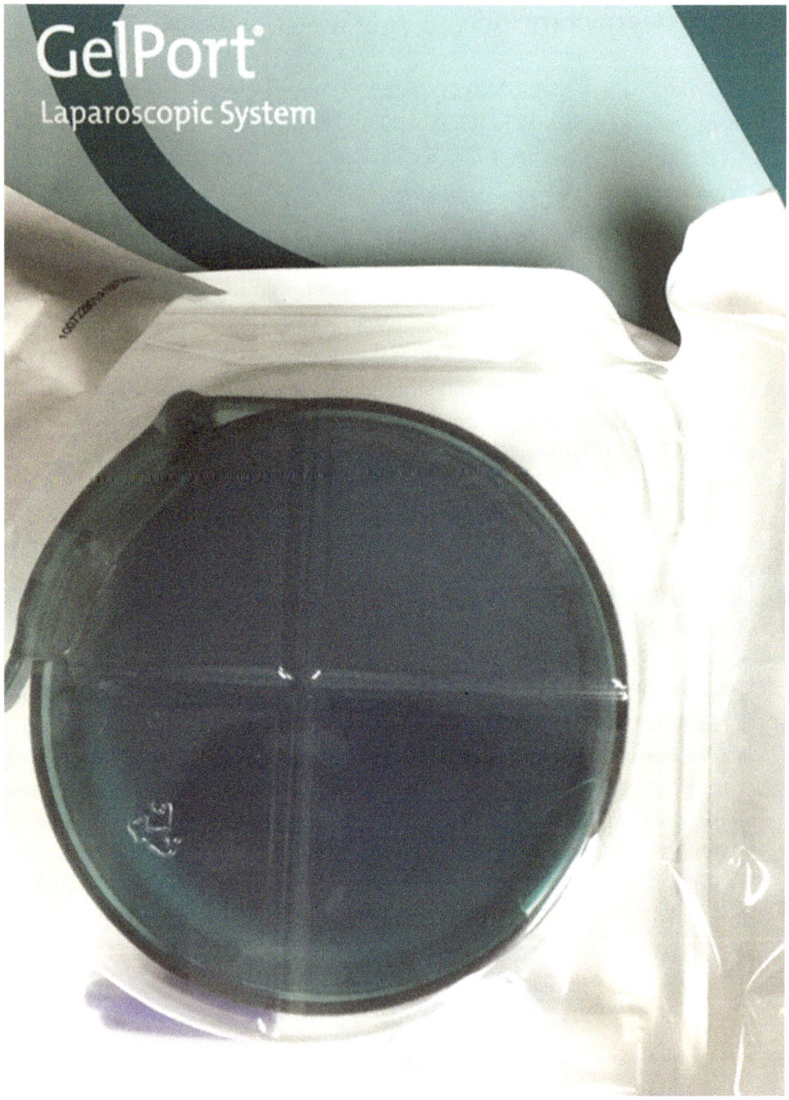

Fig. 14.11 Hand-assisted GelPort™

before full conversion to laparotomy. It has also been shown to be advantageous by reducing operating time and conversion rates while maintaining all the oncological principles and patient safety [11, 12].

14.4 Patient and Safety Monitoring

From anesthetic induction to extubation, patient safety monitoring is paramount. Laparoscopy adds new challenges both the surgeon and anesthesiologist should keep in mind. To start, initial pneumoperitoneum proceeds with a rapid stretching of the peritoneal membrane. This may lead to a vasovagal response with bradycardia and hypotension necessitating immediate desufflation and possible addition of fluids and/or a vagolytic.

Furthermore, once the abdomen is expanded to include an extra 4–6 L at a pressure of 12–16 mmHg, venous return via the inferior vena cava may become compromised. This is especially true in the patient who is positioned in reversed Trendelenburg [13]. With venous pooling within the lower extremities, a substantial and replicable risk exists for deep-venous thrombosis which should be avoided with intraoperative sequential compression devices or preoperative anticoagulation.

Mentioned earlier is the risk for gas emboli, less likely with CO_2 pneumoperitoneum, though still a serious possibility. An uncharacteristic hypotensive episode should warrant suspicion which may unfortunately be confused for the vasovagal response of pneumoperitoneum. A "mill wheel" murmur may become apparent by listening with an esophageal stethoscope, and the patient should be placed in the Trendelenburg and left lateral decubitus position to trap the gas in the apex of the right ventricle, allowing for immediate aspiration via central venous catheter access.

At the conclusion of the operation, it is imperative that all trocars are removed under direct visualization. A trocar that perhaps injured an epigastric vessel upon entry may partly mask bleeding for the duration of the surgery. Postoperative hypotension, a profound drop in hemoglobin and hematocrit, and out of proportion abdominal pain the next morning will then leave the surgeon scratching his or her head only to realize the critical error was failing to visualize each trocar removal. However, when discovered at the time of surgery, intervention may include direct pressure or full-thickness abdominal wall suture.

14.5 Special Considerations

14.5.1 Pediatrics

Laparoscopic surgery in the pediatric population is carried out very similar to that of the adult population. It is no surprise that instrumentation and insufflation should be scaled down due to size. Trocar diameters for traditional approaches rarely exceed 5 mm. Otherwise, techniques such as single-incision laparoscopic appendectomy are commonplace and employ a single, 10 mm trocar. With less abdominal wall girth and subcutaneous tissue, *usually*, pediatric laparoscopic surgery can be accomplished with insufflation pressures of 8 mmHg rather than 15 mmHg. With inguinal hernia repairs even, muscle relaxation may prove to be unnecessary, and the patient may only require laryngeal mask airway rather than conventional endotracheal tube intubation [13].

14.5.2 Pregnancy

Several factors should be considered prior to and during laparoscopic surgery in the pregnant patient. Surgical intervention should aim to ensure mother's safety without inducing a great amount of fetal risk. First and foremost, the surgeon must consider timing. Laparoscopy can be performed safely during any trimester of pregnancy, though waiting until the second trimester may reduce the rates of spontaneous abortion and preterm labor, specifically in laparoscopic cholecystectomy [14, 15].

Initial trocar placement should be based on fundal height. To avoid direct injury to the uterus, it is prudent to begin with a subcostal trocar. All three aforementioned techniques for placement, i.e., Veress, Hasson, or optical trocar, can be used when starting at the subcostal margin, and an underlying fundus is clearly not palpable. Insufflation may begin once access is safely established. Insufflation pressure between 12 and 15 mmHg is considered safe and has not increased adverse outcomes for the patient or fetus, and it should be noted the physiologic contractions of pregnancy induce a far greater intra-abdominal pressures [16].

Pregnancy inherently induces a hypercoagulable state which leads to DVT or PE in 0.5–3.0/1000 pregnancies [17]. Abdominal pressures exceeding 14 mmHg can significantly alter femoral vein hemodynamics (diameter, cross-sectional area, peak systolic flow) when compared to a low-pressure insufflation of 8 mmHg [18]. Unfortunately, studies accounting for the combined hypercoagulable effects, and subsequent adverse outcomes, of pneumoperitoneum during pregnancy are lacking at this time.

14.5.3 Elderly

Limitations for surgery in the elderly have more to do with recovery than the actual procedure.

Decreased mobility hampers recovery and allows for the milieu of postoperative risks that increase morbidity and mortality which is certainly exacerbated by a large, open incision. The advent of laparoscopic surgery has facilitated, most profoundly, the acute postoperative period where decreased pain, earlier mobility, and hastened discharge from the hospital have been repeatedly demonstrated. With this, what were once considered too dangerous of surgeries for a frail, elderly patient may be accomplished when an open incision is now out of the equation. The concern lies with whether or not the benefits gained outweigh the theoretical cost of a longer operation which may induce greater physiologic demands. Indeed, the evidence supports improved outcomes with laparoscopic surgery and the elderly; in fact, they have the most to gain from this approach [19].

14.6 Postoperative Care and Complications

14.6.1 Nausea

In laparoscopic surgery, postoperative nausea and vomiting (PONV) may be increased when compared to open surgery. The etiology is often multifactorial and can be due to anesthetic technique used, postoperative pain and pain management, and factors intrinsic to the patient. Risk factors which may lead to PONV include female gender, young age, lower ASA risk score, history of PONV or motion sickness, nonsmoking, preoperative anxiety, and increased procedure length with the use of volatile anesthetic agents. Prevention of PONV, such as with antiemetics or reduction in opioid use, can make the patient more comfortable and hasten their recovery.

14.6.2 Pain

There exist numerous studies which demonstrate reduced pain after laparoscopic surgery compared to the open approach. As with open surgery, liberal use of a liposomal based local anesthetic can prevent some of the patient's pain. The unique finding of referred shoulder pain due to diaphragmatic stretching is usually self-limited and should be treated the same as incisional pain. It is expected that this will last 1–3 days, and this may be reduced by evacuating pneumoperitoneum at the conclusion of surgery. A systematic review of 31 studies determined that low-pressure pneumoperitoneum, low insufflation rate, and active gas aspiration were effective strategies to reduce the incidence or severity of shoulder pain after laparoscopic cholecystectomy [20]. Any unusual increases in pain after hospital discharge should be evaluated to determine the etiology.

14.6.3 Diet

Resumption of a normal diet depends mostly on the patient and procedure performed rather than whether or not the surgery was laparoscopic. For routine surgeries, i.e., appendectomy or cholecystectomy, regular diet is usually tolerated as soon as postoperative day 1. Recommending a normal diet only until after demonstration of resumed bowel function is a typical rule when surgery involved anywhere along the gastrointestinal tract. Of course, this is an oversimplification, and dietary restrictions should proceed on an individualized patient basis, taking into consideration functional levels at baseline.

14.6.4 Activity

Like postoperative pain, return to normal activity is expedited with the employment of laparoscopic surgery, and the two of these go hand in hand. Use of factors that impair wound healing (steroids, chemotherapy, immunosuppression, and tobacco use) should be taken into consideration when instructing patients on when to resume normal activity. Ultimately, the best judgment for dictating activity will come from the patient listening to cues of pain and discomfort sensed by their body.

14.6.5 Wound Care

The most obvious advantage of laparoscopic surgery is the size of wound created. Incisions of

5 mm or less require only closure at the cutaneous level, which is typically achieved with one subcutaneous suture to reapproximate the edges of the wound. Larger than 10 mm, it is recommended that the peritoneum be reapproximated as well. The surgeon may also choose to use liquid adhesive and/or steri-strip bandages for reinforcement. It is important to instruct the patient to keep the skin dry for 24–48 h. Redness or discharge or increasing pain and swelling are signs that healing has gone awry, and these should be addressed promptly. These are often signs of seroma, infection, hematoma, and/or hernia. Avoidance of sun exposure and the liberal use of ultraviolet protection will reduce the darkening and subsequent visibility of scars.

14.6.6 Injuries

Many injuries may not be readily obvious at the time of surgery and only present in the postoperative period. Injuries to hollow viscera such as the stomach, small bowel, colon, bladder, or ureters can present even up to 7–10 days after surgery despite there being no visible mechanism during the procedure. Notably, thermal burns from electrocautery, anastomotic leak, and ischemia following devascularization may present hours to days following skin closure. Signs of tachycardia, anemia, or hypotension should prompt caretakers to pursuit further workup. As previously reviewed, vascular injuries such as those to the epigastric or mesenteric vessels can present postoperatively as anything from an abdominal wall hematoma to hemodynamic instability with profound anemia. Lastly, nerve injuries are best treated with prevention. This is accomplished with vigilant attention to detail such as appropriate patient positioning with judicious use of cushioning, avoidance of excessive division and traction, and awareness of anatomic structures when placing sutures, tacks, and staples.

References

1. Spaner SJ, Warnock GL. A brief history of endoscopy, laparoscopy, and laparoscopic surgery. J Laparoendosc Adv Surg Tech A. 1997;7(6):369–73.
2. Nezhat C, Nezhat C, Nezhat F. Nezhat's video-assisted and robotic-assisted laparoscopy and hysteroscopy. Cambridge: Cambridge University Press; 2013. p. 1–6.
3. Schwartz SI, Charles Brunicardi F, Andersen DK. Schwartz's principles of surgery. New York: McGraw-Hill Education; 2015.
4. Fleshman JW, Fowler DL, Whelan RL. The SAGES manual of perioperative care in minimally invasive surgery. New York: Springer; 2006. p. 25–32.
5. Grabowski JE, Talamini MA. Physiological effects of pneumoperitoneum. J Gastrointest Surg. 2009;13:1009. https://doi.org/10.1007/s11605-008-0662-0.
6. Hazebroek EJ, de Vos tot Nederveen Cappel R, Gommers D, et al. Antidiuretic hormone release during laparoscopic donor nephrectomy. Arch Surg. 2002;137:600. Discussion 605.
7. Sackier JM, Nibhanupudy B. The pneumoperitoneum-physiology and complications. In: Toouli JG, Gossot D, Hunter JG, editors. Endosurgery. New York: Churchill-Livingstone; 1996. p. 155.
8. Rivas H, Varela E, Scott D. Single-incision laparoscopic cholecystectomy: initial evaluation of a large series of patients. Surg Endosc. 2009;24(6):1403–12.
9. Antoniou SA, Pointner R, Granderath FA. Single-incision laparoscopic cholecystectomy: a systematic review. Surg Endosc. 2011;25(1):367–77.
10. Evers L, Bouvy N, Branje D, Peeters A. Single- incision laparoscopic cholecystectomy versus conventional four-port laparoscopic cholecystectomy: a systematic review and meta-analysis. Surg Endosc. 2016;31(9):3437–48.
11. Gupta P, Bhartia V. Hand-assisted laparoscopic surgery using Gelport. J Minim Access Surg. 2005;1(3):110. https://doi.org/10.4103/0972-9941.18994.
12. Marcello PW, Fleshman JW, Milsom JW, et al. Hand-assisted laparoscopic vs. laparoscopic colorectal surgery: a multicenter, prospective randomized trial. Dis Colon Rectum. 2008;51(6):818–26.
13. Holzheimer RG. Laparoscopic procedures as a risk factor of deep venous thrombosis, superficial ascending thrombophlebitis and pulmonary embolism—a case report and review of the literature. Eur J Med Res. 2004;9(9):417–22.
14. SAGES. Guidelines for diagnosis, treatment and use of laparoscopy for surgical problems during pregnancy. Surg Endosc. 2007;5(11):3479–92.
15. Glasgow R, Visser B, Harris H, Patti M, Kilpatrick S, Mulvihill S. Changing management of gallstone disease during pregnancy. Surg Endosc. 1998;12(3):241–6.
16. O'rourke N, Kodali B-S. Laparoscopic surgery during pregnancy. Curr Opin Anaesthesiol. 2006; 19(3):254–9.
17. Snow V, Qaseem A, Barry P, American College of Physicians, American Academy of Family Physicians Panel on Deep Venous Thrombosis/Pulmonary Embolism, et al. Management of venous thromboembolism: a clinical practice guideline from the

American College of Physicians and the American Academy of Family Physicians. Ann Intern Med. 2007;146(3):204–10.
18. Sharma A, Dahiya D, Kaman L, Saini V, Behera A. Effect of various pneumoperitoneum pressures on femoral vein hemodynamics during laparoscopic cholecystectomy. Updat Surg. 2016;68(2):163–9.
19. Chesney T, Acuna SA. Do elderly patients have the most to gain from laparoscopic surgery? Ann Med Surg. 2015;4(3):321–3.
20. Donatsky AM, Bjerrum F, Gögenur I. Surgical techniques to minimize shoulder pain after laparoscopic cholecystectomy. A systematic review. Surg Endosc. 2013;27(7):2275–82.

15 Fundamentals of Laparotomy Closure

William W. Hope and Michael J. Rosen

15.1 Introduction

Although not often a highlighted part of abdominal operations, secure laparotomy closure is essential to minimize the incidence of incisional hernias and infection. Despite the move to minimally invasive surgery in many common general surgical operations, the use of laparotomy is still common and has an estimated incisional hernia risk ranging from 10 to 23% and up to 69% in high-risk patient groups with long-term follow-up [1–3]. The burden of incisional hernias is a major health concern with expenditures in excess of $3 billion per year [4, 5]. Many patient-related risk factors contribute to the incidence of incisional hernia and include obesity, male gender, postoperative respiratory failure, previous wound infection, older age, reoperation, diabetes mellitus, malignancy, malnutrition, history of chemotherapy, jaundice, glucocorticosteroid use, smoking, and patients with abdominal aortic aneurysms [6–14]. While these are important factors for the surgeon to consider, they are often non-modifiable. Surgeons, however, can greatly affect the incisional hernia rate and possibly the infection rate by their choice of laparotomy closure technique. This should be an area of great focus for surgeons operating on the abdominal wall and cavity.

15.2 General Concepts

Many types of incisions for accessing the abdominal cavity have been described, and each has its particular advantage and disadvantage. The midline laparotomy (or celiotomy) incision is one of the most often used incisions for accessing the abdominal cavity. It is versatile, allows rapid access to all parts of the abdominal cavity, and is used due to the relative ease of entering the abdomen because of the lack of muscle and vasculature in this area. Although midline laparotomy is widely used, some have recommended the use of off midline incisions when possible due to incisional hernia formation [15]. Despite these recommendations, the midline laparotomy incision remains a mainstay for surgeons and is the focus of this chapter.

When discussing laparotomy closure, it is important to have a general knowledge of wound healing and abdominal wall anatomy. Healing of fascia and laparotomy incisions follow the same general principles of wound healing. This includes an inflammatory, proliferative, and maturation phase, although the aponeurosis can take longer than other tissues to heal [16].

W. W. Hope (✉)
New Hanover Regional Medical Center, University of North Carolina at Chapel Hill, Wilmington, NC, USA
e-mail: William.Hope@nhrmc.org

M. J. Rosen
Cleveland Clinic, Cleveland, OH, USA
e-mail: rosenm@ccf.org

F. Palazzo (ed.), *Fundamentals of General Surgery*, https://doi.org/10.1007/978-3-319-75656-1_15

The abdominal wall includes layers of skin, subcutaneous tissue, superficial fascia, deep fascia, muscle, extraperitoneal fascia, and peritoneum (Figs. 15.1 and 15.2). Surgeons should understand the linea alba and its surrounding structures as they relate to laparotomy closure.

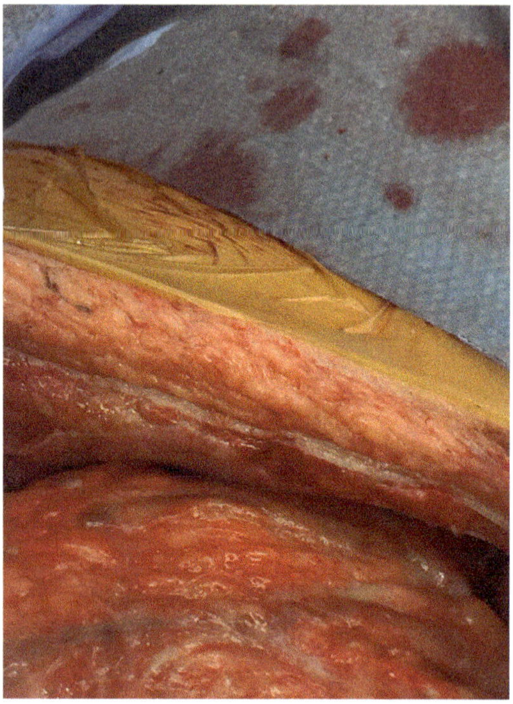

Fig. 15.1 Side view of a laparotomy incision showing the layers of the abdominal wall including skin, subcutaneous tissue, and fascia

The linea alba lies in the midline and is formed by the fusion of the anterior and posterior rectus sheath. It runs from the xiphoid process to the symphysis pubis. The rectus muscles lie lateral to the linea alba, and when the laparotomy incision veers off midline, muscle is often exposed, which can make closure more difficult (Fig. 15.3).

Certain aspects of the laparotomy closure technique can potentially make this procedure easier. The laparotomy incision should be made in the midline and should be as long as needed to provide adequate exposure. There is no clear consensus on whether to make the skin and fascial incision using a scalpel or using Bovie electrocautery. Some animal data support the use of scalpel for skin and fascial incision and report fewer wound complications and higher tensile strength [17–20]; however, the benefits have not proven clinically significant in humans, with no apparent impact on incisional hernia formation [20–25]. As previously stated, it is ideal to make the laparotomy incision through the midline, and veering off can cause bleeding and can disrupt layers of the abdominal wall often making closure more challenging and time consuming. Traditionally, a mass closure technique of suturing fascia and muscle was recommended; however, experimental and clinical studies have led to the recommendation of closure of the aponeurosis only [15, 16].

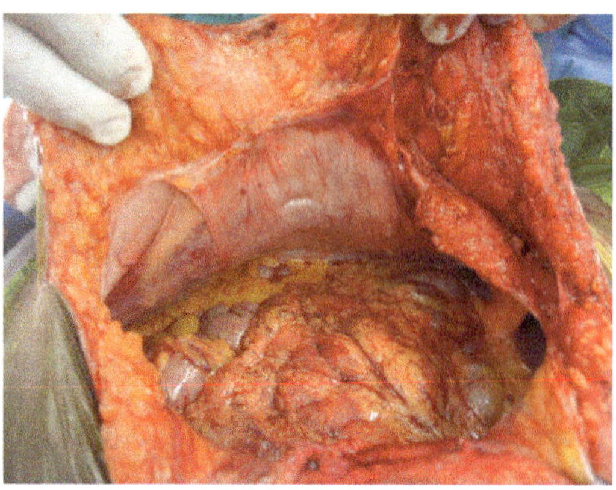

Fig. 15.2 Layers of the abdominal wall elevated to show abdominal cavity and skin, subcutaneous tissue, fascial layers, and muscle

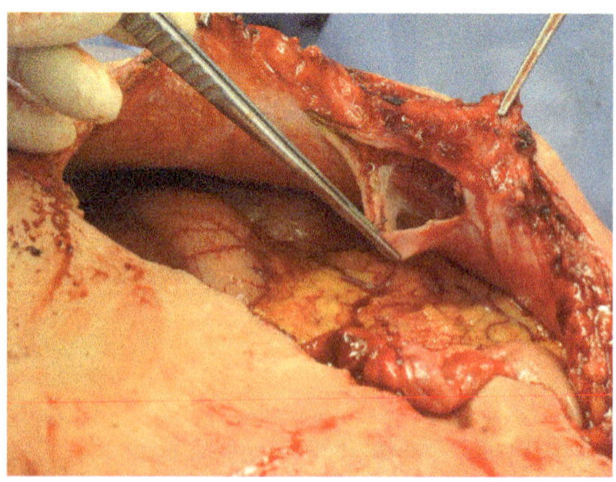

Fig. 15.3 Incision of the posterior sheath showing the anatomic makeup of the linea alba. When the midline laparotomy incision veers off midline, the rectus muscle can be exposed and complicate closure

15.3 Technical/Practical Considerations/Safety Precautions

Several technical considerations are pertinent when discussing laparotomy closure and include the type of sutures used and techniques of closure.

The suture type used for laparotomy closure has long been a subject of debate. Multiple randomized controlled trials and meta-analyses have evaluated the ideal suture for closure with differing conclusions. In general, recommendations are to use a slowly absorbing suture in a continuous fashion, because this is the most efficient technique to reduce infection and incisional hernia formation [15]. However, there is controversy on the details of the suture used. Many surgeons use a large slowly absorbing suture on a large needle that is double stranded (Fig. 15.4), while others prefer single stranded. No definitive research recommends one particular type of stitch; however, many experts have moved to using smaller suture materials/needles to facilitate a short bite technique (Fig. 15.5). For example, a 2-0 PDS Plus II (Ethicon, Somerville, NJ, USA) on a 31 mm needle was used in a recent randomized controlled trial comparing outcomes [26].

Several important points regarding closure should be highlighted. It is imperative to use meticulous suturing technique by placing the needle at a 90° angle to the desired tissue/fascia and gently follow the curve of the needle through the tissue to minimize tissue trauma (Fig. 15.6). The suture to wound length ratio is a key principle in laparotomy closure. The ratio is calculated after measuring the length of the wound and also measuring the amount of suture material used to close the wound (Figs. 15.7 and 15.8). Measuring suture material used can be done in many ways. It is usually determined by first measuring the amount of suture material available before beginning laparotomy closure and subtracting this amount from the suture remaining after closure.

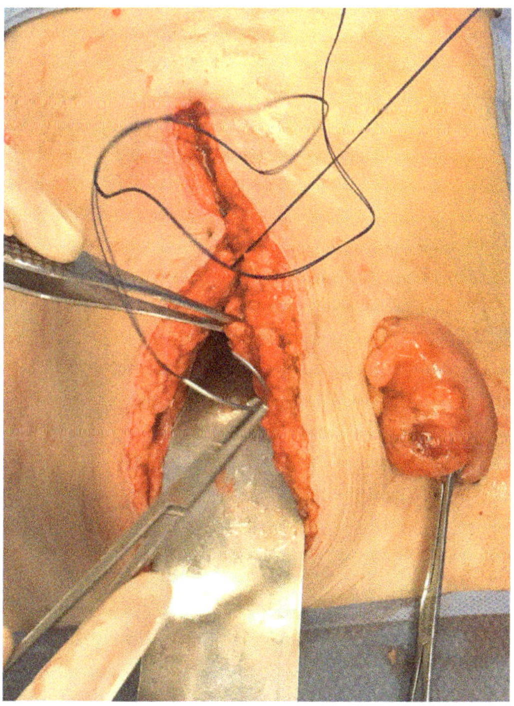

Fig. 15.4 Laparotomy closure using a double-stranded slowly absorbing suture

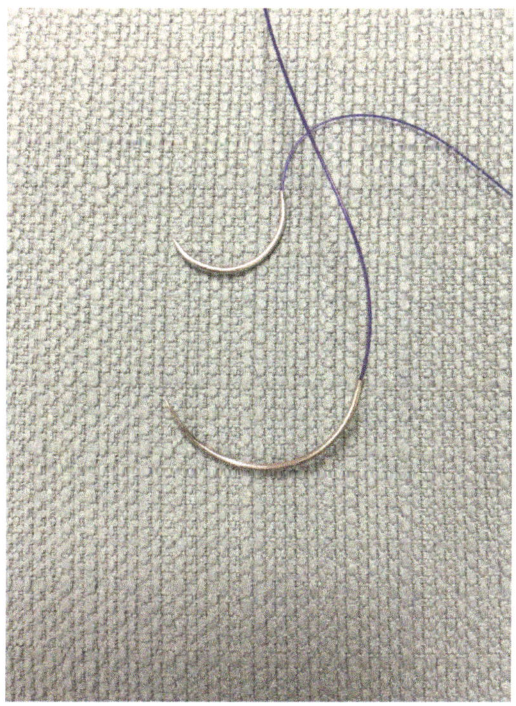

Fig. 15.5 Suture and needles. Traditionally large needles on large suture have been used, but recently smaller needles and smaller suture have been proposed

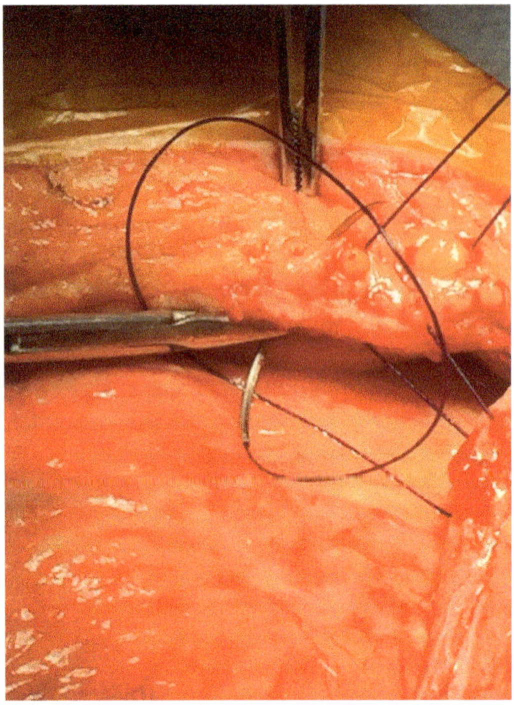

Fig. 15.6 When closing fascia, it is important to practice meticulous suturing techniques such as entering the tissue at a 90° angle and following the curve of the needle

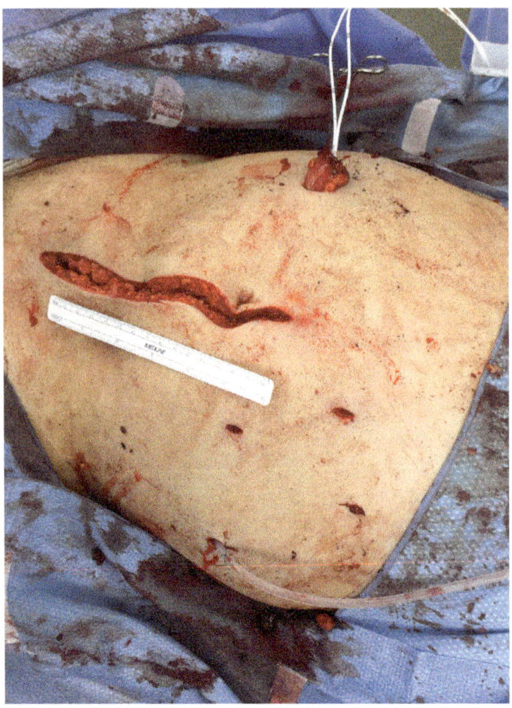

Fig. 15.7 Measuring of the laparotomy incision to calculate the suture to wound length ratio

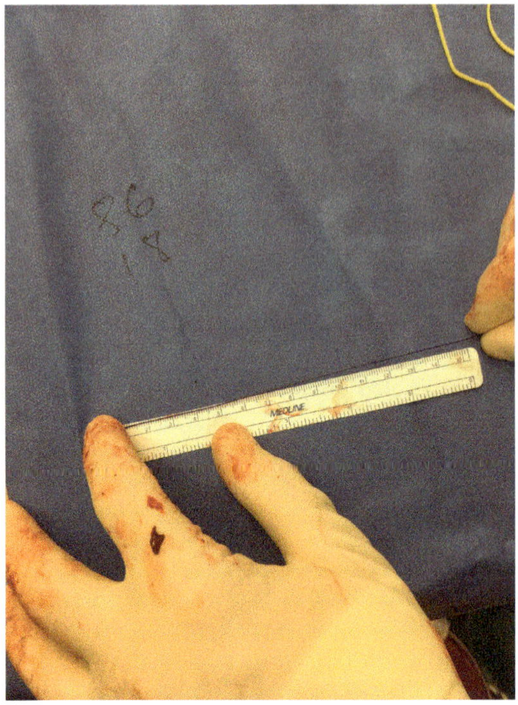

Fig. 15.8 Measuring of the remaining suture following laparotomy closure. This amount will be subtracted from the total amount of suture leaving the amount of suture used to close the fascia. This number can then be used along with the length of the fascia measurement to calculate the suture to wound length ratio

Using these numbers, the ratio is calculated. A large body of literature has long supported the notion that achieving a greater than 4:1 suture to wound length ratio decreases incisional hernia formation [27, 28]. Therefore, during laparotomy closure, the suture to wound length ratio should be calculated, and closures should be redone when they fail to meet the 4:1 target. Although the 4:1 suture to wound length ratio is generally agreed on, there are many ways to achieve this ratio, and recommendations on this have recently changed.

The traditional technique for closure involved using approximately 1 cm bites of fascia and 1 cm advances, and this was based on some experimental studies [29–31]. Recently, this technique has been challenged as new evidence shows closure with smaller bites (5–8 mm) and smaller advances (5–8 mm) produces a significantly lower incisional hernia rate [26, 32] and possibly surgical site infection rates [32] compared with the traditional closure (Figs. 15.9 and 15.10).

Recommendations vary regarding which structures should be included in abdominal closure. Traditionally, a mass closure technique of suturing fascia and muscle was recommended; however, some experimental and clinical studies recommend closure of the aponeurosis only [16], although no firm conclusions can be drawn, since there has been no clear definition of closure methods. Due to this, the European Hernia Society guidelines proposed defining mass closure as a suture bite including all layers of the abdominal wall except the skin, defining layered closure as an incision closed with more than one separate layer of fascial closure, and defining single-layer aponeurotic closure as suturing the abdominal wall fascia in one layer [15]. Whether to close the peritoneal layer separately during laparotomy closure is debated; however, no short- or long-term benefits from this technique have been reported [33], so this has not been recommended [15].

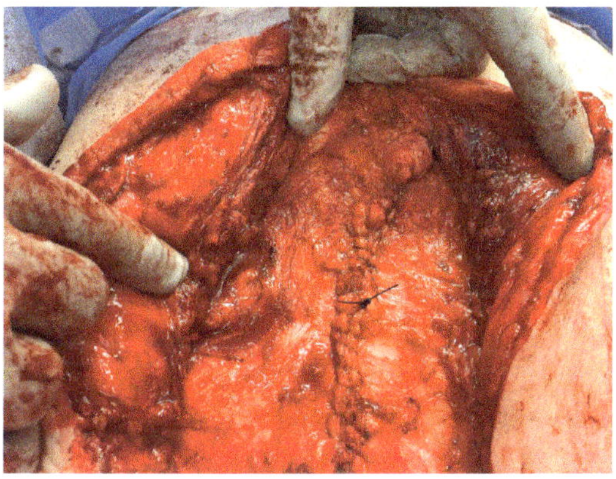

Fig. 15.9 Fascial closure using the small bites technique of 5 mm fascial bites and 5 mm advances

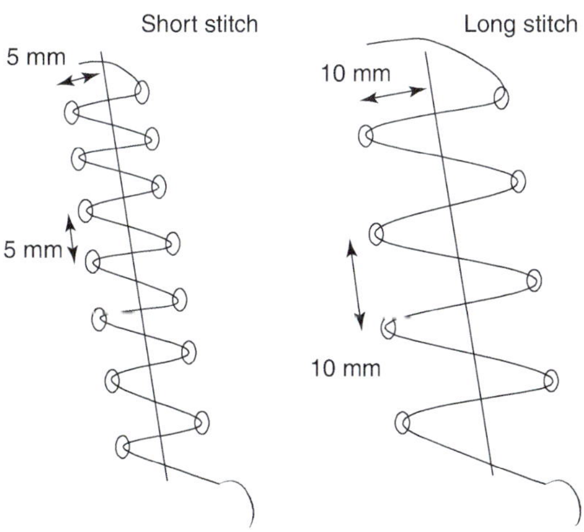

Fig. 15.10 Schematic showing two different types of laparotomy closure. Recent literature has supported the short stitch technique using 5 mm fascial bites and 5 mm advances compared with the traditional 1 cm fascial bites and 1 cm advances

15.4 Current Controversies/ Future Directions

Current laparotomy closure controversies relate to the lack of strong evidence for closure in patient groups that have not been well studied in current literature. While the evidence is convincing for the short stitch technique for laparotomy closure, one major criticism is that the data are from European studies, which include patients with a lower body mass index (BMI) compared with the United States population. Another unknown is the ideal laparotomy closure methods for patients undergoing emergency surgery. It is unknown whether the short stitch concept applies to the higher BMI patients or to patients that undergo emergency surgery. However, if you believe in the concepts related to this closure method, it makes sense that this technique would apply, although further research is needed.

One major factor related to laparotomy closure that has not been well studied is fascial tension. The amount of tension placed on the fascia during laparotomy closure may effect incisional hernia formation and ischemia development. An old adage related to the closure of fascia (or other suture closure techniques) is "approximate, don't strangulate." While many surgeons subscribe to this with regard to laparotomy closure, it is a difficult factor to measure and can be very subjective and surgeon dependent.

The future direction of laparotomy closure includes creating accurate predictive models of risk factors for incisional hernia development. Undoubtedly, some patient groups are at risk even when applying appropriate laparotomy closure principles. For these patients (such as patients with abdominal aortic aneurysms), the use of prophylactic mesh augmentation has been proposed and has shown efficacy [34]. Education will be critical, since some surgeons are still not using the short stitch technique or adhering to other principles related to laparotomy closure. Future technological advances will also have a major impact on laparotomy with the potential development of devices such as automated sewing machines to help minimize variability and improve efficiency of fascial closure techniques.

With continued advances in minimally invasive surgery, improvements in surgical techniques and education related to laparotomy closure, and the potential use of prophylactic mesh in high-risk patients, there may be a day when incisional hernias no longer exist.

Take-Home Points

- Surgeons performing laparotomies should have a basic understanding of wound healing principles and abdominal wall anatomy.
- Laparotomy closure should not be a neglected part of abdominal surgery, and evidence-based closure techniques should be taught.
- A slowly absorbable monofilament suture should be used for laparotomy closure.
- Laparotomy closure should be achieved using a 4:1 suture to wound length ratio and using a small stitch technique in appropriate patients.
- Suture to wound length ratio should be calculated following laparotomy closure to ensure an adequate 4:1 ratio is obtained.

Suggested Readings

Muysoms FE, Antoniou SA, Bury K, Campanelli G, Conze J, Cuccurullo D, de Beaux AC, Deerenberg EB, East B, Fortelny RH, Gillion JF, Henriksen NA, Israelsson L, Jairam A, Janes A, Jeekel J, Lopez-Cano M, Miserez M, Morales-Conde S, Sanders DL, Simons MP, Smietanski M, Venclauskas L, Berrevoet F, European Hernia S. European Hernia Society guidelines on the closure of abdominal wall incisions. Hernia. 2015;19:1–24. https://doi.org/10.1007/s10029-014-1342-5.

Israelsson LA, Millbourn D. Prevention of incisional hernias: how to close a midline incision. Surg Clin North Am. 2013;93:1027–40. https://doi.org/10.1016/j.suc.2013.06.009.

Hope W. Prevention of incisional hernia development. Minerva Chir. 2011;66:145–52.

Deerenberg EB, Harlaar JJ, Steyerberg EW, Lont HE, van Doorn HC, Heisterkamp J, Wijnhoven BP, Schouten WR, Cense HA, Stockmann HB, Berends FJ, Dijkhuizen FP, Dwarkasing RS, Jairam AP, van Ramshorst GH, Kleinrensink GJ, Jeekel J, Lange JF. Small bites versus large bites for closure of abdominal midline incisions (STITCH): a double-blind, multicentre, randomised controlled trial. Lancet. 2015;386:1254–60. https://doi.org/10.1016/S0140-6736(15)60459-7.

References

1. Cobb WS, Kercher KW, Heniford BT. Laparoscopic repair of incisional hernias. Surg Clin North Am. 2005;85(1):91–103.; ix. https://doi.org/10.1016/j.suc.2004.09.006.
2. Mudge M, Hughes LE. Incisional hernia: a 10 year prospective study of incidence and attitudes. Br J Surg. 1985;72(1):70–1.
3. Alnassar S, Bawahab M, Abdoh A, Guzman R, Al Tuwaijiri T, Louridas G. Incisional hernia post repair of abdominal aortic occlusive and aneurysmal disease: five-year incidence. Vascular. 2012;20(5):273–7. https://doi.org/10.1258/vasc.2011.oa0332.
4. Bower C, Roth JS. Economics of abdominal wall reconstruction. Surg Clin North Am. 2013;93(5):1241–53. https://doi.org/10.1016/j.suc.2013.06.007.
5. Reynolds D, Davenport DL, Korosec RL, Roth JS. Financial implications of ventral hernia repair: a hospital cost analysis. J Gastrointest Surg. 2013;17(1):159–66.; Discussion p. 66–7. https://doi.org/10.1007/s11605-012-1999-y.
6. Hoer J, Lawong G, Klinge U, Schumpelick V. Factors influencing the development of incisional hernia. A retrospective study of 2,983 laparotomy patients over a period of 10 years. Chirurg. 2002;73(5):474–80. https://doi.org/10.1007/s00104-002-0425-5.
7. Sorensen LT, Hemmingsen UB, Kirkeby LT, Kallehave F, Jorgensen LN. Smoking is a risk factor for incisional hernia. Arch Surg. 2005;140(2):119–23. https://doi.org/10.1001/archsurg.140.2.119.
8. Llaguna OH, Avgerinos DV, Lugo JZ, Matatov T, Abbadessa B, Martz JE, et al. Incidence and risk factors for the development of incisional hernia following elective laparoscopic versus open colon resections. Am J Surg. 2010;200(2):265–9. https://doi.org/10.1016/j.amjsurg.2009.08.044.

9. Santora TA, Roslyn JJ. Incisional hernia. Surg Clin North Am. 1993;73(3):557–70.
10. Veljkovic R, Protic M, Gluhovic A, Potic Z, Milosevic Z, Stojadinovic A. Prospective clinical trial of factors predicting the early development of incisional hernia after midline laparotomy. J Am Coll Surg. 2010;210(2):210–9. https://doi.org/10.1016/j.jamcollsurg.2009.10.013.
11. Franchi M, Ghezzi F, Buttarelli M, Tateo S, Balestreri D, Bolis P. Incisional hernia in gynecologic oncology patients: a 10-year study. Obstet Gynecol. 2001;97(5 Pt 1):696–700.
12. Sugerman HJ, Kellum JM Jr, Reines HD, DeMaria EJ, Newsome HH, Lowry JW. Greater risk of incisional hernia with morbidly obese than steroid-dependent patients and low recurrence with prefascial polypropylene mesh. Am J Surg. 1996;171(1):80–4. https://doi.org/10.1016/S0002-9610(99)80078-6.
13. Takagi H, Sugimoto M, Kato T, Matsuno Y, Umemoto T. Postoperative incision hernia in patients with abdominal aortic aneurysm and aortoiliac occlusive disease: a systematic review. Eur J Vasc Endovasc Surg. 2007;33(2):177–81. https://doi.org/10.1016/j.ejvs.2006.07.009.
14. Hope W. Prevention of incisional hernia development. Minerva Chir. 2011;66(2):145–52.
15. Muysoms FE, Antoniou SA, Bury K, Campanelli G, Conze J, Cuccurullo D, et al. European Hernia Society guidelines on the closure of abdominal wall incisions. Hernia. 2015;19(1):1–24. https://doi.org/10.1007/s10029-014-1342-5.
16. Israelsson LA, Millbourn D. Prevention of incisional hernias: how to close a midline incision. Surg Clin North Am. 2013;93(5):1027–40. https://doi.org/10.1016/j.suc.2013.06.009.
17. Rappaport WD, Hunter GC, Allen R, Lick S, Halldorsson A, Chvapil T, et al. Effect of electrocautery on wound healing in midline laparotomy incisions. Am J Surg. 1990;160(6):618–20.
18. Kim H, Brunner E, Ritter E, Thompson D, Devereux D. Relevance of methods of skin incision technique on development of wound infection. Am Surg. 1991;57(2):129–30.
19. Ozgun H, Tuncyurek P, Boylu S, Erpek H, Yenisey C, Kose H, et al. The right method for midline laparotomy: what is the best choice for wound healing? Acta Chir Belg. 2007;107(6):682–6.
20. Allan SN, Spitz L, van Noort R, Black MM. A comparative study of scalpel and electrosurgical incision on subsequent wound healing. J Pediatr Surg. 1982;17(1):52–4.
21. Franchi M, Ghezzi F, Benedetti-Panici PL, Melpignano M, Fallo L, Tateo S, et al. A multicentre collaborative study on the use of cold scalpel and electrocautery for midline abdominal incision. Am J Surg. 2001;181(2):128–32.
22. Kearns SR, Connolly EM, McNally S, McNamara DA, Deasy J. Randomized clinical trial of diathermy versus scalpel incision in elective midline laparotomy. Br J Surg. 2001;88(1):41–4. https://doi.org/10.1046/j.1365-2168.2001.01625.x.
23. Shamim M. Diathermy vs. scalpel skin incisions in general surgery: double-blind, randomized, clinical trial. World J Surg. 2009;33(8):1594–9. https://doi.org/10.1007/s00268-009-0064-9.
24. Ziv Y, Brosh T, Lushkov G, Halevy A. Effect of electrocautery vs. scalpel on fascial mechanical properties after midline laparotomy incision in rats. Isr Med Assoc J. 2001;3(8):566–8.
25. Garcia A, Nascimento JE, Darold EM, Pimentel RE, Curvo EA, Daud FO. Healing of abdominal wall aponeurosis of rats after incision with either cold scalpel or electrocautery. Acta Cir Bras. 2007;22(Suppl 1):12–5.
26. Deerenberg EB, Harlaar JJ, Steyerberg EW, Lont HE, van Doorn HC, Heisterkamp J, et al. Small bites versus large bites for closure of abdominal midline incisions (STITCH): a double-blind, multicentre, randomised controlled trial. Lancet. 2015;386(10000):1254–60. https://doi.org/10.1016/S0140-6736(15)60459-7.
27. Jenkins TP. The burst abdominal wound: a mechanical approach. Br J Surg. 1976;63(11):873–6.
28. Israelsson LA, Jonsson T, Knutsson A. Suture technique and wound healing in midline laparotomy incisions. Eur J Surg. 1996;162(8):605–9.
29. Leaper DJ, Pollock AV, Evans M. Abdominal wound closure: a trial of nylon, polyglycolic acid and steel sutures. Br J Surg. 1977;64(8):603–6.
30. Hogstrom H, Haglund U, Zederfeldt B. Suture technique and early breaking strength of intestinal anastomoses and laparotomy wounds. Acta Chir Scand. 1985;151(5):441–3.
31. Sanders RJ, DiClementi D, Ireland K. Principles of abdominal wound closure. I. Animal studies. Arch Surg. 1977;112(10):1184–7.
32. Millbourn D, Cengiz Y, Israelsson LA. Effect of stitch length on wound complications after closure of midline incisions: a randomized controlled trial. Arch Surg. 2009;144(11):1056–9. https://doi.org/10.1001/archsurg.2009.189.
33. Gurusamy KS, Cassar Delia E, Davidson BR. Peritoneal closure versus no peritoneal closure for patients undergoing non-obstetric abdominal operations. Cochrane Database Syst Rev. 2013;7:CD010424. https://doi.org/10.1002/14651858.CD010424.pub2.
34. Muysoms FE, Detry O, Vierendeels T, Huyghe M, Miserez M, Ruppert M, et al. Prevention of incisional hernias by prophylactic mesh-augmented reinforcement of midline laparotomies for abdominal aortic aneurysm treatment: a randomized controlled trial. Ann Surg. 2016;263(4):638–45. https://doi.org/10.1097/SLA.0000000000001369.

16 Fundamentals of Robotic Surgery

Tomoko Mizota, Victoria G. Dodge, and Dimitrios Stefanidis

16.1 Introduction

16.1.1 The Advent of Robotic Surgery

Advancements in technology have revolutionized surgery, first with the introduction of laparoscopic surgery and more recently with the advent of robotic surgery. The original idea of the current robotic surgery system began with the concept of "telepresence" at the National Aeronautics and Space Administration (NASA) [1]. NASA researchers created a virtual reality system that could be remotely controlled to operate in space. This system displayed a three-dimensional (3D) graphic image, which seemed to surround the viewer in an imaginary environment [2]. This idea was introduced to surgery in the 1980s allowing surgery to be performed remotely by an expert surgeon transferring his/her skill techniques to the patient site. In 1997, the first telepresence surgery cholecystectomy was performed in Belgium [3]. After being approved for clinical use in the USA in 2000, robotic surgery has been applied to diverse surgical procedures in a variety of disciplines, such as urology, general surgery, gynecology, neurosurgery, orthopedics, and cardiac surgery [4]. The number of procedures performed by robotic surgery has been constantly increasing since its introduction. According to the annual report of Intuitive Surgical Inc. (Sunnyvale, CA), which has developed the da Vinci® Surgical System, approximately 563,000 procedures were performed across specialties in the USA in 2016 [5] up from just under 300,000 procedures in 2011 for an approximate 190% increase in case volume over the past 5 years [5].

T. Mizota · V. G. Dodge · D. Stefanidis (✉)
Department of Surgery, Indiana University School of Medicine, Indianapolis, IN, USA
e-mail: dimstefa@iu.edu

16.2 Features of Robotic Surgery

16.2.1 Advantages of Robotic Surgical Systems Over Laparoscopic Surgery

Several technological limitations in laparoscopic surgery have made the learning curve long and difficult. A robotic surgical system has been developed to address constraints of laparoscopy in addition to enabling telepresence surgery [6, 7]. Table 16.1 lists specific features of robotic surgery, which address limitations of laparoscopy and make difficult tasks easier, resulting in improved operator workload.

16.2.2 Three-Dimensional Imaging

Traditional laparoscopes show surgeons the operating field in two-dimensional (2D) images on a

F. Palazzo (ed.), *Fundamentals of General Surgery*, https://doi.org/10.1007/978-3-319-75656-1_16

Table 16.1 Advantages of robotic surgical systems over laparoscopic surgery

	Laparoscopic surgery	Robotic surgery
Image quality	Two-dimensional	Three-dimensional
Movements	Reversal/fulcrum effect	Natural intuition
Motion scaling	Amplified	Favorable
Tremor	Amplified	Eliminated
Degrees of freedom (DOF)	5 DOF	7 DOF
Camera platform	Unstable, held by assistant	Stable, controlled by operator
Ergonomics	Restricted	Improved

screen. Surgeons are required to recognize 3D anatomy from 2D images, which makes laparoscopic surgery challenging and highly demanding. In contrast, the camera system in robotic surgery is stereoscopic, allowing surgeons to perform procedures watching 3D images. The binocular imaging system reduces surgeon workload and improves depth perception and precision during surgery [8].

16.2.3 Elimination of Motion Reversal

Due to leverage around a trocar site (fulcrum), laparoscopic instrument tips move opposite of the surgeon's hand motions. This juxtaposition can interfere with a surgeon's performance during laparoscopy. Conversely, robotic instruments translate surgeon's hand motions into identical instrument tip movements. This simplifies operating tasks and improves surgeon's performance by mimicking natural hand motions.

16.2.4 Favorable Motion Scaling and Tremor Elimination

The fulcrum effect has another influence on instrument handling. The motions of instrument tips are amplified greater than surgeon's hand motions, which complicates the learning curve of laparoscopic surgery. Robotic surgery overcomes this issue with motion amplification adjustments. Robotic systems have several levels of motion scaling for both instruments and the visual field, so that surgeons can select a preferable scaling. For instance, when a 3:1 ratio scale is selected, the motion of the instrument tip is reduced by one third of the surgeon's hand motion.

In addition to motion scaling, a high-performance computer eliminates the effect of tremors in a surgeon's hands. It also enables more precise and delicate movement of the robotic instruments.

16.2.5 Increased Degrees of Freedom

Since laparoscopic instruments are straight, the degrees of freedom (DOF) are limited to five: pitch, jaw, rotation, insertion/extraction, and actuation of the instrument. The 5 DOF restricts the mobility of a surgeon's technical performance and makes laparoscopic procedures difficult. The robotic system has a joint at the end of the end-effector, which moves like a human wrist (7 DOF) [7]. This then reflects a surgeon's complex performance in the tips of the instruments.

16.2.6 Stable Camera Platform

During laparoscopic surgery, an assistant handles a camera and is required to manually adjust the camera position and orientation frequently. Since an operating view of laparoscopic surgery completely depends on images captured by a camera, the assistant's skill in camera handling and communication with the primary surgeon has a large impact on procedure performance. On the other hand, a robotic surgery camera system can be handled by a primary surgeon, which aids in tremor elimination. This enables operating view stability and comfort for a surgeon.

16.2.7 Ergonomic Positioning

Ergonomic equipment for surgeons is essential to maximize surgeon performance. Laparoscopy has been demonstrated to lead to surgeon fatigue and pain in the neck, back, shoulders, elbows and hips, because surgeons are required to stand throughout a laparoscopic procedure, sometimes in contorted positions [9]. To overcome these issues, the robotic system is equipped with an adjustable console. Thus, a surgeon can adjust his/her visualization system and padded forearm rest to the most favorable height. This may facilitate improved surgeon performance in his/her most comfortable position [10].

16.2.8 Safety Mechanisms

Equipment problems can cause critical injury to patients. Unlike laparoscopic equipment, the robotic surgery system has multiple sensing mechanisms to prevent patient injury. When the system senses an error during a procedure, the surgeon is alerted in order to avoid a patient injury. In addition, when a malfunction occurs in one component, other backup components work to maintain the operation safely. If the system still needs to be shut down, it occurs stepwise, but not immediately.

16.3 Effective and Safe Use of the Robotic System

This section describes a stepwise practical usage guide of the robotic surgery system. Although robotic systems have built-in safety mechanisms for the automatic detection of errors, they introduce new challenges for the operating room (OR) team that need to be addressed. For example, the remote position of the operating surgeon to the patient bed introduces team communication issues that need to be addressed. In the following paragraphs, we will provide some practical tips for trainees new to robotic surgery that can help them master this promising technique faster.

16.3.1 Preoperative Phase

- Setting up the robotic system
- While the robotic system is typically set up by OR personnel prior to case start, it is still important for surgeons to understand the basic steps of its setup; this may prove valuable in some occasions where personnel experience may be lacking. The camera, for example, needs to be calibrated appropriately prior to case start. Inappropriate calibration will cause problems with visualization at the surgeon console; therefore, if problems are encountered with the image quality, camera recalibration should be considered. Attention to system maintenance is also required to keep the system working efficiently.
- The robotic arms should be draped before the case starts.
- Setting up the robotic room for best efficiency (positioning of the patient and operating table)
- Utilizing gravity is essential not only in laparoscopic surgery, but in robotic surgery as well. To maximize its advantage, surgeons should be familiar with how to use gravity while maintaining patient safety. A patient can easily slide or move during the procedure if he/she is poorly positioned. To prevent improper patient positioning, surgeons need to secure the patient well on the operating table, and test table manipulations before draping the patient to ensure that the patient does not slide or move. Additionally, surgeons need to make sure the operating table is locked to prevent movement during the procedure. This is particularly important with the older generation of existing systems (da Vinci® Si) as motion of the patient during the procedure can lead to injuries. The newer generation of robotic systems (da Vinci® Xi), however, has addressed this issue by allowing the robot to move with the operating table.

16.3.2 Intraoperative Phase

- Trocar placement
- Trocar placement is one of the significant differences between robotic and laparoscopic systems, primarily with regard to distance between trocars and the target. Surgeons should be thoroughly knowledgeable and plan where to place trocars safely. A common error is to place trocars too close to each other, thus allowing robotic arms to collide during the procedure. Additionally, trocars should typically be placed a bit further away from the target than is necessary for laparoscopy.

- A robotic trocar has a thick black line near the tip (Fig. 16.1). This line should be positioned at the internal surface level of the cavity (i.e., peritoneum, pleura, etc.). This minimizes friction between the trocars and the cavity wall (i.e., abdomen, chest wall, etc.) during motion of the arms.
- Docking of robot cart and arms
- The orientation of the surgical cart depends on the type of procedure performed (Fig. 16.2, 16.3, and 16.4). Generally, the robotic cart is positioned near the target side, so that its robotic arms can more easily reach the target, i.e., at the feet for pelvic procedures (Fig. 16.2) or over the head for upper abdominal procedures (Fig. 16.3). Robotic arm docking sequence varies from case to case, but either starts from one side and goes to the other or starts with the

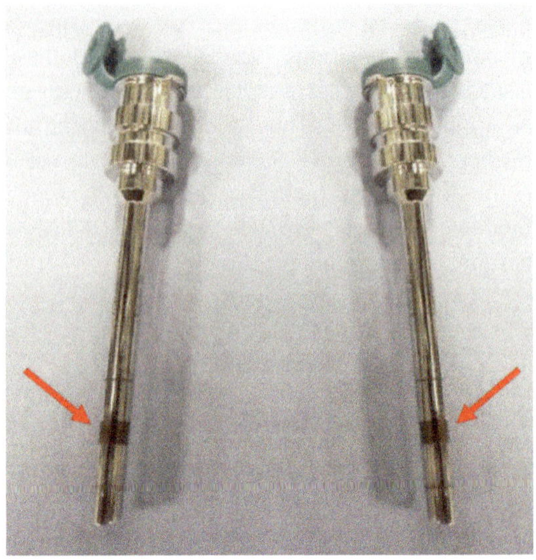

Fig. 16.1 Robotic trocars

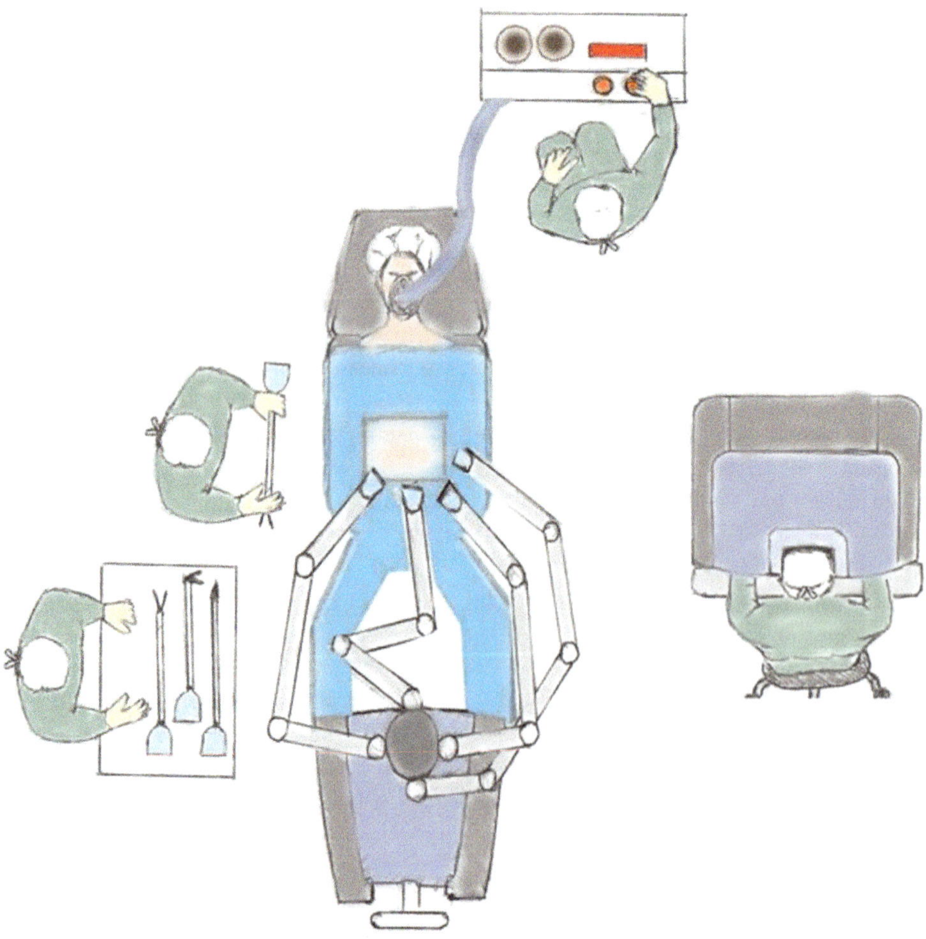

Fig. 16.2 Pelvis—at the feet, between the legs, or side-docked (i.e., prostate, colon, and rectum)

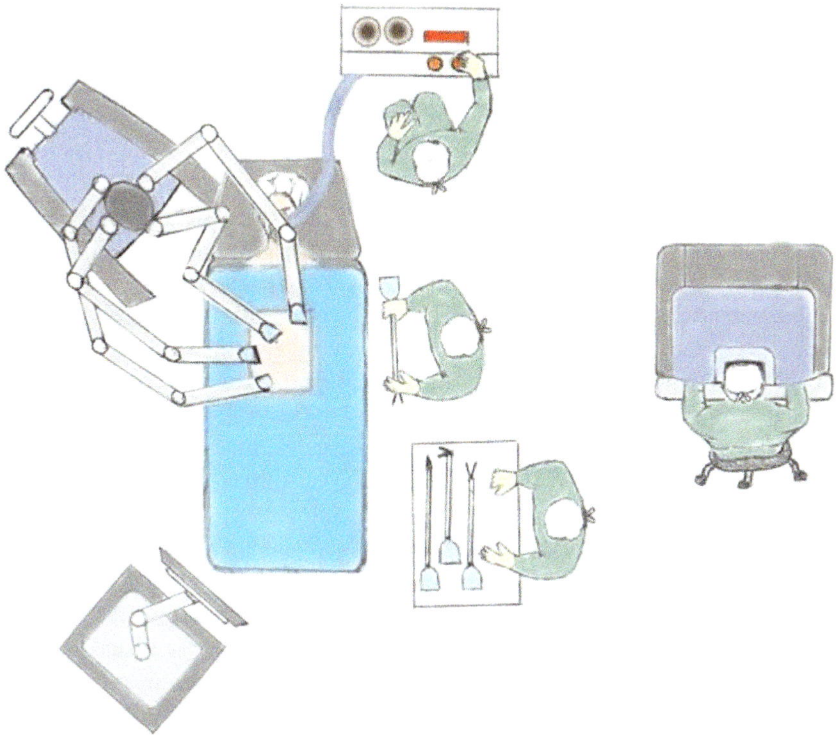

Fig. 16.3 Upper abdomen—over the shoulder (i.e., foregut)

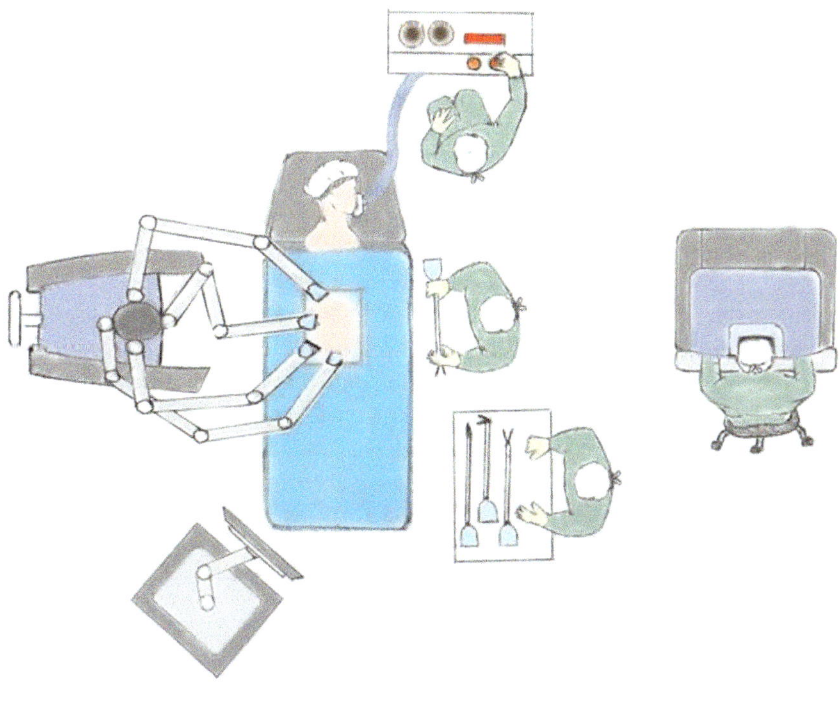

Fig. 16.4 Flanks—beside patient (i.e., kidney)

camera arm and continues to the rest of the arms. Once all arms are docked, surgeons should confirm that the arms can move without collisions. If not given proper attention, this may limit instrument motion during the procedure. The newer generation da Vinci® Si has automated this process as it aligns the arms automatically in reference to the target tissue so that collisions are minimized.

- Most novices find it very challenging to attach the robotic arms to the trocars (this is mostly true for the Si system and easier for the Xi). To facilitate docking, align the axis of the trocar with the axis of the arm. Once the trocars have been attached to the arms, the arm can be elevated to some degree using the clutch button, so that the abdominal wall can be pulled further away from the intra-abdominal organs. This may be particularly useful in cases where working space is limited due to patient anatomy. This maneuver may enhance the ability to dissect.
- Instrument insertion
- Upon the first instrument insertion, the clutch button needs to be depressed to slide the instrument in and place it in the desired position. Clutch button depression should be quick and temporary. A common mistake made by unfamiliar users is to keep their finger on the clutch button too long, which causes inadvertent repeat depression and locking of the arm, preventing further movement. Similar to laparoscopic surgery, any further instruments need to be visualized when inserted into a cavity to avoid preventable injuries. Further, the camera should be set at a wide-angle view to improve visualization of any structures in the cavity as well as the instrument tip. Additionally, when an instrument is removed, the surgeon and the bedside assistant should confirm that the instrument is not attached to tissue. Communication between the surgeon and the bedside assistant is therefore vital during this step.
- Importantly, during an instrument exchange (i.e., after the instrument has been placed and used), the clutch button should not be depressed; the instrument should just be pulled out and the desired instrument inserted in its place. The arm light will turn green, and the instrument can be safely reintroduced to its prior position by pushing the instrument in. This is a safety mechanism of the robotic system, which allows efficient instrument exchange without the need for visual monitoring of the insertion process. If, however, the robotic arm is clutched during an instrument exchange, this safety mechanism is canceled, and instrument insertion needs to be visually monitored.
- Setting up the surgeon console
- The surgeon console can be adjusted to an ergonomically comfortable position which will minimize surgeon stress and fatigue during the procedure. A surgeon can adjust the height of the viewer, the level of the handrest, and the position of foot controls.

Next, the visual field should be set up. For safety, the instruments should always be kept within the visual field as instrument movements in the absence of visualization can lead to injuries. The placement of a surgeon's head inside the forehead rest of the console is required to activate the robotic instruments. The surgeon can control instruments when his/her fingers are placed in the controllers. If too much pressure is applied on the controllers, the instrument will be temporarily locked. In this case, the surgeon needs to release the pressure and move the controllers gently again. If the surgeon takes his/her fingers off the controllers after activation, uncontrollable movement may occur which can lead to injury and must be avoided. If this occurs inadvertently, the best approach is for the surgeon to immediately remove his/her head from the viewer (which will immobilize the instruments). If he/she attempts to reinsert the fingers into the controllers, this may likely lead to further movement and additive risk since it is done blindly (as the surgeon cannot directly visualize his/her fingers with his/her head inside the viewer).

16.3.3 Postoperative Phase

- Undocking the robot
- After confirming that the instruments are not attached to any organs of the patient, they can be removed, the arms can be detached from the trocars, and the robot can be safely undocked. After this process, the robotic patient-side cart should be moved away from the patient. The surgeon should always pay attention to both the patient and the robot so that no injury occurs. In emergency situations, the arms can be removed quickly with the trocars attached.

16.4 Robotic Skill Acquisition

16.4.1 Issues with Robotic Surgery with Focus on Surgeon Competency

While new technology has revolutionized patient care in many instances, its introduction is often associated with poorer patient outcomes. This issue became evident during the introduction of laparoscopic techniques in surgery. Despite multiple benefits of laparoscopy over laparotomy on patient outcomes, an increased incidence of technical complications was observed related to inadequate training of surgeons on this new technique [11]. To overcome this issue, the Society of American Gastrointestinal and Endoscopic Surgeons (SAGES) and the American College of Surgeons (ACS) developed the Fundamentals of Laparoscopic Surgery (FLS), a simulation-based curriculum for the acquisition of basic laparoscopic skills outside the OR [12]. Training on FLS has been demonstrated to improve surgeon proficiency in laparoscopy [13], and currently FLS certification is a requirement for residents to obtain board certification in general surgery.

Similar to the experience with laparoscopy, robotic surgery has come under scrutiny due to a number of reported adverse events resulting in lawsuits against the manufacturer. One of the main plaintiffs' allegations has been inadequate training of surgeons [14–16]. Several authors have therefore recommended that standardized curricula for the training and assessment of robotic surgery skills should be developed [17–19]. Accordingly, surgeons should be required to possess an appropriate skill level utilizing the robotic system prior to performing an operation on a patient.

To address this need, the Fundamentals of Robotic Surgery (FRS) [20] was developed as a simulation-based curriculum to help surgeons acquire basic knowledge and skills crucial to performing robotic surgery.

16.4.2 Fundamentals of Robotic Surgery (FRS)

FRS is a proficiency-based progression curriculum (course) of basic robotic surgery skills which was developed using a full life-cycle curriculum development method by over 80 robotic surgery experts, behavioral psychologists, medical educators, statisticians, and psychometricians from around the world. The Department of Defense and Intuitive Surgical, Inc. funded its development. The main aim was to develop a standardized curriculum that would help ensure that surgeons safely and efficiently perform robotic surgery [21].

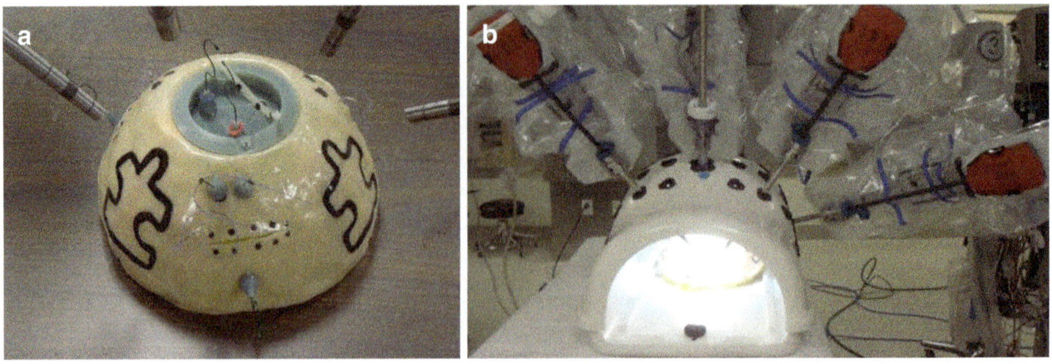

Fig. 16.5 FRS physical model with dome (**a**) and torso box trainer (**b**)

Proficiency-based training is recognized as an effective method in surgical education [22, 23]. In contrast to traditional training, which arbitrarily defines training duration and/or number of practice sessions, proficiency-based training sets expert-derived performance goals for trainees to achieve. Thus, it enables training to be tailored to individual needs and ensures the acquisition of the desired level of performance upon completion.

The FRS curriculum consists of an online curriculum that provides fundamental knowledge of robotic surgery and a dry lab training module for psychomotor skills with tasks specific to robotic surgery (www.frs.casenetwork.com/lms/). The online curriculum includes basic instructions on the use of the robot from preoperative preparation to postoperative debriefing. It also includes a team training component, which is a vital skill, especially in robotic surgery, to facilitate communication between surgeons and other medical professionals in the OR. The psychomotor module contains basic tasks of robotic surgery on a physical model (Fig. 16.5) or virtual reality simulators (Fig. 16.6), ring tower transfer (Fig. 16.7a), knot tying (b), railroad track (c), fourth arm cutting (d), puzzle piece dissection (e), and vessel energy dissection (f). In addition to these training materials, the FRS includes assessment tools in each module to assess surgeon technical and nontechnical competency, which ensures skills to perform safe and successful robotic surgery.

The development process of the FRS curriculum is available online at www.frsurgery.org.

Take-Home Points

- Robotic surgery can enhance surgical capabilities but requires a new skill set, which needs to be mastered.
- All trainees/surgeons who will be performing robotic surgery need to become familiar with the features and nuances of currently available robotic surgery systems.
- Similar to other areas of surgical practice, engagement in deliberate practice is paramount to become proficient in robotic surgery and to optimize patient outcomes. Simulation-based skills curricula, such as the Fundamentals of Robotic Surgery, have been developed to promote this goal.

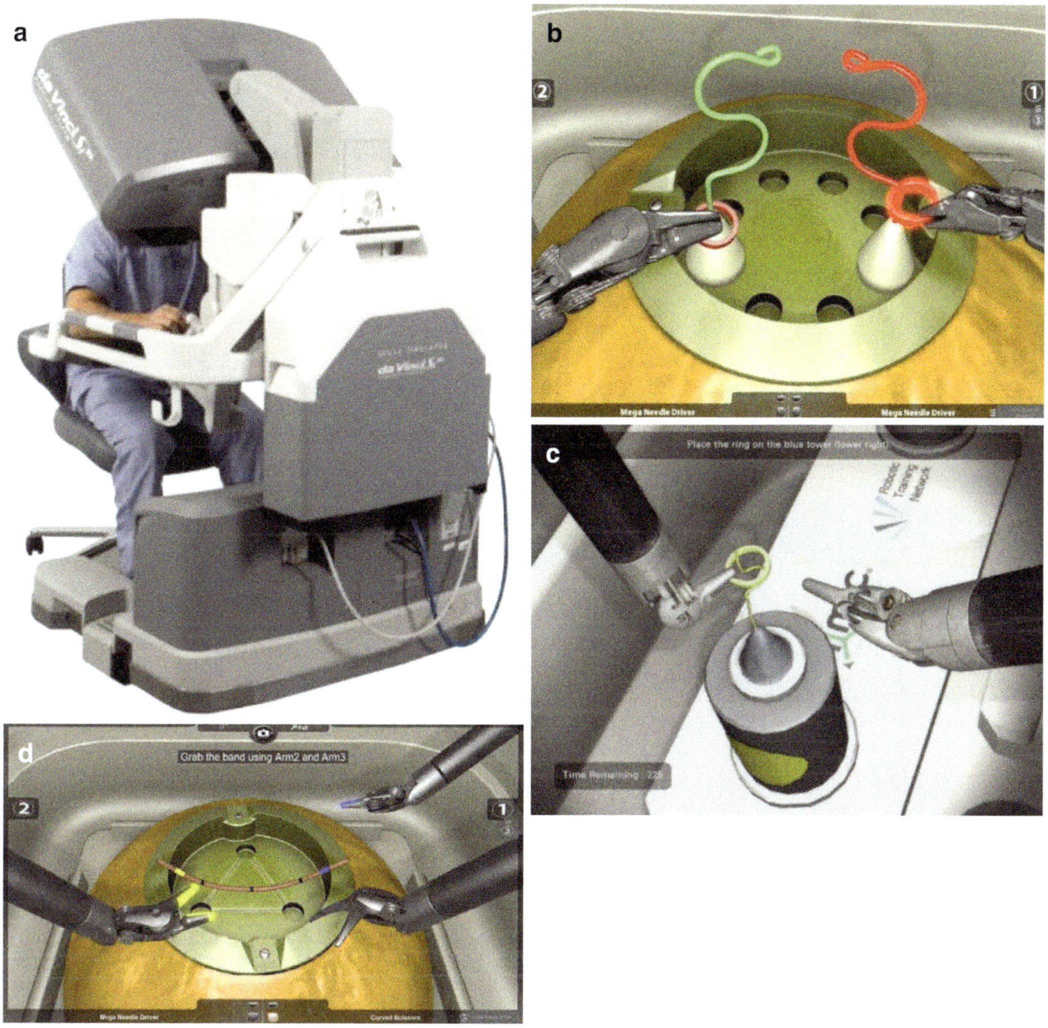

Fig. 16.6 da Vinci Skills Simulator® (dVSS) (**a**) and virtual reality simulation of the FRS dome: dVSS dome (**b**+**c**) with different skill testing units and RobotiX Mentor virtual reality simulation (**d**)

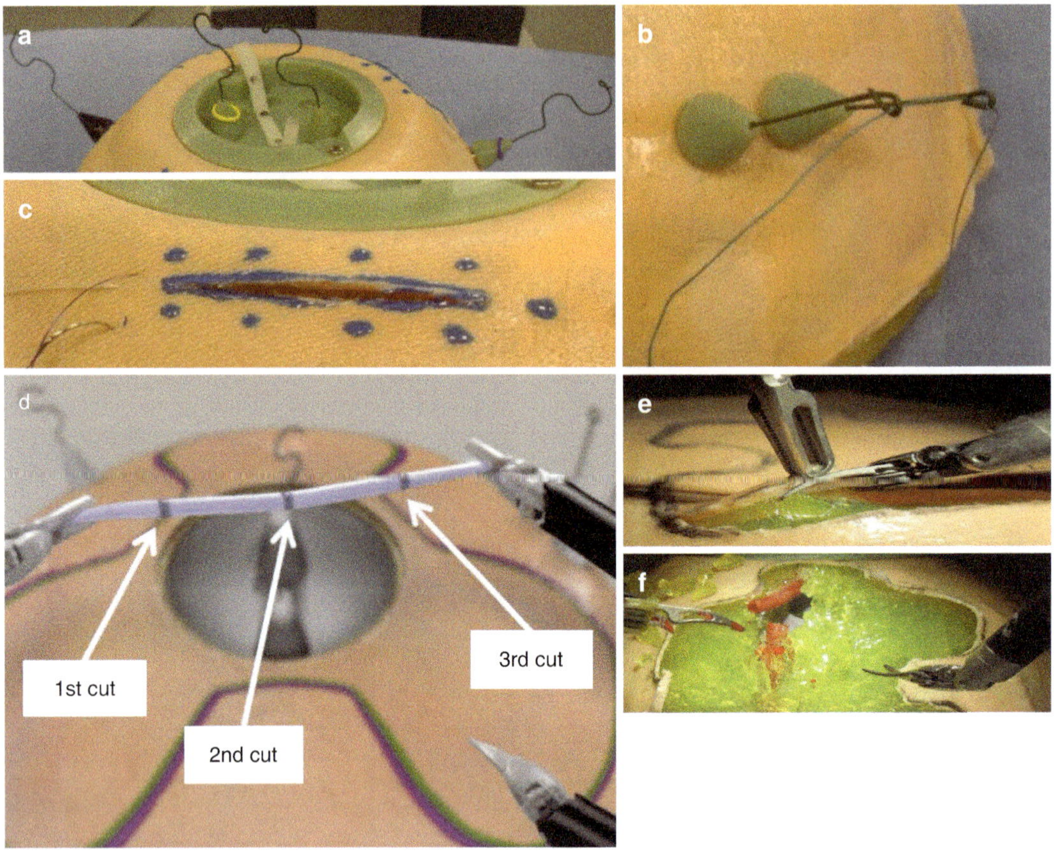

Fig. 16.7 Simulation tasks on a physical model. Ring tower transfer (**a**), knot tying (**b**), railroad track (**c**), fourth arm cutting (**d**), puzzle piece dissection (**e**), and vessel energy dissection (**f**)

Suggested Readings

Lendvay TS, Hannaford B, Satava RM. Future of robotic surgery. Cancer J. 2013;19(2):109–19.

Smith R, Patel V, Satava R. Fundamentals of robotic surgery: a course of basic robotic surgery skills based upon a 14-society consensus template of outcomes measures and curriculum development. Int J Med Robot. 2014;10(3):379–84.

Chang L, Satava RM, Pellegrini CA, Sinanan MN. Robotic surgery: identifying the learning curve through objective measurement of skill. Surg Endosc. 2003;17(11):1744–8.

References

1. Satava RM. Surgical robotics: the early chronicles: a personal historical perspective. Surg Laparosc Endosc Percutan Tech. 2002;12(1):6–16.
2. Fisher S, McGreevy M, Humphries J, Robinett W. Virtual environment display system. In: Crow F, Pizer S, editors. Proceedings of the workshop on interactive 3-dimensional graphics. New York: ACM; 1986. p. 1–12.
3. Himpens J, Leman G, Cadiere G. Telesurgical laparoscopic cholecystectomy. Surg Endosc. 1998;12(8):1091.
4. Wormer BA, Dacey KT, Williams KB, Bradley JF 3rd, Walters AL, Augenstein VA, et al. The first nationwide evaluation of robotic general surgery: a regionalized, small but safe start. Surg Endosc. 2014;28(3):767–76.
5. Annual report 2016. Intuitive Surgical Inc. http://phx.corporate-ir.net/phoenix.zhtml?c=122359&p=irol-irhome. Accessed 12 Apr 2017.
6. Valverde A, Goasguen N, Oberlin O. Fundamentals of robotic surgery or of robotic-assisted telemanipulated laparoscopy. J Visc Surg. 2014;151(3):213–21.
7. Kenngott HG, Muller-Stich BP, Reiter MA, Rassweiler J, Gutt CN. Robotic suturing: technique and benefit in advanced laparoscopic surgery. Minim Invasive Ther Allied Technol. 2008;17(3):160–7.

8. Bhayani SB, Andriole GL. Three-dimensional (3D) vision: does it improve laparoscopic skills? An assessment of a 3d head-mounted visualization system. Rev Urol. 2005;7(4):211–4.
9. Hubert N, Gilles M, Desbrosses K, Meyer JP, Felblinger J, Hubert J. Ergonomic assessment of the surgeon's physical workload during standard and robotic assisted laparoscopic procedures. Int J Med Robot. 2013;9(2):142–7.
10. van der Schatte Olivier RH, Van't Hullenaar CD, Ruurda JP, Broeders IA. Ergonomics, user comfort, and performance in standard and robot-assisted laparoscopic surgery. Surg Endosc. 2009;23(6):1365–71.
11. Shah SR, Mirza DF, Afonso R, Mayer AD, McMaster P, Buckels JA. Changing referral pattern of biliary injuries sustained during laparoscopic cholecystectomy. Br J Surg. 2000;87(7):890–1.
12. Fundamentals of Laparoscopic Surgery. http://www.flsprogram.org/. Accessed 5 Jun 2017.
13. Sroka G, Feldman LS, Vassiliou MC, Kaneva PA, Fayez R, Fried GM. Fundamentals of laparoscopic surgery simulator training to proficiency improves laparoscopic performance in the operating room-a randomized controlled trial. Am J Surg. 2010; 199(1):115–20.
14. da Vinci Robot Lawsuit. Surgical Watch. http://surgicalwatch.com/davinci-robot/lawsuit/. Accessed 15 May 2017.
15. Alemzadeh H, Raman J, Leveson N, Kalbarczyk Z, Iyer RK. Adverse events in robotic surgery: a retrospective study of 14 years of FDA data. PLoS One. 2016;11(4):e0151470.
16. Ferrarese A, Pozzi G, Borghi F, Marano A, Delbon P, Amato B, et al. Malfunctions of robotic system in surgery: role and responsibility of surgeon in legal point of view. Open Med (Wars). 2016;11(1):286–91.
17. Chang L, Satava RM, Pellegrini CA, Sinanan MN. Robotic surgery: identifying the learning curve through objective measurement of skill. Surg Endosc. 2003;17(11):1744–8.
18. Zorn KC, Gautam G, Shalhav AL, Clayman RV, Ahlering TE, Albala DM, et al. Training, credentialing, proctoring and medicolegal risks of robotic urological surgery: recommendations of the society of urologic robotic surgeons. J Urol. 2009;182(3): 1126–32.
19. Lendvay TS, Hannaford B, Satava RM. Future of robotic surgery. Cancer J. 2013;19(2):109–19.
20. Fundamentals of Robotic Surgery. http://frsurgery.org/. Accessed 15 Apr 2017.
21. Smith R, Patel V, Satava R. Fundamentals of robotic surgery: a course of basic robotic surgery skills based upon a 14-society consensus template of outcomes measures and curriculum development. Int J Med Robot. 2014;10(3):379–84.
22. Brunner WC, Korndorffer JR Jr, Sierra R, Dunne JB, Yau CL, Corsetti RL, et al. Determining standards for laparoscopic proficiency using virtual reality. Am Surg. 2005;71(1):29–35.
23. Seymour NE, Gallagher AG, Roman SA, O'Brien MK, Bansal VK, Andersen DK, et al. Virtual reality training improves operating room performance: results of a randomized, double-blinded study. Ann Surg. 2002;236(4):458–63.

Fundamentals of Gastrointestinal Anastomoses

17

Talar Tatarian, Andrew M. Brown, Michael J. Pucci, and Francesco Palazzo

17.1 Introduction

The creation of a gastrointestinal anastomosis is a fundamental skill essential to general surgery. As surgical techniques have evolved over the centuries, key concepts critical to the success of an anastomosis hold true. This chapter will detail the history of gastrointestinal anastomoses, will provide general principles for creation of a viable and successful anastomosis, and will review key technical considerations and current controversies.

17.2 Historical Perspective

Writings on gastrointestinal wound healing date as far back as the early nineteenth century. In 1812 Benjamin Travers affirmed, "the union of a divided bowel requires the contact of the cut extremities in their entire circumference…the species of suture employed is of secondary importance if it secures the contact" [1, 2]. A decade later, the French surgeon Antoine Lembert further specified the importance of serosal apposition with mucosal inversion [1, 2]. It took until the late nineteenth century for William Stewart Halsted to identify the submucosa as the strongest layer of the intestinal wall [1–3]. Through most of the twentieth century, it became standard practice to perform a two-layer, inverting anastomosis.

Controversy arose in the 1960s and 1970s when studies on canine models found everted anastomoses to have increased edema and tensile strength in the first 21 days after surgery [4]. This was quickly refuted by several animal studies which strongly recommended against mucosal eversion after finding inverted anastomoses to have superior strength and decreased adhesion formation [5–7].

Further debate arose in 1966 with the introduction of automatic stapling devices. Ravitch et al. were the first to report on the benefits of the "Ligating-Dividing-Stapling Instrument," citing versatility, dependability, and a decrease in bowel wall trauma [8]. Initial randomized controlled trials (RCTs) comparing stapled versus hand-sewn gastrointestinal anastomoses found no difference in the rate of anastomotic leak, morbidity, or mortality [9]. Since these early RCTs, newer studies have found there are differences depending on the specific situation and location within the gastrointestinal tract.

In 1993, Choy et al. published a large RCT demonstrating that stapled ileocolonic anastomoses after elective right hemicolectomy had decreased

T. Tatarian · A. M. Brown · M. J. Pucci
F. Palazzo (✉)
Department of Surgery, Sidney Kimmel Medical College, Thomas Jefferson University, Philadelphia, PA, USA
e-mail: Francesco.Palazzo@jefferson.edu

F. Palazzo (ed.), *Fundamentals of General Surgery*, https://doi.org/10.1007/978-3-319-75656-1_17

fecal contamination and a trend toward a decreased anastomotic leak rate [10]. This was later supported by a 2011 Cochrane report comparing 441 stapled versus 684 hand-sewn anastomoses. Stapled ileocolonic anastomoses had a significantly lower rate of anastomotic leak, particularly in patients with malignancy [11]. Studies of trauma patients after penetrating bowel injury have found lower leak rates with hand-sewn anastomoses [12, 13].

Data regarding colorectal anastomoses has been mixed [9]. A 2001 meta-analysis included nine trials studying 1233 patients randomized to a hand-sewn versus stapled colorectal anastomosis [14]. The authors found a higher incidence of anastomotic strictures in the stapled group; however, the overall, radiological, and clinical leak rates were similar. As such, current guidelines recommend the surgeon use their clinical judgment in deciding which type of technique to use.

17.3 Physiology of Wound Healing and Anatomy of the Intestinal Wall

In order to understand the basic principles guiding the construction of a gastrointestinal anastomosis, it is important to understand the basic physiology of gastrointestinal wound healing and anatomy of the intestinal wall.

Creation of an enterotomy leads to initial hemostatic vasoconstriction followed by secondary vasodilation and increased capillary permeability, mediated by kinins. This results in edema and swelling at the tissue ends [15, 16]. The appearance of granulation tissue in the anastomosis commences the proliferative phase of healing during which collagen undergoes lysis and synthesis [15, 17, 18]. Studies in rabbits have shown that between days three and five of healing, there is an abundance of undifferentiated mesenchymal cells in the healing muscle layers along with capillary invasion. These cells transform into smooth muscle cells and phagocytic histiocytes. This transformation is thought to be responsible for the establishment of smooth muscle tissue [15, 19].

The serosa consists of a thin layer of connective tissue covering the muscularis externa. It is covered on its outer aspect by the mesothelial lining of the peritoneal cavity. Good serosal apposition is necessary to minimize the risk of leakage [4, 15, 20, 21] and is best achieved by using an inverting type of suture technique. Extraperitoneal segments of the GI tract without a serosal covering lack this component of anastomotic protection and are at a higher risk of complications, as seen in the esophagus and lower third of the rectum [15, 22].

The submucosa provides the GI tract with the majority of its tensile strength and is responsible for anchoring the sutures that hold an anastomosis together [15, 23]. The submucosa is composed of loosely interwoven collagenous, elastic, and nerve fibers in addition to blood and lymphatic vessels. This layer has a predominance of type I collagen [15, 24].

Intestinal mucosa is repaired by migration and hyperplasia of epithelial cells which cover the granulation tissue of the wound and seal the defect, creating a watertight barrier [15, 25]. This sealing can occur in as little as three days if the layers of the bowel wall are directly apposed. Any inversion or eversion of specifically the mucosa will delay this process [15, 26].

17.4 General Concepts and Considerations

17.4.1 Factors Determining Anastomotic Healing

Both local and systemic factors impact anastomotic wound healing. These are highlighted in Table 17.1.

The key local factors encouraging healing include adequate intrinsic blood supply and the avoidance of undue tension on the anastomosis [15, 27, 28]. These affect oxygen delivery to the tissue which is required for the hydroxylation of lysine and proline during collagen synthesis [15, 27, 29, 30]. During the explorative, resective, and reconstructive steps of any procedure, the surgeon must employ meticulous technique in order to avoid excessive or rough handling of tissues. Additionally, excessive effort aimed at mobiliz-

Table 17.1 Local and systemic factors affecting anastomotic healing [7, 10]

	Local	Systemic
Positive	Adequate blood supply Healthy tissue edges Seromuscular apposition	Adequate nutritional status Hemodynamic stability
Negative	Tension on the anastomosis Presence of infected or necrotic tissue Hematoma formation Radiation to involved bowel distal obstruction	Anemia/blood transfusion Liver/kidney failure Medications (immunosuppressant, NSAIDs, steroids) Sepsis

ing the limbs to bring together can damage the primary blood vessels and impact perfusion [15, 31, 32]. Conversely, inadequate mobilization can leave tension on the anastomosis, compromising microperfusion leading to inflammatory cell infiltrates [15, 33]. The effect of tension on the microcirculation at the anastomotic site is least tolerated in the colon [15, 34].

Systemically, the presence of hypotension, hypovolemia, or sepsis affects blood flow and subsequent oxygen delivery. Patient factors such as malnutrition, immunosuppression, and the use of certain medications (i.e., steroids, NSAIDs) can also impair wound healing.

17.4.2 Anastomotic Configuration

Gastrointestinal anastomoses are classically described by the alignment of lumens being anastomosed (end-to-end, end-to-side, side-to-side) and the relative direction of peristalsis in the two segments (isoperistaltic vs antiperistaltic). In deciding which configuration to choose, one must take into consideration the segments of bowel being anastomosed, size discrepancy between the two segments, and any tension that may exist across the anastomosis. Anastomosis to the "side" of a segment is useful in situations where there is a size discrepancy between two loops, such as a gastroenteric or ileocolonic anastomosis. A side-to-side configuration also creates a wider anastomosis, minimizing the risk of narrowing or stricturing. An isoperistaltic anastomosis is thought to promote emptying and is generally preferred; however, an antiperistaltic anastomosis may be considered if delayed emptying is desired (i.e., short gut).

17.4.3 Choice of Suture Material or Stapling Device

The choice of suture material is generally dependent on the location within the GI tract and the enteric layer being anastomosed [35]. Sutures are typically 2-0 or 3-0 gauge in caliber and connected to a narrow, *tapered* needle of similar size. Suture may be monofilament, braided, or barbed. When performing a two-layer anastomosis, the inner layer traditionally utilizes an absorbable suture material (i.e., polyglactin [Vicryl]). The outer seromuscular layer is composed of nonabsorbable suture such as silk or polyester (Ethibond). For single-layer intestinal anastomoses, a long-lasting absorbable suture (e.g., polydioxanone [PDS]) or a nonabsorbable suture may be used. In creating a bilioenteric anastomosis, an absorbable synthetic monofilament suture is preferred to prevent infection or stone formation.

If the surgeon opts for a stapled anastomosis, important considerations include choice of stapling device and staple height. For a more in-depth look at stapling devices, you may refer to Chapter 10. In general, linear cutting staplers are preferred for a side-to-side anastomosis, whereas circular staplers are useful for end-to-side or end-to-end anastomoses. Staplers are available in various lengths and diameters depending on intestinal location and use. Staple cartridges are color coded to correspond to the height of the staples [36]. For intestinal anastomoses, a cartridge with an open/closed stapled height of 3.5/1.5 mm is commonly used. For thicker tissues (i.e., gastric tissue) a 3.8/1.8 mm or 4.1/2.0 mm cartridge may be used.

17.5 Technical Considerations: Review of Specific Anastomoses

Fundamental to the success of any intestinal anastomosis is the adherence to a few key principles, aimed to minimize the risk of leak or disruption [2]. First, the surgeon must employ good surgical technique, minimizing trauma to the tissues through gentle handling with atraumatic instruments. All sutures should incorporate the submucosa, which is the strength layer of the small intestine. Care should be taken to approximate the mucosa while preventing it from extruding from the suture line. Sutures should be placed 2–3 mm apart in order to create a watertight, airtight, leakproof closure. Finally, all segments of bowel being joined must have healthy blood supply with adequate hemostasis and avoidance of tension on the anastomosis. As it applies to any anastomosis, be it gastrointestinal or vascular, one key tenet is that no distal stricture or obstruction should exist; otherwise, the anastomosis healing and lifespan are doomed.

With these general concepts in mind, we will highlight the technical aspects of creating a few common anastomoses.

17.5.1 Hand-Sewn Gastrojejunostomy

This section will review a hand-sewn end-to-side isoperistaltic gastrojejunostomy in both a double-layer and single-layer fashion. It is important to note that this technique can be adapted to construct an enteroenteric, ileocolonic, or colocolonic anastomosis.

17.5.1.1 Double-Layer Hand-Sewn Gastrojejunostomy

The cut end of each enteric segment is brought together and aligned in an isoperistaltic orientation. The cut ends are secured by a staple line, non-crushing bowel clamp, or a series of Babcock clamps. For the purposes of this chapter, we will assume the cut end is secured by a staple line. Stay sutures are placed at the proximal and distal ends of the anastomosis, 5 mm from the staple line, incorporating a seromuscular bite using 3-0 silk. These sutures are left untied and are secured with a small clamp.

The posterior outer layer is created first using interrupted seromuscular (Lembert) stitches of 3-0 silk (Fig. 17.1). On the jejunal side, bites should be taken along the posterior wall, 5 mm away from the antimesenteric border. On the gastric side, bites should be taken on the posterior wall, ending 5 mm away from the staple line. Stitches should be placed 3–4 mm apart. Care should be taken to take good seromuscular bites, avoiding full thickness bites incorporating the mucosa. Sutures can be tied sequentially or once all stitches have been placed. All knots are then cut with the exception of the most proximal and distal knots, which serve to maintain traction.

With the posterior outer layer complete, the gastric staple line is excised, and a jejunal enterotomy is made to expose the mucosa. The posterior inner layer is then created using 3-0 absorbable braided sutures in a running locking fashion (Fig. 17.2). Two separate full thickness sutures are placed starting at the midpoint of the anastomosis. Each suture is tied down and then tied to the tail of the other. Full thickness running locking bites should be taken, advancing 5 mm with each bite while remaining 2–3 mm above the posterior Lembert stitches. Once at the apices, the same sutures are used to "turn the corner" as you transition to the anterior inner layer. A full thickness bite is taken from the gastric lumen toward the corner stitch on the gastric side (in to out). The next bite is then taken from the corner stitch on the jejunal side into the jejunal lumen (out to in). Once back in the lumen, the next stitch crosses over to the gastric side. This continues around the corners, advancing only a few millimeters until you reach the anterior layer.

The anterior inner layer is constructed using a "Connell" stitch, passing the suture from outside in, then inside out on one side, then crossing directly across and passing from outside in to inside out on the other side (Fig. 17.3). (Common saying for the Connell Stitch: "Go into the bar, then out of the bar, cross the street and go into the next bar, go out of the bar, cross the street, etc.") The bites should incorporate a relatively larger bite of serosa and smaller bites of mucosa to ensure good inversion of the mucosa and aposition of the serosa. Once the two sutures meet at the midpoint of the anterior wall of the anastomosis, they are tied together to complete the anterior inner layer. As this step is completed, it is important for the assistant to keep constant tension on this running suture.

The anterior outer layer is constructed using 3-0 silk Lembert sutures traversing the length of the anastomosis. Seromuscular bites should be taken 3–4 mm apart and then tied. Once the anastomosis is complete, it should be examined and palpated to ensure patency and integrity.

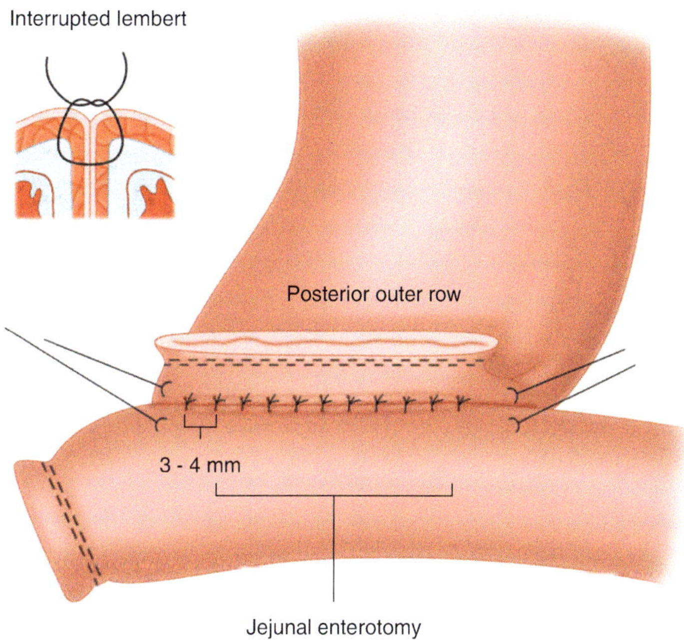

Fig. 17.1 Hand-sewn two-layer gastrojejunostomy: the posterior row is composed of interrupted Lembert sutures (inset) using 3-0 silk. Stitches should be placed 3–4 mm apart, taking good seromuscular bites. Once all knots have been tied, the gastric staple line is excised, and a jejunal enterotomy is made using surgical energy

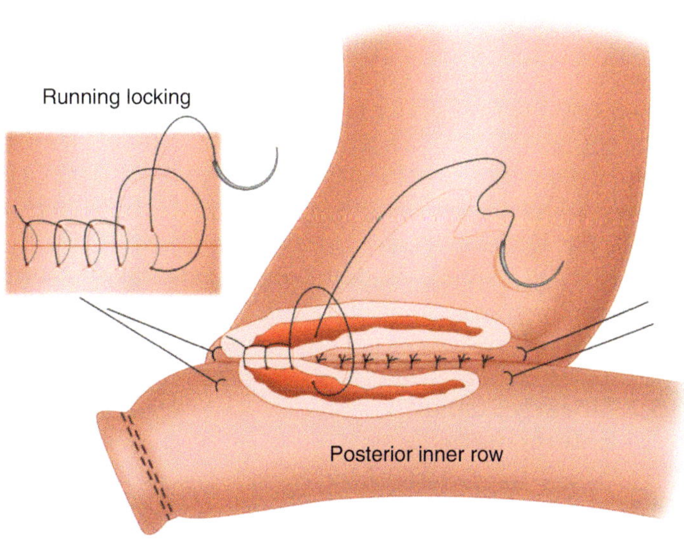

Fig. 17.2 Hand-sewn two-layer gastrojejunostomy: the posterior inner row is performed using 3-0 Vicryl in a running locking fashion. Bites should remain 2–3 mm above the posterior Lembert suture while advancing 5 mm with each bite

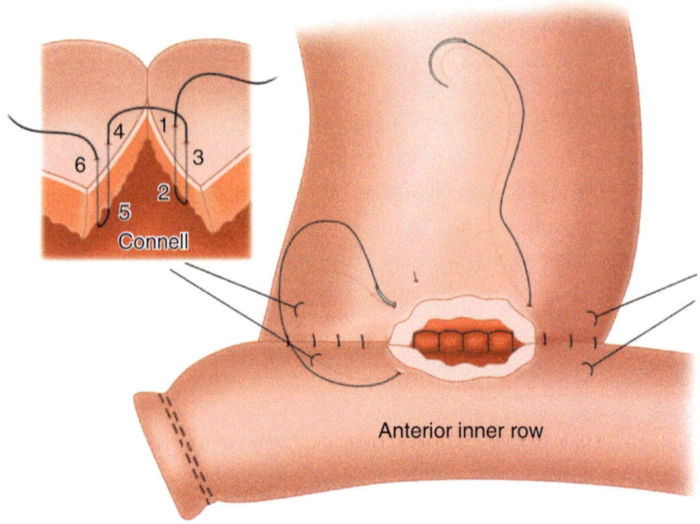

Fig. 17.3 Hand-sewn two-layer gastrojejunostomy: the anterior inner row is constructed using a Connell stitch, passing the suture from outside in and then inside out on one side, then crossing directly across, and passing from outside in to inside out on the other side (inset). The bites should incorporate a larger bite of serosa and smaller bite of mucosa to ensure good inversion of the mucosa, as well as aposition of the serosa

17.5.1.2 Single-Layer Hand-Sewn Gastrojejunostomy

The single-layer anastomosis begins similar to the double-layer anastomosis by bringing both the cut end of the jejunum to the cut end of the stomach. While generally a slowly absorbable suture is utilized, the techniques that have been described for a single-layer anastomosis can employ multiple different knots: some of these advocate the use of running near full thickness sutures (avoiding mucosa), some employ the use of interrupted vertical mattress inverting sutures (Gambee stitch), and others support the use of the Halstead stitch (editor's note: some of these basic stitches can be found in Chap. 3).

With any suturing technique utilized, the same general concepts apply: the cut ends are aligned with interrupted sutures, and the posterior wall is the first one created (in a running or interrupted fashion); when using a running suture, generally three quarters of the anastomosis are sutured together prior to switching to a series of interrupted sutures to complete the final millimeters of the anterior wall.

17.5.2 Linearly Stapled Enteroenterostomy

A linear stapler is commonly used to create a side-to-side, functional end-to-end enteroenterostomy. To begin, the cut ends of the segments being anastomosed are placed side by side. If the cut ends are stapled off, a small enterotomy is made proximally along the antimesenteric border of each segment (Fig. 17.4). Alternatively, the corner of each staple line can be cut off at the antimesenteric border. One fork of the automatic stapling device is placed through each enterotomy. The two forks are then connected and the intestinal lumens manipulated to ensure good antimesenteric to antimesenteric apposition (Fig. 17.4). If creating an enterocolonic anastomosis, the stapler should be aligned along the tinea as opposed to the true antimesenteric border. The stapling device is then fired to create a single common channel. The staple line within the lumen should be inspected to ensure hemostasis. The common enterotomy is brought together with clamps to create a temporary linear closure. Here it is important to adjust the staple lines within the intestinal lumen so they are not directly crossing. A second firing of the linear stapler directly below the clamps permanently closes the enterotomy. The staple line should be inspected for bleeding.

While not necessary, some surgeons opt to further reinforce the staple line along the common enterotomy by "dunking" it with a series of Lembert sutures. The distal end of the interior staple line can also be reinforced with a single 3-0 silk Lembert stitch. This step—advocated by many—has also been heavily criticized for its paradoxical potential of weakening the staple line. Finally, the resulting mesenteric defect should be closed.

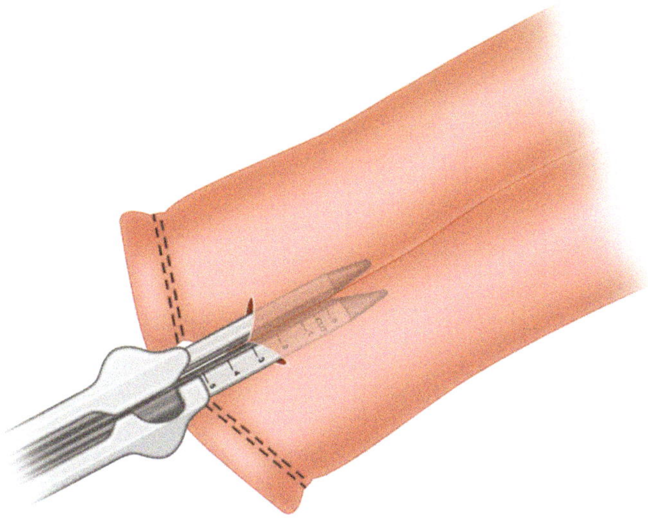

Fig. 17.4 Stapled enteroenterostomy: the two forks of the stapler are placed through enterotomies made along the respective antimesenteric borders. Before the stapling device is closed, the intestinal lumens should be manipulated to ensure good antimesenteric to antimesenteric apposition. The common enterotomy is approximated with clamps before being closed with a second firing of the stapler (not shown)

17.5.3 Circular Stapled Colorectal Anastomosis

A colorectal anastomosis can be created in an end-to-end or end-to-side fashion using a circular end-to-end anastomosis (EEA) stapler. This requires the patient to be positioned in lithotomy. Generally, the proximal colonic margin and distal rectal margin are divided first with a linear stapler.

The proximal (colonic) end of the anastomosis is prepared first. The linear staple line is cut off, and the lumen diameter is measured using a series of sequential dilators in order to select the appropriately sized stapling device. The anvil head is then placed within the lumen of the bowel. A single purse-string suture using 3-0 silk or polypropylene is placed along the cut end of bowel either freehand or using an automatic purse-stringing device (Fig. 17.5). The suture is tied around the anvil above the tying notch, securing the anvil in place. The tails of this suture should be kept very short.

The trans-anal portion of the anastomosis begins with gentle dilation of the anus, first manually, then with sequential dilators. This is performed by the assistant who is no longer within the sterile field. The shaft of the EEA stapler is placed through the anus and into the rectum. The surgeon helps to guide the EEA stapler to the very end of the rectal stump. When the face of the EEA stapler shaft is flush with the rectal staple line, the assistant turns the knob of the stapler in a counterclockwise fashion to extend the trocar through the rectal wall. The anvil's shaft is mated with the trocar until it snaps into place (Fig. 17.5). At this point, the surgeon should ensure that the colon and rectum are aligned without twisting of the mesentery. The EEA stapler is closed by turning the knob in a clockwise direction until the ends are perfectly apposed. A marker on the EEA device will guide the surgeon to ensure the anastomosis isn't too tight or too loose. The stapler is then fired and removed by turning the knob counterclockwise for three half-turns and then rotating the stapler itself counterclockwise for a half-turn to then remove it from the anus. The stapler should be inspected on the back table to ensure there are two intact "doughnuts," confirming that the stapler fired correctly. The anastomosis is then interrogated by instilling air in the rectum, while the pelvis is filled with saline, watching for air bubbles.

17.6 Current Controversies

17.6.1 Closure of Mesenteric Defects

It is well accepted that routine closure of mesenteric defects after Roux-en-Y gastric bypass surgery reduces the rate of internal hernia formation. This has been supported by both retrospective and prospective randomized controlled trials [37, 38]. To date, there is no consensus on the ideal method of primary closure. Surgeons use a variety of techniques including stapled closure and

Fig. 17.5 Stapled end-to-end colorectal anastomosis: the anvil head is secured within the proximal colonic lumen using a purse-string (inset). This is then mated with the trocar, which is seen extending out of the stapler shaft and through the rectal wall

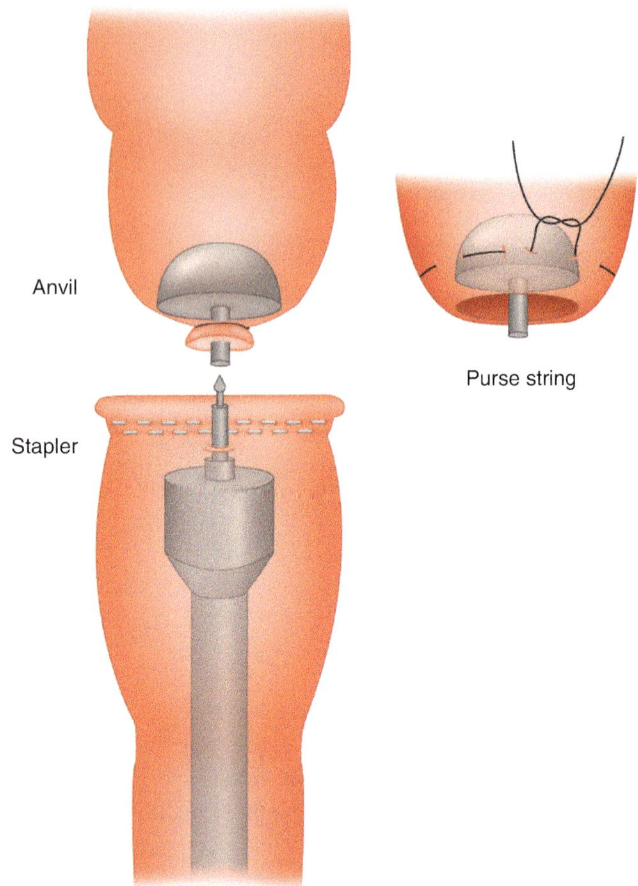

interrupted versus running closure using nonabsorbable or barbed suture [38, 39].

Routine closure of mesenteric defects during colon surgery is more controversial. In the era of laparoscopic surgery, routine closure has been limited by technical difficulty given the small surgical space, proximity to mesenteric blood supply and underlying ureter, and the increase in operative time [40]. On the other hand, leaving the defect open poses a risk of internal herniation and subsequent small bowel obstruction or strangulation. Unlike with laparoscopic Roux-en-Y gastric bypass, the incidence of symptomatic internal herniation after laparoscopic colon resection is relatively low. A retrospective review of 530 consecutive patients found a 0.8% incidence of internal herniation, recommending against routine closure of the mesenteric defect [41]. Larger, prospective randomized trials are needed.

17.6.2 Use of Barbed Suture

Unidirectional barbed suture has been used in general surgery for cruroplasty and for the closure of peritoneal defects created during gastrointestinal and hernia surgery [42, 43]. Barbed suture provides the surgeon with the ability to anchor the filament in a knotless manner and allows for tension to be evenly distributed across a wound as the barbs serve as fixation points [44]. The surgeon is thus able to operate independently with more technical ease.

Studies evaluating the use of barbed suture in creating gastrointestinal anastomoses have been more limited. Recent studies have compared the use of barbed suture to traditional interrupted sutures in creating or closing the gastrojejunostomy during laparoscopic Roux-en-Y gastric bypass [44–46]. All have found a significantly shorter suture time and decreased cost associated with barbed suture;

however, two of the studies reported a case of anastomotic leak with barbed suture. Larger randomized trials are needed in both laparoscopic and open cases before its use in gastrointestinal anastomoses can be more widely adopted.

17.6.3 Intraoperative Indocyanine Fluorescence Green Angiography

Adequate blood supply is the most critical factor impacting anastomotic healing. Several methods for objectively measuring blood perfusion have been proposed including pulse oximetry, Doppler ultrasound, spectrophotometry, and others [47, 48]. In the last decade, there has been an emergence of fluorescence angiography (FA) using indocyanine green and near-infrared light to assess bowel perfusion. This tool has demonstrated accuracy in assessing microperfusion and has been associated with improved outcomes in hepatobiliary, foregut, transplant, and plastic surgery [49–55].

Recent studies looking at anastomotic leaks in intestinal anastomoses have focused on colonic surgery. The 2015 PILLAR II study was a prospective, multicenter study looking at 139 patients who had a colonic anastomosis. The authors found that FA changed the operative plans in 11 (8%) patients, and while the whole cohort had two (1.4%) anastomotic leaks, there were no leaks in the 11 patients who had their operative plan changed as a result of FA [49]. A 2017 retrospective, case-matched study found that surgeons changed the planned anastomotic level of the colon in two of 42 patients in the FA group (4.7%). There were no anastomotic leaks in the FA group and two in the historical control group [47].

While fluorescence angiography may be a promising adjunct to aid in intraoperative perfusion assessment, randomized controlled trials are needed to truly establish its efficacy.

Take-Home Points

- Care should be taken to employ good surgical technique and to minimize tissue trauma through gentle handing with atraumatic instruments.
- The success of the anastomosis is dependent upon healthy blood supply with adequate hemostasis and avoidance of tension.
- All sutures should incorporate the submucosa (strength layer of the small intestine) and approximate the mucosa while preventing it from extruding from the suture line.
- The choice of suture material or staple is generally dependent on the location within the GI tract and the enteric layer being anastomosed.

Suggested Readings

Shackelford RT, Zuidema GD, Bickham WS. Surgery of the alimentary tract. 2d ed. Philadelphia: Saunders; 1978.

Ravitch MM, Rivarola A. Enteroanastomosis with an automatic instrument. Surgery. 1966;59(2):270–7.

Choy PY, Bissett IP, Docherty JG, et al. Stapled versus handsewn methods for ileocolic anastomoses. Cochrane Database Syst Rev. 2011(9):CD004320.

Thornton FJ, Barbul A. Healing in the gastrointestinal tract. Surg Clin North Am. 1997;77(3):549–73.

Stenberg E, Szabo E, Agren G, et al. Closure of mesenteric defects in laparoscopic gastric bypass: a multicenter, randomized, parallel, open-label trial. Lancet. 2016;387(10026):1397–404.

References

1. Ravitch MM, Canalis F, Weinshelbaum A, et al. Studies in intestinal healing. 3. Observations on everting intestinal anastomoses. Ann Surg. 1967;166(4):670–80.
2. Shackelford RT, Zuidema GD, Bickham WS. Surgery of the alimentary tract. 2d ed. Philadelphia: Saunders; 1978.
3. Halsted WS. Practical circular suture of the intestines; an experimental study. Am J Med Sci. 1887;94:436–61.
4. Getzen LC, Roe RD, Holloway CK. Comparative study of intestinal anastomotic healing in inverted and everted closures. Surg Gynecol Obstet. 1966;123(6):1219–27.
5. Goligher JC. Visceral and parietal suture in abdominal surgery. Am J Surg. 1976;131(2):130–40.
6. Trueblood HW, Nelsen TS, Kohatsu S. Wound healing in the colon: comparison of inverted and everted closures. Surgery. 1969;65:919.
7. Gill W, Fraser SJ, Carter DC. Everted intestinal anastomosis. Surg Gynecol Obstet. 1969;128:1297.
8. Ravitch MM, Rivarola A. Enteroanastomosis with an automatic instrument. Surgery. 1966;59(2):270–7.

9. Goulder F. Bowel anastomoses: the theory, the practice and the evidence base. World J Gastrointest Surg. 2012;4(9):208–13.
10. Kracht M, Hay JM, Fagniez PL, et al. Ileocolonic anastomosis after right hemicolectomy for carcinoma: stapled or hand-sewn? A prospective, multicenter, randomized trial. Int J Color Dis. 1993;8(1): 29–33.
11. Choy PY, Bissett IP, Docherty JG, et al. Stapled versus handsewn methods for ileocolic anastomoses. Cochrane Database Syst Rev. 2011(9):CD004320.
12. Brundage SI, Jurkovich GJ, Hoyt DB, et al. Stapled versus sutured gastrointestinal anastomoses in the trauma patient: a multicenter trial. J Trauma. 2001; 51:1054–61.
13. Demetriades D, Murray JA, Chan LS, et al. Handsewn versus stapled anastomosis in penetrating colon injuries requiring resection: a multicenter study. J Trauma. 2002;52:117–21.
14. Lustosa SA, Matos D, Atallah AN, et al. Stapled versus handsewn methods for colorectal anastomosis surgery. Cochrane Database Syst Rev. 2001(3):CD003144.
15. Thornton FJ, Barbul A. Healing in the gastrointestinal tract. Surg Clin North Am. 1997;77(3):549–73.
16. Mall F. A study of intestinal contraction. Healing of intestinal sutures. Reversal of the intestine. Boston: U Holzer; 1887. p. 77.
17. Jibom H, Ahonen J, Zederfeldt B. Healing of experimental colonic anastomoses. III. Collagen metabolism in the colon after left colon resection. Am J Surg. 1980;139:398.
18. Stromberg BV, Klein L. Collagen formation during the healing of colonic anastomoses. Dis Colon Rectum. 1982;25:301.
19. Mori N, Doi Y, Hara K, et al. Role of multipotent fibroblasts in the healing colonic mucosa of rabbits. Ultrastructural and immunocytochemical study. Histol Histopathol. 1992;7:583.
20. diZerega GS. The peritoneum and its response to surgical injury. Prog Clin Biol Res. 1990;358:1.
21. LaCalle JP, Sole JM, Pey GC, et al. Rotated intestinal anastomoses. Surg Gynecol Obstet. 1982;154:662.
22. Goligher JC, Graham NG, De Dombal ET. Anastomotic dehiscence after anterior resection of rectum and sigmoid. Br J Surg. 1970;57:109.
23. Halsted WS. Circular suture of the intestine: an experimental study. Am J Med Sci. 1887;94:436.
24. Graham MF, Diegelmann RF, Elson CO, et al. Collagen content and types in the intestinal strictures of Crohn's disease. Gastroenterology. 1988;94:257.
25. Graham MF, Blomquist P, Zederfeldt B. The alimentary canal. In: Wound healing: biochemical and clinical aspects. Philadelphia: WB Saunders; 1992. p. 433.
26. Ellison G. Wound healing in the gastrointestinal tract. Semin Vet Med Surg. 1989;4:287.
27. Hunt TK, Zederfeldt B, Goldstick TK. Oxygen and healing [review]. Am J Surg. 1969;118:521.
28. Wise L, McAlister W, Stein T, et al. Studies on the healing of anastomoses of small and large intestines. Surg Gynecol Obstet. 1975;141:190.
29. Carrico TJ, Mehrhof AJ, Cohen IK. Biology of wound healing [review]. Surg Clin North Am. 1984;64:721.
30. Udenfriend S. Formation of hydroxyproline in collagen [review]. Science. 1966;152:1335.
31. Chung R. Blood flow in colonic anastomoses. Effect of stapling and suturing. Ann Surg. 1987;206:335.
32. Schrock T, Cerra F, Hawley PR, et al. Wounds and wound healing (clinical conference). Dis Colon Rectum. 1982;25:1.
33. Hogstrom H, Haglund U, Zederfeldt B. Tension leads to increased neutrophil accumulation and decreased laparotomy wound strength. Surgery. 1990;107:215.
34. Shikata J, Shida T. Effects of tension on local blood flow in experimental intestinal anastomoses. J Surg Res. 1986;40:105.
35. Yeo CJ. Shackelford's surgery of the alimentary tract. 7th ed. Philadelphia: Elsevier/Saunders; 2013.
36. Chekan E, Whelan RL. Surgical stapling device-tissue interactions: what surgeons need to know to improve patient outcomes. Med Devices. 2014;7: 305–18.
37. Brolen RE, Kella VN. Impact of complete mesenteric closure on small bowel obstruction and internal mesenteric hernia after laparoscopic Roux-en-Y gastric bypass. Surg Obes Relat Dis. 2013;9(6): 850–4.
38. Stenberg E, Szabo E, Agren G, et al. Closure of mesenteric defects in laparoscopic gastric bypass: a multicenter, randomized, parallel, open-label trial. Lancet. 2016;387(10026):1397–404.
39. Aghajani E, Nergaard BJ, Leifson BG, et al. The mesenteric defects in laparoscopic Roux-en-Y gastric bypass: 5 years follow-up of non-closure versus closure using the stapler technique. Surg Endosc. 2017;31:3743–8. https://doi.org/10.1007/s00464-017-5415-.
40. Sim WH, Wong KY. Mesenteric defect after laparoscopic left hemicolectomy: to close or not to close? Int J Color Dis. 2016;31(7):1389–91.
41. Cabot JC, Lee SA, Yoo J, et al. Long-term consequences of not closing the mesenteric defect after laparoscopic right colectomy. Dis Colon Rectum. 2010; 53(3):289–92.
42. Wade A, Dugan A, Plymale MA, et al. Hiatal hernia cruroplasty with a running barbed suture compared to interrupted suture repair. Am Surg. 2016;82(9):271–4.
43. Takayama S, Nakai N, Shiozaki M, et al. Use of barbed suture for peritoneal closure in transabdominal preperitoneal hernia repair. World J Gastrointest Surg. 2012;4(7):177–9.
44. Bautista T, Shabbir A, Rao J, et al. Enterotomy closure using knotless and barbed suture in laparoscopic upper gastrointestinal surgeries. Surg Endosc. 2016;30(4):1699–703.
45. Blasi VD, Facy O, Goergen M, et al. Barbed versus usual suture for closure of the gastrojejunal anastomosis in laparoscopic gastric bypass: a comparative trial. Obes Surg. 2013;23(1):60–3.
46. Marco Milone M, Di Minno MN, Galloro G, et al. Safety and efficacy of barbed suture for gastrointestinal suture: a prospective and randomized

study on obese patients undergoing gastric bypass. J Laparoendosc Adv Surg Tech A. 2013;23(9):756–9.
47. Boni L, Fingerhut A, Marzorati A, et al. Indocyanine green fluorescence angiography during laparoscopic low anterior resection: results of a case-matched study. Surg Endosc. 2017;31(4):1936–840.
48. Urbanavicius L, Pattyn P, de Putte DV, et al. How to assess intestinal viability during surgery: a review of techniques. World J Gastrointest Surg. 2011;3(5):59–69.
49. Jafari MD, Wexner SD, Martz JE, et al. Perfusion assessment in laparoscopic left-sided/anterior resection (PILLAR II): a multi-institutional study. J Am Coll Surg. 2015;220(1):82–92.
50. Holm C, Tegeler J, Mayr M, et al. Monitoring free flaps using laser-induced fluorescence of indocyanine green: a preliminary experience. Microsurgery. 2002;22(7):278–87.
51. Hutteman M, Van Der Vorst JR, Mieog JSD, et al. Near-infrared fluorescence imaging in patients undergoing pancreaticoduodenectomy. Eur Surg Res. 2011;47(2):90–7.
52. Rodriguez-Hernandez A, Lawton MT. Flash fluorescence with indocyanine green videoangiography to identify the recipient artery for bypass with distal middle cerebral artery aneurysms: operative technique. Neurosurgery. 2012;70(2):209–20.
53. Shimada Y, Okumura T, Nagata T, et al. Usefulness of blood supply visualization by indocyanine green fluorescence for reconstruction during esophagectomy. Esophagus. 2011;8(4):259–66.
54. Still J, Law E, Dawson J, et al. Evaluation of the circulation of reconstructive flaps using laser induced fluorescence of indocyanine green. Ann Plast Surg. 1999;42(3):266–74.
55. Waseda K, Ako J, Hasegawa T, et al. Intraoperative fluorescence imaging system for on-site assessment of off-pump coronary artery bypass graft. JACC Cardiovasc Imaging. 2009;2(5):604–12.

18 Fundamentals of Vascular Anastomosis

Selena G. Goss and Dawn M. Salvatore

18.1 Introduction and Historical Background

The history of vascular repair and anastomotic creation is relatively recent in the surgical field. While vessel ligation and cauterization had been the mainstays of vascular control for centuries, attempts at suture repair of blood vessels date back only to the late eighteenth century. In fact, the first successful end-to-end arterial anastomosis was performed by Dr. John Murphy of Chicago in 1896. Only in the twentieth century did the field of vascular surgery experience a series of leaps and bounds, transporting us to our current methods of practice.

While vascular surgeons can usually be called upon to aid in challenging vascular emergencies, it is still imperative that every general surgeon possesses among their armamentarium of skills the ability to perform a vascular repair or anastomosis. In this chapter we present the equipment required, the general principles of vascular procedures, and the fundamental techniques of performing vessel repair and vascular anastomoses.

The basic instruments needed for creation of a vascular anastomosis are listed in Table 18.1. The specific uses of each of these are discussed throughout the chapter. Most of the instruments listed will be very familiar to the general surgeon, as they are utilized in other areas of surgical practice.

In this chapter, we will refer to the creation of a vascular anastomosis, where the term "vascular" can be applied to either venous or arterial vessels. Furthermore, though we may refer to an "arteriotomy," it is important to note that the discussion can often be applicable to the venous system as well. Likewise, the term "anastomosis" can refer to the connection of any conduit, whether venous or arterial. Finally, the term "conduit" can be considered as describing any vessel (autologous, autogenous, or synthetic) or graft that is being anastomosed to any target vessel.

18.2 General Concepts in Vascular Surgery

18.2.1 Exposure

The key to performing any vascular anastomosis is adequate exposure of the vessels involved, along with protection of adjacent structures. Electrocautery is used to dissect away overlying and surrounding soft tissues. Conversion to sharp dissection with Metzenbaum scissors is most appropriate once the vessel is in close proximity. Knowledge of the anatomy is imperative.

S. G. Goss · D. M. Salvatore (✉)
Department of Surgery, Sidney Kimmel Medical College, Thomas Jefferson University, Philadelphia, PA, USA
e-mail: selena.goss@jefferson.edu

F. Palazzo (ed.), *Fundamentals of General Surgery*, https://doi.org/10.1007/978-3-319-75656-1_18

Table 18.1 Basic instruments used for performing a vascular anastomosis (see Appendix)

Forceps
DeBakey forceps
Right angle forceps
Gerald forceps (or other atraumatic, vascular forceps)
Vascular clamps or alternatives
Large vessel clamps (DeBakey peripheral vascular, renal, profunda, etc.)
Bulldog clamps
Yasargil clamps
Medi-Loops (vessel loops)
Metal clips (small, medium, large)
11-blade scalpel
Scissors
Metzenbaum scissors
DeBakey-Potts scissors
Potts scissors ("pinch" Potts)
Vascular needle holders (fine-tipped needle holders)
Castroviejo needle holder
Ryder needle holder
Mayo-Hegar needle holder
Sutures
3-0, 4-0, 5-0, 6-0, 7-0 Prolene
4-0, 5-0, 6-0 PTFE suture
Irrigation catheter
DeBakey heparin injector ("olive tip") catheter
Stoney heparin injector
Patch/grafts (as required by clinical scenario)
Autologous vein patch/graft
Allograft (CryoGraft, cadaveric graft)
Xenograft (bovine pericardial patch)
Synthetic patch/graft
Polyester (Dacron)
Polytetrafluoroethylene (PTFE, Gore-Tex)
Misc
Syringes
Felt pledgets
Rubber shods
Sklar Bakes or Garrett dilators

Dissection down to the vessel is facilitated by the fact that there are typically no (or very few) anterior branches of almost all arterial and venous vessels. Thus, once a vessel is identified, sharp dissection along the anterior surface is performed with a fair amount of ease. It is important to clear all tissue away from the adventitia so that a clean, precise anastomosis can be constructed. The vessel should be handled with care, using non-traumatic vascular forceps (i.e., DeBakey forceps) to grasp only the adventitia. Whenever possible, grasping of the entire vessel or the intima should be avoided. The exposure should allow for sufficient distance to allow clamp placement for proximal and distal control of the vessel as well as provide enough working room to fashion the anastomosis (Fig. 18.1).

18.2.2 Proximal and Distal Vascular Control

Once the vessel has been sufficiently exposed, vessel loops are placed proximal and distal to the anticipated site of anastomosis. Vessel loops can be placed on larger side branches as well. These loops allow for control and manipulation of the vessel for clamp placement. The loop can also be used for vascular control. There are a variety of tools that can be used to gain vascular control (Fig. 18.2).

Most small arterial and venous branches can be ligated with clips or silk ties without clinical sequelae. However in certain situations, for example, in a limb with chronic vascular occlusion and extensive collaterals, preservation of even small branches should be prioritized. Small arterial branches (1–3 mm) can be controlled with small- or medium-sized clips, with clips removed once the anastomosis is completed. Yasargil vascular clamps are often used for temporary control of small vessels (Fig. 18.2). Healthy small- and medium-sized vessels (3–6 mm) can be easily controlled with vessel loops by a double-loop (Potts) technique. For control of larger vessels, various sizes of angled and curved clamps have been developed to provide vascular control while minimizing interference to the operative field.

It is important to take note of the degree of atherosclerotic calcification of the vessel wall being clamped, as this may alter the degree to which clamping is effective. A heavily calcified vessel is often coexistent with an irregular and plaque-laden lumen and thus may not occlude completely when clamped.

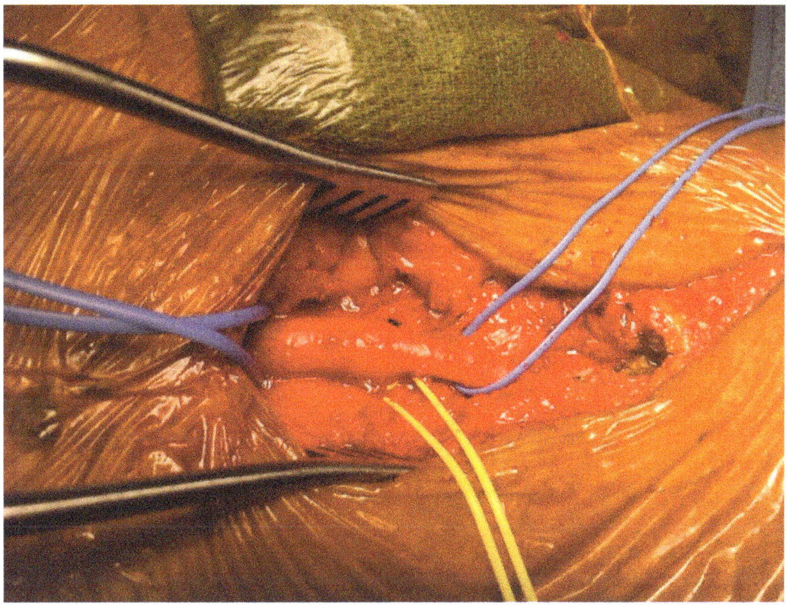

Fig. 18.1 Exposure of the femoral vessels, to allow for adequate proximal and distal control and subsequent anastomosis creation. Blue vessel loops are placed around the CFA (*left*), the SFA (*right*), and a yellow vessel loop is placed around the PFA in Potts fashion

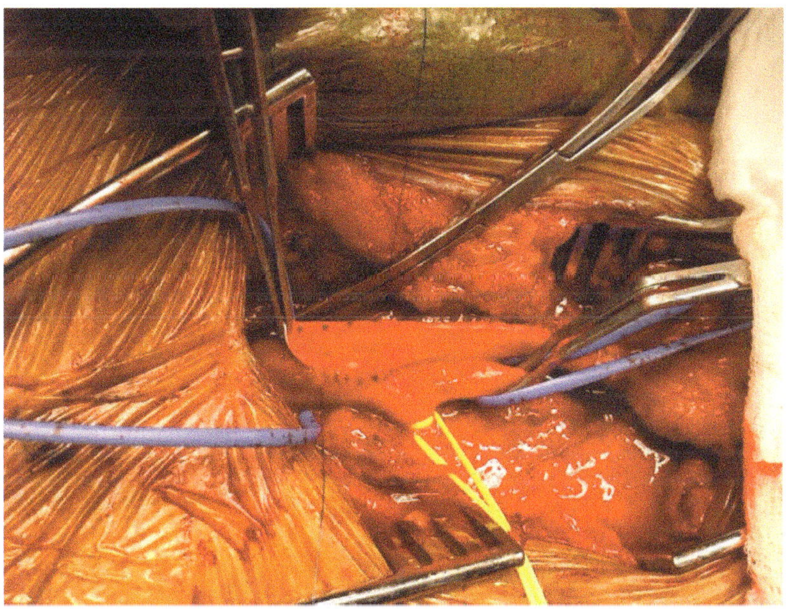

Fig. 18.2 A PTFE graft being sutured onto the distal common femoral artery (CFA). A variety of tools can be used to gain vascular during creation of an anastomosis. A femoral artery clamp is placed on the CFA (*left*), while a profunda artery clamp has been placed on the SFA (*right*). Blue vessels loops lay loosely open on the CFA (*left*) and SFA (*right*). A yellow vessel loop has been placed in Potts fashion around a PFA branch

Furthermore, clamping such a vessel may cause inadvertent damage, such as vessel wall tear or luminal disruption, requiring more extensive dissection, endarterectomy, or even excision of the vessel and reconstruction (beyond the scope of this chapter). In these instances, another option for proximal and distal control is balloon catheter occlusion.

Once the vessels are adequately exposed and vessel loops are in place, appropriate vascular clamps can be chosen for control of each involved vessel. It is important to have the operative field and vessels involved prepared in such a way that vascular control can be obtained at the appropriate time, specifically after anticoagulation and vessel and conduit preparation.

18.2.3 Anticoagulation

Once adequate proximal and distal control has been achieved, the patient is systemically anticoagulated, most commonly by intravenous administration of heparin (heparin sodium 50–100 units/kg). Generally, 3–5 min of circulation time is allowed prior to vessel clamping. Anticoagulation is performed to prevent thrombosis, and accumulation of platelet aggregates in the involved vessels during their manipulation and exposure to surrounding, thrombotic tissues. A 1000 unit bolus dose of heparin is then administered every hour thereafter until the anastomosis is complete and uninterrupted circulation is reestablished.

In certain situations, such as with a trauma victim of polytrauma who suffers a major extremity vessel transection and a concomitant intracranial hemorrhage, systemic anticoagulation may be contraindicated. Direct intravenous or intra-arterial heparin instillation is an acceptable alternative method to provide anticoagulation.

Once the anastomosis has been completed, the effects of the anticoagulant are allowed to wear off or can be inhibited by administration of a reversal agent. Protamine sulfate, used to reverse the effects of heparin, is given at a dose of 1 mg per every 100 units of heparin administered during the previous few hours of surgery. As protamine has been shown to have serious side effects, including hypotension and anaphylactoid reactions, it is administered slowly and is not to exceed 50 mg in total.

18.2.4 Conduit and Target Vessel Preparation

An anastomosis can be constructed by sewing a patch onto a target vessel, by primarily sewing vessels together in end-to-end fashion, or by insertion of a conduit onto a target vessel in end-to-side fashion. If a conduit is used, preparation is relatively straightforward. The surgeon must ensure that there is proper orientation of the conduit without twisting, kinking, or redundancy, especially during tunneling the conduit in an anatomic or subcutaneous plane.

An autologous vein graft is prepared by sequentially flushing the vein, which is dilated against resistance in order to detect areas of leakage or stenosis. This serial dilation is performed by compressing the vein manually or with a soft vascular clamp, while it is actively flushed with heparinized saline. An autogenous or synthetic graft is inherently without defects and can be utilized immediately once available. Regardless of the type of conduit being used, it is important to ensure that the conduit lies without kinking or twisting.

18.2.5 Arteriotomy/Venotomy

Once the graft is prepared and heparin has systemically circulated, the previously prepared vascular clamps and previously placed vessel loops are applied, and a longitudinal arteriotomy (for the purpose of this chapter, arteriotomy and venotomy are used interchangeably) is created. An 11-blade scalpel is ideal for creating a 2–3 mm longitudinal arteriotomy, with care taken to not violate the back wall of the vessel. The arteriotomy is elongated proximally and distally to the desired length using DeBakey-Potts or Potts scissors. In general, the size of the arteriotomy can range from 8 to 20 mm depending on the clinical situations. In similarity to the sizing of a bowel anastomosis, the appropriate sizing of a vascular anastomosis is dictated in some part by experience and gestalt; however, the ultimate goal is to have a patent anastomosis that allows for laminar flow into the target vessel.

Inadequate vascular control is generally apparent by continuous bleeding from the arteriotomy. In controlled and elective situations, it is ideal to investigate ongoing bleeding promptly. Creating the anastomosis with ongoing bleeding, though necessary in certain circumstances, is cumbersome and can lead to an imperfect anastomosis. The most common reasons for ongoing bleeding are incomplete vascular clamp application; inadequate control due to a missed, usually posterior, branch vessel; and non-compressible, often calcified vessels that cannot be adequately controlled with clamping.

18.2.6 Anastomosis

The conduit is brought into the field and positioned for anastomosis creation. In general, permanent, monofilament suture (i.e., Prolene) with the size of the suture (3-0, 4-0, 5-0, 6-0, or 7-0) is chosen depending upon vessel caliber. For example, a common femoral artery anastomosis will generally require a 5-0 Prolene suture, while a tibial artery may require a 6-0 or 7-0 Prolene suture. The anastomosis can be created in standard running fashion (most common) or interrupted sutures placed in simple or horizontal mattress fashion.

Certain principles of anastomotic creation should be followed for proper construction to prevent luminal narrowing and ensure hemostasis. First, the securing knots are tied down on the outside of the vessel, not within the lumen. Second, the securing knots should be placed at or near the 9 o'clock or 3 o'clock position on the longitudinal axis of the arteriotomy (Fig. 18.3). Ensuring that the knots are not located at the "toe" or "heel" position of the anastomosis prevents narrowing of the anastomosis at these critical points. Furthermore, proper placement of the suture at these two locations is most critical as inadequate technique results in anastomotic leaks that can be difficult and awkward to repair once the anastomosis is complete.

During creation of the anastomosis, it is important to verify patency of the inflow and outflow vessels. Sklar Bakes or Garrett dilators may be passed proximally and distally to ensure that the inflow and outflow vessels are not compromised by the anastomosis.

18.2.7 Completing the Anastomosis and Reperfusion

Just prior to completion of the anastomosis, with one or two suture throws remaining, the anastomosis is flushed by sequentially releasing and re-clamping the inflow and outflow vessels. This allows any stagnant and potentially clotted blood and intraluminal debris to be purged from the vessel. The arteriotomy is then forcefully, but carefully, flushed with heparinized saline to allow any remaining platelet aggregates, debris,

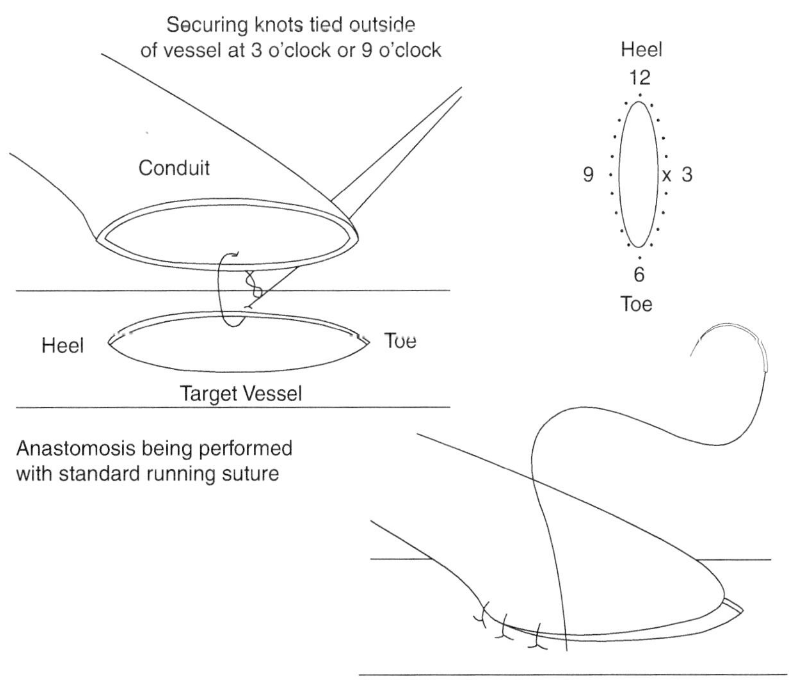

Fig. 18.3 The anatomy of a vascular anastomosis. Depicting face of a clock, toe, heel, etc.

and air to be evacuated from the vessel lumen. The anastomosis is then completed as the monofilament suture is tied down and secured with 6–8 knots.

While completing the anastomosis, it is important to carefully release the vascular clamps in a deliberate and sequential manner so as to allow any potential debris to be carried into the least vital outflow vessel. Notably, it is often useful to leave the clamps released but in place, should there be uncontrolled bleeding from the arteriotomy that requires re-clamping. This allows ease of obtaining immediate vascular control again, in order to inspect the anastomosis, with less concern for injuring a vessel by having to reposition and replace the vascular clamp.

This sequence involves unclamping then re-clamping a distal vessel first to allow back-bleeding into the anastomosis and evacuation of any debris or clot. Next, the proximal inflow vessel (or vessels) is unclamped such that any potential debris would flow forward out of the circulatory system and through the unfinished anastomosis, while the outflow vessels remain clamped. Once the anastomosis is completed, the least vital outflow vessel, for example, a branch vessel or a vessel which is not supplying an end-organ structure, is unclamped allowing for any possible remaining debris to be flushed downstream to a non-vital location. The inflow vessel is unclamped, and, finally, the main outflow vessel is unclamped, and forward flow is reestablished with all vessels now unclamped.

18.2.8 Hemostasis and Suture Repair

Once the anastomosis is completed and vascular control removed, the suture line is checked for hemostasis. Reasons for continued bleeding from a freshly created anastomosis are the presence of a defect in the suture line (i.e., poorly placed, improperly spaced, or loose sutures), needle hole bleeding, and generalized oozing from systemic anticoagulation.

Bleeding from suture needle holes is common and can usually be controlled with placement of topical hemostatic agents and a short period of gently applied pressure. Surgicel® (Ethicon Inc., Cincinnati, Ohio), Surgicel® Fibrillar™ (Ethicon Inc., Cincinnati, Ohio), and Floseal hemostatic matrix (Baxter International Inc., Deerfield, IL) are some commonly used topical hemostatic agents. Removal, irrigation, and repeat use of these agents can be performed as necessary, especially during reversal (i.e., protamine administration) of systemic anticoagulation.

A true defect in the anastomosis will result in persistent, vigorous bleeding from the suture line. There are a number of maneuvers that can be used to achieve hemostasis in these situations. First, a simple figure-of-eight repair stitch using monofilament suture will often stanch the bleeding from a suture line defect. If the vessel wall is fragile, a pledgeted suture placed in horizontal mattress fashion can help support the suture repair. Although manufactured felt pledgets are often available and typically used, a pledget can be formed from a piece of autologous muscle, an excess piece of vein graft, or a spare piece of prosthetic graft.

A Word on Shunting

Occasionally, one encounters a situation where vascular control is required; however, simultaneous preservation of forward flow is essential. Such scenarios are most commonly encountered in traumatic injury to the carotid, vena cava, or extremity vessels. When ongoing distal perfusion is needed, flow through the severed vessel can be maintained by the use of a shunt. A variety of vascular shunts exist (beyond the scope of this chapter); however, any sterile tubing can be fashioned to provide this function so long as the ends are securely anchored to the inflow and outflow vessels. Anchoring can be accomplished with externally placed umbilical tape (i.e., Rommel clamps) or specifically designed, circular (i.e., Javid) vessel clamps.

18.3 Physiology of a Vascular Anastomosis

The ideal consequence of creating an anastomosis is forward flow without unnecessary loss of energy as blood is propelled forward. The decision to create an end-to-end anastomosis versus an end-to-side (or side-to-end) anastomosis has physiological consequences. Generally, an end-to-end anastomosis will have less physiologic disturbance as blood is flowing forward without a flow divider or significant change in angle in the direction of flow, namely, blood will flow more or less to follow a straight path.

In creating an end-to-side anastomosis, however, one must consider the angle between the graft and the native vessel. The greater the angle between the graft and native vessel, the more energy is lost in the transition at the anastomosis. In general, one should aim to create a 45° (end-to-side) anastomosis in order to minimize the energy loss and thus decrease the pressure gradient across the connection (Fig. 18.4).

When an end-to-side fashion anastomosis is created, there are inherent physiologic consequences, including flow disturbance, turbulence, and areas of stagnation, that have implications for the involved vessel walls. The areas of the anastomotic connection that are impacted most heavily include the "floor," the "toe," and the "heel" of the anastomosis (Fig. 18.4). The "floor" describes the recipient vessel wall that lies opposite to the opening of an end-to-side anastomosis. The "toe" of the anastomosis denotes the distal most end of the anastomosis, which sits furthest along the recipient vessel. The "heel" of the anastomosis designates the most proximal end of the anastomosis, which sits closest along the recipient vessel.

These three areas, which are prone to fluctuating or low shear stress, constitute the regions that are most conducive to development of intimal hyperplasia and atherosclerosis. Unfortunately, the long term consequences of these structural changes are anastomotic compromise which can lead to vessel stenosis or occlusion. Thus, precise and intentional fashioning of an anastomosis is of paramount importance.

18.4 Technical and Practical Considerations for Creating Vascular Anastomoses

18.4.1 Primary and Patch Repair

The principles of patch repair are similar to the creation of any vascular anastomosis. A patch can be composed of an autologous vessel (vein patch), an autogenous vessel (cryopreserved

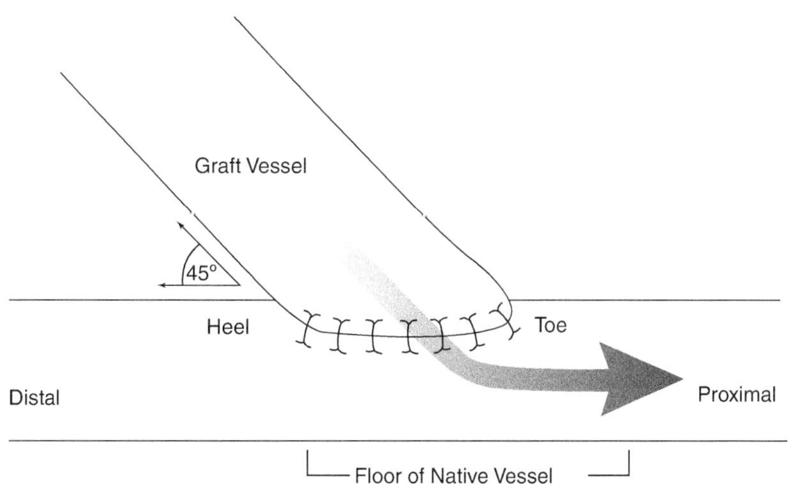

Fig. 18.4 Physiology of an end-to-side anastomosis. Side view of an anastomosis, depicting flow through, angle, floor, toe, heel, etc.

cadaveric vein), a xenographic vessel (bovine pericardial patch), or synthetic material. If it is anticipated that a patch repair will be required, an astute surgeon will prepare and drape a patient's groin in anticipation of greater saphenous vein harvest as this vessel is readily identified and easily procured. The patch is fashioned to the appropriate size and shape of the target vessel defect. Construction of the repair is most commonly performed with either single running or four-quadrant suture repair (see below Sects. 18.4.2 and 18.4.3).

Oftentimes, a small iatrogenic or traumatic defect in a vessel can be repaired with a monofilament suture in figure-of-eight or horizontal mattress fashion, without compromising the lumen. If, however, the defect encompasses a significant portion of the vessel wall, patch repair may be necessary to simultaneously repair the injury and maintain adequate vessel lumen. Likewise, a longitudinal arteriotomy, which may be performed for endarterectomy, thrombectomy, or vessel exploration, is generally repaired with a patch to prevent luminal narrowing.

18.4.2 Single Running Suture

An anastomosis can be fashioned with a single, continuous, monofilament suture, with extra care taken to ensure that the lumen is not narrowed. This anastomosis is useful for superficial surgical fields, where the operator has ease of access to the target vessel.

A double-barreled, monofilament suture is placed at either the 9 o'clock or 3 o'clock position, with one needle traveling inside-out on the artery and the other needle traveling inside-out on the conduit. With both sutures held at equivalent lengths, three knots are tied down to secure the conduit down onto the artery. You will notice that having traveled inside-out on both vessels, the knot will land, appropriately, on the outside of the vessel. One suture is then protected with a shodded clamp, and the other suture becomes the working suture. Starting from the knot at the 3 o'clock position, the first suture should be threaded outside-in on the conduit and then inside-out on the target vessel. The suture can be sewn in continuous running fashion from the knot (at 3 o'clock) to the opposite side, 180° from the original knot (9 o'clock). Once halfway around the anastomosis (9 o'clock), this initial suture , is protected with a shodded clamp, and the previously protected suture is then run in similar fashion in the opposite direction. With both sutures meeting at the 9 o'clock position, the anastomosis can be flushed and completed.

18.4.3 Four-Quadrant Repair (Diamond-Shaped Arteriotomy)

Four-quadrant repair is another method for creating an anastomosis that can be utilized when the operator has easy access to the target vessel, such as in a superficial extremity vessel. One arm of a double-barreled monofilament suture is sewn inside-out at the heel (12 o'clock) of the target vessel, and the other arm is sewn inside-out on the conduit. Each arm of the suture is made to be of even length, and three knots are tied down, fastening the conduit securely to the target vessel. One arm of the suture is protected with a shodded clamp, and the other is run in continuous fashion, beginning with an outside-in throw on the conduit followed by an inside-out throw on the target vessel and so on.

When initiating suture at the heel or the toe, it is important to remember that sutures should be thrown radially outward, like the spokes of a bicycle wheel, with a millimeter or two *more* progress made on the target vessel than on the conduit. This will provide optimal apposition at the suture line with less risk of anastomotic defects. The suture is continued until the 3 o'clock position and then protected with a shodded clamp. The other arm of the suture is then sewn in similar fashion to the 9 o'clock position and then protected once again with a shodded clamp.

Ensuring the conduit is sized and spatulated appropriately to the arteriotomy (or target vessel), a second double-barreled monofilament suture is begun, in similar fashion to the first, but

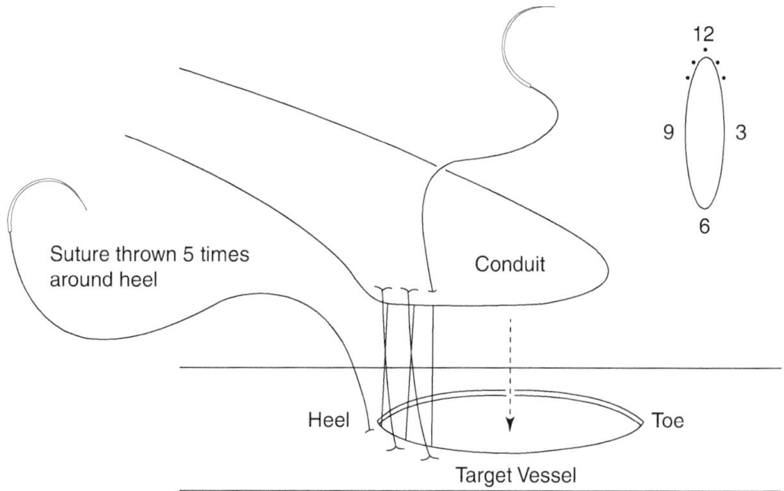

Fig. 18.5 Parachute technique for anastomosis creation

this time at the toe (6 o'clock) of the anastomosis. Suturing is performed in similar fashion such that each end of this second suture meets the shodded sutures at the 3 o'clock and 9 o'clock positions. The sutures are tied down at the 3 o'clock and 9 o'clock positions for anastomosis completion.

18.4.4 Parachute Technique

It is not uncommon to be required to create an anastomosis in a deep wound or narrow surgical field. In order to facilitate creation of an anastomosis in such a situation, the "parachute technique" aids in ensuring proper placement of sutures in the toe and heel of the anastomosis in an "open" technique. As previously discussed, this is of distinct mention as the toe and heel are the two areas of the anastomosis most likely to be disadvantaged by suture defects or anastomotic narrowing. These are coincidentally the most difficult areas to properly repair once creation of the anastomosis is underway.

The parachute technique is begun with the conduit a short distance from the target vessel. The operator sews a double-barreled, monofilament suture outside-in on the conduit a few millimeters away from the heel, bringing just over half of the suture through; the other half of the suture if protected to the edge of the surgical wound with a shodded clamp. The suture is then sewn inside-out on the target vessel, progressively toward the heel, without bringing the conduit down onto the target vessel. Keeping the conduit a short distance from the target vessel while continuing to sew creates the appearance of so-called parachute strings between the conduit and target vessel (Fig. 18.5). In general, the suture is thrown a total of five times, effectively placing two sutures on one side of the heel, one suture at the apex (12 o'clock) of the heel, and another two sutures on the opposite side of the heel.

Once these five throws have been completed at the heel, the operator and the assistant gently and simultaneously pull tension on both ends of the suture bringing the conduit down onto the target vessel. From here, the remainder of the anastomosis is generally more straightforward and can be performed by single running suture technique or with a second running suture, as in the four-quadrant repair technique as discussed earlier in this chapter.

18.5 Complications of Vascular Anastomosis

Early complications of vascular anastomosis creation include surgical bleeding and conduit thrombosis, which may due to technical deficiency at the anastomosis or inadequacy of the conduit, the latter of which is beyond the scope of this chapter. Generally, when a problem occurs within the first 7 days after intervention, a technical error must be assumed. The most common reasons for failure are undue tension on the conduit, poor lie of the conduit with kinking or twisting, and improper construction of the anastomosis with luminal narrowing.

Postoperative bleeding can be mild, moderate, or severe, with the latter usually requiring take-back and exploration to control bleeding. Some degree of oozing from a fresh anastomosis can be attributed to bleeding from needle holes, though this is usually self-limited and readily controlled with topical hemostatic agents or reversal of anticoagulation, as previously discussed.

When bleeding is more significant and the aforementioned maneuvers are ineffective, all aspects of the anastomosis should be carefully inspected. Any obvious defects between the target vessel and the graft can readily be repaired with a single 5-0 Prolene horizontal mattress or figure-of-eight suture. Occasionally, a pledgeted suture can be used to reinforce a suture repair, especially if the target vessel wall is thin or weakened.

One of the most feared early complications of creating a vascular anastomosis is thrombosis of the conduit or target vessel. Unfortunately, vessel thrombosis is sometimes not discovered until post-assessment, on clinical exam, and then confirmed with noninvasive studies. Expedient reoperation is necessary to investigate the anastomosis and all vessels involved, as a technical error must be ruled out as the culprit. In the absence of finding a technical problem at reoperation, one must consider a coagulopathy or other hematologic issues as a possible cause for thrombosis.

Anastomotic narrowing is a complication that can develop months or years after surgery. Luminal compromise can result from intimal hyperplasia. This thickening of the intimal layer is a natural response to violation of the vessel wall and surgical manipulation. Bypass grafts and major vessels that have undergone repair or reconstruction are thus followed with serial imaging, in order to identify any flow limitation or anastomotic site complication that may require intervention to maintain vessel or conduit patency.

18.5.1 Emergency Maneuvers for Obtaining Vascular Control

Occasionally, a traumatic or iatrogenic vascular injury proves uncontrollable despite attempts at repair. In these situations, there are emergency maneuvers that can be performed to allow for control of life-threatening hemorrhage. The simple act of applying direct, manual pressure at the site of hemorrhage, without the application of gauze or other packing material, will be sufficient to halt profuse bleeding. Likewise, vascular clamp application is the preferred maneuver.

In deep surgical wounds, such as in the pelvis or retroperitoneum, where visualization and access may be difficult, ongoing hemorrhage can preclude any real attempt at suture repair. In these events, it is safest to use direct pressure with a sponge stick, proximal and distal to the defect than to attempt a blind repair, where surrounding structures could inadvertently become injured thus worsening the situation. If an extremity vessel is injured and vascular control cannot be obtained, application of a tourniquet to the proximal extremity can provide temporary control. Ongoing distal extremity bleeding is generally less severe and can be controlled with direct manual pressure.

When vessels are exposed and vascular control or direct repair is not feasible, the use of Fogarty balloon occlusion catheters can be employed. These catheters are available in multiple sizes and lengths and can be advanced into a vessel through the defect with balloon inflation providing cessation of flow. For example, 5–8 mm caliber vessels can generally be controlled with #4, #5, or #6 Fogarty balloon catheters.

The use of any of these aforementioned maneuvers is of course temporary, and they should provide partial, if not complete, control of hemorrhage. The patient can then undergo active resuscitation, allowing time to call for the assistance of a vascular surgeon.

18.6 Current Controversies and Future Directions

The techniques for creating a vascular anastomosis have not changed significantly in the recent decades, though emerging technology has developed exploring the creation of a sutureless anastomosis. A Hybrid Vascular Graft (W. L. Gore & Associates, Newark, DE) has been developed that merges endovascular and open surgical techniques, allowing for a hybrid approach to creating a vascular anastomosis.

The hybrid graft is composed of standard expanded polytetrafluoroethylene (ePTFE), commonly used in vascular surgery, attached to a short segment of ePTFE that is reinforced with nitinol. This latter segment, which compacted to allow for ease of intraluminal insertion, comprises the so-called sutureless anastomosis of the graft. The compacted section of graft is manually inserted into the inflow portion of the anastomosis, and a trigger wire is released, allowing for deployment of the compacted section of the graft and apposition to the inflow vessel wall. The radial force of the graft against the inflow vessel wall precludes the need for suturing the graft to the inflow vessel. The remainder of the graft is then available for traditional anastomosis creation to the outflow vessel.

The Hybrid Vascular Graft has found its niche in difficult to access vessels, where extensive dissection may not be feasible or safe. Studies are currently being conducted on the utility and safety of using this graft in complicated carotid artery disease.

Take-Home Points

- A basic understanding of the techniques involved in creating a vascular anastomosis is necessary for every general surgeon.
- Adequate exposure of the vessels involved is paramount to obtaining vascular control and creating vascular anastomoses.
- Having adequate inflow, an appropriate conduit, and adequate outflow are the key components of a successful vascular anastomosis or repair.
- Understanding the physiology of a vascular anastomosis can aid in its creation.
- Vascular anastomoses can be created using a multitude of techniques.
- Obtaining hemostasis at a vascular anastomosis can be challenging but is usually achievable with diligent anastomotic creation and the aid of topical hemostatic agents.
- If vascular control is not achievable by direct means of repair, a number of maneuvers can be used to prevent catastrophic bleeding, allowing for time to call in the assistance of a vascular surgeon.

Appendix

Below is a compilation of photos demonstrating basic instruments used in vascular surgery for creating an anastomosis. This is by no means an exhaustive list but rather serves as a general overview of instruments that can be utilized.

A variety of vascular clamps are used to gain vascular control on peripheral blood vessels.

A variety of instruments are used to obtain vascular control on small and delicate vessels. Bulldogs clamps (top row) of different sizes are made in metal and plastic and can be useful in controlling side branches of major vessels. Gold Yasargil clamps (bottom, right) are placed with a Yasargil applier (bottom row).

Locking and non-locking Castroviejo needle holders (top row) are generally used for suture 5-0 or smaller. Ryder needle holders can be used for more sturdy needles and suture.

Castroviejo needle holders are used to perform vascular suturing with small caliber needles and suture.

An olive tip (top) or Stoney (bottom) heparin injector can be used to flush blood vessels and anastomoses prior to repair or closure, to ensure evacuation of air and debris.

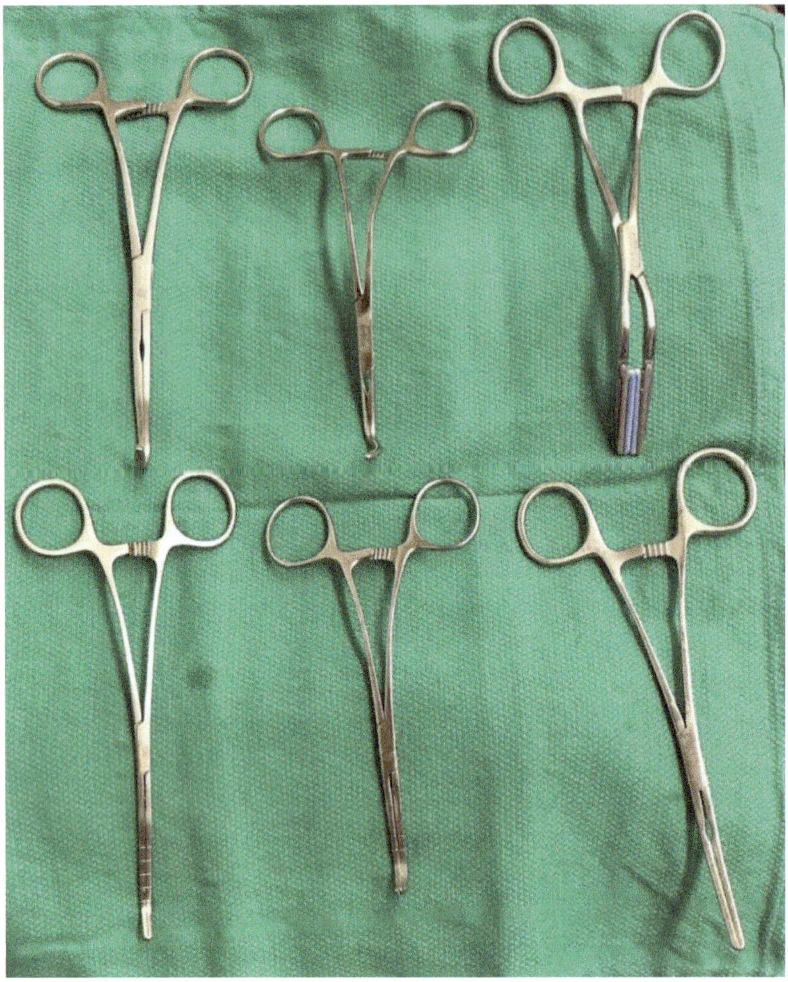

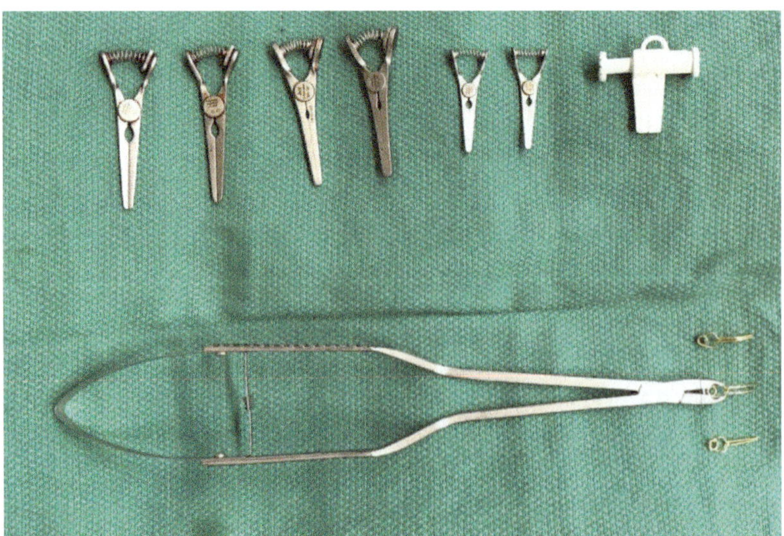

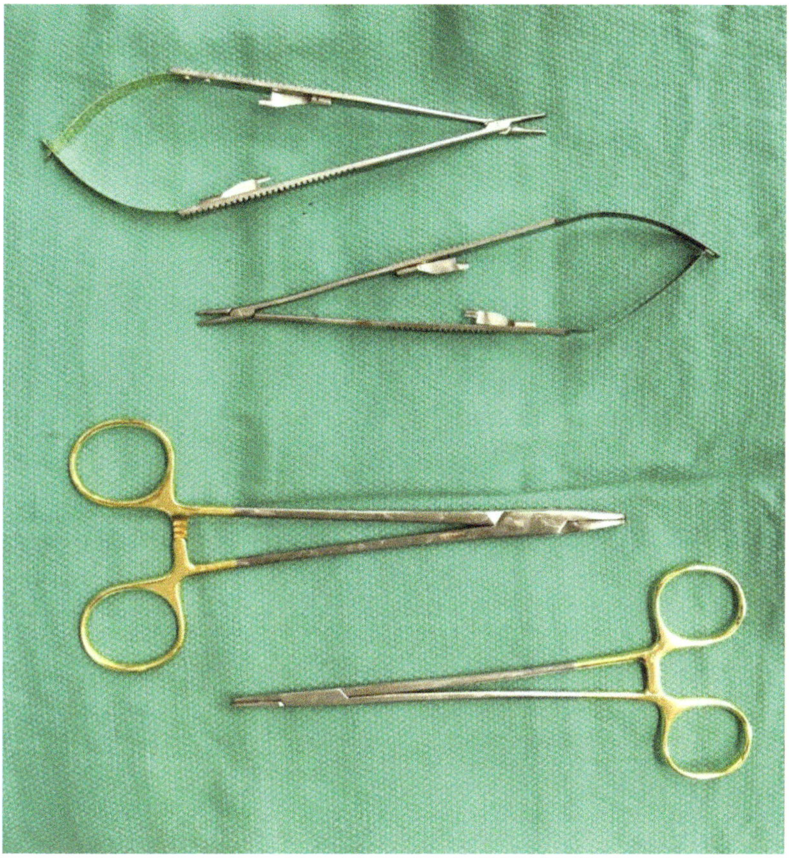

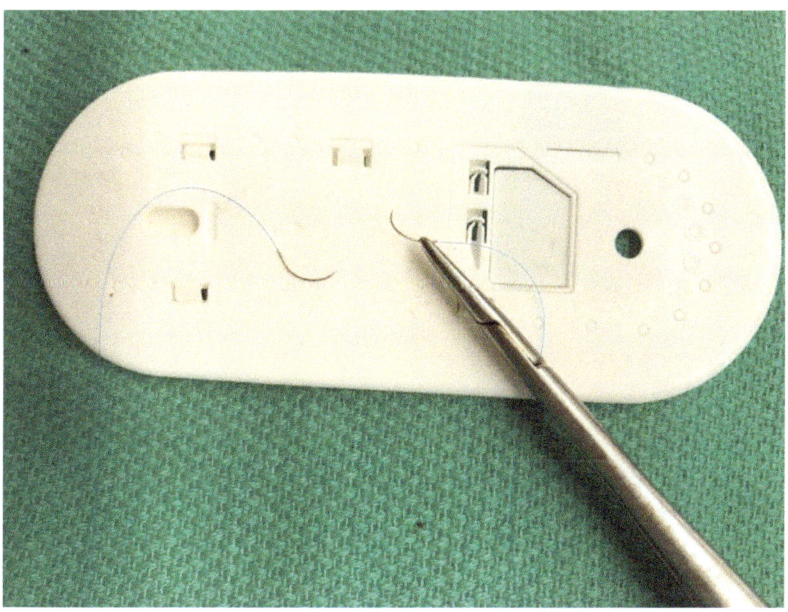

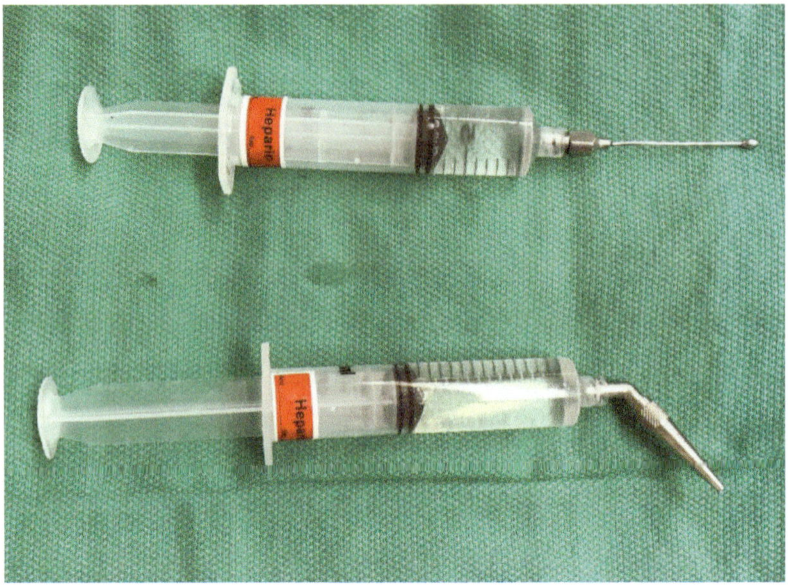

Suggested Readings

Cronenwett JL, Johnston KW. Chapter 87: Technique: open surgical. In: Rutherford's vascular surgery. 8th ed. Philadelphia: Saunders; 2014. p. 1284–303.

Hoballah JJ. Chapters 1–11 in Vascular reconstructions. Anatomy, exposures, and technique. New York: Springer; 2000.

Friedman SG. A history of vascular surgery. 2nd ed. Hoboken: Wiley-Blackwell; 2005.

Gore® Hybrid Vascular Graft. 2017, August. Retrieved from http://www.goremedical.com/products/hybrid.

Stanley JC, Veith F, Wakefield TW. Current therapy in vascular and endovascular surgery. 5th ed. Philadelphia: Saunders; 2014.

Valenti D, et al. Carotid bypass using the gore hybrid vascular graft as a rescue technique for on-table failed carotid endarterectomy. J Vasc Surg. 2016;64:229–32.

Fundamentals of Exploratory Laparotomy for Trauma

19

Chia-jung K. Lu and Joshua A. Marks

19.1 Introduction

19.1.1 Historical Background

The exploratory laparotomy for trauma focuses on efficient surgical techniques to control hemorrhage and contamination prior to the onset of the deadly triad: hypothermia, coagulopathy, and acidosis. Stone et al. first introduced the concept of intra-abdominal pack tamponade in 1983. In their study, trauma laparotomies were aborted at the first sign of coagulopathy, intra-abdominal packs were placed to achieve tamponade, and patients returned to the operating room for definitive surgery after the correction of coagulopathy [1].

Rotondo et al. refined the techniques and introduced the concept of damage control laparotomy in their landmark paper published in 1993. The damage control laparotomy is divided into three phases:

C.-j. K. Lu
Department of Surgery, Division of Acute Care Surgery, Sidney Kimmel Medical College at Thomas Jefferson University, Philadelphia, PA, USA

J. A. Marks (✉)
Department of Surgery, Sidney Kimmel Medical College, Thomas Jefferson University, Philadelphia, PA, USA
e-mail: Joshua.Marks@jefferson.edu

1. An abbreviated index operation focused on the rapid surgical control of hemorrhage and contamination followed by intra-abdominal packing and temporary closure
2. Intensive care unit (ICU) resuscitation to correct hypothermia, coagulopathy, and acidosis
3. Re-exploration with definitive surgical repair and reconstruction of all injuries once hemodynamic stability is achieved [2]

The continued application of damage control principles in treating severely injured trauma patients has led to improved survival with penetrating abdominal trauma and has been utilized in other fields including emergency general, thoracic, urologic, and vascular surgery [3].

19.1.2 Indications and Goals

Trauma patients presenting to the emergency department are evaluated using the Advanced Trauma Life Support (ATLS) protocol. Regardless of a patient's physiology or mechanism of injury, the ABCDEs of trauma resuscitation are always applied. Primary survey including assessment of airway, breathing, circulation, disability, and exposure followed by secondary survey and adjuncts to the survey, such as plain film radiographs and bedside ultrasound, helps identify patients who require emergent laparotomy

F. Palazzo (ed.), *Fundamentals of General Surgery*, https://doi.org/10.1007/978-3-319-75656-1_19

and provides clues for the necessity of damage control surgery.

Indications for trauma laparotomy include patients with hemodynamic instability, peritonitis, and trajectory suggesting abdominal injury such as transabdominal penetrating wounds or abdominal wounds that violate the anterior rectus fascia. There may be a role for nonoperative management of certain penetrating wounds; however, such discussion is beyond the scope of this chapter. In general, trajectory determination yields injury identification and frequently requires exploration. The unstable trauma patient belongs in the operating room, and the abdomen is often the source.

Once the trauma laparotomy is under way, one of the most challenging aspects is knowing when to employ damage control techniques. This is a difficult decision even in the hands of the most experienced trauma surgeon. Waiting for the deadly triad to set in is too late. The surgeon must identify early cues including bowel edema, dusky serosal surfaces, tissues cold to touch, noncompliant swollen abdominal wall, and diffuse oozing. The three main indications for damage control surgery include:

1. Exsanguinating, hypothermic, and coagulopathic patient dying on the operating table
2. Inability to control hemorrhage with direct hemostasis (large liver laceration, ruptured retroperitoneal hematomas)
3. Inability to close the abdomen (tension due to visceral edema, noncompliant abdominal wall) [4]

The goals of damage control laparotomy are to stop potential life-threatening bleeding, to identify the injuries, to control contamination, and to provide temporary abdominal closure [4]. Regardless of the mechanism and extent of injury, adhering to these basic principles will allow the surgeon to maneuver through a damage control surgery in a calm and systematic fashion. This chapter focuses on key maneuvers of damage control laparotomy for trauma, potential pitfalls associated with each maneuver, and available bailout techniques. The objective is to simplify each maneuver to its bare essentials so that a surgeon at any level of training can confidently execute the steps of an exploratory laparotomy for trauma.

19.2 General Concepts

Successful exploratory laparotomy in trauma begins with preoperative setup and ends with transportation to the surgical ICU for continued resuscitation. This section highlights the general concepts and key steps to the trauma laparotomy. The details of specific exposures and maneuvers for the retroperitoneal vessels and individual organ systems are discussed in the Technical Approaches section.

19.2.1 Preoperative Essentials

The team must minimize the "door to cut" time. The initial resuscitation should follow a fast orderly tempo that must continue through to the OR and beyond until surgical control of injury and physiologic capture has been obtained. Multiple tasks need to happen simultaneously as the patient is being transported to the OR. The blood bank should be alerted of a potential activation of the massive transfusion protocol. The OR staff is notified to adjust the room temperature to 75–80 °F and to ensure the availability of a rapid transfuser (delivers large volume warm fluid and blood products to the patient) and a cell saver in the room. Although cell savers are extremely useful in the setting of hemorrhage, intra-abdominal contamination is a contraindication for their use.

19.2.2 Positioning and Prepping (Fig. 19.1)

Do not delay positioning and prep once the patient is on the OR table. Remember, minimize the "door to cut" time! Work concurrently with anesthesiologists as they secure the airway and begin preparations for resuscitation. Position the patient supine with both arms out. This allows anesthesia access to bilateral upper extremities for intravenous lines and monitoring purposes

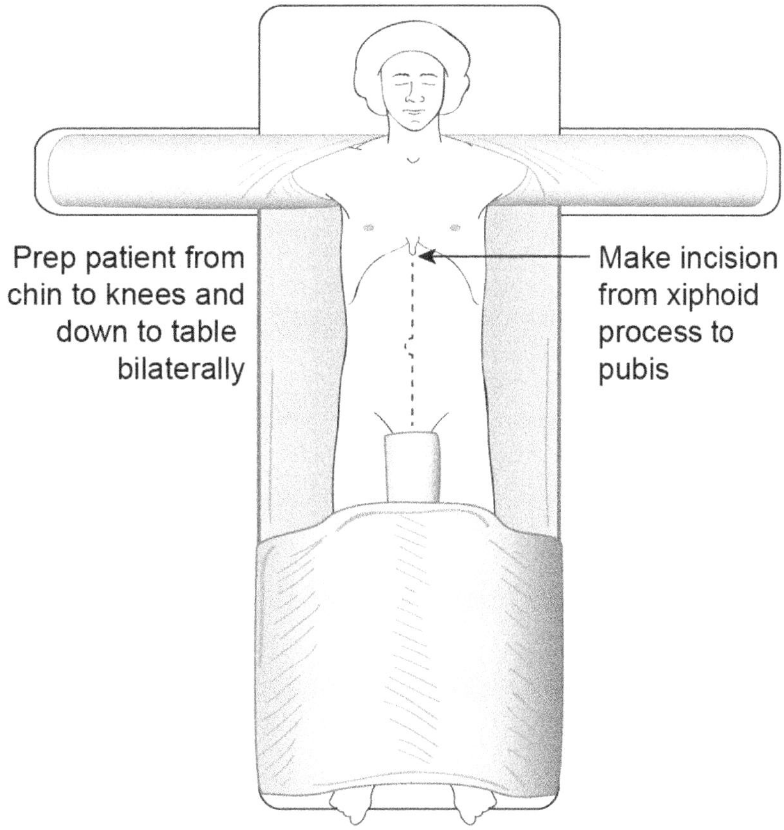

Fig. 19.1 Patient positioning and prepping (supine, arms out, and areas to prep)

and the surgeon access to the chest. Place a Foley catheter to monitor urine output as well as to triage the genitourinary system. Prep the patient from the chin to knees and down to the operating table bilaterally. This permits the surgeon access to the abdomen for laparotomy, to the chest for potential sternotomy or thoracotomy, to the groin for additional central lines, and to the lower extremities for saphenous vein graft harvest as vascular conduit. A groin towel is placed to ensure sterility.

19.2.3 Incision

The trauma laparotomy incision is midline from the xiphoid to the pubis.

19.2.3.1 Key Maneuvers

- Make a single incision with a #10 scalpel from the xiphoid to the pubic symphysis.
- The peritoneal cavity should be entered after three decisive strokes of the scalpel:
  - The first stroke of the scalpel divides the skin and dermis to expose the subcutaneous fat.
  - The second stroke of the scalpel divides the subcutaneous fat to expose the linea alba of the midline fascia.
  - The third stroke of the scalpel divides the fascia and opens the peritoneum.

    Be ready to encounter a gush of blood as the abdominal tamponade is released.

    Do not forget to communicate with the anesthesiologists prior to releasing the abdominal tamponade so that they can prepare their resuscitation.

19.2.3.2 Potential Pitfalls

A trauma patient with multiple previous abdominal procedures presents as a challenge due to a potentially hostile abdomen. Midline incisions in these circumstances may not permit the rapid access needed and may cause additional damage to underlying structures due to dense adhesions. An alternative approach is the bilateral subcostal incision through which most of the abdomen still can be explored.

19.2.4 Hemorrhage Control: Packing the Four Quadrants of the Abdomen

Once the abdomen is entered, the next move is eviscerating the small bowel and packing the abdomen to help control hemorrhage.

19.2.4.1 Key Maneuvers

- Pack the four quadrants of the abdomen with folded, radiopaque laparotomy pads in a clockwise fashion starting in the right upper quadrant.
- Packing the right upper quadrant and liver (Fig. 19.2):
  - Divide the falciform ligament between two Kelly clamps and ligate with 0-silk sutures.
  - Surgical assistant retracts the abdominal wall upward and away from the liver.
  - Position your non-dominant hand over the liver to protect and retract it inferiorly.
  - Use your dominant hand to position dry packs above the liver.
  - Reposition your non-dominant hand under the liver to retract it superiorly, and position packs below the liver.

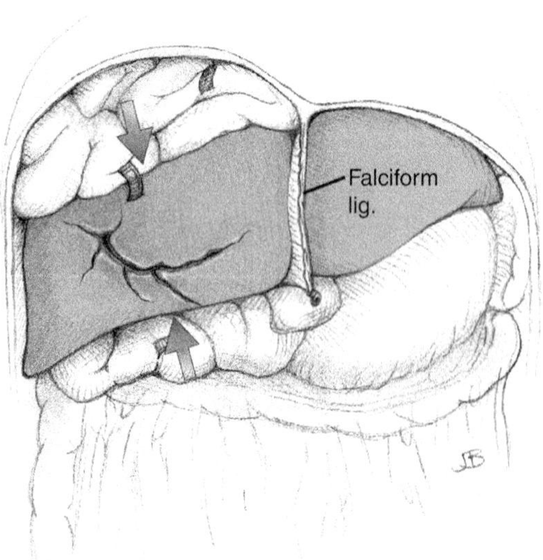

Fig. 19.2 Packing of the RUQ—liver packing

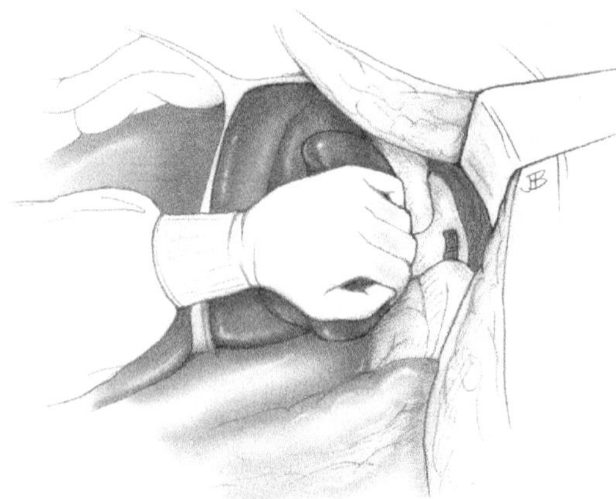

Fig. 19.3 Packing of the LUQ—spleen packing

  - The liver is now compressed anteriorly and posteriorly to achieve hemostasis.
- Packing the left upper quadrant and spleen (Fig. 19.3):
  - Surgical assistant retracts the left abdominal wall outward away from the spleen.
  - Position your non-dominant hand over the spleen to protect and elevate it toward the midline.
  - Use your dominant hand to position dry packs posterior to the spleen.
  - Release the spleen and place dry packs anterior to the organ.
- Packing the left lower quadrant and pelvis:
  - Surgical assistant retracts the abdominal wall laterally and away from the colon.
  - Sweep the small bowel and left colon superomedially.
  - Pack the left paracolic gutter and pelvis with dry packs.
- Packing the right lower quadrant and pelvis:
  - Surgical assistant retracts the abdominal wall laterally and away from the colon.
  - Sweep the small bowel and right colon superomedially.
  - Pack the right paracolic gutter and pelvis with dry packs.
- Once the four quadrants are packed and hemorrhage is temporarily controlled, inform the anesthesiologist and allow adequate resuscitation before proceeding.
- Abdominal retractors such as Bookwalter, Thompson, or Balfour should be set up at this time to assist in abdominal wall retraction.

19.2.4.2 Potential Pitfalls

In terms of packing, quality is more important than quantity! Under-packing results in continued hemorrhage, while over-packing can compress the inferior vena cava (IVC), cause decrease in venous return, and result in hypotension.

19.2.5 Hemorrhage Control: Identifying Retroperitoneal Hematomas (Fig. 19.4)

The retroperitoneum is divided into three zones, each containing vital structures that may require exploration during a trauma laparotomy:

- Zone 1 encompasses the central region of the retroperitoneum and extends from the diaphragm to the aortic bifurcation. It contains the abdominal aorta, celiac axis, superior mesenteric artery (SMA), IVC, proximal renal vasculatures, pancreas, and portions of the duodenum.

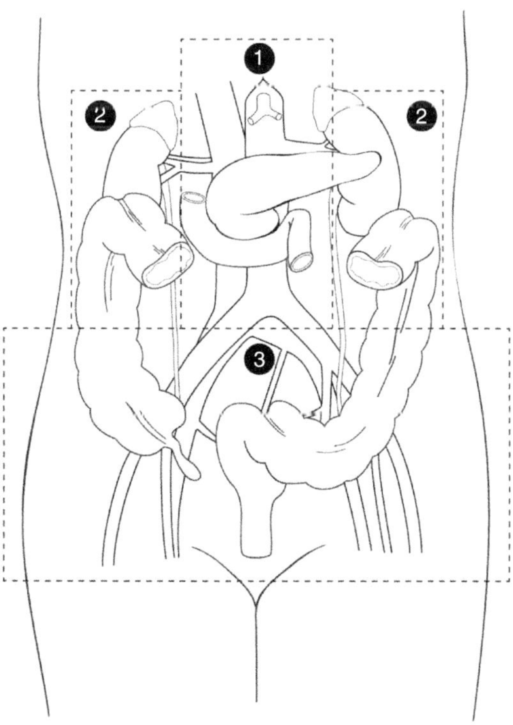

Fig. 19.4 Retroperitoneal hematoma zones 1, 2, and 3

Table 19.1 Exploration of retroperitoneal hematomas

Zone	Penetrating injury	Blunt injury
1 (central)	Explore	Explore
2 (perinephric)	Explore	Observe if not pulsatile/expanding
3 (pelvic)	Explore	Observe if not pulsatile/expanding

- Zone 2 encompasses the lateral regions of the retroperitoneum and contains the renal hilum vasculature, kidney, adrenal gland, ureter, and colon.
- Zone 3 is the pelvic retroperitoneum containing the iliac vessels and portions of the colon and rectum.

Indications for exploration vary with each zone and the mechanism of injury (Table 19.1). In general, all penetrating, pulsatile, and expanding hematomas require exploration. All zone 1 retroperitoneal hematomas are explored regardless of mechanism of injury. The vascular surgery tenet of obtaining proximal and distal control remains true during exposure and exploration of retroperitoneal hematomas.

19.2.6 Injury Identification

19.2.6.1 Key Maneuvers

- Remove packs one quadrant at a time, starting from t.ctive bleeding, retroperitoneal hematomas, bile staining, succus leakage, and diaphragmatic injuries.
- Running the small bowel:
  - Identify the ligament of Treitz by lifting up the transverse colon and following the transverse mesocolon to its base.
  - Flip the small bowel back and forth between your hands to evaluate the bowel wall and its mesentery.
  - Examine the entire small bowel from the ligament of Treitz to the terminal ileum.
- Assessing the colon:
  - Identify the cecum and examine the ascending, transverse, descending, and sigmoid colon for bowel wall and mesocolon injuries.

- Follow the sigmoid colon to the rectosigmoid junction and evaluate the intraperitoneal rectum.
- A digital rectal exam and rigid proctosigmoidoscopy should be performed in all patients with high index of suspicion for rectal injury (pelvic fractures, truncal gunshot and stab wounds, penetrating wounds of the lower abdomen, buttocks, or perineum).

- Diaphragmatic injuries are difficult to diagnose and must be repaired once identified:
  - Reduce any abdominal contents from the intrathoracic cavity.
  - Surgical assistant retracts the liver or spleen inferiorly to provide diaphragmatic exposure.
  - Reapproximate the diaphragmatic defect with hemostats.
  - Primarily repair the diaphragm with running or interrupted nonabsorbable sutures over a red rubber catheter inserted into the pleural space.
  - Place the catheter to suction to evacuate the pneumothorax.
  - The assistant removes the catheter as the surgeon ties down the suture repair.
  - Insert chest tube on injured side.

19.2.6.2 Pitfalls

Do not forget to evaluate the gastroesophageal junction, the anterior and posterior aspects of the stomach, and the pancreas via the lesser sac. Expose the gastroesophageal junction by dividing the left triangular ligament of the liver and retracting the left lobe of the liver laterally. To enter the lesser sac, first retract the stomach superiorly and the greater omentum inferiorly. Make a transverse incision in the thin portion of the omentum with Bovie cautery just inferior and parallel to the greater curvature of the stomach. The posterior aspect of the stomach is assessed through the lesser sac. The anterior surface of the body and tail of the pancreas can be visualized and palpated through the lesser sac as well.

19.2.7 Contamination Control

The goal is to limit the amount of intra-abdominal contamination as quickly as possible and plan for definitive repair at a later time. Bowel injuries can be controlled and contained via several techniques:

- Grasp and close opposing bowel walls with Babcock or Allis clamps.
- Suture closure (interrupted or running) the bowel injury with any suture on a non-cutting needle.
- Skin staples to reapproximate the bowel edges.
- Tie off the proximal and distal ends of the injured bowel with umbilical tape (effectively isolating the area of injury).
- Resect the injured bowel segment with a gastrointestinal anastomosis (GIA) stapler, and leave the bowel in discontinuity.

19.2.8 Temporary Abdominal Closure

At this point of the operation, ongoing hemorrhages are halted, major injuries are identified, and intra-abdominal contaminations are controlled. It is time to determine whether the patient is stable for definitive repair or unstable and requires damage control procedures. Contraindications to immediate reconstruction include hemodynamic instability; physiologic derangements including hypothermia, acidosis, and coagulopathy (be vigilant during the operation and look for these signs before they actually appear); and multisystem injuries. Competing priorities such as concomitant head injury may require an abbreviated damage control operation. In addition, visceral edema, abdominal noncompliance, and the need for a second-look laparotomy preclude definitive abdominal closure in trauma patients.

A few common techniques for temporary abdominal closure are listed below, and a more detailed analysis of such techniques is offered in Chap. 20:

- Rapid skin closure with towel clamps sequentially applied to skin edges 1–2 cm apart [4]
- Negative pressure/vacuum-assisted closure (such as the ABThera system, KCI Medical)
- Bogota bag or mesh closure

19.2.8.1 Potential Pitfalls

Abdominal compartment syndrome (ACS) can occur in the setting of an open abdomen! ACS is defined as intra-abdominal pressure ≥20 mmHg with organ dysfunction [5]. Signs include elevated peak airway pressure, hypotension, oliguria, and bowel ischemia. Treat ACS by removing the temporary abdominal closure device and releasing the pressure via a laparotomy. In some instances, tight or excessive intra-abdominal packings may also need to be removed.

19.2.9 Transport from the OR to the SICU

This is a crucial yet often overlooked and underrated step of trauma laparotomy [4]. The transportation process should be a well-orchestrated event with constant communication between the surgeon, anesthesiologist, OR staff, and SICU team. Prior to leaving the controlled setting, ensure the availability of an ICU bed, monitoring devices, Ambu bag, blood products, and vasopressor medications. A thorough sign-out from the surgeon and anesthesiologist and a clear understanding of the patient's condition are keys to a successful ICU resuscitation.

19.3 Technical Approaches

19.3.1 Exposing the IVC

19.3.1.1 Key Maneuver: Cattell-Braasch Maneuver (Fig. 19.5)

- *Right-sided visceral medial rotation* with the surgeon positioned on the patient's left side.
- Retract the right colon medially with your left hand to expose the white line of Toldt.
- Holding the cecum in your left hand, bluntly dissect the white line of Toldt with your left index finger, and travel superiorly from the cecum to the hepatic flexure (the correct plane consists of loose areolar tissue that should easily divide).
- Continue mobilization of the right colon medially and superiorly to the transverse colon until the IVC, right kidney, and iliac vessels are visualized.

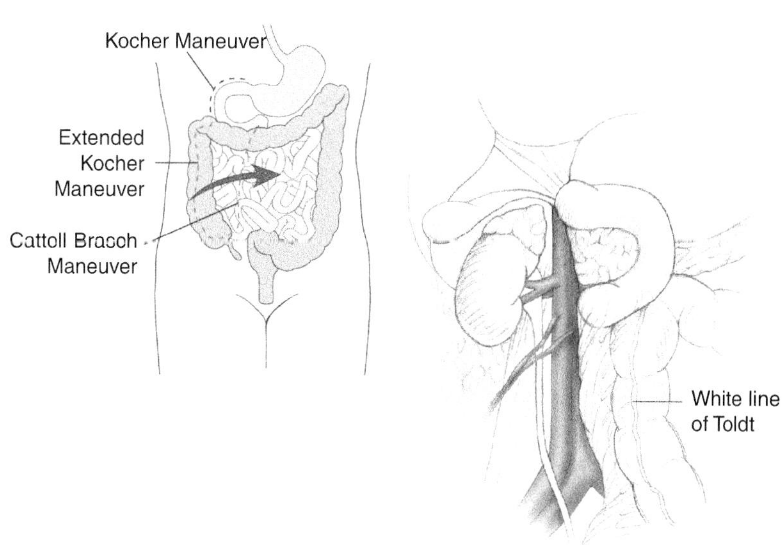

Fig. 19.5 Cattell-Braasch maneuver

19.3.1.2 Potential Pitfalls

The correct plane of dissection can be more difficult to identify in the presence of a retroperitoneal hematoma. However, hematomas often create a dissection plane and may help guide your maneuver. Dissecting in a plane deep to the white line of Toldt will result in elevation of the right kidney. Identify and protect the duodenum as it is exposed with the mobilization of the hepatic flexure of the colon.

19.3.1.3 Key Maneuver: Kocher Maneuver

- Medial visceral rotation of the duodenum to expose the posterior aspect of the pancreatic head.
- The c-loop of the duodenum is exposed after the hepatic flexure is mobilized.
- Gently retract the duodenum medially with your left hand.
- Using a combination of blunt and sharp dissection, divide the peritoneal attachments to the lateral wall of the duodenum with your right hand from the first portion, and move inferiorly to the third/fourth portion.
- The maneuver is complete when the aorta is visualized.

19.3.2 Exposing the Abdominal Aorta

19.3.2.1 Key Maneuver: Mattox Maneuver (Fig. 19.6)

- *Left-sided visceral medial rotation* with the surgeon positioned on the patient's right side.
- Retract the left colon medially with your left hand to expose the white line of Toldt.
- Bluntly dissect the white line of Toldt with your right index finger and travel superiorly from the sigmoid colon to the splenic flexure.
- Identify the spleen, retract the spleen medially in your left hand, and divide the peritoneal attachments to the spleen with your right hand.
- Rotate the left colon, spleen, tail of the pancreas, and stomach medially and superiorly to expose the abdominal aorta and the iliac vessels.

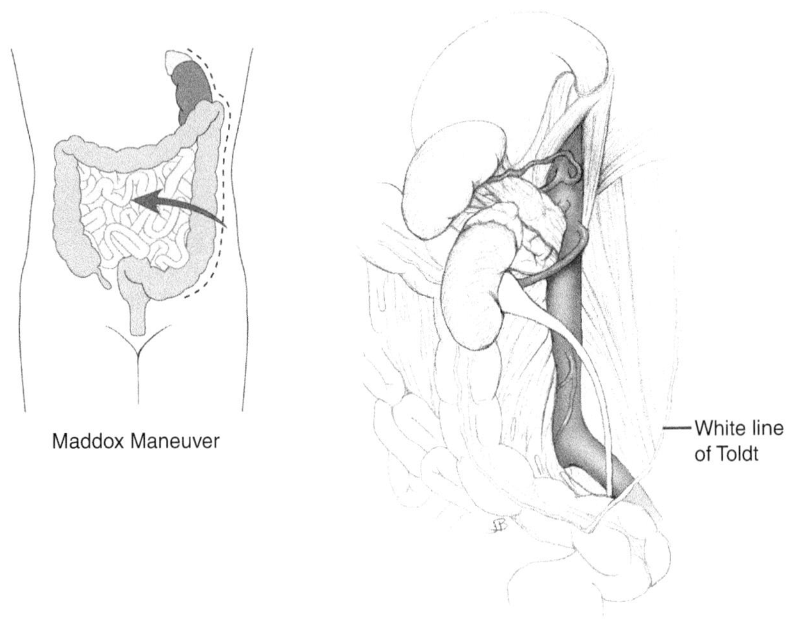

Fig. 19.6 Mattox maneuver

19.3.2.2 Potential Pitfalls

The Mattox maneuver may be too time-consuming for patients who require immediate supraceliac aortic control in the setting of an expanding retroperitoneal hematoma. To expose the aorta above the celiac axis, retract the stomach laterally, and sharply divide the gastrohepatic ligament vertically. Retract the distal esophagus/proximal stomach laterally and the left hepatic lobe to the right (the left triangular ligament may need to be divided) to expose the left crus of the diaphragm. Use your dominant index finger to bluntly dissect the loose tissue around the aorta superiorly and inferiorly until an aortic clamp can be placed along the aorta. An orogastric tube placed by the anesthesiologist will help differentiate the esophagus from the potentially flaccid, empty aorta.

19.3.3 Liver Injuries

Hepatic injuries range from small parenchymal lacerations that are easily treated with pressure and hemostatic agents to large avulsions or retrohepatic vena cava hemorrhage that require full liver mobilization and vascular control. Regardless of the extent of the injury (and you likely will not know the full extent initially), the first step is to pack the liver. Hemorrhage not well controlled by packing will require further mobilization and exploration. Three commonly utilized techniques for treating liver injuries/bleeding are discussed below. Several additional techniques are listed, but detailed descriptions are beyond the scope of this chapter.

19.3.3.1 Key Maneuver: Hepatic Packing

- Recreate the anatomy by packing above and below the liver.
- Anterior hepatic packing:
  - Divide the falciform ligament as previously described.
  - Retract the liver inferiorly with one hand, and place packs over the retracting hand between the anterior surface of the liver and the diaphragm.
- Lateral hepatic packing:
  - Retract the liver medially one hand, and place packs over the retracting hand between the right lateral surface of the liver and the abdominal sidewall.
- Posterior hepatic packing:
  - Retract the liver superiorly with one hand, and place packs under the retracting hand between the posterior surface of the liver and the infra-hepatic structures.
- If bleeding stops after packing, leave the packs in place! Premature removal of the packing may result in further bleeding from peeling the packs off the injured parenchyma.
- To remove the packing, slowly irrigate with water to loosen the packs.
- Localize and control residual areas of bleeding.

19.3.3.2 Potential Pitfalls

Excessive packing can compress the IVC and jeopardize venous return. Too much packing can also limit diaphragmatic movement and cause increase peak airway pressure and hypoventilation. Full mobilization of the liver by dividing the triangular and coronary ligaments may improve exposure of the injury and allow more effective packing. However, if a retrohepatic injury is suspected, mobilization of the right liver lobe may unroof the tamponade and cause severe hemorrhage.

19.3.3.3 Key Maneuver: Pringle Maneuver

- Retract the anterior edge of the liver superiorly and to the right.
- Insert the left index finger into the foramen of Winslow.
- Pinch the thumb on top of the index finger to control the portal triad (hepatic artery, portal vein, common bile duct).
- A vascular clamp can replace the fingers for long-term control.
- Release the clamp intermittently to limit total ischemia time.

19.3.3.4 Potential Pitfalls

The Pringle maneuver is ineffective in patients with a replaced left hepatic artery (most commonly off the left gastric artery) or injuries to the hepatic veins and retrohepatic IVC. A replaced right hepatic artery (off the SMA) commonly travels posterior to the portal vein. Feel for a pulsatile structure posterior to the portal vein to help identify this vessel. Be careful not to injure the artery when placing a vascular clamp during the Pringle maneuver.

19.3.3.5 Key Maneuver: Suture Repair

- Reapproximate the liver parenchymal lacerations with sutures (0-chromic) on a large blunt needle.
- Take large bites incorporating the uninjured liver parenchyma and capsule.
- Place figure-of-eight or horizontal mattress sutures.

19.3.3.6 Potential Pitfalls

Taking too small of a bite of the liver parenchyma can cause the suture to tear through and result in more bleeding. When tying down the sutures, apply just enough tension to reapproximate the lacerated edges. Excessive tension during knot tying will further avulse the liver and exacerbate the injury.

19.3.3.7 Additional Hemostatic Agents and Techniques

Learn the available topical hemostatic agents available at your institution. Commonly utilized topical agents include thrombin Gelfoam, Surgicel, Combat Gauze, and fibrin glue. Argon beam coagulator can be used for hemostasis by creating an eschar on the bleeding liver surface. Omental packing is useful in deep liver lacerations and needs to be secured with sutures. Through-and-through liver injuries can be controlled via balloon tamponade by using a Blakemore tube or a homemade balloon constructed from a Penrose drain over a hollow rubber catheter. A hepatotomy can be performed after adequate vascular inflow control with the Pringle maneuver. Using the finger fracture technique, parenchymal defects are opened to expose the injured vessels/ducts. Bleeding vessels are then controlled with direct suture ligation, clips, or electrocautery. Atrial caval shunts and hepatic venovenous bypass are rarely used (and also rarely successful) and beyond the scope of this chapter.

19.3.4 Splenic Injuries

Indications for splenectomy in a trauma patient include active bleeding, hemodynamic instability, and concurrent moderate to severe brain injury that can exacerbate with ongoing hypotensive episodes. Due to its posterior location, the spleen must be mobilized to the midline to allow better exposure and control. Splenorrhaphy is rarely performed during a trauma laparotomy. When in doubt, the spleen should come out!

19.3.4.1 Key Maneuver: Splenectomy

- Surgeon is positioned on the patient's right side.
- Place the left hand posterior to the spleen and retract the spleen medially and anteriorly.
- Medial retraction of the spleen exposes the retroperitoneal splenic attachments.
- Dissect and divide (blunt, sharp, or cautery) the superior lienophrenic, lateral lienocolic, and posterior lienorenal attachments with the right hand.
- Lift the spleen off the right kidney and toward the abdominal midline.
- Place laparotomy pads posteriorly in the splenic fossa to prevent the spleen from falling back into its original position.
- Divide the short gastric vessels (suture ligation, stapler, energy device) to expose the splenic hilum.
- Ligate and divide the hilar vessels:
  - Individually dissect out the splenic artery and vein, place two hemostats on each vessel, divide between the hemostats with scissors, and suture ligate the two ends with 2-0 silk ties.
  - An alternative is to divide the artery and vein with a vascular stapling device.

19.3.4.2 Potential Pitfalls

Excessive retraction during mobilization can tear the splenic capsule and cause more bleeding.

Identify and protect the tail of the pancreas to prevent pancreatic leak and fistulas. Protect the stomach during division of the short gastric vessels. Care must be taken to ensure that all of the short gastric vessels are adequately ligated to prevent postoperative bleeding.

19.3.5 Pancreatic and Duodenal Injuries

The pancreas and duodenum are surrounded by numerous vital structures. Adequate assessment of these two organs requires multiple maneuvers, and detection of any pancreatic and duodenal injuries should raise suspicion for associated injuries to adjacent structures.

19.3.5.1 Key Maneuver: Exposure of the Duodenum

- The first portion is inspected by following the distal stomach to the pylorus and continuing distally.
- The second and third portions are exposed with the Kocher maneuver, which also allows examination of the posterior aspect of the c-loop.
- The fourth portion is exposed by dividing the ligament of Treitz.
- The third and fourth portion of the duodenum can be further mobilized with a Cattell-Braasch maneuver by carrying the dissection to the root of the small bowel mesentery.

19.3.5.2 Key Maneuver: Exposure of the Pancreas

- Expose the superior border of the pancreas by dividing the gastrohepatic ligament.
- Exposing the anterior surface:
  - Open the lesser sac and retract the stomach superiorly.
  - Sharply incise and divide the peritoneal covering of the pancreas to examine its anterior surface.
  - Continue the dissection to the right of the patient to expose the entire anterior aspect of the pancreas from the tail to the head.
- Exposing the posterior surface:
  - A Kocher maneuver exposes the posterior aspect of the head and neck of the pancreas.
  - Medial mobilization of the spleen by dividing the lienocolic and lienorenal ligaments exposes the posterior aspect of the body and tail of the pancreas.

19.3.6 Kidney Injuries

Renal injuries are most commonly identified on CT scan during a trauma work-up. Indications for exploration include active bleeding, hemodynamic instability, expanding or pulsatile hematoma, and injury to the ureters or bladder. Renal salvage is rarely indicated if the patient has a normal contralateral kidney.

19.3.6.1 Key Maneuver

- Exposure of the right kidney:
  - Perform a right-sided medial visceral rotation to mobilize the right colon.
  - Perform a Kocher maneuver to mobilize the duodenum.
- Exposure of the left kidney:
  - Perform a left-sided medial visceral rotation to mobilize the left colon, spleen, and distal pancreas.
- Vascular control:
  - Obtain proximal renal vascular control prior to entering Gerota's fascia.
  - Lift the transverse colon and follow the mesocolon to its base.
  - Sharply open and enter the retroperitoneum at this level.
  - Extend the opening from the ligament of Treitz to the aortic bifurcation to allow full exposure of the renal vessels.
  - Identify the right renal vein as it enters the right lateral edge of the IVC, and isolate it with a vessel loop.
  - Retract the right renal vein superiorly to expose the underlying right renal artery, and isolate the artery with a vessel loop.
  - Identify the left renal vein as it crosses the aorta laterally and enters the left lateral

  - edge of the IVC, and isolate it with a vessel loop.
  - Retract the left renal vein superiorly to expose the underlying right renal artery, and isolate the artery with a vessel loop.
- Nephrectomy:
  - Once vascular control is obtained, open Gerota's fascia sharply at the lateral edge of the kidney.
  - Right nephrectomy: place the left hand posterior to the kidney, mobilize it medially and anteriorly into the midline abdomen, and ligate and divide the renal vessels.
  - Left nephrectomy: place the left hand posterior to the kidney, mobilize it medially and anteriorly into the midline abdomen, and ligate and divide the renal vessels.

19.3.6.2 Potential Pitfalls

When isolating and dividing the renal veins, remember that the right adrenal vein drains directly into the IVC, while the left adrenal vein drains into the left renal vein. Prior to performing a nephrectomy, always confirm the presence of a contralateral kidney! If prior imaging is unavailable, an intraoperative on-table IV pyelogram can be performed to assess the contralateral kidney.

19.3.7 Vascular Injuries: What Can and Cannot Be Ligated!

The abdominal aorta cannot be ligated! Suprarenal aortic injuries may need repair with a graft, even in the face of contamination. Injuries to the aortic bifurcation can be repaired with extra-anatomical bypasses. All infrarenal IVC injuries can be ligated if necessary. Suprarenal IVC injuries cannot be ligated and may require shunting and repair with greater saphenous vein patch. The celiac trunk can be ligated due to extensive collaterals. The SMA cannot be ligated and should be repaired with a saphenous vein or internal iliac artery conduit. The SMV and portal vein can be ligated; however, a second-look laparotomy to evaluate bowel edema and viability is appropriate. The IMA and IMV can be ligated.

Take-Home Points

- Once the decision is made to take a trauma patient to the OR, notify the anesthesiologist, blood bank, and OR staff, and move quickly. Minimize the "door to cut" time.
- Communicate with the anesthesiologist before releasing the abdominal tamponade.
- Be vigilant with abdominal packing; underpacking results in continued hemorrhage, while over-packing can compress the IVC and decrease venous return.
- Run the entire length of the bowel and quickly control any contamination. Reserve definitive repair for a later time.
- Constantly evaluate the patient for physiological derangements including hypothermia, coagulopathy, and acidosis.
- Decision for damage control surgery should be made prior to the onset of the lethal triad.
- Abdominal compartment syndrome can occur in patients with an open abdomen.

References

1. Stone H, Strom P, Mullins R. Management of the major coagulopathy with onset during laparotomy. Ann Surg. 1983;197(5):532–5.
2. Rotondo M, Schwab C, McGonigal M, Phillips G, Fruchterman T, Kauder D, Latenser B, Angood P. 'Damage control': an approach for improved survival in exsanguinating penetrating abdominal injury. J Trauma. 1993;35(3):375–82.
3. Johnson J, Gracias V, Schwab C, Reilly P, Kauder D, Shapiro M, Dabrowski G, Rotondo M. Evolution in damage control for exsanguinating penetrating abdominal injury. J Trauma. 2001;51(2):261–71.
4. Hirshberg A, Walden R. Damage control for abdominal trauma. Surg Clin N Am. 1997;77(4):813–20.
5. Jacobs L, Luk S. Advanced trauma operative management. Woodbury: Cine-Med; 2010.

20 Fundamentals of Temporary Abdominal Wall Closure

Shelby Resnick and Niels D. Martin

20.1 Introduction

In contemporary surgical practice, a fair amount of surgical jargon surrounds temporary abdominal wall closure. To clarify, a "temporarily closed" abdominal wall is often described as an abdominal wall that has been "left open." In fact, in the surgical literature, management of a temporary abdominal wall closure is synonymous with management of the "open abdomen" or often termed a "damage control closure" (to be described below), understanding the various nomenclatures will alleviate future confusion.

There are many clinical scenarios that can lead to a temporary abdominal wall closure [1]. While ultimately the techniques of temporary closure are similar, it is important to understand the underlying pathophysiology of each patient to optimize care. In fact, the underlying pathology often drives the decision-making for abdominal wall closure.

Temporary abdominal wall closure was first widely described in the latter part of the twentieth century by vascular surgeons whose patients developed abdominal compartment syndrome following major abdominal aortic aneurysm surgery [2]. These patients underwent massive volume resuscitation, and only by leaving the abdomen open, with a temporary dressing, could the lethality of compartment syndrome be overcome.

In the early 1990s, this technique was combined with the surgical "temporization" of other intra-abdominal injuries in the trauma literature; together, it was called "damage control." The term originated with the US Navy and describes the process of temporizing damage to a ship, just enough to maintain sea and battle worthiness, until the vessel could return safely for full repairs. Surgically, damage control temporizes traumatic abdominal injuries to allow for a stabilization of patient physiology and hemodynamics [3]. Only the most immediately life-threatening issues are addressed at the index operation. The final step of the damage control index operation is creation of a temporary abdominal closure.

The temporary abdominal wall closure in damage control allows for shunting of vascular injuries, packing of solid organ injuries, and controlling contamination that may result in bowel discontinuity. The ultimate destination of the damage control patient is the intensive care unit,

S. Resnick • N. D. Martin (✉)
Trauma and Surgical Critical Care,
University of Pennsylvania, Philadelphia, PA, USA
e-mail: shelby.resnick@uphs.upenn.edu;
niels.martin@uphs.upenn.edu

F. Palazzo (ed.), *Fundamentals of General Surgery*, https://doi.org/10.1007/978-3-319-75656-1_20

where hemodynamic and physiologic stabilization occurs prior to definitive surgical treatment. Therefore, the temporary abdominal closure is primarily managed outside of the operating room.

Beyond vascular and trauma surgery, temporary abdominal closures may be necessary following any abdominal surgery where the patient suffers a significant base deficit, low pH, hypothermia, large blood loss or requirement for blood transfusion, hypotension, high lactate, coagulopathy, or high degree of contamination [4]. The etiologies of these patients include intra-abdominal sepsis, abdominal compartment syndrome, pending abdominal compartment syndrome, hemorrhagic pancreatitis, and ruptured abdominal aortic aneurysms. Temporary abdominal wall closure also facilitates "second-look" surgery for reexamination in the setting of mesenteric ischemia. Finally, occasionally the abdomen is either opened or left open to treat extra-abdominal pathology such as refractory elevated intracranial pressure [5]. In this setting, the open abdomen lowers central venous pressure and allows for improved venous outflow from the brain. In total, these general surgery indications for temporary abdominal wall closure occur at a higher frequency than trauma. A 2017 multicenter study ordered the indication from most to least frequent as peritonitis, trauma, vascular emergencies, ischemia, pancreatitis, and abdominal compartment syndrome [6].

Regardless of indication, the methods and techniques of temporary abdominal closure are similar, based on the concept that the fascial edges and skin are not approximated leaving the intra-abdominal viscera exposed. This temporary anatomy requires unique technical and medical management knowledge and skills. Understanding the various options and their specific advantages and disadvantages and recognizing potential complications are now a necessary component of surgical training.

20.2 General Concepts

Techniques for temporary abdominal wall closure have evolved in the past three decades to optimize the function and safety of the temporary closure. Beyond providing a "dressing" to the abdominal wall defect, the technique has several other goals. This includes protecting the abdominal viscera from desiccation and infection while allowing for fluid control. Abdominal fluids should optimally be prevented from pooling in the recesses of the peritoneum and also be adequately quantified upon removal. Peritoneal fluid often contains cytotoxic inflammatory mediators and endotoxins, including IL-6, IL-10, TNF-alpha, TNF-beta, and CRP, which have been thought to play a contributing role in the development of multiple organ dysfunction syndrome. Animal studies have suggested that reducing the concentration of these mediators can help prevent inflammatory progression; however this mechanism has not been definitively shown in clinical studies [7, 8].

An ideal temporary abdominal wall closure system would also facilitate eventual formal fascial closure and minimize the chances of long-term ventral hernia formation. This is generally achieved by preserving fascial integrity, preventing fascial retraction (without creating pathologic tension), and decreasing the risk of adhesion and fistula formation. Additionally, the technique should be easy to use by practitioners in the operating room and at the bedside in the intensive care unit. It should allow for rapid removal and placement and be valuably priced.

The most frequently employed temporary abdominal wall closure methods include patch techniques and/or negative pressure therapy systems. Older methods which include simple skin closure or silo methods are mentioned here for thoroughness; however, for the above optimization reasons, both the skin only and silo techniques are generally avoided if possible.

20.2.1 Skin Only

Skin-only closures utilize penetrating towel clamps or staples to close the skin. This technique provides few of the advantages achieved with more sophisticated temporary closure techniques and leaves the patient at a much higher risk for development of abdominal compartment syndrome.

20.2.2 Silo Techniques ("Bogota Bag")

The silo technique is commonly known as the "Bogota bag" named after the Colombian surgeon who introduced it in the 1980s. It refers to the use of any translucent, nonadherent, sterile bag used to cover the abdominal cavity. Commonly, an IV, dialysate, or irrigation bag is used for this technique and is sewn to the skin edge, circumferentially around the wound. The silo technique does allow for visual inspection of the abdominal viscera at the bedside. It is also inexpensive and requires few materials, making it a reasonable option in resource-poor environments. However, it lacks the capabilities of more advanced temporary closure systems in terms of fluid control and the ability to accommodate for increasing intra-abdominal pressures.

20.2.3 Patch Techniques

Patch techniques involve the use of a prosthetic material sewn to the edges of the fascia effectively "bridging" the defect. This allows for easy reentry on subsequent explorations and in theory prevents fascial retraction. At each reoperation, the fascial edges can be more closely approximated and the patch progressively trimmed to allow for eventual primary closure of the fascia, at which time the patch is completely cut out of the fascia. A disadvantage of using this method is that each time the fascia is sutured to the patch, there is a potential to damage the fascial layers which need to stay intact for primary closure to be possible. The potential for fascial damage is further accentuated in hypotensive, critically ill, and/or malnourished patients where the puncturing of suture holes through the fascia can lead to fascial ischemia and necrosis, especially when repeated tightening of the patch is performed. Patch options include synthetic materials such as polytetrafluoroethylene and Vicryl mesh. There are patch techniques that minimize fascial manipulation during serial explorations, such as the Wittmann Patch [9] (Fig. 20.1). Patch techniques can be combined with negative pressure therapy to help control and quantify peritoneal effluent.

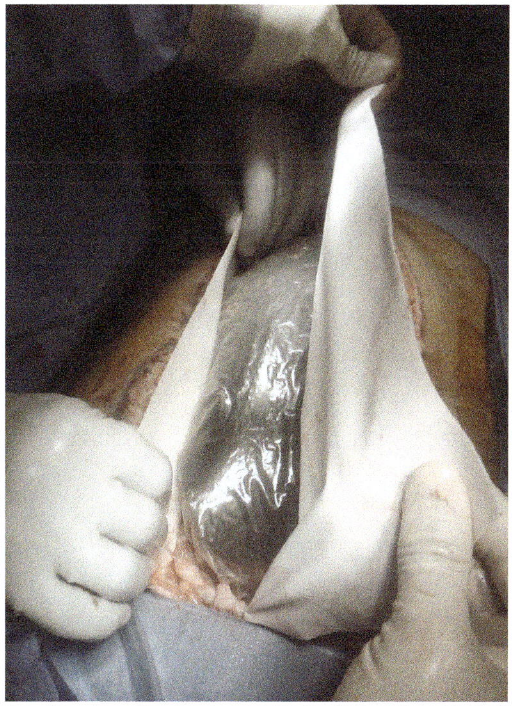

Fig. 20.1 Patch technique. A Wittmann Patch is sewn to the fascia and then closed over the protective layer with a Velcro®-like closing technique

20.2.4 Negative Pressure Therapy Systems

The most common contemporary techniques in temporary abdominal wall closure involve a negative pressure therapy system (NPTS). Most applications are commercial in nature and are highly utilized, in part, due to ease of use. Additionally, there is increasing literature supporting a higher primary fascial closure rate, even after long-term applications. NPTS allow for control of the abdominal fluid effluent and its quantification. The dressings themselves are relatively compliant, thus minimizing (but *not* negating) progression of increased abdominal hypertension to frank abdominal compartment syndrome. There are two main types of NPTS, towel-based and sponge-based. NPTS employs the use of a nonadherent protective layer opposing the bowel that is perforated to allow for fluid effluent, combined with an overlying sponge, gauze, or other porous materials in the subcutaneous space, and an outer, occlusive dressing. Once sealed, controlled suction can be placed on the porous layer to create the negative pressure and draw off accumulating fluids and toxic metabolites. Noncommercial methods can be performed with products commonly found in most operating rooms.

20.3 Technical Considerations

20.3.1 Patch Technique

The commercially available Wittmann Patch™ is comprised of two sheets of biocompatible material which attach to each other using a Velcro®-like closing technique, one with micro hooks and the other with loops. Each sheet is sutured to the abdominal fascia. The abdominal wound can then be easily opened and closed by pulling them apart or pressing them together, respectively. The entire patch is then covered with a hypobaric wound shield (HWS) to help prevent contamination and promote removal of fluid. The classically described HWS is similar to the towel-based NPTS, the Barker VAC (see below), where a sterile gauze is used to cover the wound and the patch. A drain is then placed across the gauze and placed to wall suction. Finally, the entire wound site is covered with a plastic adhesive drape to seal it. In lieu of a hypobaric wound shield as described above, some surgeons opt to use a commercial negative pressure wound system for more robust fluid management and measurement.

In a similar manner to the Wittmann Patch™, polytetrafluorethylene (PTFE) patches can be used to accomplish the same goals. Sewn to the edges of the abdominal fascia, the patch is then sewn together down the center, cut to reopen and resewn at each subsequent closing of the abdomen.

20.3.2 Towel-Based NPTS (Barker VAC)

The Barker VAC is a towel-based NPTS. A three-layered occlusive dressing is used to apply negative pressure and can be formed quickly and inexpensively with materials found in most operating rooms. In one of the original papers by Barker, the technique was estimated to cost $126, though likely higher now due to inflation [10] (Table 20.1).

The Barker Drain System provides to some degree the same advantages as the commercial negative therapy systems. It is generally much less expensive than commercial products and can be created with simple materials. However, it does not remove fluids as efficiently as the commercially available products [11].

Table 20.1 Materials and steps for placement of the Barker VAC

Materials	Placement steps
• Polyethylene drape: Barker initially described the use of the 3 M™ Steri-Drape™ large towel drape 1010; however, in a pinch, a sterile X-ray cassette cover will also suffice • Surgical towels • Two 10 mm flat silicone drains with bulb • Y adapter • Adhesive drape (Ioban) • Skin adhesive (Mastisol® or tincture of benzoin)	1. Obtain a polyethylene drape 2. Cut 1 cm slits in a polyethylene sheet to allow for drainage of the peritoneal fluid 3. Place the sheet between the viscera and anterior abdominal wall (Fig. 20.2) 4. Place moist surgical towels over the drape in the subcutaneous space 5. Lay the two flat drains over the towels 6. The skin is dried and prepped with an adhesive 7. An adhesive sheet is placed across the wound and adhered to the skin (Fig. 20.3) 8. The drains are connected via the y-connecting adapter and placed to wall suction

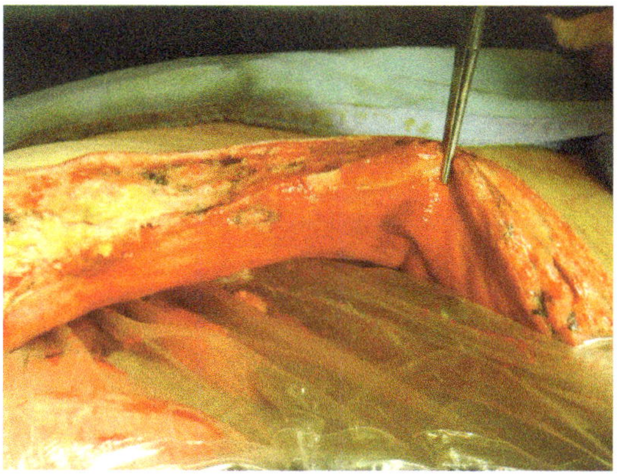

Fig. 20.2 Visceral protection. All contemporary forms of temporary abdominal closure involve the placement of a nonadherent sterile covering to protect the abdominal viscera and prevent adhesion formation

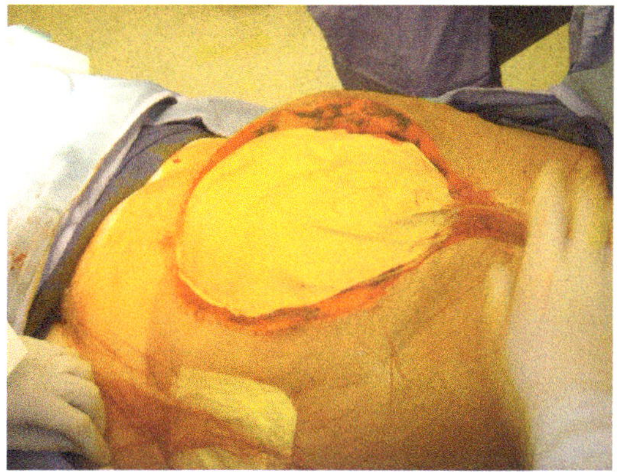

Fig. 20.3 Towel-based negative pressure therapy system (Barker VAC). Using materials found in most operating rooms, the Barker VAC creates an inexpensive, three-layered occlusive dressing to which negative pressure is then applied

Table 20.2 Placement steps for the commercial negative pressure therapy system (ABThera™)

1. Place the protective layer over the abdominal contents. The layer may need to be trimmed to fit the abdomen. If this is the case, it is important to not leave any exposed foam sponge so as to prevent any direct exposure of the sponge to the bowel which may cause injury
2. The football-shaped foam piece is then sized to the dimensions of the subcutaneous space. It should be in contact with all wound edges but not overlapping the skin, which will help to apply medial tension
3. Prep the skin with an adhesive, i.e., Mastisol® or tincture of benzoin, to promote adhesion, especially in areas of skin overlap or high moisture, like groin creases
4. The adhesive drape is then placed to cover the foam and surrounding skin. The importance of this step cannot be underestimated. For people with a large body habitus, an assistant to help hold back the skin, so a good seal with no gaps can be achieved, is paramount. Any gaps will create subsequent challenges for the device and care team. Cutting the large adhesive sheet into smaller more manageable sheets can help in more heavily creased areas. Additionally, shaving off excessive body hair will be appreciated by the patient at the time of removal and can help with achieving a better seal
5. A 2.5 cm hole is cut in the adhesive and foam where the interface suction pad will be placed. Choose a location that will be most effective for flow and the position of the tube; this is generally centrally on the device. Adhere the suction pad over the cut hole (Fig. 20.4)
6. Connect the NPT machine and canister. Initial settings should be set based on the physiology of the patient. The usual set pressure is 125 mmHg continuous

20.3.3 Sponge-Based NPTS (ABThera™)

In contrast to the Barker VAC, commercially available, sponge-based abdominal NPTS are designed to more evenly distribute the negative pressure and to better drain the recesses and dependent portions of the abdomen [11]. Some studies have indicated that use of an instillation feature available on some commercial NPTS can decrease the number of intestinal adhesions, help prevent dehydration, and facilitate re-exploration [4] (Table 20.2).

If a NPTS is used in the setting of significant bleeding and/or coagulopathy, the suction should be placed at a lower level (~75 mmHg) for the first 48 h to avoid persistent hemorrhage and allow clotting of blood vessels. The output canister should be closely monitored for signs of ongoing bleeding. Suction should also not be in direct contact with bowel. Any anastomosis created during surgery should be placed in the abdomen away for the NPTS.

20.4 Practical/Safety Precautions

Damage control laparotomy has decreased mortality rates in emergency surgery, but morbidity following the technique is still significant. Complications following an open abdomen are divided into early

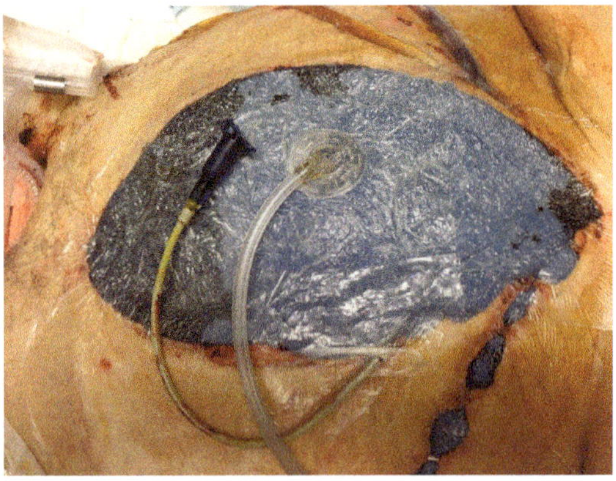

Fig. 20.4 Commercial negative pressure therapy system (ABThera™). A suction pad is placed in a location that will be most effective for flow and the position of the tube. An open abdomen is not a contraindication to enteral feeding, and temporary abdominal closures can be used in conjunction with feeding tubes

and late complications. Prevention and early recognition of complications can be facilitated with a high level of suspicion, comprehensive postoperative critical care, and optimal nutritional support.

20.4.1 Early Complications

Patients requiring temporary abdominal closure often require massive volume resuscitation and intra-abdominal packing or have continued hemorrhage making them an at-risk population for the development of abdominal compartment syndrome. Even with an open abdomen, patients can develop intra-abdominal hypertension and compartment syndrome and should therefore be monitored closely. Monitoring options include bladder pressure transduction as well as physiologic assessments of urine output, airway pressures, and blood pressure. Development of abdominal compartment syndrome with a temporary abdominal closure in place requires immediate attention. The temporary abdominal closure should be immediately released or removed. Every attempt should be made to keep the abdominal viscera covered to prevent further damage or desiccation of the bowel, often a new dressing can be fashioned to the dimensions of the larger wound.

Patients with temporary abdominal closure are also at high risk for malnutrition for multiple reasons including critical illness, lack of enteral feeding secondary to intestinal injury or held for procedures, and high-volume protein loss from the peritoneal cavity fluid effluent. Peritoneal fluid is estimated to contain 3 g/dL of protein, with net daily losses frequently quantified in liters, placing patients at an extremely high risk for protein-calorie malnutrition [12]. This additional protein loss should be taken into account when calculating caloric needs for repletion in a patient with an open abdomen.

20.4.2 Postoperative Care

Patients with a temporary abdominal wall closure should be monitored in the intensive care unit. Optimal care of the underlying pathology in combination with management targeted at the open abdomen, including controlled volume resuscitation and appropriate ratios of blood products, has been associated with a survival advantage [13].

Hypertonic saline has been suggested in the literature to help facilitate earlier abdominal wall closure. While the exact mechanism in humans has not been well described, the concept is that the higher concentration of saline functions to decrease overall fluid administered and additionally may shift fluid into the vascular system and decrease the capillary leak that occurs, thus preventing visceral edema. In a study of 23 patients who received 3% sodium chloride at 30 mL/h immediately after damage control surgery through postoperative day 3 or fascial closure (whichever occurred sooner), there was a 100% abdominal wall closure rate by day 7 [14].

Enteral nutrition is encouraged in all critically ill patients, especially those with an open abdominal wall. Studies have demonstrated that the use of enteral feeds in patients with an open abdomen is associated with decreased morbidity and mortality and increased rates of fascial closure [15]. Additionally, patients with a temporary abdominal closure do not require paralysis or deep sedation. Standard sedation goals are acceptable in this population. In fact, if the patient meets the usual pulmonary criteria, extubation is also acceptable with an open abdominal wall.

20.4.3 Late Complications

While the abdomen should not be closed if the patient remains at a significantly high risk for development of abdominal compartment syndrome, once the required surgical procedures have been completed, every attempt should be made to close the abdomen in a timely fashion. The sooner the abdomen is closed after the initial operation, the lower the likelihood of complications, including fistula formation and loss of domain leading to hernia formation.

While the ideal timeline for return to the operating room has not been fully described, it is well agreed upon that delays in returning to the operating room are associated with a decrease in the ability to achieve primary fascial closure. Pommerening et al. found that for each additional hour beyond 24 that a patient was delayed returning to the operating room was associated with a 1.1% decrease in the likelihood of primary fascial closure [16]. This same study found that complication rates were increased in patients who returned beyond 48 h. Additionally, functional outcomes, including quality of life, pain, and return to work, are improved in a patient who undergoes abdominal wall closure within the first 7 days [17].

Primary closure of the abdominal fascial edges is usually possible when the fascial edges are 3–7 cm apart. Separations any greater than this require more complex surgical techniques to achieve definitive closure. Some cases may require component separation with myofascial flaps if adequate skin coverage is unavailable. In cases of severe contamination or in abdomens unable to be closed beyond 8 days, consideration of a planned ventral hernia is necessary. To create a planned ventral hernia, a synthetic absorbable mesh, frequently Vicryl, is sewn to the fascial edges to encourage granulation tissue formation over the bowel while preventing further loss of domain. Once granulation has occurred, a split-thickness skin graft is placed for ultimate coverage. This results in a ventral hernia that can be repaired 6–12 months later.

20.4.4 Enterocutaneous Fistula (ECF)

Enterocutaneous fistulas are a dreaded complication after an open abdomen, the incidence of which can run from 5 to 15% [11]. Not only do ECFs create a significant reduction in quality of life, but they also carry a significant mortality risk given the increased incidence of sepsis, malnutrition, dehydration, and electrolyte imbalances. A correlation exists between the number of days of temporary closure and ECF development [6, 18]. Other risk factors for fistula formation include bowel injuries and anastomoses, colon resections, large volume resuscitation, intra-abdominal sepsis, increased number of repeat explorations, and use of a permanent mesh directly in contact with the bowel [18]. NPTS can be used to control ECF effluent and prevent breakdown and further contamination of surrounding tissues. Additionally, skin grafting around the fistula can allow for ultimate placement of a wound manager device. ECFs often create complex wounds, and whenever possible, a skilled wound therapist should be involved in planning and creating the appropriate wound managing systems.

20.5 Future Directions/ Current Controversies

Temporary abdominal wall closure along with the associated care models such as damage control has become lifesaving tools for the acute care surgeon. As the indications for leaving an abdominal wall open have expanded beyond the trauma patient, there is increasing concern that this valuable technique is being over utilized, leading to unnecessarily high rates of complications. Patients are now surviving their initial insult, and many will face complications and repeat surgeries stemming from the temporary closure. For some, the mortality benefit has been traded in for long-term morbidity. In a single-center retrospective study of a Houston trauma center, the authors found that 20% of patients who underwent a damage control laparotomy did not meet traditional indications [19]. The same group subsequently instituted a quality improvement project which decreased the number of traumatic open abdomens by 16% without changing mortality rates [20]. Future efforts will likely continue to redefine the appropriate indications for temporarily closing the abdominal wall in both trauma and emergency surgery populations.

Take-Home Points

- Temporary abdominal closure is a frequently employed technique in trauma and other aspects of emergency surgery that require a "damage control" approach.
- Temporary abdominal closure techniques should control fluid losses and minimize loss of domain, in addition to providing coverage/protection of the bowel and intra-abdominal contents.
- There are many options available to the surgeon for temporary abdominal closure, which include silo techniques, patch techniques, and negative pressure therapy systems. Each has advantages and disadvantages associated with them.
- A patient with a temporary abdominal closure can still develop an abdominal compartment syndrome and should be closely monitored.
- When using NPTS, low suction should be used for the coagulopathic patient. The canister should be carefully monitored for signs of ongoing surgical bleeding.
- When using temporary abdominal closure devices, care must be taken to avoid injury to the bowel. If a negative pressure system is used, a barrier to protect the bowel from direct suction should be employed.
- All attempts to decrease the amount of time the patient has an open abdomen should be made. Patients should return for initial attempt at closure within 48 h, if possible.
- Delay in closure increases complications including fluid loss, protein loss, fistula formation, and ventral hernias.
- Temporary abdominal closure alone does not necessitate paralysis or deep sedation nor prevent liberation from mechanical ventilation or enteric feeding from occurring. These elements of care should be evaluated on a case-by-case basis.

Suggested Readings

Rotondo MF, Schwab CW, McGonigal MD, et al. 'Damage control': an approach for improved survival in exsanguinating penetrating abdominal injury. J Trauma. 1993;35:375–82; discussion 382–3.

Kron IL, Harman PK, Nolan SP. The measurement of intra-abdominal pressure as a criterion for abdominal re-exploration. Ann Surg. 1984;199(1):28–30.

Wittmann DH, Aprahamian C, Bergstein JM, Edmiston CE, Frantzides CT, Quebbeman EJ, Condon RE. A burr-like device to facilitate temporary abdominal closure in planned multiple laparotomies. Eur J Surg. 1993;159(2):75.

Chiara O, Cimbanassi S, Biffl W, et al. International consensus conference on open abdomen in trauma. J Trauma. 2016;80:173–83.

Kirkpatrick AW, Roberts DJ, Faris PD, et al. Active negative pressure peritoneal therapy after abbreviated laparotomy: the intraperitoneal vacuum randomized controlled trial. Ann Surg. 2015;262(1):38–46.

References

1. Weber DG, Bendinelli C, Balogh ZJ. Damage control surgery for abdominal emergencies. Br J Surg. 2014;101(1):e109–18.
2. Kron IL, Harman PK, Nolan SP. The measurement of intra-abdominal pressure as a criterion for abdominal re-exploration. Ann Surg. 1984;199(1):28–30.
3. Rotondo MF, Schwab CW, McGonigal MD, et al. 'Damage control': an approach for improved survival in exsanguinating penetrating abdominal injury. J Trauma. 1993;35(3):375–82; discussion 382-3.
4. Chiara O, Cimbanassi S, Biffl W, et al. International consensus conference on open abdomen in trauma. J Trauma. 2016;80:173–83.
5. Joseph DK, Dutton RP, Aarabi B, Scalea TM. Decompressive laparotomy to treat intractable intracranial hypertension after traumatic brain injury. J Trauma. 2004;57(4):687–93.
6. Coccolini F, Montori G, Ceresoli M, et al. IROA: International Register of Open Abdomen, preliminary results. World J Emerg Surg. 2017;12:10.

7. Kubiak BD, Albert SP, Gatto LA, et al. Peritoneal negative pressure therapy prevents multiple organ injury in a chronic porcine sepsis and ischemia/reperfusion model. Shock. 2010;34(5):525–34.
8. Kirkpatrick AW, Roberts DJ, Faris PD, et al. Active negative pressure peritoneal therapy after abbreviated laparotomy: the intraperitoneal vacuum randomized controlled trial. Ann Surg. 2015;262(1):38–46.
9. Wittmann DH, Aprahamian C, Bergstein JM, et al. A burr-like device to facilitate temporary abdominal closure in planned multiple laparotomies. Eur J Surg. 1993;159(2):75–9.
10. Brock WB, Barker DE, Burns RP. Temporary closure of open abdominal wounds: the vacuum pack. Am Surg. 1995;61(1):30–5.
11. Demetriades D. Total management of the open abdomen. Int Wound J. 2012;9(Suppl 1):17–24.
12. Hourigan LA, Linfoot JA, Chung KK, et al. Loss of protein, immunoglobulins, and electrolytes in exudates from negative pressure wound therapy. Nutr Clin Pract. 2010;25(5):510–6.
13. Duchesne JC, Kimonis K, Marr AB, et al. Damage control resuscitation in combination with damage control laparotomy: a survival advantage. J Trauma. 2010;69(1):46–52.
14. Harvin JA, Mims MM, Duchesne JC, et al. Chasing 100%: the use of hypertonic saline to improve early, primary fascial closure after damage control laparotomy. J Trauma. 2013;74(2):426–30; discussion 431-2.
15. Burlew CC, Moore EE, Cuschieri J, et al. Who should we feed? Western Trauma Association multi-institutional study of enteral nutrition in the open abdomen after injury. J Trauma. 2012;73(6):1380–7; discussion 1387-8.
16. Pommerening MJ, DuBose JJ, Zielinski MD, et al. Time to first take-back operation predicts successful primary fascial closure in patients undergoing damage control laparotomy. Surgery. 2014;156(2): 431–8.
17. Fox N, Crutchfield M, LaChant M, Ross SE, Seamon MJ. Early abdominal closure improves long-term outcomes after damage-control laparotomy. J Trauma. 2013;75(5):854–8.
18. Bradley MJ, DuBose JJ, Scalea TM, et al. Independent predictors of enteric fistula and abdominal sepsis after damage control laparotomy: results from the prospective AAST Open Abdomen registry. JAMA Surg. 2013;148(10):947–54.
19. Hatch QM, Osterhout LM, Podbielski J, et al. Impact of closure at the first take back: complication burden and potential overutilization of damage control laparotomy. J Trauma. 2011;71(6):1503–11.
20. Harvin JA, Kao LS, Liang MK, et al. Decreasing the use of damage control laparotomy in trauma: a quality improvement project. J Am Coll Surg. 2017;225:200. [Epub ahead of print].

21 Fundamentals of Exploratory Thoracotomy for Trauma

Deepika Koganti and Alec C. Beekley

21.1 Introduction

Thoracotomy for trauma can be classified into four categories:

1. Thoracotomy for resuscitative maneuvers only
2. Thoracotomy for both identification and treatment of thoracic injuries and resuscitative maneuvers
3. Thoracotomy for treatment of identified injuries in stabilized patients
4. Delayed thoracotomy for treatment of sequelae of traumatic injuries

The distinction is important since the first two categories involve operations on unstable patients. Time for extensive preoperative work-up, discussion on approaches, and recruitment of specialists is not available. Simplicity, speed, flexibility, and boldness are required for a successful outcome in these patients. In contrast, the last two categories of patients are often stable enough that advanced imaging, consultation with specialists, and careful operative planning can occur before going to the operating room. In addition, minimally invasive, image-guided radiologic therapies and endovascular techniques are increasingly utilized in the setting of stable trauma patients with injuries that require surgical intervention. The distinction between the third and second categories of patients is not as clear, in that some trauma patients with thoracic injuries may be stable on presentation but deteriorate rapidly and require more prompt intervention. For the purpose of this chapter, the focus will be primarily on the first two categories of thoracotomy listed above. Although the treatment of specific injuries will be touched upon, a complete discussion of the treatment of cardiac, pulmonary, esophageal, and thoracic great vessel injury is beyond the scope of this chapter.

The exploratory thoracotomy for trauma is historically one of the most controversial surgical procedures performed. The first reported successful prehospital thoracotomy was done on a kitchen table in Montgomery, Alabama, in 1902 [1]. While the execution of the procedure has certainly evolved since the early 1900s, the quoted survival rates of emergency thoracotomy in the literature are extremely variable, contributing to the controversy over the topic. Rates have been reported from 0% to 70%. This large variation is largely due to the fact that different traumatic mecha-

D. Koganti
Department of Surgery, Sidney Kimmel Medical College, Thomas Jefferson University, Philadelphia, PA, USA
e-mail: deepika.koganti@jefferson.edu

A. C. Beekley (✉)
Department of Surgery, Division of Acute Care Surgery, Division of Bariatric Surgery, Sidney Kimmel Medical College at Thomas Jefferson University, Philadelphia, PA, USA
e-mail: alec.beekley@jefferson.edu

F. Palazzo (ed.), *Fundamentals of General Surgery*, https://doi.org/10.1007/978-3-319-75656-1_21

nisms have different outcomes. For penetrating chest trauma, the survival rates are approximately 18–33%. For stab wounds causing cardiac tamponade only, survival rates reach 70%. However, for blunt trauma, survival rates are 0–2.5%. Yet, some blunt trauma patients have a higher chance of survival based on presence or absence of vital signs [2]. The likelihood of survival is the leading factor in determining the indications for an emergency thoracotomy. Due to varying practices for performance of emergency department thoracotomy (EDT), the Eastern Association for the Surgery of Trauma (EAST) published evidence-based guidelines in 2015. A strong recommendation was made for EDT for a pulseless patient after a penetrating injury with signs of life. EDT was conditionally recommended for patients who present pulseless with no signs of life after penetrating thoracic or extra-thoracic injury, for patients who present pulseless with signs of life after penetrating extra-thoracic injury, and for patients who present pulseless with signs of life after blunt injury. A recommendation was made against EDT for patients who present pulseless with no signs of life after blunt injury [3].

The goal of the EDT is to obtain access to the chest to achieve direct hemorrhage control, release cardiac tamponade, control air embolism, perform internal cardiac massage, and optimize flow to the brain and heart to keep the patient alive for further definitive management in the operating room.

21.2 Resuscitative vs. Exploratory Thoracotomy

The above criteria outline indications for or against immediate thoracotomy. However, patients who arrive in more stable condition after thoracic trauma may not need an immediate thoracotomy and have time to undergo further evaluation. As always, the algorithm of airway, breathing, and circulation should be followed for each trauma patient, and interventions such as intubation, placement of chest tubes, and insertion of large bore IVs should be done as appropriate. A chest x-ray should be obtained once the patient is stabilized. This simple and quick study provides an extensive amount of information on potential life-threatening injuries including presence of tension pneumothorax, hemothorax, bony injury, and mediastinal injury such as widened mediastinum and pneumomediastinum. Another valuable and quick study is the Focused Assessment with Sonography for Trauma (FAST). The FAST includes evaluation of the pericardial and peritoneal cavities. The eFAST, or extended FAST, has been established to further evaluate the pleural spaces using ultrasonography. This study can pick up hemothoraces and pneumothoraces requiring chest tube placement [4]. As stated in the guidelines above, if a chest tube is placed and 1500 cc of blood is immediately drained or 200 cc/h over 4 h, an emergency thoracotomy is indicated.

21.3 Technique for Emergency Thoracotomy

Since an emergency thoracotomy is never a planned procedure, all equipment should be readily available and easily accessible. Most importantly, all providers should know where these instruments are located in the trauma bay or operating room prior to an emergency. The following is a list of equipment to successfully perform an emergency thoracotomy [5, 6]:

1. Personal protective equipment: gloves, sterile gloves, gown, scrub cap, face mask, and shoe covers
2. Prepping the chest: povidone-iodine and sterile drapes
3. Access to the chest: scalpel with no. 10 blade, curved Mayo scissors, rib spreader, Lebsche knife, Gigli saw, and/or trauma shears
4. Control of hemorrhage and injury repair: Metzenbaum scissors, DeBakey vascular forceps, DeBakey aortic clamp, Satinsky vascular clamps, artery clips, long and short needle holders, high-volume suction, 3-0 nonabsorbable suture (nylon, polypropylene) on round-bodied needle, 2-0 absorbable ties, laparotomy packs, Teflon pledgets, suture scissors, Foley catheter 20F with 30 cc balloon, chest tube 30F, internal defibrillator, and ACLS medications

Once the decision to proceed with emergency or resuscitative thoracotomy has been made, time is of the essence. There is no time for placement of a double-lumen endotracheal tube or bronchial blocker. Furthermore, establishment of large bore intravenous lines, while ultimately necessary for success, can be performed by other providers in parallel to surgical opening of the chest. Optimal positioning of the patient is supine with the arms out to the sides. This position allows access to both chest cavities but can allow additional providers access to the upper extremities for antecubital intravenous line placement by either percutaneous techniques or direct cutdown. If the equipment is immediately available, a rolled towel or blanket can be stuffed behind the chest to slightly elevate the operative (usually left) side (~20°). This positioning can allow better posterior extension of the thoracotomy incision and increased exposure to the posterior aspect of the hemithorax, without compromising access to other body cavities. The entire chest from the chin to at least midway between xiphoid process and umbilicus and laterally from bed to bed should be prepped. If the surgeon's setting is a trauma operating room, a complete prep from the chin to knees may be continued, while initial access to the chest is gained. Since emergency or resuscitative thoracotomy is frequently initiated with a left anterolateral approach, the left side of the chest is prepped first, so the primary surgeon can begin the thoracotomy incision as soon as possible.

The goal is entry into the pleural cavity through the fourth or fifth intercostal space. Counting of the ribs is generally not recommended, and many providers use the inferior edge of the nipple/areola complex as a landmark in nonobese males. Surgeons should realize that the nipple may *not* be a reliable anatomic landmark in obese patients or females. In this instance, the inframammary crease and/or xiphoid process may serve to provide surgeons with a better idea of where to place the initial incision in such patients. Superior retraction of the breast should be performed prior to incision in these instances.

The incision may begin at the left lateral edge of the sternum. Some surgeons recommend beginning on the *right* lateral edge of the sternum, as this maneuver may save time for additional skin opening if division across the sternum is required (as it frequently is). In nonobese males, the incision may track along the inferior border of the left nipple/areola complex and then follow a gentle superior curve toward (but not into) the axilla. This incision placement mimics the natural anatomic contour of the ribs and may make pleural entry easier.

The incision is performed boldly with a no. 10 blade scalpel (Fig. 21.1). The skin, subcutaneous tissue, and chest wall musculature are frequently divided, and the chest wall is exposed on the initial swipe of the blade. Intercostal incision may continue with the scalpel, although some surgeons prefer a curved Mayo scissors to open the intercostal musculature and pleura above the rib. One side of the scissors is inserted into the pleural cavity and one side left out; with respirations temporarily held by anesthesia, the scissors can be pushed along the rib medially and then laterally to open the intercostal muscles and pleura. It is frequently better to err a little high on the incision and intercostal space rather than err too low. The intercostal incision should be opened as widely as possible to allow both of the surgeon's hands access to the chest. For petite individuals with relatively small thoracic cages, the surgeon should not hesitate to open the intercostal incision all the way medially to the sternum and divide the sternum for better exposure. Sternal

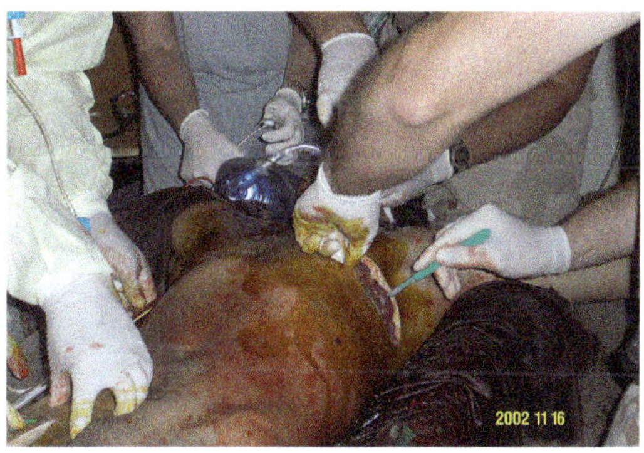

Fig. 21.1 Initial incision for the left anterolateral (resuscitative) thoracotomy. Note simultaneous performance of right tube thoracostomy and right femoral venous cutdown

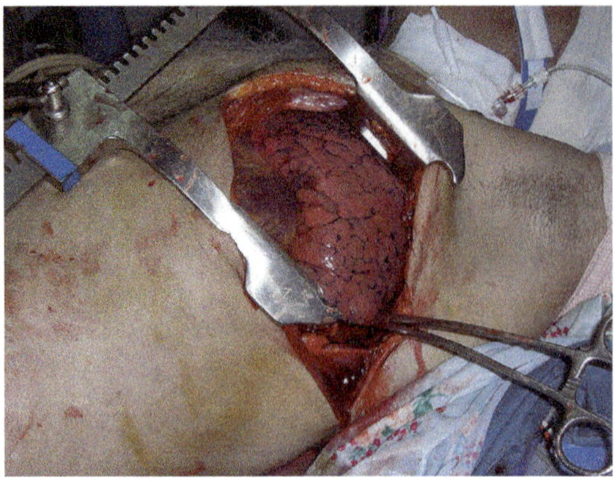

Fig. 21.2 Left anterolateral thoracotomy with Finochietto retractor cross bar on the medial side and hand crank inferior and medial. Note that the cross bar would interfere with clamshell extension and hand crank would be in the way of superior aspect of laparotomy incision. Note cross clamp is in place and well away from retractor

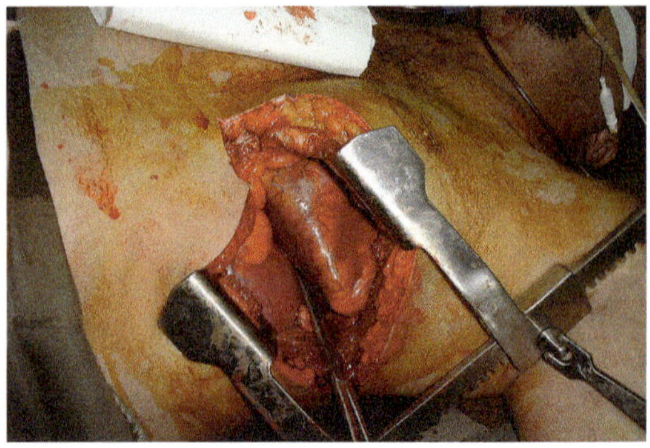

Fig. 21.3 Left anterolateral thoracotomy with Finochietto retractor cross bar on the lateral side and hand crank superior and lateral. Note extension to a clamshell incision would be unobstructed but hand crank is sitting in axilla. Note cross clamp is in place but almost sitting on retractor

division can be done with a Lebsche knife, trauma shears, bandage scissors, or Gigli saw.

A rib spreader (Finocchietto retractor) is now placed in the intercostal incision to provide retraction. This device is a rack-and-pinion retractor. The "rack" side, or crossbar, can be placed medially, which has the advantage of easy access to the hand crank on the inferior and medial side of the field and clearer access to the posterior portions of the pleural cavity for maneuvers like aortic cross clamping or treatment of lung injuries. The disadvantage of this placement is that the hand crank and cross bar can obstruct access to the heart, right side of the chest, or superior aspect of the abdomen if midline laparotomy is performed (Fig. 21.2). Placement of the rack laterally has the advantage of an unobstructed view of the heart and unimpeded access to the sternum and right chest for "clamshell" extension of the thoracotomy incision. With lateral rack placement, the hand crank resides superiorly and laterally (Fig. 21.3); surgeons should be aware that this positioning can result in the hand crank catching clothing, blankets, or the patient's shoulder skin and tissues as the crank is turned.

Access to and exposure of the pleural and pericardial cavities should generally take less than 2 min. While surgical access to the left chest is initiated, the surgeon should direct other members of the trauma team to empirically place a chest tube in the right chest. This can provide some information on pathology in the right chest and guide secondary steps.

Upon entry into the pleural cavity, several possible scenarios may be encountered:

1. A large rush of air under pressure is released. The patient may or may not have return or improvement in vital signs. The lung injury that was the source of the tension pneumothorax may be large or small, but it should be sought out for evaluation, as some may require surgical treatment. In patients who have clinically improved, with release of tension pneumothorax, methodical exploration of the chest may be performed once other body cavities have been evaluated for injuries. In patients who do not improve, surgeons should evaluate for another problem, such as tamponade or hemorrhage in another body cavity.
2. A massive rush of blood under pressure is released. This frequently represents a difficult challenge as it can indicate a great vessel, proximal lung hilum, or cardiac injury. Treatment of these various injuries will be discussed below.
3. Neither blood nor air is released. This may indicate a contained pericardial tamponade or a hemorrhage source in another body cavity.

If opening the pericardium reveals no injury but an empty or near-empty heart, resuscitative measures (such as application of aortic cross clamp) should be instituted, and a rapid search for hemorrhage sources in other cavities must begin.

21.4 Pericardiotomy

After the chest is opened, exposure obtained, and obvious intrathoracic hemorrhage sources controlled or temporized, the pericardium should be opened. This generally should be done relatively early in the steps of resuscitative thoracotomy. This is typically done with a longitudinal incision along the left lateral aspect of pericardium, usually anterior and parallel to the left phrenic nerve. A tense pericardium can be difficult to grasp or lift with forceps. In this instance, a scalpel blade can be used to make a small (5–10 mm) nick in the pericardium to then allow Metzenbaum scissors to be inserted to open the pericardiotomy widely. Obviously, care must be taken such that the scalpel does not injure the underlying heart. In the absence of blood or fluid in the pericardium sac, the pericardium may be loose enough to grasp and elevate with forceps to simply make the initial cut with the Metzenbaum scissor tips.

The pericardium should be opened for the majority of its longitudinal dimension (thoracic inlet to the diaphragm). The heart can then be delivered and inspected for injury. Treatment of cardiac injuries is briefly addressed below. In the absence of organized cardiac activity, open cardiac compression should be initiated. The technique for open cardiac massage is to place the bases of the surgeon's palms together at the inferior apex of the heart. The left hand is typically positioned right and anterolateral and the right hand left and posterolateral. The flat aspects of the palms are then closed together around the heart from the base of the palm toward the fingertips. One-handed compressions or angling of the fingertips into the myocardium should be avoided, as direct perforation of the heart can occur with this technique.

In settings where the heart is empty and the suspected hemorrhage source is below the diaphragm, application of an aortic cross clamp as described below should probably occur before prolonged open cardiac massage or delivery of intracardiac medications and/or electric shocks. In settings where a cardiac injury is present, the injury should be repaired or temporized before attempting to restore cardiac activity. Surgeons should realize that successful restoration of perfusing cardiac activity will not occur in the setting of an empty heart, profound acidosis, or profound hypothermia.

There is no accepted algorithm for delivery of intracardiac medications. Surgeons have tried epinephrine, atropine, calcium chloride, sodium bicarbonate, vasopressin, and likely a host of other vasoactive medications in attempts to restart the heart, with varying degrees of success. Surgeons should be wary of the typical vasoactive medication ampules such as epinephrine or atropine. The needles associated with these ampules are typically large and can actually result in a cardiac injury that will continue to bleed in a coagulopathic patient. Successful salvage after resuscitative thoracotomy has more to do with the reversibility of the underlying insult rather than the technique or medications employed. At the conclusion of a successful resuscitative procedure, it is rare that the pericardium can be closed due to cardiac congestion from resuscitation and treatment.

Critical to the success of the procedure is the teamwork of all involved. The surgeon can perform the fastest and smoothest resuscitative thoracotomy, but without concomitant establishment of large bore intravenous lines, initiation of damage control resuscitation strategies, and in-parallel triage of other body cavities for injury and/or treatment of other hemorrhage sources, success will not be possible.

21.4.1 Application of Aortic Cross Clamp

Before rushing to cross clamp the descending aorta, the surgeon should consider what he is trying to accomplish by the maneuver. If there is known or suspected uncontrolled hemorrhage above the diaphragm, aortic cross clamping makes no sense and may actually worsen bleeding. The settings where application of an aortic cross clamp may help are as follows:

1. The patient is in extremis with multiple injuries. The bleeding source or sources have not been clearly identified. The initial thoracotomy has not demonstrated a source, and the goal is to restore perfusion at least to the heart, lungs, and brain until hemorrhage sources can be identified and controlled.
2. The patient is in extremis with a cardiac or intrathoracic injury which has been repaired or controlled. The goal is to restore perfusion at least to the heart, lungs, and brain to allow time for continued blood product resuscitation.
3. The patient is in extremis with a known or suspected injury below the diaphragm. Application of the cross clamp is a temporizing measure to allow resuscitation to begin and allow the surgical team time to find and control the hemorrhage source.

In all instances, the cross clamp is a temporizing measure, and the surgeon should realize that once applied, the clock is ticking. After about 30 min (or less), the patient will become "cross clamp dependent," and successful salvage becomes highly unlikely.

The cross clamp should be applied to the descending aorta as close to the diaphragm as possible. Nevertheless, surgeons should not hesitate to use the most accessible place on the descending aorta to place their clamp based on their initial incision and the patient's habitus and anatomy. Division of the inferior pulmonary ligament can assist with superior and anterior retraction of the lung, but this maneuver is not always necessary. Once the lung is retracted anteriorly, the surgeon should slide her knuckles along the posterior aspect of the rib cage until she feels them curve anteriorly to the articulation with the vertebral column. Typically, the first tubular structure encountered will be the descending aorta. It is often flaccid in patients who have hemorrhaged to arrest or near-arrest. If an orogastric tube has been placed, the surgeon can often use its presence to help distinguish the flaccid aorta from the esophagus. If it can be visualized, the parietal pleura overlying the aorta should be spread with a scissors or clamp and the aorta partially encircled with the surgeon's nondominant thumb and index finger. A pitfall with this step is that complete encirclement of the aorta can result in avulsion of an intercostal artery (which behaves like a hole in the aorta and can result in substantial bleeding). With gentle traction of the aorta, the surgeon can apply the cross clamp (Figs. 21.2 and 21.3). Failure to open the parietal pleura overlying the aorta often results in the clamp slipping off the aorta or incompletely occluding it.

Once the clamp is in place, if possible the surgeon should request a timer be started and callouts at 10 min intervals instituted. The surgeon should not release the cross clamp until in a position to control hemorrhage and when some hemodynamic stability is restored. Patients requiring cross clamp for more than 30 min almost uniformly develop fatal physiology. Therefore, if normo- or hypertensive blood pressures are achieved and hemorrhage is controlled, the surgeon should consider removal of the clamp in a slow, controlled fashion and be willing to tolerate some permissive hypotension. Furthermore, if a hemorrhage source below the diaphragm is identified and controlled or the clamp can be moved to a more distal location proximal to an injury, this should be done as soon as possible. Infrarenal aortic cross clamping may be tolerated for a longer period of time than descending thoracic cross clamping.

21.4.2 Clamshell Thoracotomy

The clamshell extension into the opposite pleural cavity provides excellent exposure to the heart, both pulmonary hilum and even (to some degree) the proximal great vessels. This maneuver should be done anytime additional exposure is needed for surgery on the heart, pulmonary hilum, or great vessels. It is recommended that the incision extension from the left chest to the right chest be curved gently superior, as the right hemidiaphragm is higher and the right pulmonary hilum may be better exposed with this maneuver. The sternum can be divided with a heavy scissor, Lebsche knife, or Gigli saw. This move severs the internal mammary arteries. Once the patient is resuscitated, these will bleed quite vigorously and will need to be controlled, which is fortunately relatively easy to do. The use of a Finocchietto retractor can assist with maximal exposure to both thoracic cavities (Figs. 21.4 and 21.5).

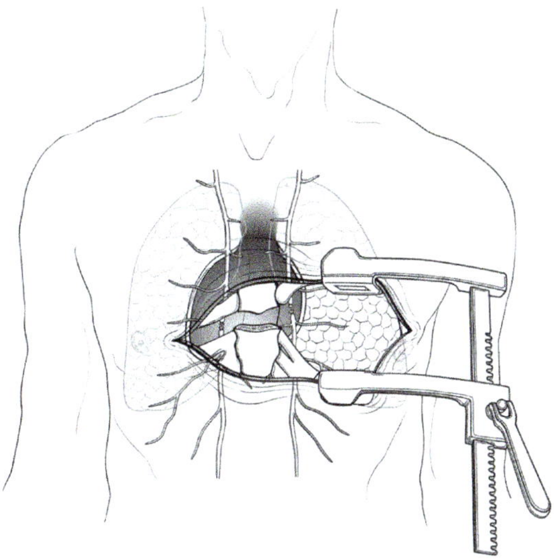

Fig. 21.4 Diagram showing extension of anterolateral thoracotomy into clamshell extension with division of sternum and ligation of internal mammary arteries (Reprinted with permission from Chapter 13: Choice of Thoracic Incision, from *Front Line Surgery: A Practical Approach* Edited Martin M and Beekley A. Springer; New York, 2011)

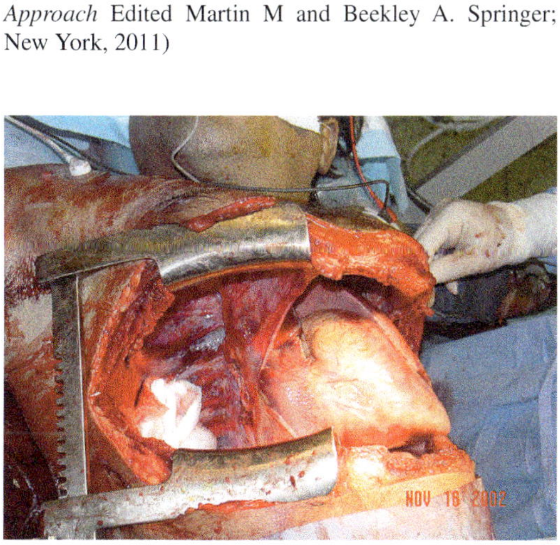

Fig. 21.5 Clamshell thoracotomy incision exposure. Right pneumonectomy has been completed

21.4.3 Median Sternotomy

In certain instances, the median sternotomy may afford superior exposure and be the incision of choice. Examples of trauma scenarios where median sternotomy may be superior to thoracotomy include isolated stab wounds within a few centimeters of midline in the setting of obvious clinical tamponade (distended neck veins, hypotension, and clear breath sounds bilaterally). In these cases, the likelihood of anterior cardiac injury and pericardial tamponade is so high and the exposure via sternotomy so ideal that this should be the incision of choice. Gunshot wounds in the same area are more variable in terms of trajectory and energy transfer, and hence thoracotomy may be better in those instances. The median sternotomy affords exposure to the heart, ascending aorta, proximal aortic arch and arch vessels (except left subclavian artery), innominate vein, superior vena cava, and pulmonary artery and hilum. The median sternotomy may also be useful for injuries to the thoracic inlet, as the incision may be easily extended up either side of the neck or out above or below either clavicle. With planning, practice, experience, and proper equipment, the median sternotomy can also be accomplished in minutes.

The median sternotomy incision is begun just above the jugular or suprasternal notch and taken to just below the xiphoid process. Cautery can be used to divide the subcutaneous tissues and strap musculature just above the jugular notch and the subcutaneous tissues just below the xiphoid process. With continued dissection, the surgeon can carefully insert his index finger in the retrosternal plane at these locations to create the initial dissection plane for either an electric sternal saw or the Lebsche knife (Fig. 21.6). The sternum can be opened fairly rapidly with either of these instruments. Ventilation should be held during sternal division. Care should be taken to stay as close to the middle of the sternum as possible.

Bone wax, if available, can be used on bleeding sternal edges, but the goal is to get after the injury that is killing the patient. A rack-and-pinion sternal retractor can then be placed; some cautery dissection of filmy retrosternal attachments may

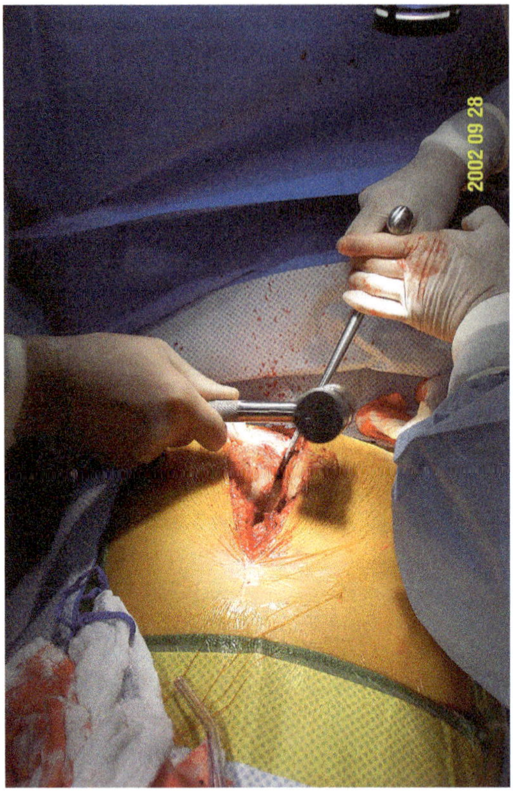

Fig. 21.6 Median sternotomy being performed with Lebsche knife (Photo courtesy of Dr. Peter G. Deveaux and Dr. Garth Lecheminant)

be necessary to facilitate this retraction. Exposure to the superior mediastinum requires division of the thymus; care should be taken to avoid injury to the innominate vein with this maneuver. The pericardium should then be opened longitudinally, using techniques as described in the resuscitative thoracotomy section. Once the pericardium is incised enough to get a finger in, the remainder can quickly and safely be dissected by dividing the pericardium over the surgeon's finger or suction tip (Fig. 21.7). Although techniques to create a "pericardial well" are described, this is not always necessary or helpful unless extensive work on the heart is required. If there is difficult exposure to a cardiac injury, multiple heavy silk stitches can be placed on either side of the cut edges of pericardium and draped over the retractor or actually affixed to the drapes with a clamp under some tension (Figs. 21.8 and 21.9). This elevates the heart slightly into the field and helps

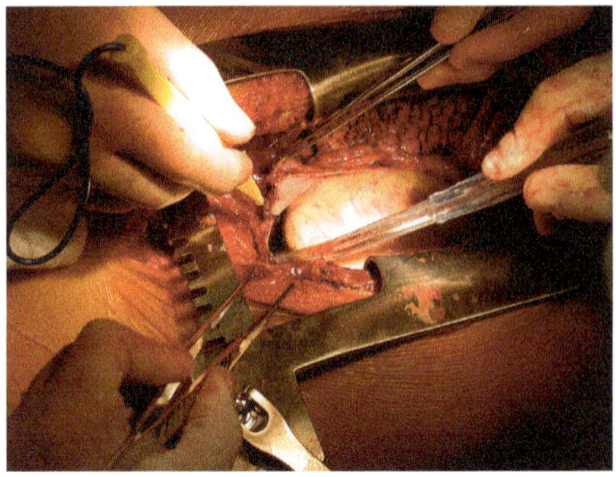

Fig. 21.7 Pericardium being opened through median sternotomy incision (Photo courtesy of Dr. Peter G. Deveaux and Dr. Garth Lecheminant)

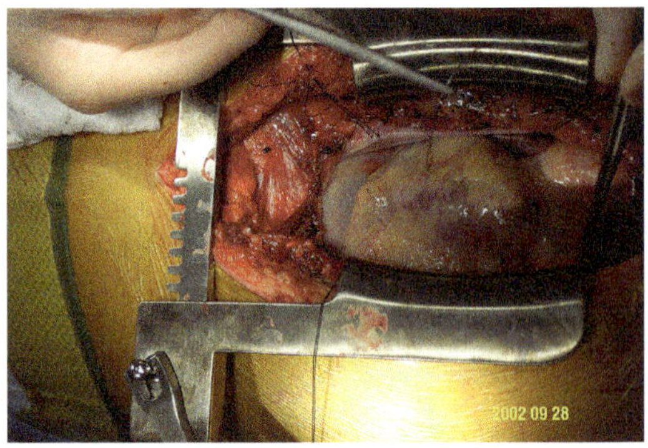

Fig. 21.8 "Pericardial well" being created with heavy silk sutures secured to cut edges of the pericardium (Photos courtesy of Dr. Peter G. Deveaux and Dr. Garth Lecheminant)

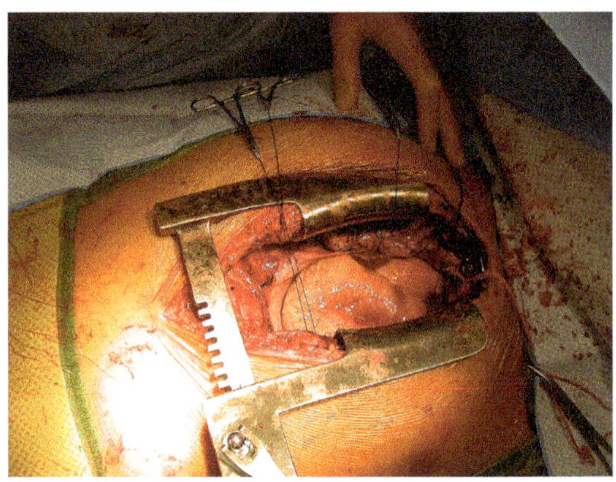

Fig. 21.9 Complete "pericardial well" created with heavy silk sutures secured to cut edges of pericardium (Photos courtesy of Dr. Peter G. Deveaux and Dr. Garth Lecheminant)

keep the ventilating lungs from pushing into view. Patients with tamponade physiology will often have immediate correction of their hypotension, unless they are in full arrest already. The surgeon should initially seek simple digital control of cardiac injuries exposed. Treatment of these injuries is briefly discussed below.

21.4.4 "Trapdoor" Incision

The anterolateral thoracotomy incision and the median sternotomy can be combined, although doing so increases morbidity and makes closure more challenging. The combination of these surgical approaches never occurs based on initial plans but arises out of necessity. One can anticipate a scenario where a patient in extremis with penetrating thoracic trauma or combined mediastinal and cervical trauma had an initial surgical approach with a left anterolateral thoracotomy but then had operative findings (proximal great vessel, e.g., left subclavian) that could not be adequately exposed by the anterolateral thoracotomy approach. Combination of the anterolateral thoracotomy, median sternotomy, and even an additional clavicular extension into a "trapdoor" exposure allows access to the proximal great vessels including the left subclavian artery and vein. This is obviously a more morbid procedure, but surgeons should remember it is being done to save a life.

21.4.5 Initial Steps in the Blood-Filled Chest

If upon opening the chest a significant amount of blood is encountered, the first step is to ensure adequate exposure by maximizing length of incision and self-retained retraction. Rather than go directly to full packing of the thoracic cavity like in a trauma laparotomy, scoop or sweep the blood out of the chest through the incision, and then use dry lap pads and suction to try to rapidly clean up the remaining blood and fluid. If the inflated lung is continually in the way, a technique to deflate the lung without using a double-lumen tube or bronchial blocker is to have the anesthesia team briefly disconnect the ventilator circuit, then compress the lung with laparotomy pads, and keep it compressed with lap pads and a lung retractor, while mechanical ventilation is reinstituted. Use dry lap pads to soak up or blot up any blood, and try to hone in on the bleeding source. Once the bleeding is controlled, systematically explore for other injuries.

21.4.6 Lung Injuries

Lung injuries range from small lacerations to destructive lesions requiring anatomic resection. Small lacerations can be oversewn or stapled off; through-and-through penetrating wounds with hemorrhage can be exposed through the technique of stapled tractotomy, where an anvil of the linear stapler is passed through the wounds and the other half of the stapler is closed over it exteriorly. Firing the stapler safely opens the superficial lung above the injury to allow direct visualization and suture control of the hemorrhage or air leaks (Fig. 21.10). The majority of lung injuries can be managed with this technique or nonanatomic stapled resection (Fig. 21.11). Major hemorrhage from the middle of the lung parenchyma or near the hilum can be temporized with either a "hilar twist" maneuver (Fig. 21.12), manual compression of the hilum in the surgeon's hand, or vascular clamping (Fig. 21.13). The goal in this setting is speed and simplicity. Anatomic resections, such as lobectomy, can be challenging even in elective settings. In unstable trauma patients, they are even more so. A thorough understanding of lobar anatomy and variations in segmental and subsegmental variability is necessary for safe resection. Pneumonectomy for trauma can be successfully performed, but the need for it must be recognized as early as possible, and close coordination with anesthesia is required (Fig. 21.14).

21.4.7 Cardiac Injuries

Small cardiac injuries can be oversewn with 3-0 to 5-0 monofilament suture. The heart can be partially stabilized by the surgeon's nondominant

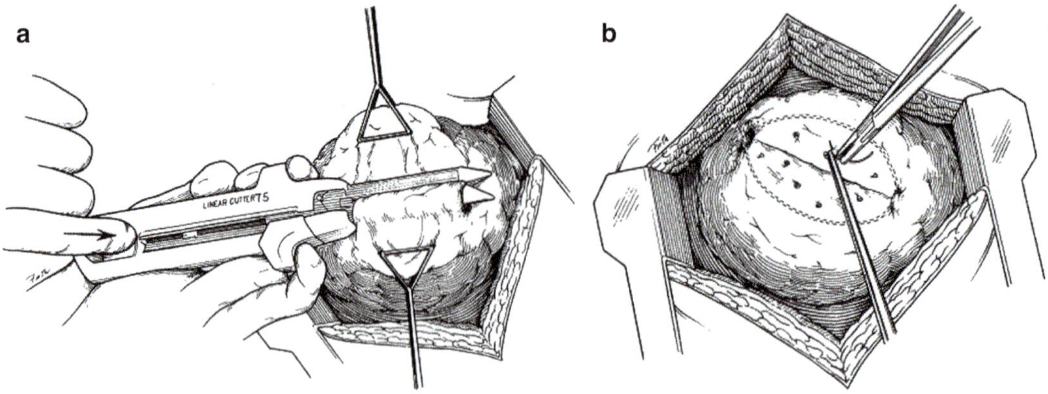

Fig. 21.10 Stapled tractotomy technique for control of bleeding from through-and-through pulmonary wounds. A linear stapler is passed through the defect and fired (**a**) opening the tract and exposing the underlying injured lung tissue for direct suture control (**b**) (Reprinted with permission from Asensio J et al., J Am Coll Surg 1997;185:486–487)

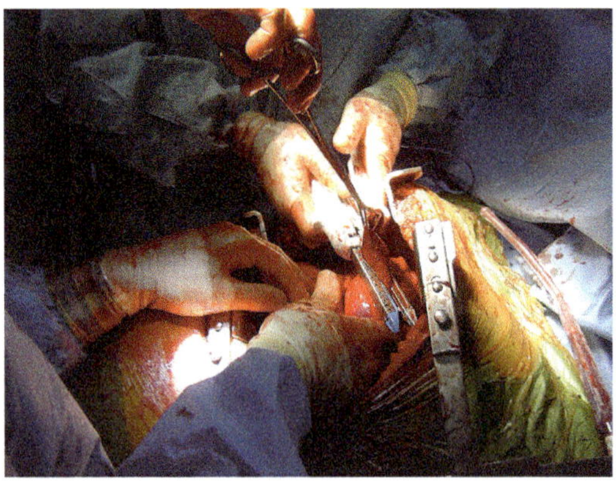

Fig. 21.11 Nonanatomic stapled lung resection for control of pulmonary injury (Photo courtesy of Dr. Adam Hamawy and Dr. Dennis Chambers)

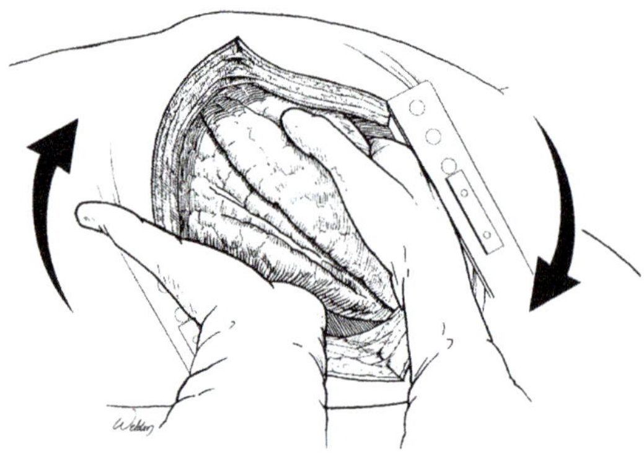

Fig. 21.12 "Hilar twist" technique for rapid and temporary control of pulmonary hilar hemorrhage (Reprinted with permission from Chapter 14: Lung Injuries in Combat, from *Front Line Surgery: A Practical Approach* Edited Martin M and Beekley A. Springer; New York, 2011)

hand or an assistant. The use of pledgets is generally recommended, and surgeons should be careful that suture placement does not encircle or injure coronary vessels (Fig. 21.15). The presence of penetrating injury to the heart necessitates a complete inspection of all surfaces of the heart. Through-and-through injuries are rarely survivable but, if present in a living patient, require closure of external holes with subsequent evaluation for septal or valvular injury.

21.4.8 Esophageal Injury

The proximal two-thirds of the esophagus are best accessed through the right chest and the distal esophagus through the left chest. If possible, the devitalized tissue should be debrided and a primary repair in layers performed. More destructive lesions may require esophagectomy and immediate or delayed reconstruction, depending on patient status.

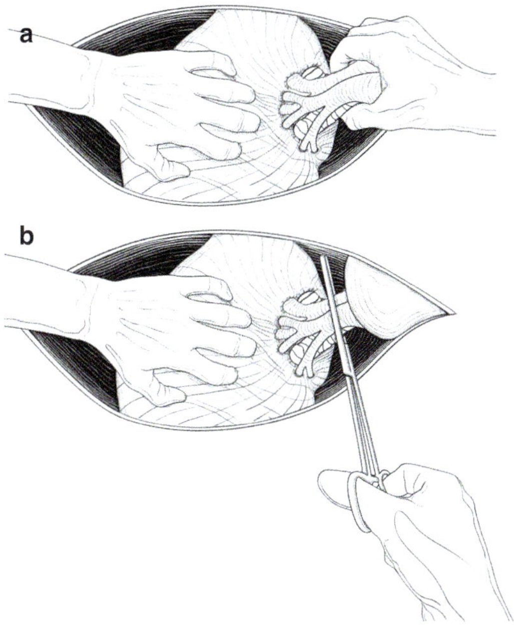

Fig. 21.13 Control of pulmonary hilm, initially with the surgeon's hand (**a**) and then with a vascular clamp (**b**). Note lateral retraction of the lung with opposite or assistant's hand (Reprinted with permission from Chapter 14: Lung Injuries in Combat, from *Front Line Surgery: A Practical Approach* Edited Martin M and Beekley A. Springer; New York, 2011)

21.4.9 Great Vessel Injury

Due to the high lethality of these injuries, there are few individual surgeons who have extensive experience with their treatment. Standard vascular principles of adequate exposure, proximal and distal control, debridement of devitalized vessel ends, and tension-free reconstruction with interposition generally apply. Subclavian vessels can frequently

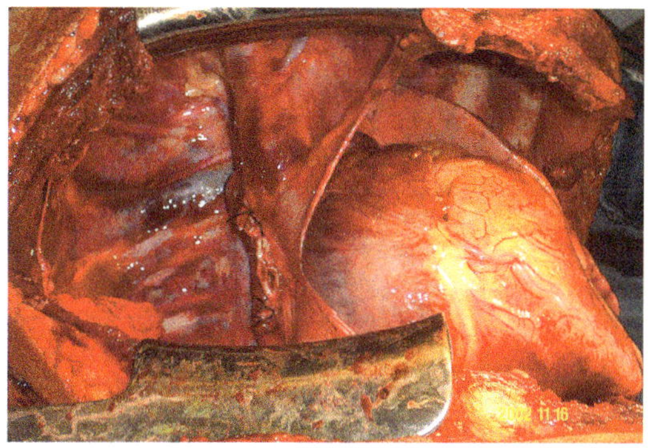

Fig. 21.14 Close-up of hilum remnant after control and division with TA 60 mm stapler for rapid pneumonectomy

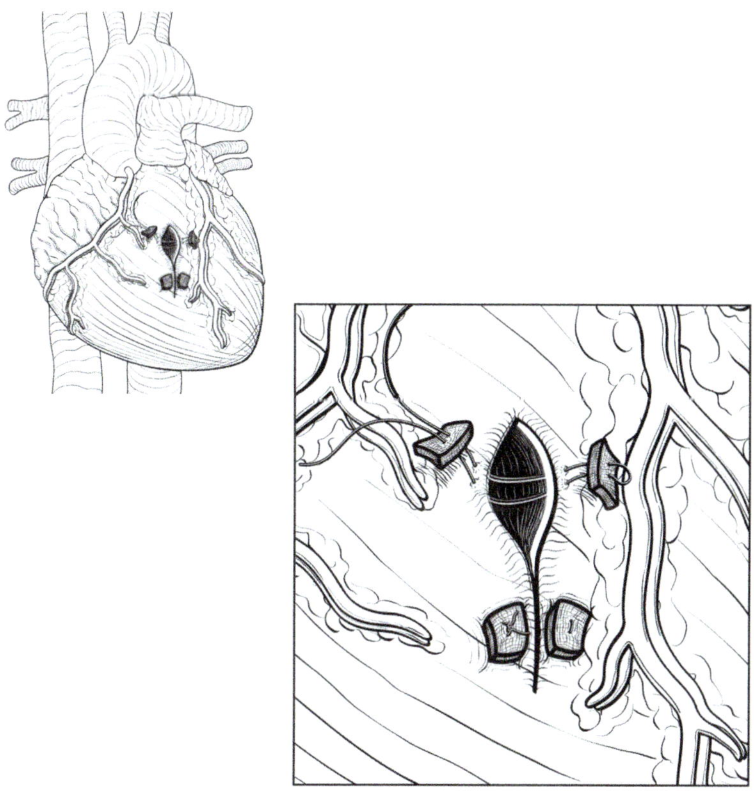

Fig. 21.15 Suture repair of cardiac wound utilizing pledgets (Reprinted with permission from Chapter 15: Diagnosis and Management of Penetrating Cardiac Injury, from *Front Line Surgery: A Practical Approach* Edited Martin M and Beekley A. Springer; New York, 2011)

be ligated, which will be well tolerated and can be bypassed or reconstructed when the patient is more stable. Vascular shunts can also be placed as a temporizing damage control measure. Major venous structures such as the superior vena cava and suprahepatic inferior vena cava should have lateral repair (*not* ligation) if possible. Although anterolateral thoracotomy may be the utility incision for patients in extremis, surgeons should learn alternate incisions or extensions which may provide optimal exposure to various injuries (Table 21.1).

Table 21.1 Six evidence-based recommendations for EDT from the Eastern Association for the Surgery of Trauma (J Trauma. 79(1):159–73, 2015)

Question	Recommendation
PICO #1	In patients who present pulseless to the emergency department *with signs of life* after *penetrating thoracic injury*, we **strongly recommend** resuscitative emergency department thoracotomy. **Strong recommendation**
PICO #2	In patients who present pulseless to the emergency department *without signs of life* after *penetrating thoracic injury*, we **conditionally recommend** resuscitative emergency department thoracotomy. **Conditional recommendation**
PICO #3	In patients who present pulseless to the emergency department *with signs of life* after *penetrating extra-thoracic injury*, we **conditionally recommend** resuscitative emergency department thoracotomy. **Conditional recommendation**
PICO #4	In patients who present pulseless to the emergency department *without signs of life* after *penetrating extra-thoracic injury*, we **conditionally recommend** resuscitative emergency department thoracotomy. **Conditional recommendation**
PICO #5	In patients who present pulseless to the emergency department *with signs of life* after *blunt injury*, we **conditionally recommend** resuscitative emergency department thoracotomy. **Conditional recommendation**
PICO #6	In patients who present pulseless to the emergency department *without signs of life* after *blunt injury*, we **conditionally recommend** *against* resuscitative emergency department thoracotomy. **Conditional recommendation**

21.5 Complications and Future Directions

The emergency thoracotomy, like any other procedure, is not without complications. Injury to other thoracic structures including lacerations of the heart, coronary arteries, aorta, phrenic nerves, esophagus, and lungs can occur [7]. Ischemia to other organs distal to the aortic cross clamping, including the spinal cord and brain, can occur as well [8, 9]. Of the patients who survive EDT, a reported 15% are noted to have severe neurological impairment. The most common postoperative complications include atelectasis, pneumonia, recurrent bleeding, diffuse intravascular coagulation, empyema, infections, and sternal dehiscence [10].

The risk to the healthcare team must also be taken into consideration. Trauma patients tend to have a higher rate of infectious diseases, placing trauma providers at high risk, especially in an emergency setting. For example, one study found a 7% incidence of either HIV or hepatitis B in an urban trauma population [11, 12], while another study found that 26% of acutely injured patients had evidence of exposure to HIV (4%), hepatitis B (20%), or hepatitis C virus (14%) [13], emphasizing the importance of personal protection.

While the emergency thoracotomy has had its place in the surgical world for over a hundred years, it continues to elicit controversy. However, no other alternative procedure has challenged the EDT until recently. The resuscitative endovascular balloon occlusion of the aorta (REBOA) is a temporary endovascular catheter inserted via the common femoral artery into the aorta to provide aortic occlusion. Like aortic cross clamping during a thoracotomy, the goal of the balloon is to stop the hemorrhage and perfuse the heart and brain until definitive hemostasis can be obtained. REBOA is seen as the preferred procedure by some surgeons since it is much less invasive and has been associated with fewer complications [14, 15]. However, there is no published consensus on the indications for REBOA use. It currently has mainly been utilized in blunt and penetrating abdominal or pelvic injuries [16]. Despite the promising role of the REBOA, its clinical benefit still remains unclear with some studies showing no clear reduction in hemorrhage-related mortality, and it is not without complications [17]. However, Rhee et al. found in an autopsy study that REBOA use would have been potentially beneficial in 50.0% of blunt thoracic and 33.3% of penetrating thoracic trauma patients [18]. While new, innovative procedures such as REBOA continue to find their place in the trauma setting, the emergency thoracotomy continues to remain the "go to" for surgeons.

Take-Home Points

- Indications for an emergency thoracotomy include patients who present pulseless and have suffered penetrating trauma with or without signs of life *or* have suffered blunt trauma with signs of life within 5 min of arrival.
- Start with an anterolateral thoracotomy in an unstable or arrested patient.
- Median sternotomy may be a better initial choice if the patient has isolated clinical signs of cardiac tamponade from an anterior low-velocity wound.
- If the hemorrhage source is not obviously in the left pleural space, a pericardiotomy along with exploration of other body cavities for identifying hemorrhage should be done.
- Indications for cross clamp of the aorta include hemodynamic instability with unidentified hemorrhage, hemodynamic instability after repair of intrathoracic injury, or hemodynamic instability with known hemorrhage below the diaphragm.
- The aortic cross clamp should be removed as soon as possible after hemorrhage control is established; survival after 30 min of cross clamp time is rare.
- If the chest is filled with blood, first maximize exposure and then evacuate the blood. Hold respirations briefly to pack, and ultimately retract the deflated lung.
- The resuscitative endovascular balloon occlusion of the aorta (REBOA) may be an alternative to emergency thoracotomy done for hemorrhage control and should be considered in certain cases.

Suggested Readings

Front Line Surgery: A Practical Approach, Editors: Martin M. and Beekley, A.

Top Knife: Art and Craft of Trauma Surgery by Hirschberg and Mattox.

ASSET: Advanced Surgical Skills for Exposure in Trauma by American College of Surgeons Committee on Trauma.

Advanced Trauma Operative Management (ATOM): Surgical Strategies for Penetrating Trauma, Editors: Jacobs, L. and Luk, S.

References

1. Brohi K. trauma.org. 2006. Retrieved from http://www.trauma.org/index.php/main/article/361/.
2. Brohi K. trauma.org. 2001. Retrieved from http://www.trauma.org/archive/thoracic/EDTrationale.html.
3. Eastern Association for the Surgery of Trauma. An evidence-based approach to patient selection for emergency department thoracotomy: a practice management guideline from the Eastern Association for the Surgery of Trauma. J Trauma Acute Care Surg. 2015; 79(1):159–73.
4. Hammada S, et al. Integrating eFAST in the initial management of stable trauma patients: the end of plain film radiography. Ann Intensive Care. 2016;6:62.
5. Brohi K. trauma.org. 2001. Retrieved from http://www.trauma.org/archive/thoracic/EDTindications.html.
6. Feliciano D. Thoracotomy in the emergency department. (A. C. Trauma, Producer). 2004. Retrieved from https://www.facs.org/~/media/files/quality%20programs/trauma/publications/thoracotomy.ashx.
7. Cothren C, Moore E. Emergency department thoracotomy for the critically injured patient: objectives, indications, and outcomes. World J Emerg Surg. 2006;1:4.
8. Connery C, et al. Paraparesis following emergency room thoracotomy: case report. J Trauma. 1990; 30:362.
9. Brohi K. trauma.org. 2001. Retrieved from http://www.trauma.org/archive/thoracic/EDToperative.html.
10. Dizon V, et al. Trauma reports. 2003. Retrieved from https://www.ahcmedia.com/articles/25786-ed-thoracotomy-revisited-a-complete-reassessment-of-its-past-present-and-future.
11. Baker J, et al. Unsuspected human immunodeficiency virus in critically ill emergency patients. JAMA. 1987;257:2609.
12. Sloan EP, et al. Human immunodeficiency virus and hepatitis B virus seroprevalence in an urban trauma population. J Trauma. 1995;38:736.
13. Caplan E, et al. Seroprevalence of human immunodeficiency virus, hepatitis B virus, hepatitis C virus, and rapid plasma reagin in a trauma population. J Trauma. 1995;39:533.

14. Moore L, et al. Resuscitative endovascular balloon occlusion of the aorta for control of noncompressible truncal hemorrhage in the abdomen and pelvis. Am J Surg. 2016;212:1222–30.
15. Brenner M. A clinical series of resuscitative endovascular balloon occlusion of the aorta for hemorrhage control and resuscitation. J Trauma Acute Care Surg. 2013;75:506–11.
16. Barnard E, et al. Resuscitative endovascular balloon occlusion of the aorta (REBOA): a population based gap analysis of trauma patients in England and Wales. Emerg Med J. 2015;32(12):926.
17. Morrison J, et al. A systematic review of the use of resuscitative endovascular balloon occlusion of the aorta in the management of hemorrhagic shock. J Trauma Acute Care Surg. 2016;80:324–34.
18. Joseph B, et al. Identifying potential utility of resuscitative endovascular balloon occlusion of the aorta: an autopsy study. J Trauma Acute Care Surg. 2016; 81:128–32.

22 Fundamentals of Becoming a Safe and Independent Surgeon (From First Assistant to Skilled Educator)

Nabeel R. Obeid and Konstantinos Spaniolas

22.1 Introduction

Primum Non Nocere This Latin phrase is known to all in the medical profession and translates to "First, do no harm." It is a guiding principle for physicians throughout the world and holds especially true in the practice of surgery. The surgeon must, at every level for every intervention, decide if the potential risks outweigh its proposed benefits. This thought process occurs on a daily basis in clinical practice, when reviewing a surgical consent with a patient or discussing an invasive procedure with the family of a critically ill patient.

This core principle is just one of the many elements that shape a surgeon, leading to safe and independent care of the surgical patient. One must obtain the proper set of skills and specialty training in order to be proficient with providing such care. This education begins in medical school with rigorous courses and clinical rotations and advances into specialty training with graduated responsibility in the form of residency training. William Halsted is credited with establishing the first American surgical education program at Johns Hopkins in 1889, which was an apprenticeship, pyramidal residency model intended to produce a single, well-trained surgeon scientist [1]. However, it was Edward Churchill of the Massachusetts General Hospital who introduced the rectangular concept of a surgical residency program in 1938, where trainees would learn from multiple expert surgical educators and would be given increasing levels of responsibility with demonstration of competence. This has stood the test of time and remains the basis for surgical training today.

22.2 General Concepts

Surgical training in the United States is governed by the Accreditation Council for Graduate Medical Education (ACGME). Their program requirements specifically outline competency-based goals and delineation of resident responsibilities and highlight six core competencies including patient care and procedural skills [2]. Despite the graded responsibility and structured nature of these programs, there have been concerns regarding passive advancement of residents from year to year without demonstration of competence. Therefore, the ACGME and American Board of Surgery (ABS) jointly instituted the General Surgery Milestone Project [3]. This program was designed as a more effective way to evaluate residents in the core competencies and to improve transparency for how the resident is

N. R. Obeid • K. Spaniolas (✉)
Department of Surgery, Stony Brook Medicine, Stony Brook, NY, USA
e-mail: Konstantinos.Spaniolas@stonybrookmedicine.edu

F. Palazzo (ed.), *Fundamentals of General Surgery*, https://doi.org/10.1007/978-3-319-75656-1_22

evaluated, ultimately ensuring advancement based on these milestones of achievement.

The ACGME, in collaboration with the ABS and Association of Program Directors in Surgery (APDS), has also released updated case minimum requirements for each category, effective for the 2017–2018 academic year, which parallel the changing patterns of surgical care [4]. These include a higher case number for basic and complex laparoscopic procedures and reflect the emphasis on appropriate and relevant training for today's surgeon. In addition, there is now a requirement to log 25 cases, at a minimum, in the role of teaching assistant as a chief resident. This is intended to help residents develop the skills necessary to safely and effectively teach junior residents, a skill that will be invaluable in their future practice.

Another step taken to ensure competence and promote safety is the intraoperative assessment requirement of the ABS. The board now requires a minimum of six operative and six clinical performance assessments to be eligible for certification [5]. These assessments consist of procedure- or encounter-specific evaluations by faculty of resident performance, both intraoperatively and in the outpatient setting. The strict accreditation process of the ACGME for surgical training programs and the arduous certification process administered by the ABS help to ensure that graduating residents attain the essential knowledge and skills necessary to make the safe transition to surgical practice.

Despite the efforts to ensure resident competency and readiness for practice, a recent report suggested a shortcoming in this regard for those entering general surgery subspecialty fellowship training [6]. This widely referenced and highly publicized study reported the results of a comprehensive survey administered by the Fellowship Council, which was sent to program directors in minimally invasive, bariatric, colorectal, hepatobiliary, and thoracic surgery fellowships. The results were surprising to many, including the fact that one in five new fellows was unprepared for the operating room, 30% were unable to perform a laparoscopic cholecystectomy independently, and almost one quarter of fellows were unable to recognize early signs of complications. Additionally, lack of confidence by surgical residents has been shown to be a significant factor in choosing to pursue a fellowship in the first place [7]. Another study evaluated the relationship between surgeon status and rate of complications among newly trained ophthalmologists and found that surgeons in their first year of practice were nine times more likely to have high complication rates (defined as >2%) as compared to surgeons in their tenth year in practice [8]. Each year of independent practice found a 10% drop in patient risk of adverse event. Although these findings seem intuitive, they are alarming nonetheless, and the patient safety issues are evident.

While concerning in many regards, this deficiency appears to dissipate by the time the trainee completes their respective fellowship (if pursued), with one study reporting 95% of respondents being highly satisfied with operative experience and feeling competent in completing 85% of procedures [9]. In fact, the methods of assessment for procedural training in surgical fellowships have been studied and appear to be successful from both the director and trainee perspectives [10]. Overall, it appears that the fellowship year(s) may help to bridge the gap from residency to enter independent practice as a competent and well-prepared surgeon.

The transition from training to surgical practice is a difficult one. The challenges are many, including independent patient care, operating room autonomy, as well as less obvious issues such as practice management skills, which have been shown to be absent from most surgical training program curriculums [11]. For a new surgeon, hospitals will review privilege requests and, once approved, may require formal proctoring or a focused professional practice evaluation during a provisional period. This involves the newly hired surgeon to be evaluated by an experienced physician as a quality control measure, ensuring that the surgeon possesses the appropriate and expected technical skills to safely care for patients.

22.3 Practical Considerations

Formal Programs The American College of Surgeons (ACS) initiated a 1-year transition to practice program in 2013, the goals of which are to help surgeons establish autonomy in decision-making, both in and out of the operating room, mentorship, and familiarity with practice management [12]. This program has had initial success and is expanding nationwide in diverse practice settings, serving as an excellent platform to provide a smooth transition for the young, independent surgeon.

Mentorship Whether part of a formal program or not, one of the keys to success for newly established surgeons is to find an effective mentor. This individual should serve as an advisor for such a transition, investing time and effort to help guide and support the surgeon early in his career. For many, this takes the form of a senior partner or a division chief, but most importantly, this role should be filled by someone who expresses a dedication and commitment to ensuring the success of the young surgeon. With time and experience, the surgeon may take on more complex cases, and having an effective mentor is invaluable in this setting.

Seeking Out Opinions In addition to finding a quality mentor, it is important to develop collaborative relationships with other surgeons. This can be quite helpful when faced with a diagnostic dilemma and unique patient presentation or, perhaps most notably, for intraoperative consultations [13]. In such times, seeking the opinion of others is vital to one's success. Many times, these relationships are with former mentors or other faculty at teaching institutions. Participating in mortality and morbidity conferences and other hospital-wide venues will allow a new surgeon to promptly familiarize with a new practice environment and importantly identify surgeon-experts in different fields. In addition, unconventional but increasingly popular approaches such as the ACS Communities online forums and social media outlets, like the International Hernia Collaboration or Bariatric Surgery Masters Facebook group, can facilitate interactions between a young surgeon and other expert surgeons while overcoming geographic limitations [14, 15].

Choose Wisely One of the basic principles that should be adhered to is to create an environment for success early on by modifying the variables that are under one's control in the practice setting. Surgical outcomes, both at the individual and department level, are increasingly being used to measure quality and value. These can be used for metrics as part of institutions' quality improvement programs but also help to make sure individual surgeons are meeting the expected benchmarks. In this light, for the young surgeon, it is important to "start smart." Early in one's independent clinical practice, it is wise to begin with low-complexity cases to maximize the potential for favorable outcomes while still refining on technical skills and familiarizing with a new environment. Success is more likely when choosing to perform routine operations early on, those that the surgeon can perform with comfort and confidence, rather than high-complexity cases (e.g., revisional bariatric, hepatopancreatobiliary, or low rectal cancer cases). With increased case volume, the learning curve becomes less steep and outcomes tend to improve. This is well demonstrated for many surgical procedures, from hernia repair to complex gastrointestinal or subspecialty surgery [16–19]. Once experience is established, vigilance and careful planning are paramount to venture into more complex clinical cases, in order to avoid the pitfall of overconfidence. As care complexity increases, seeking out opinions, intraoperative assistance, and detailed preoperative planning can increase the chances of operative and long-term success. In re-operative surgery, this includes getting all the required information (e.g., imaging, liberal use of endoscopy, previous operative reports) prior to walking into the operating room.

Prepare for Success Patient complexity is also a significant factor, and the newly independent surgeon should likely avoid the medically complex patient with multiple major comorbidities or risk factors for complications (e.g., end-organ failure, extremes of age) during the early stage of practice. One study comparing outcomes among surgeons in various stages of their careers found that for cardiovascular procedures, early-stage surgeons had higher morbidity and mortality rates than later-stage surgeons, but the reverse was true for digestive procedures, possibly due to an appropriate selection of less complex patients by the early-stage surgeons [20]. A list of common surgical complications with associated risk factors is shown in Table 22.1, which may serve as a guide in selecting appropriate and low-risk surgical patients [21–32]. Risk factor optimization and patient preparedness for surgery will also allow for better postoperative outcomes.

Look Around You The independent surgeon should also be mindful of the environment in which they practice. Despite being well-trained or experienced with high-risk procedures, one's hospital infrastructure may not have the capacity or resources for these procedures to be done in a safe manner without jeopardizing patient outcomes. If such operations or high-risk patients are to be taken on, a planned, measured approach should be used with careful review of the steps and details; assembly of a specialized, experienced team; and even consideration for a practice run with a cadaver or animal laboratory.

Finally, the newly trained surgeon entering practice should adhere to safe practice patterns and society guidelines. This will help the surgeon establish a credible reputation of practicing evidence-based medicine consistent with current standards of care, thereby delivering optimal care to the patient. Examples of popular society guidelines include the clinical practice guidelines of the American Society of Colon and Rectal Surgeons (ASCRS) or the practice management guidelines of the Eastern Association for the

Table 22.1 Common complications among varying surgical subspecialties with associated risk factors

Morbidity (procedure)	Risk factor(s)
General surgery	
Incisional hernia (abdominal procedure)	Laparotomy, COPD, increased BMI[a]
Surgical-site infection (ventral hernia repair)	OR time $\geq$ 4 h, lack of vacuum dressing[b]
Mortality (open ventral hernia repair)	Functional status, liver disease, malnutrition, age > 65 years, ASA $\geq$ 4, contamination[c]
Colorectal surgery	
Surgical-site infection (elective colectomy)	Contaminated or dirty case, female gender, open surgery[d]
Anastomotic leak (laparoscopic low anterior resection)	Male gender, BMI $\geq$ 25 kg/m^2, ASA > 2, tumor size >5 cm, preoperative chemotherapy, longer OR time, number of staple firings $\geq$3, intraoperative blood loss/transfusions, anastomosis within 5 cm of anal verge[e]
Incisional hernia (sigmoidectomy)	Wound packing, infection, previous hernia[f]
Vascular	
Acute kidney injury (elective abdominal aortic aneurysm)	Active smoker, HTN, CKD, open repair, arrhythmias[g]
Groin wound infection (lower extremity revascularization)	Previous groin dissection, female gender, increased BMI, ESRD, malnutrition, urgent/emergent procedure[h]
Bariatric surgery	
Venous thromboembolism (bariatric)	Male gender, higher BMI, CHF, HTN, age $\geq$ 60 years, African-American race, COPD[i]
Leak (laparoscopic sleeve gastrectomy)	Male gender, BMI $\geq$ 50 kg/m^2, OR time, conversion to open, intraoperative complications, HTN, degenerative joint disease[j]

Table 22.1 (continued)

Morbidity (procedure)	Risk factor(s)
Surgical oncology	
Pancreatic leak (pancreaticoduodenectomy)	Soft pancreatic texture, intraoperative blood transfusion ≥4 units[k]
Bile leak (hepatectomy)	Bevacizumab use, major hepatectomy, two-stage hepatectomy, selective clamping, R1 or R2 resection[l]

COPD chronic obstructive pulmonary disease, *BMI* body mass index, *OR* operating room, *ASA* American Society of Anesthesiologists classification, *HTN* hypertension, *CKD* chronic kidney disease, *ESRD* end-stage renal disease, *CHF* congestive heart failure
[a]Goodenough et al. [21]
[b]Poruk et al. [22]
[c]Basta et al. [23]
[d]Pedroso-Fernandez et al. [24]
[e]Qu et al. [25]
[f]Connelly et al. [26]
[g]Castagno et al. [27]
[h]Bennett et al. [28]
[i]Haskins et al. [29]
[j]Benedix et al. [30]
[k]Fathy et al. [31]
[l]Guillaud et al. [32]

Surgery of Trauma (EAST) [33, 34]. The surgeon should also be familiar with society safety initiatives, like the Safe Cholecystectomy Program of the Society of American Gastrointestinal and Endoscopic Surgeons (SAGES) [35].

22.4 Current Controversies/ Future Directions

Training of the general surgeon continues to evolve over time, as specific initiatives and adaptations occur frequently with the primary goal of ensuring competent surgeons that are capable of providing optimal surgical care to the patient. It is likely that future efforts will focus on ways to make the transition to independent practice more seamless and may make these formalized transition programs more widespread and readily available. For the new surgeon, proficiency-based credentialing may be the way of the future, using both simulation and submission of intraoperative videos of individual performance for review.

Take-Home Points

- General surgery residency aims to graduate competent surgeons; despite this, evidence suggests that training may be inadequate for independent practice.
- Subspecialty fellowship training may be a way to close the gap, producing surgeons who are capable of practice in an environment of autonomy.
- Formal transition to practice programs exists to aid new surgeons in settling into practice.
- Finding an effective mentor who is committed to the success of the surgeon is paramount.
- Developing a collaborative relationship with peers, senior faculty or partners, or joining online forums can help the surgeon in complex or challenging situations.
- "Start smart" by choosing low-complexity cases in low-acuity patients to help maximize early success and positive outcomes.
- Understanding practice environment and hospital capabilities/resources can guide the surgeon to select appropriate patients; it is critical to prepare in advance and ensure an experienced team is available for more complex procedures.
- Familiarity with society guidelines will allow the surgeon to practice the most up-to-date, evidence-based medicine and provide optimal care to the surgical patient.

Suggested Readings

Mattar SG, Alseidi AA, Jones DB, Jeyarajah DR, Swanstrom LL, Aye RW, et al. General surgery residency inadequately prepares trainees for fellowship: results of a survey of fellowship program directors. Ann Surg. 2013;258:440–9.

Cogbill TH, Shapiro SB. Transition from training to surgical practice. Surg Clin North Am. 2016;96:25–33.

Klingensmith ME, Cogbill TH, Luchette F, Biester T, Samonte K, Jones A. Factors influencing the decision of surgery residency graduates to pursue general surgery practice versus fellowship. Ann Surg. 2015;262:449–55.

References

1. Grillo HC. Edward D. Churchill and the "rectangular" surgical residency. Surgery. 2004;136:947–52.
2. Accreditation Council for Graduate Medical Education. ACGME Program Requirements for Graduate Medical Education in General Surgery. Accreditation Council for Graduate Medical Education. 2017. http://www.acgme.org/Portals/0/PFAssets/ProgramRequirements/440_general_surgery_2017-07-01_TCC.pdf. Accessed 13 Mar 2017.
3. Accreditation Council for Graduate Medical Education: Milestones. 2017. http://www.acgme.org/What-We-Do/Accreditation/Milestones/Overview. Accessed 13 Mar 2017.
4. Review Committee for Surgery. Defined Category Minimum Numbers: General Surgery Effective for Program Graduates Beginning Academic Year 2017–2018. Accreditation Council for Graduate Medical Education. 2016. https://www.acgme.org/Portals/0/UPDATED_DEFINED_CATEGORY_MINIMUM_NUMBERS_EFFECTIVE_ACADEMIC_YEAR_2017-2018_GENERAL_SURGERY.pdf. Accessed 13 Mar 2017.
5. The American Board of Surgery: General Surgery: Training Requirements. 2017. http://www.absurgery.org/default.jsp?certgsqe_training. Accessed 13 Mar 2017.
6. Mattar SG, Alseidi AA, Jones DB, Jeyarajah DR, Swanstrom LL, Aye RW, et al. General surgery residency inadequately prepares trainees for fellowship: results of a survey of fellowship program directors. Ann Surg. 2013;258:440–9.
7. Klingensmith ME, Cogbill TH, Luchette F, Biester T, Samonte K, Jones A. Factors influencing the decision of surgery residency graduates to pursue general surgery practice versus fellowship. Ann Surg. 2015;262:449–55.
8. Campbell RJ, El-Defrawy SR, Gill SS, Whitehead M, Campbell EL, Hooper PL. New surgeon outcomes and the effectiveness of surgical training: a population-based cohort study. Ophthalmology. 2017;124:532–8.
9. Watanabe Y, Madani A, Bilgic E, McKendy KM, Enani G, Ghaderi I, et al. Don't fix it if it isn't broken: a survey of preparedness for practice among graduates of Fellowship Council-accredited fellowships. Surg Endosc. 2016. https://doi.org/10.1007/s00464-016-5231-0.
10. Gearhart SL, Wang MH, Gilson MM, Chen B, Kern DE. Teaching and assessing technical proficiency in surgical subspecialty fellowships. J Surg Educ. 2012;69:521–8.
11. Klingensmith ME, Cogbill TH, Samonte K, Jones A, Malangoni MA. Practice administration training needs of recent general surgery graduates. Surgery. 2015;158:773–6.
12. Cogbill TH, Shapiro SB. Transition from training to surgical practice. Surg Clin North Am. 2016;96:25–33.
13. Novick RJ, Lingard L, Cristancho SM. The call, the save, and the threat: understanding expert help-seeking behavior during nonroutine operative scenarios. J Surg Educ. 2015;72:302–9.
14. American College of Surgeons: ACS Communities. 2017. http://acscommunities.facs.org/home. Accessed 9 Apr 2017.
15. International Hernia Collaboration Facebook group. 2017. https://www.facebook.com/groups/herniacollab/. Accessed 9 Apr 2017.
16. Mathur S, Lin SY. The learning curve for laparoscopic inguinal hernia repair: a newly qualified surgeon perspective. J Surg Res. 2016;205:246–51.
17. Celio AC, Kasten KR, Brinkley J, Chung AY, Burruss MB, Pories WJ, et al. Effect of surgeon volume on sleeve gastrectomy outcomes. Obes Surg. 2016;26:2700–4.
18. Celio AC, Kasten KR, Burruss MB, Pories WJ, Spaniolas K. Surgeon case volume and readmissions after laparoscopic Roux-en-Y gastric bypass: more is less. Surg Endosc. 2017;31:1402–6.
19. Hata T, Motoi F, Ishida M, Naitoh T, Katayose Y, Egawa S, et al. Effect of hospital volume on surgical outcomes after pancreaticoduodenectomy: a systematic review and meta-analysis. Ann Surg. 2016;263:664–72.
20. Studnicki J, Fisher JW, Tsulukidze MM, Taylor YJ, Salandy S, Laditka JN. Career phase of board-certified general surgeons: workload composition and outcomes. Arch Surg. 2011;146:1307–13.
21. Goodenough CJ, Ko TC, Kao LS, Nguyen MT, Holihan JL, Alawadi Z, et al. Development and validation of a risk stratification score for ventral incisional hernia after abdominal surgery: hernia expectation rates in intra-abdominal surgery (the HERNIA project). J Am Coll Surg. 2015;220:405–13.
22. Poruk KE, Hicks CW, Trent Magruder J, Rodriguez-Unda N, Burce KK, Azoury SC, et al. Creation of a novel risk score for surgical site infection and occurrence after ventral hernia repair. Hernia. 2017;21:261–9.
23. Basta MN, Fischer JP, Wink JD, Kovach SJ. Mortality after inpatient open ventral hernia repair: developing a risk stratification tool based on 55,760 operations. Am J Surg. 2016;211:1047–57.
24. Pedroso-Fernandez Y, Aguirre-Jaime A, Ramos MJ, Hernández M, Cuervo M, Bravo A, et al. Prediction of surgical site infection after colorectal surgery. Am J Infect Control. 2016;44:450–4.
25. Qu H, Liu Y, Bi DS. Clinical risk factors for anastomotic leakage after laparoscopic anterior resection for

rectal cancer: a systematic review and meta-analysis. Surg Endosc. 2015;29:3608–17.
26. Connelly TM, Tappouni R, Mathew P, Salgado J, Messaris E. Risk factors for the development of an incisional hernia after sigmoid resection for diverticulitis: an analysis of 33 patients, operative and disease-associated factors. Am Surg. 2015;81:492–7.
27. Castagno C, Varetto G, Quaglino S, Frola E, Scozzari G, Bert F, et al. Acute kidney injury after open and endovascular elective repair for infrarenal abdominal aortic aneurysms. J Vasc Surg. 2016;64:928–33.
28. Bennett KM, Levinson H, Scarborough JE, Shortell CK. Validated prediction model for severe groin wound infection after lower extremity revascularization procedures. J Vasc Surg. 2016;63:414–9.
29. Haskins IN, Amdur R, Sarani B, Vaziri K. Congestive heart failure is a risk factor for venous thromboembolism in bariatric surgery. Surg Obes Relat Dis. 2015;11:1140–5.
30. Benedix F, Poranzke O, Adolf D, Wolff S, Lippert H, Arend J, et al. Staple line leak after primary sleeve gastrectomy-risk factors and mid-term results: do patients still benefit from the weight loss procedure? Obes Surg. 2017. https://doi.org/10.1007/s11695-017-2543-7.
31. Fathy O, Wahab MA, Elghwalby N, Sultan A, EL-Ebidy G, Hak NG, et al. 216 cases of pancreaticoduodenectomy: risk factors for postoperative complications. Hepato-Gastroenterology. 2008;55:1093–8.
32. Guillaud A, Pery C, Campillo B, Lourdais A, Sulpice L, Boudjema K. Incidence and predictive factors of clinically relevant bile leakage in the modern era of liver resections. HPB. 2013;15:224–9.
33. American Society of Colon and Rectal Surgeons Clinical Practice Guidelines. 2017. https://www.fascrs.org/physicians/clinical-practice-guidelines. Accessed 9 Apr 2017.
34. Eastern Association for the Surgery of Trauma Practice Management Guidelines. 2017. https://www.east.org/education/practice-management-guidelines. Accessed 9 Apr 2017.
35. Society of American Gastrointestinal and Endoscopic Surgeons Safe Cholecystectomy Program. 2017. https://www.sages.org/safe-cholecystectomy-program/. Accessed 9 Apr 2017.

23 Fundamentals of Acceptable Behavior in the Operating Room (Etiquette)

Annie P. Ehlers and Andrew S. Wright

23.1 Introduction

> *Nothing is less important than which fork you use. Etiquette is the science of living. It embraces everything. It is ethics. It is honor.*
>
> —Emily Post

As much as the culture and practice of surgery have changed and evolved over the last several hundred years, it remains true that the operating room (OR) can be an intimating place for medical students or junior residents. In the past, surgeons have often had the reputation of being arrogant or demeaning, with frequent stories akin to hazing of junior residents in the OR, or of impulsive, disruptive behavior aimed at team members such as nursing staff, anesthesia team, and support personnel. In fact, this type of "old-school" behavior is no longer acceptable, for many reasons. The OR is a special place, but it is still in the end a workplace, and workplace norms of mutual respect and polite behavior must apply. In the modern era, it is clear that surgeons must work in a respectful and collaborative fashion with all members of the patient care team. It is incumbent on the surgeon to create an atmosphere of mutual respect, trust, and communication.

It is increasingly clear that a culture of safety and respect in the operating room leads to improved patient outcomes. This same culture of respect also improves team communication, enhances professionalism, and allows for a better educational experience for all. This chapter aims to be an introduction to the fundamentals of behavior and communication in the OR. This is often called "OR etiquette," as etiquette is defined as a code of conduct among a group or professionals that should dictate how we act and work with others. This is related to but distinct from manners—which are behaviors (good or bad) that reflect our attitude toward others. Etiquette, therefore, creates the structure within which manners exist.

We begin with a discussion of the evidence behind the increased understanding of the importance of behavior and communication in the OR. We describe the key team members that are encountered and then move forward with a discussion focused on communication, skills of leadership and followership, methods of giving and receiving feedback, and a discussion of available programs for improving team communication and culture. Finally, we will end with a few pointers for how good manners in the operating room can enhance the OR experience for all.

A. P. Ehlers • A. S. Wright (✉)
Department of Surgery, University of Wisconsin, Madison, WI, USA
e-mail: awright2@uw.edu

F. Palazzo (ed.), *Fundamentals of General Surgery*, https://doi.org/10.1007/978-3-319-75656-1_23

23.2 The Importance of Team Culture in the OR Environment

Analysis of medical errors has shown that more than two-thirds involve issues of team communication [1], and these are contributed to by issues of institutional and team culture. These errors can include missed communication, inaccurate communication, or inability or unwillingness of team members to speak up—all of which can be related to the culture of a team or institution and which are dramatically affected based on the tone and climate set by surgeon leaders, both in and out of the operating room.

Every team and institution have a "safety culture"—the attitudes, behaviors, and expectations that affect patient outcomes for good or for ill. There is increasing evidence that this safety culture directly affects both morbidity and mortality. For example, in a study of 31 hospitals in South Carolina, institutional safety culture was directly related to patient death [2]. For every 1-point change (on a 7-point scale) in the hospital-level scores for respect, clinical leadership, and assertiveness, 30-day mortality after surgery decreased from 29% to 14%. In another example, measures of safety culture across 22 hospitals in Michigan directly predicted patient outcomes after bariatric surgery [3]. In that study, when nurses rated coordination of OR teams as acceptable, rather than excellent, serious complications were 22% more likely.

23.3 The Operating Room Team

The act of surgery is inherently team-based. Each operation requires the surgeon to work closely and effectively with their assistants, anesthesia providers, nursing staff, surgical technologists, and ancillary staff members to make the OR function. Team members frequently move in and out of the OR, with change of shift or for breaks, and additional team members may be required for specialty or emergency care. The key is to remember that the patient is at the center of the team, thus the phrase "patient-centered care." Always keep in mind that patient safety and well-being are at the heart of all our efforts. It is especially important that all members of the team have a "shared mental model"—a common understanding of the issues, both medical and logistical, which might affect the course of an operation. This allows for improved efficiency, better situational awareness, and better ability to recognize and respond to issues. Here we describe the individuals commonly encountered in the operating room.

23.3.1 The Surgeons

Every surgical team will consist of an attending surgeon, usually accompanied by one or more assistants. In the private practice setting or for particularly complex cases involving multiple organ systems, this assistant may be a second attending surgeon. Alternatively, surgeons in private practice may operate with certified surgical assistant (CSA) or physician assistant (PA), with various regulations regarding scope of practice based on relevant state law.

In the academic setting, the assistants may include medical students, residents, or fellows. Fellows are fully trained surgeons who have completed residency and who are doing 1–3 years of additional subspecialty training. They may be in an ACGME-accredited program, in which case they are usually not licensed to practice independently, or may be in a non-ACGME fellowship, in which case they may be (but are not always) licensed and credentialed to practice independently.

In the learning environment, it is important for the surgeons to discuss roles and responsibilities as well as educational goals for the case, which may vary depending on the level of training and experience of the team members. An important concept in surgical education is "progressive autonomy," in which learners are allowed to take on more and more responsibility in an operation based on their level of competency. A preoperative discussion between the surgeon and the resident is critical to clear understanding of which parts of the operation the learner can be expected to perform and when the attending might need to take control of the case.

It is the responsibility of every member of the surgeon's team to review the patient's case in detail to understand their past medical and surgical history, their current disease and how it has been managed to date, relevant medications, and review of all diagnostic studies to anticipate difficulties that may be encountered during the operation. Secondarily, it is incumbent on each member to discuss the case with other members of the team to ensure that all individuals have a shared mental model of the operative plan, the postoperative plan, and any anticipated difficulties.

During the operation, the patient is the focus of the team. Each individual is expected to do their part to advance the operation while helping other team members to do the same. Following the operation, it is important to discuss postoperative care such as pain management, dietary restrictions, venous thromboembolism prophylaxis, and the need for new or existing prescription medications.

23.3.2 The Surgical Technologist or Scrub Nurse

Working closely with every surgical team is the surgical technologist or scrub nurse, often referred to as the "scrub." This individual will have various levels of training depending on their background—he or she may be a certified surgical technician or a nurse with extra training. The scrub is an integral part of the team as they are responsible for ensuring that all necessary equipment is open or readily available prior to the case starting, anticipating the needs of the surgeon to maximize efficiency, and troubleshooting when there are equipment problems or failures. Depending on the scope of practice as defined by state law and regulations, the scrub may or may not be authorized to assist with limited surgical tasks. It is the responsibility of the surgeon (or surgical resident in their place) to meet with the scrub ahead of time, confirm that all necessary equipment is available, and confirm this during the surgical pause or "time-out." Doing so will foster a collegial environment while also helping the case run more smoothly.

23.3.3 The Circulator

The circulator is typically a nurse by training who is responsible for maintaining the flow of the OR, while the surgeons are sterilely gowned and gloved. It is important (especially for new residents) to introduce yourself to the circulator to open the flow of communication for the day and to give them a baseline understanding of your skill level so that they can assist you as necessary. For example, the circulator may pay extra close attention to the medical student as they don their sterile gown and glove to ensure that they do not break the sterile field. Throughout the case, the circulator works to maintain the flow of the OR. As such, the circulator is not always available to assist in tasks not related to the direct care of the patient.

23.3.3.1 The Anesthesia Team

Without the anesthesia team, the surgeon cannot operate. The anesthesia team consists of either an attending anesthesiologist who is present for the duration of the case or an anesthesia resident or certified registered nurse anesthetist (CRNA) who is supervised by an attending anesthesiologist who may be overseeing several operations at once. In some states, depending on state law, a CRNA can also practice independently. The anesthesia provider is often helped by an anesthesia technician, much like the surgeon is helped by a surgical technician.

The anesthesia team is responsible for providing pain control and sedation, managing the airway, medical and fluid management throughout the case, and monitoring the patient for any physiologic derangements that may or may not be related to the operation at hand. They should meet the patient ahead of time to evaluate for any risk factors such as underlying cardiovascular or pulmonary disease.

Communication with the anesthesia team is critical for maintaining the safety and well-being of the patient. One of the most important tools to promote this communication is the surgical pause or "time-out," which will be discussed in greater detail later on in the chapter. Throughout the case, the surgical team must also alert the anesthesia team if they anticipate significant hemodynamic changes for the patient. This can range from events as common as insufflation of pneumoperitoneum during a laparoscopic operation to more uncommon events such as unexpected, significant hemorrhage. Conversely, it is imperative that the anesthesia team communicates with the surgeon about any significant changes in hemodynamic status or about other issues that may impact patient care.

Finally, it is important to debrief with anesthesia at the end of the case, to ensure that all members of the team have the same situational awareness and understanding of the patient's intraoperative course and postoperative plan. This includes issues such as fluid and electrolyte management, expected or potential postoperative issues, and a plan for pain management.

23.3.4 Additional Support Personnel

Depending on the case, there may be many other support personnel in the operating room. This often includes perfusionists, pharmacists and pharmacy technicians, and IT support. Other specialty physicians such as pathologists, gastroenterologists, or pulmonologists may come into the OR to analyze samples, assist or perform joint procedures, or discuss unusual situations. The housekeeping personnel are often neglected and ignored but are critical for OR operations and efficiency. As discussed in the "manners" section below, a kind word and helping hand to housekeeping can go a long way.

A special mention should be made of industry representatives, who may often be present in the operating room during a case. A complete analysis of the relationship between surgeons and industry is beyond the scope of this chapter. In brief, the role of an industry representative is to be an unobtrusive resource for the safe and effective implementation of technology. They should respond to questions when asked and can give advice about the specific techniques for devices or implants. They should not provide clinical advice or guidance. Their presence should also be limited to only those portions of the case where their services are needed and should never be in the OR prior to or during anesthesia induction or during positioning or prepping and draping in the operating room. They should not directly interface with the patient or provide clinical care, except as necessary for device interrogation or programming when needed.

23.4 Communication

One of the most important determinants of a successful operation is ongoing effective communication between all members of the surgical team. The goal is for each member of the team to have a common understanding about the patient, the proposed operation, and the expected flow of the case—the "shared mental model." One of the most common communication tools used in this setting is the surgical pause or "time-out." While many institutions use a time-out, many of these are unstructured and therefore miss an opportunity to ingrain a culture of communication.

In order to combat this, we strongly recommend using a structured and formalized checklist as part of the surgical pause. The prototype for this type of structured process is the World Health Organization Surgical Safety Checklist. The Surgical Safety Checklist, introduced in 2008, is a 19-point checklist to be used at 3 time points—immediately when the patient enters the operating room (prior to induction of anesthesia), just before the skin incision and just before the patient leaves the operating room [4, 5]. The checklist was tested in eight cities throughout the world to test its impact on patient morbidity and mortality. In a before-after study design, the investigators found that implementation of the checklist was associated with a significant reduction in mortality rate (1.5% vs. 0.8%, $p < 0.01$) and inpatient complications (11.0% vs. 7.0%, $p < 0.01$) [4]. While the checklist has largely been heralded as a success, some critics have asserted that it is not the checklist itself that reduces complications but rather the fact that the checklist provides an opportunity for the team to come together and discuss critical elements that are not to be missed [6]. It is our opinion that it does not matter how the checklist works, only that it does.

Several additional studies have shown other benefits to introduction of a formalized checklist, including reduced mortality, morbidity, and hospital length of stay as demonstrated in a recent randomized controlled study that showed reduction in complications from 19.9% to 11.5% with introduction of the checklist [7]. Despite this, some other studies of surgical checklists have shown no improvement in outcomes [8, 9]. This seems to be due to implementation issues, with wide variations in implementation between institutions and even between different specialties within an institution, with suboptimal implementation being common [10, 11]. Institutions who adopt a checklist in name only, but whose team members ignore or minimize the process, are unlikely to reap the benefits. On the other hand, institutions that develop a strong culture of safety with robust and mandatory implementation will see better results [12]. This speaks to the importance of the etiquette of the OR—the code of conduct that regulates our actions.

In order to derive the most benefit from the surgical safety checklist, all team members must be present and actively engaged in the process. Music should be turned off, side conversations stopped, and all attention should be focused on the checklist items and how they relate to the patient. Typically it is the role of the surgical attending, fellow, or resident to lead the checklist. As the designated leader, it is important to review and discuss each individual item on the checklist. This includes ensuring that every team member has introduced themselves and making it clear that all individuals in the OR are empowered to speak up if they become aware of a potentially unsafe situation.

The checklist can be modified by individual hospitals or services to include relevant items specific to their patient population. For example, if a specific surgical team has additional items that must not be forgotten (e.g., processes regarding cardiopulmonary bypass in cardiac surgery), this can be included. Many checklists also include a debriefing section for use at the end of the case including items such as specimen processing, communication with the patient's family, and who will accompany the patient to the postanesthesia or intensive care unit.

23.5 Leadership and Followership

Although the OR may seem like a highly regimented environment, each member of the surgical team will serve as both a "leader" and a "follower" at different points during the operation. This includes everyone from the most senior attending surgeon to the most junior medical student.

Within the OR, the surgical attending has ultimate responsibility for the patient. However, surgical residents will often act as leaders to junior residents and medical students. In the setting of "progressive autonomy" for surgical trainees, the attending surgeon may also formally or informally cede control of the case to the resident or fellow and may take a follower role him or herself. In fact, more often than not, the surgical attending will assist a senior resident through a case, rather than perform the operation with the resident's assistance.

In the OR, the team leader is responsible for setting the tone. It is up to the leader to make sure that all team members have a shared understanding of how the day will proceed as well as any potential problems that may arise. In many cases, the surgical attending does not arrive to the OR until the patient has arrived, been intubated, and prepped and draped. In this case, it is up to the senior-most resident to lead the team. A resident who arrives early, completes the surgical timeout in a thorough but efficient manner, and moves the room forward is much more effective than one who arrives late or is not familiar with the patient or the case. While an extensive discussion of successful leadership traits is outside of the realm of this chapter, *in general a good leader is one who outlines a clear vision of the work that needs to be accomplished while also empowering those around them to take ownership over their individual work.*

While leadership is a commonly discussed topic, what is less commonly discussed is the importance of "followership." While there are several different descriptions of the various types of "followers" on any given team, many focus on a spectrum from passive to active and from dependent, uncritical thinking to independent, critical thinking [13, 14]. Compared to the field of leadership, the study of followership is relatively new, but it is generally agreed that effective followers are those who are paying attention to what is going on around them, taking an active interest in the process, and questioning or challenging leadership or the status quo when necessary. This last point is especially critical.

In the OR, being a good follower is a crucial component to maintaining patient safety as it is incumbent upon the followers (including residents, medical students, nursing staff, and all other participants) to speak up if they notice that something is going wrong or that the environment has become unsafe. Especially for more junior members of the team, it can be intimidating to alert the attending that he or she may be making a mistake or misjudging the situation. However, it is important to remember that such actions, when carried out with tact and respect, are in the best interest of the patient and may actually prevent serious harm from occurring.

23.6 Giving and Receiving Feedback

Feedback has gained an increasingly important role in surgical education. Feedback may be summative and/or formative. Summative feedback is often given at discrete time points such as the end of a rotation and is a culmination of observations of performance. Formative feedback involves an ongoing assessment of skills or knowledge and may be given throughout an education experience.

There is an often misunderstood distinction between teaching and feedback. As an example, teaching is when the attending surgeon corrects the resident's needle angle during a bowel anastomosis. Feedback is when the attending surgeon and resident meet after the case and discuss performance—either technical or nontechnical. For example, a feedback session might discuss room setup, efficiency, technical maneuvers, and communication.

Giving and receiving feedback are distinct skills that require both parties to be attentive and open. To facilitate this process, several methods have been described that turn feedback into an active process for both parties. Ideally, the mentor and the trainee have a briefing prior to the case in order to set learning objectives and then formally debrief after the case to discuss how well the learning objectives were met as well as ways to improve this in the future. In the press of clinical concerns and the drive toward efficiency, the debrief session is often skipped or missed. It is incumbent on the learner, therefore, to specifically seek out and ask the attending surgeon for feedback and if necessary to schedule formal meeting times. It is also important for feedback to flow both ways, and the attending surgeon should ask for feedback from the residents as well.

A good methodology for providing feedback is to ask an open-ended question such as "How did you think that operation went?" Which can be followed with "What went well?" and "What could have gone better?" This allows the person providing feedback with a baseline to start from and allow for self-reflection on the part of the learner. This can be followed with specific feedback about one to two actionable items, preferably relating back to the goals stated during the initial briefing.

23.7 Improving Communication Skills

While a number of high-quality tools exist to augment the surgical education provided in a residency program, most focus on pathophysiology of disease or surgical technique. A less commonly discussed yet increasingly important component of surgical education is the nonoperative skills that are required for safe and effective patient care. A common term for this is "Nontechnical Skills for Surgeons" or NOTSS. Developed in Europe by a team of surgeons, anesthesiologists, and psychologists, the

NOTSS curriculum aims to identify important nontechnical skills needed by surgeons for successful practice. Each element or skill is categorized as being related to situation awareness, decision-making, leadership, or communication and teamwork [15].

There are four core categories within the NOTSS curriculum. The first is situational awareness, which focuses on gathering information and assimilating it for use in the current and future time. An example of this would be the surgeon who learns that their patient has chronic pain understands that this may lead to difficulty controlling postoperative pain and subsequently works with the anesthesia team prior to the case to formulate a plan. The second category is decision-making. This skill can build on "situation awareness" as it requires the surgeon to take in all of the available information to formulate their options and then select the best option for the patient. Intrinsic in this is that the surgeon also communicates the selected option, formulates a plan, and then later analyzes their choice. The third category is leadership, which has been previously discussed in this chapter. The fourth is communication and teamwork. Surgeons who excel at this skill actively engage their team to develop a shared mental model that can then be used to mount a more coordinated effort [15]. Surgical safety checklists are one way to improve communication and teamwork, as discussed above. While NOTSS is a relatively new concept, there is evidence to suggest that these nontechnical skills can improve surgeon performance overall [16].

Another great resource for training and development in leadership, followership, and team communication skills is the TEAM STEPPS program developed by the Agency for Healthcare Quality and Research [17]. This includes basic skills such as establishing roles, communication techniques including cross-checks, checkbacks, and callouts, as well as more advanced skills such as team huddles, briefing and debriefing, and strategies for managing conflicts or disagreements. Many institutions have adopted TEAM STEPPS training, and the course is available online for individuals through the AHRQ website.

23.8 Manners in the Operating Room

If OR etiquette represents a code of conduct—respect, communication, shared mental model, and teamwork—then manners represent the behaviors that embody this code of behavior. These seem like simple rules that should have been learned at an early age, but a few pointers will go a long way toward integrating junior residents and students into the OR team.

1. Be polite.
2. Be respectful.
3. Be humble.
4. Learn everyone's name.
5. Offer help without being asked.
6. Ask for help when needed.
7. Thank your colleagues.
8. Keep the patient at the center of all you do.

Rude, disruptive, or disrespectful behavior is not tolerated. Do not yell or make sarcastic comments. Do not make jokes with sexual or racial themes. Do not gossip or denigrate others. Many surgeons enjoy listening to music in the operating room, but in choosing a playlist, be aware that some music may have offensive lyrics that should not be played in the workplace. It is most polite to ask before playing music and to check in with music preferences, as not everyone in the OR may appreciate loud death metal. Music should be turned off during critical times such as the initial time-out.

Surgeons use social media like many others, but the OR is not the place to check Facebook or Instagram. When posting to social media, be professional anything posted to the Internet can be screen captured and spread, no matter what privacy settings you may have turned on. A recent study of publicly accessible Facebook posts showed 14.1% of surgery residents had posted potentially unprofessional content, and 12.2% had clearly unprofessional content, with violations of patient privacy being one of the most common problems, along with description of binge drinking and racially or sexually offensive material [18]. Specific to the OR, be aware that social media postings with potentially identified patient information are absolutely forbidden. This does not need to include a name of a patient to be identifiable information—a few details of a particularly unique case and a timestamped posting can be enough to cause trouble.

Conclusion

In this chapter, we have reviewed the fundamentals of acceptable behavior in the OR. While nothing can substitute the value of spending time in the OR learning these skills firsthand, understanding these basic tenets is an important first step for medical students and residents beginning their surgical training.

Take-Home Points

- Effective communication improves patient safety and may reduce medical errors.
- Identifying and understanding the roles of each member of the surgical team is an important starting point for new medical students and residents.
- The use of surgical safety checklists can improve the safety culture by promoting a shared mental model.
- All members of the surgical team should strive to act as effective leaders and followers while participating in the operation.
- Teaching and feedback are two distinct entities that are important aspects in the development of a surgeon.
- Keep the patient at the center of all you do in the OR.

Recommended Readings

Gawande A. The checklist manifesto: how to get things right. New York: Metropolitan Books; 2010.

Institute of Medicine (IOM). To err is human: building a safer health system. Washington, DC: The National Academies Press; 2000.

Yule S, Paterson-Brown S. Surgeons' non-technical skills. Surg Clin North Am. 2012;92(1):37–50.

"TeamSTEPPS." Available at https://www.ahrq.gov/teamstepps.

References

1. Institute of Medicine (IOM). To err is human: building a safer health system. Washington, DC: The National Academies Press; 2000.
2. Molina G, Berry WR, Lipsitz SR, Edmondson L, Li Z, Neville BA, et al. Perception of safety of surgical practice among operating room personnel from survey data is associated with all-cause 30-day postoperative death rate in South Carolina. Ann Surg. 2017;266(4):658–66.
3. Birkmeyer NJ, Finks JF, Greenberg CK, McVeigh A, English WJ, Carlin A, et al. Safety culture and complications after bariatric surgery. Ann Surg. 2013;257(2):260–5.
4. Haynes AB, Weiser TG, Berry WR, Lipsitz SR, Breizat AH, Dellinger EP, et al. A surgical safety checklist to reduce morbidity and mortality in a global population. N Engl J Med. 2009;360(5):491–9.
5. WHO surgical safety checklist and implementation manual. Available from, http://www.who.int/patientsafety/safesurgery/ss_checklist/en/.
6. Pugel AE, Simianu VV, Flum DR, Patchen Dellinger E. Use of the surgical safety checklist to improve communication and reduce complications. J Infect Public Health. 2015;8(3):219–25.
7. Haugen AS, Softeland E, Almeland SK, Sevdalis N, Vonen B, Eide GE, et al. Effect of the World Health Organization checklist on patient outcomes: a stepped wedge cluster randomized controlled trial. Ann Surg. 2015;261(5):821–8.
8. Erestam S, Haglind E, Bock D, Andersson AE, Angenete E. Changes in safety climate and teamwork in the operating room after implementation of a revised WHO checklist: a prospective interventional study. Patient Saf Surg. 2017;11:4.
9. Zingiryan A, Paruch JL, Osler TM, Hyman NH. Implementation of the surgical safety checklist at a tertiary academic center: Impact on safety culture and patient outcomes. Am J Surg. 2016;214(2):193–7.
10. Biffl WL, Gallagher AW, Pieracci FM, Berumen C. Suboptimal compliance with surgical safety checklists in Colorado: a prospective observational study reveals differences between surgical specialties. Patient Saf Surg. 2015;9(1):5.
11. Russ S, Rout S, Caris J, Mansell J, Davies R, Mayer E, et al. Measuring variation in use of the WHO surgical safety checklist in the operating room: a multicenter prospective cross-sectional study. J Am Coll Surg. 2015;220(1):1–11.e4.
12. Gitelis ME, Kaczynski A, Shear T, Deshur M, Beig M, Sefa M, et al. Increasing compliance with the World Health Organization surgical safety checklist-a regional health system's experience. Am J Surg. 2017;214(1):7–13.
13. Gibbons A, Bryant D. Followership: the forgotten part of doctors' leadership. BMJ Careers. 2012;19:2012.

14. Klingensmith ME. Leadership and followership in surgical education. Am J Surg. 2016;213(2):207–11.
15. Yule S, Paterson-Brown S. Surgeons' non-technical skills. Surg Clin North Am. 2012;92(1):37–50.
16. Hull L, Arora S, Aggarwal R, Darzi A, Vincent C, Sevdalis N. The impact of nontechnical skills on technical performance in surgery: a systematic review. J Am Coll Surg. 2012;214(2):214–30.
17. Team STEPPS. Available from, https://www.ahrq.gov/teamstepps/index.html.
18. Langenfeld SJ, Cook G, Sudbeck C, Luers T, Schenarts PJ. An assessment of unprofessional behavior among surgical residents on Facebook: a warning of the dangers of social media. J Surg Educ. 2014;71(6):e28–32.

Fundamentals of the Daily Routine as a Surgeon: Philosophy, Mentors, Coaches, and Success

24

Charles J. Yeo

24.1 Introduction

We are all stimulated, prompted, and pushed by others to achieve what we can in life. Many of us will reflect back to the lessons from our parents, our siblings, and our many teachers along life's course, all of whom have given us some measure of direction and focus toward our careers. This chapter is designed to be a bit philosophical and a personal testimony to some of the things that I believe are important in creating a successful surgical career.

First, I would like to commence with a top ten list, somewhat in the tradition of the David Letterman show "Daily Top Ten List." This list however was composed by Dr. Richard C. Thirlby, given as his presidential address to the Western Surgical Association in 2006, and published in the *Archives of Surgery* in 2007 (Fig. 24.1). I have used this top ten list for many years when talking about surgical careers to our medical students at the Thomas Jefferson University. Dr. Thirlby starts with #10 and counts down to his #1 reason for going into general surgery. At #10, he commences with "training is fun (you'll never forget it) and training never stops." Certainly this is an important issue, focusing on the importance of lifelong learning, and the change that accompanies surgical careers. At #9, we have "job security," which refers to the fact that general surgeons are necessary and much needed commodity and that on the national level, there are many open positions for general surgeons, often not in urban centers but in more rural areas. At #8 we have "the pay is not bad," making reference to the fact that the compensation of general surgeons is comfortable and well-above societal averages. At #7 we have the entry "your mother will be proud of you." I would add that fathers, aunts, and many other family members are often proud and pleased with having a surgeon in the family. At #6, "surgeons have panache: the surgical personality and the culture of surgery." Very true—some of the TV and movie stereotypes of surgeons are true. There is doubtless a certain culture, ambiance, and feel of a surgical group. At #5 we have "you will have heroes; you will be a hero." I doubt there is any surgeon who has trained and who does not have a litany of stories about those that have influenced them, driven them, motivated them, and done amazing things with surgical patients. Additionally, the assistance we render to patients often leads them to be thankful, grateful, and consider you a hero. At #4, "there is spirituality if you want it." There can be no doubt about this. At times, patients will miraculously recover from

C. J. Yeo
Professor and Chairman, Department of Surgery, Senior Vice President and Chair, Enterprise Surgery, Jefferson Health, Jefferson University Hospital, Philadelphia, PA, USA
e-mail: charles.yeo@jefferson.edu

F. Palazzo (ed.), *Fundamentals of General Surgery*, https://doi.org/10.1007/978-3-319-75656-1_24

Fig. 24.1 The top ten list of Dr. Richard Thirlby. Arch Surg 2007; 142: 423–429

TOP TEN LIST

1. I love to cut
2. Patients will change your life
3. You will change patients' lives
4. There's spirituality if you want it
5. You will have "heroes"; you will be a hero
6. Surgeons have panache: the surgical personality and the culture of surgery
7. Your mother will be proud of you
8. The pay is not bad
9. Job security
10. Training is fun (you'll never forget it) and training never stops

Fig. 24.2 The *Ten Commandments* from the *New King James Version* of the *Holy Bible*

The Ten Commandments (Exodus 20:2-17 NKJV)

1. I am the Lord your God. You shall have no other gods before Me.
2. You shall not make for yourself a carved image or bow down to it. For I am the Lord your God.
3. You shall not take the name of the Lord your God in vain.
4. Remember the Sabbath day, to keep it holy.
5. Honor your father and your mother.
6. You shall not murder.
7. You shall not commit adultery.
8. You shall not steal.
9. You shall not bear false witness against your neighbor.
10. You shall not covet your neighbor's house; you shall not covet your neighbor's wife, nor anything that is your neighbors.

major interventions or trauma, often inexplicably, and out of the bounds of statistical predictions. At #3, "you will change patients' lives." Without a doubt this is one of the most personally satisfying end points for me. I still tingle when I get a simple "thank you for saving my life 5 years ago." At #2, "patients will change your life," an important, almost daily occurrence and a truism. We learn from our patients' daily, exhibit non-judgmentalism and become better human beings due to our interactions with our many patients. Lastly, at #1, "I love to cut," reflecting the joy that comes from performing a procedure with perfection, detail, and a minimum of motions, all for the good of the patient. How can you not love this top ten list! Thank you Dr. Thirlby.

24.2 Two Other Ten Commandments

Not to be overly dramatic, but there is another list of ten items which I believe are equally important in the daily life of a surgeon. Taken from the *New King James Version* of the *Holy Bible*, these are referred to as the well-known Ten Commandments (Fig. 24.2). In my mind, these ten commandments, now several thousand years old, represent important lessons regarding one's higher power, the sanctity of the Sabbath day, respecting one's parents, and prohibiting actions such as murder, adultery, theft, lying, and coveting others' belongings. Inarguably, these are appropriate ideals to live by.

Remaining on the theme of top ten lists or Ten Commandments, I have always had affection for a list of ten items proposed by Dr. James D. Hardy, MD, the longtime outstanding chair at the University of Mississippi in Jackson, Mississippi. Perhaps I am partial to Dr. Hardy's list because he took the time to phone me back in 1986, as a young faculty member at Johns Hopkins, having heard me speak at a meeting, to ask me to write a book chapter for his famous text book *Hardy's Textbook of Surgery*, 2nd edition, published in 1988. I worked hard on this chapter, as it was on the topic of "The Pancreas," quite a broad and extensive topic in a clinical domain that ended up

Fig. 24.3 Hardy's Ten Commandments

Hardy's Ten Commandments

1. Honor thy Faculty and Administration
2. Always remember who you are and what you represent
3. Continue to improve work habits, efficiency and excellence
4. Educational and professional growth must be continued throughout a career
5. Treasure and preserve your clinical integrity
6. Prepare for leadership
7. Admire and nourish professional relationships
8. On achieving immortality: Great teachers live on
9. Nurture your family: "plan for, and spend time alone with each child; the greatest thing a parent can do for the children is to love the spouse; take quiet time alone for creative thinking"
10. Enjoy your work: "There is nothing more sustaining through the vicissitudes of life, than the daily pursuit of important work that you truly enjoy"

being quite important to me in my career. Dr. Hardy presented his personal ten commandments at the University of Pennsylvania Medical School commencement on May 24, 1992, as he was the invited speaker at what was the 50th anniversary of his graduation from Penn Medical School. His list was published in the *Journal of the Mississippi State Medical Association*, and it reflects a fascinating combination of personal and cultural values (Fig. 24.3). Dr. Hardy spoke of honoring the faculty and the entire administration of the institution, remembering who you are and what you represent, and constantly striving to improve work habits, efficiency, and excellence. He goes on to discuss the importance of educational and professional growth throughout a career and the importance of preserving one's integrity. He speaks of preparation for leadership and nourishing professional relationships. He notes the importance of teachers and how they live on in the lives of their learners. He then, for numbers nine and ten, takes a more personal tone, speaking about family and specifically stating in #9 "plan for, and spend time alone with each child; the greatest thing a parent can do for the children is to love the spouse; take quiet time alone for creative thinking." Lastly (#10), he talks about enjoyment of one's work and ends with "there is nothing more sustaining through the vicissitudes of life, than the daily pursuit of important work that you truly enjoy." In my mind, these remarkable ten items provide a very meaningful mixture of both organizational and personal suggestions to achieve satisfaction in one's personal and professional life.

24.3 Lesson from a Coach: Part One

While the training of a general surgeon is lengthy (4 years of medical school, followed by at least 5 years of surgical residency), there are many fundamentals imbued within the training paradigm that become important on a day-to-day basis for those of us that practice the field of surgery. Surgery itself requires knowledge, technical skill, and stamina but, ultimately, teamwork. The surgeon does not function alone. Within the complex framework of the current healthcare delivery system, the surgeon is one of many professionals who provides care to patients. Consider the nurses, anesthesiologists, support staff, administrators, dietary staff, etc., all of whom must work in unison to provide safe and effective care. On a smaller scale, this is quite similar to the workings of a team; let's take, for example, a college basketball team.

One of my heroes in life is Pete Carril, former basketball coach at Princeton University, who, in his tenure there, won 514 games and 13 Ivy League men's basketball championships. For 29 years Carril's teams won because he knew how to teach basketball, perhaps better than others of his era. He knew how to explain the sound fundamentals and basic strategies that make up the game to generations of young scholar athletes participating on the national stage. A short but wonderful book authored by Pete Carril and Dan White and introduced by Bobby Knight is entitled *The Smart Take from the Strong* (Fig. 24.4). In this

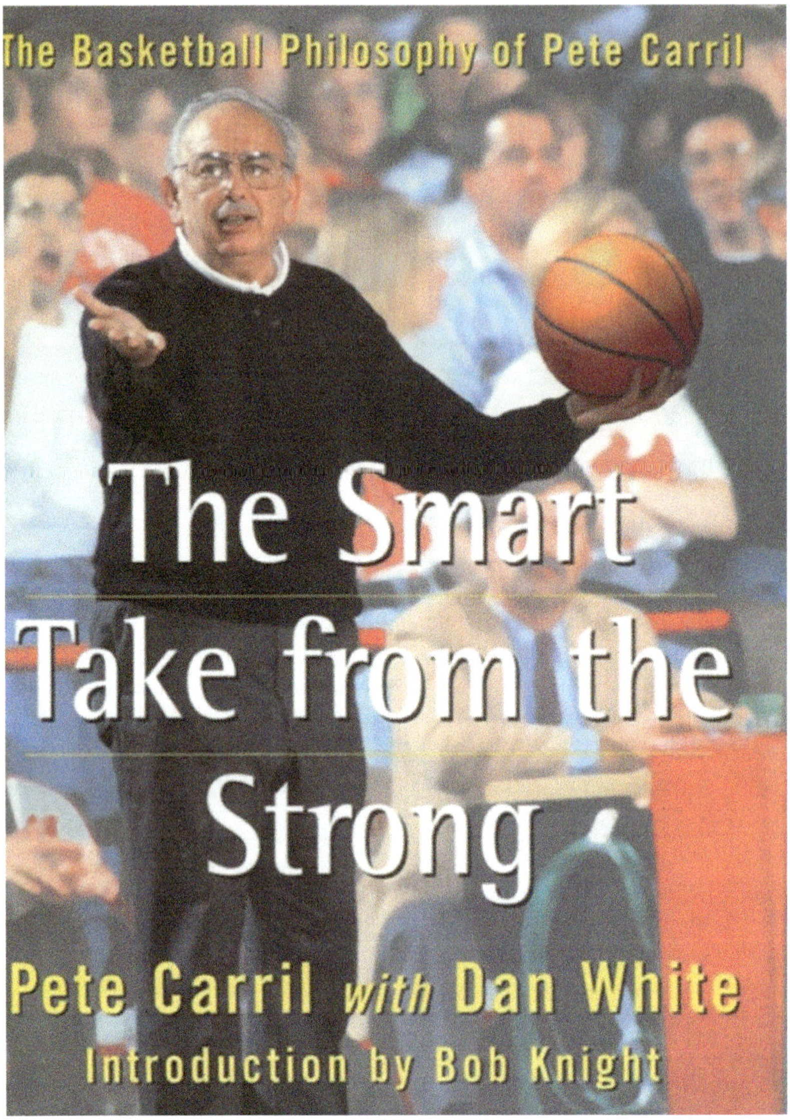

Fig. 24.4 Pete Carril: *The Smart Take From The Strong*

book, Coach Carril lays bare his philosophy for basketball success. At the end of the book, he provides a few pages entitled "25 little things to remember." While these little things are quite relevant to basketball, they are also relevant to life and surgery. For example #1, "every little thing counts. If not, why do it?" Or, #13, "you want to be good at those things that happen a lot." Or, #17, "in trying to do a specific thing, the specific thing is what you must practice. There is little transfer of learning." In addition to those three selected ones, there are two others that I particularly enjoy, #19, "anyone can be average", and #23, "the way you think affects what you see and do." Yes I am a big fan of Coach Carril. Thankfully, to this day he remains a common presence at Jadwin Gym, in Princeton, watching the new generation of Ivy League basketball players (both men and women) compete, strive to win, and mature both on and off the basketball court (the actual hardwood floor has been named "Carril Court" in his honor). Teamwork, vision, anticipation, and dedication to one's personal effort are important not only in basketball but in surgery.

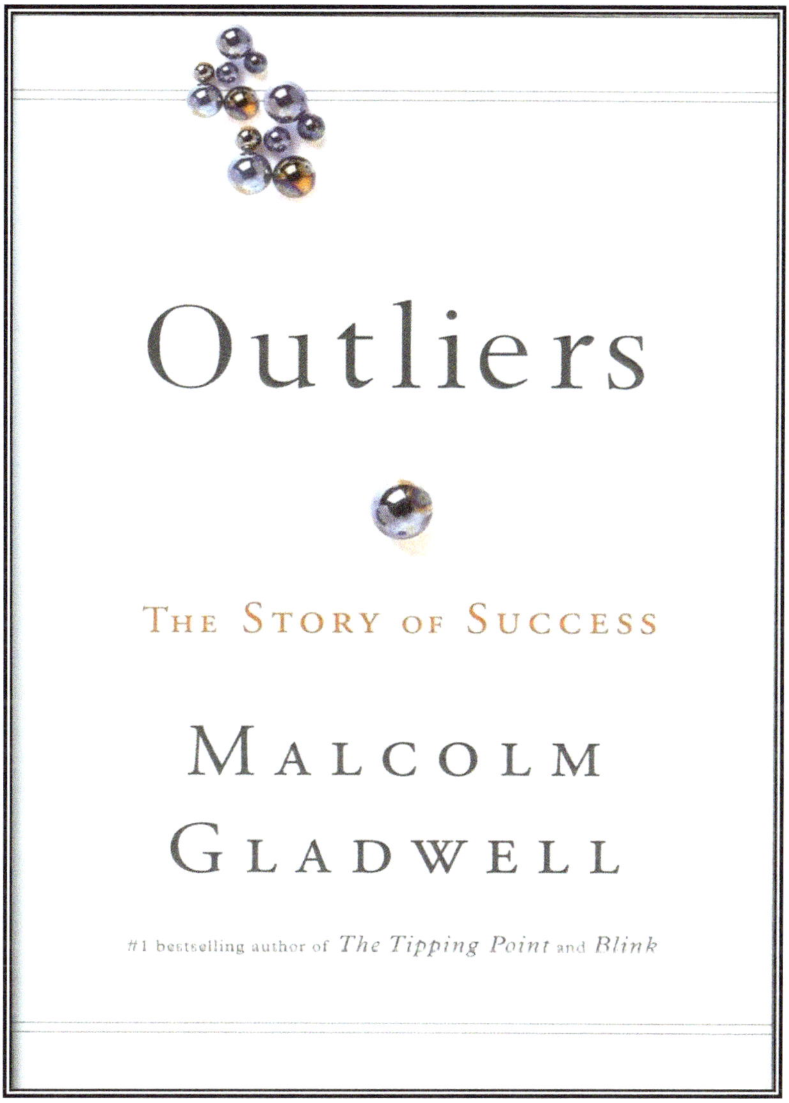

Fig. 24.5 Malcolm Gladwell, *Outliers: The Story of Success*

24.4 Malcolm Gladwell

Keeping on those same topics of teamwork, repetitive action, and success, Malcolm Gladwell, the bestselling author of various books including *The Tipping Point*, *Blink* and others, provides a nice synopsis of these points in his book entitled *Outliers: The Story of Success* (Fig. 24.5). In this book, Gladwell discusses the now well-known theme supported by neurologist Daniel Levitin, that is, the 10,000 hours of practice dogma. Gladwell writes "In study after study, of composers, basketball players, fiction writers, ice skaters, concert pianists, chess players, master criminals, and what have you, this number comes up again and again." That is, that 10,000 hours of practice are required to achieve the level of mastery associated with being a world-class expert in anything. Contrast this with the current 850 cases needed for a graduating surgical chief resident to document when submitting his or her credentials to the American Board of Surgery. Let's take this number—850 cases. Let's make the assumption that the average case that a chief resident scrubs on is perhaps 2 hours in duration, noting that many cases such as breast biopsies and endoscopies are short, well less than 1 hour, and others certainly exceed 3–4 hours. However, 2 hours appears to be a reasonable guesstimate. If one multiplies 850 hours times 2, the result is merely 1700 hours, far short of the 10,000 hours of practice needed to achieve mastery. Also, some of that 1700 hours may not actually be spent in actual performance of the operation, such as suturing, dissecting, or firing staplers, but rather may involve set up, closure, or waiting for pathology results. Hence, we have additional support for the premise of Coach Carril. Carril stresses teamwork, paying attention, focus on the basics, and his #18, "whatever you are doing is the most important thing that you are doing while you are doing it." In those 850 cases, residents need to focus on deliberate practice and learning correct technique.

In *Outliers*, Gladwell goes on to stress the three qualities that employment or work needs to have if it is to be considered satisfying to the employee. Stated another way, these are the three attributes that our profession must have in order to give satisfaction in the field of surgery: autonomy, complexity, and a connection between effort and reward. In my mind, surgery offers all three. There certainly is autonomy when it comes to surgical decision-making, surgical skills, and performance of surgical procedures. Complexity is obvious, as even the most straightforward inguinal hernia repair, bowel resection, or endovascular intervention has elements that are complex and challenging. Lastly, the connection between effort and reward can be seen at two levels: first, surgical effort in a difficult scenario may lead to the reward of a patient surviving a difficult disease. Second, a surgeon's overall effort (by this I mean operations performed, patients seen, or even work relative value units (wRVUs) achieved) is typically linked to personal compensation and salary. While this may not be true in surgical residency, it tends to be true after completion of residency in both academic practice and in private practice.

24.5 William Stewart Halsted

It is impossible for me to contribute a chapter regarding the daily routine of a surgeon without mentioning arguably the most famous of all American surgeons, Dr. William Stewart Halsted. A recent biography by Gerald Imber (Fig. 24.6) makes use of many past works and synthesizes them nicely into a modern-day biography entitled *Genius on the Edge: The Bizarre Double Life of Dr. William Stewart Halsted.* William Stewart Halsted was born on September 23, 1852, in New York City, educated at Andover and Yale, and went to medical school at the College of Physicians and Surgeons in New York City, graduating in 1878. He took his internship at Bellevue Hospital and was the first "Professor of Surgery in the Johns Hopkins Hospital" as stated on his grave stone. He died on September 7, 1922, at the Johns Hopkins Hospital, a post-op death. Halsted's career highlights are numerous and include his work with cocaine leading to its use as a topical anesthetic; his contributions to the "radical cure" of the inguinal hernia; his use of Listerian principles to dramatically decrease wound infections; his operations for gallbladder disease, thyroid disease, periampullary cancer, aneurysm, and breast cancer; and his embracing the role of the surgeon as a clinician-scientist. The Halsted residency program was renowned for its final product that of generating 17 chief residents in a total of 33 years. Imber writes: "Halsted was a complex and isolated man, forbidding and nurturing; rigid, proper, and secretive; compulsive and negligent; stimulating and reclusive; addicted and abstemious;… and always concerned with advancing the science of surgery… if a single person can be considered the father of modern surgery, the only contender is William Stewart Halsted."

Interestingly, much like the story that I discussed earlier of Dr. Hardy returning to his medical school graduation to deliver an address at the 50th anniversary of his medical school graduation, Halsted was invited back to his undergraduate

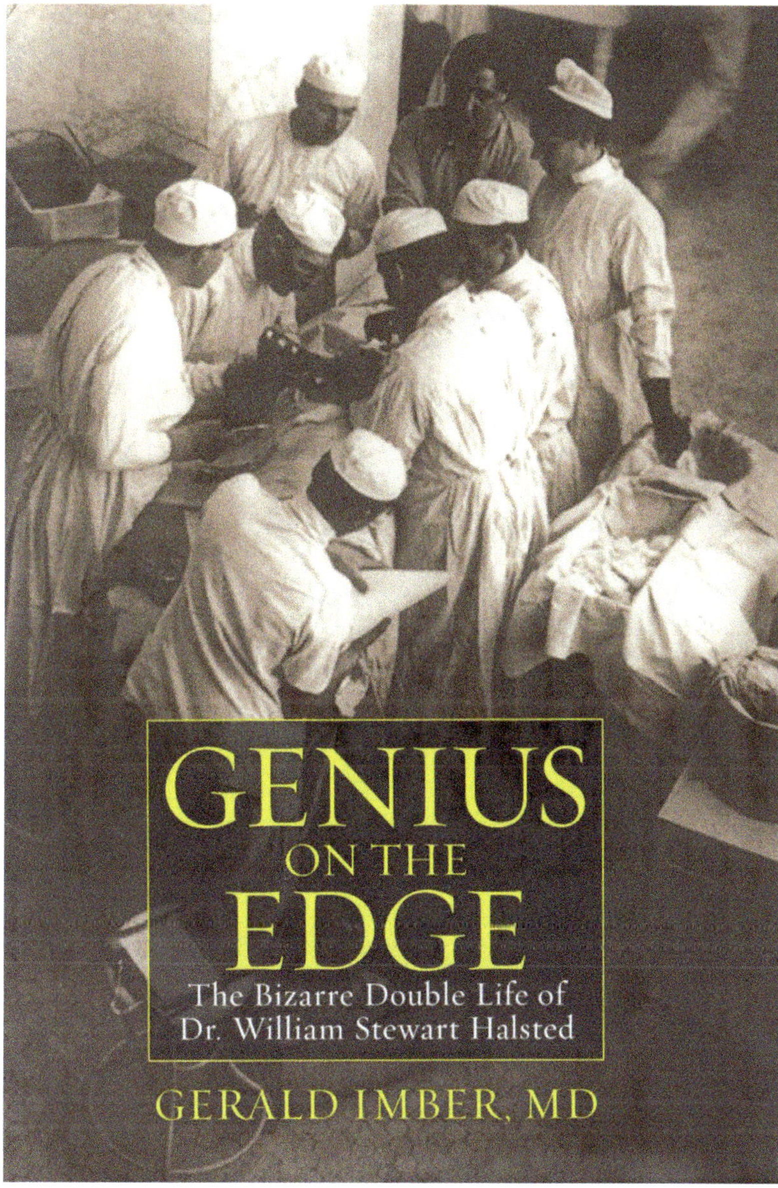

Fig. 24.6 Gerald Imber, *Genius on the Edge: The Bizarre Double Life of Dr. William Stewart Halsted*

university, Yale, where on June 27, 1904, he addressed the graduates 30 years after his own college graduation and reflected upon the progress of surgery. Halsted writes: "Pain, hemorrhage, infection- the three great evils which had always embittered the practice of surgery and checked its progress, were, in a moment, in a quarter of a century (1846–1873) robbed of their terrors. A new era has dawned; and in the 30 years which have elapsed since the graduation of the class of 1874 from Yale, probably more has been accomplished to place surgery on a truly scientific basis than in all the centuries which had preceded this wondrous period." I must say I love these two great sentences delivered by Halsted in New Haven, CT. Halsted then goes on to be somewhat critical of the status quo, particularly in the USA,, and lauds the medical education in "the well-supported medical departments of European universities." He further goes on to discuss "the problem of the education of our surgeons," stating that it is still unsolved, and not sufficient for adequate training. He then delivers two of the most off-quoted sentences ever composed in surgery: "We need a system, and we shall surely have it, which will produce not only surgeons but surgeons of the highest type, men (women) who will stimulate the first youths of our country to study surgery and devote their energies and their lives to raising the standards of surgical science. Reforms, the need of which must come on the side both of the hospital and the university. unhampered by traditions… providing the requisite opportunities for the prolonged and thorough training of those preparing for the higher careers in medicine and surgery…"

Following Halsted's death in 1922, one of his colleagues and admirers, Dr. Rudolph Matas, the professor of surgery at Tulane, delivered a speech on the occasion of the first memorial meeting for Dr. Halsted, held in Baltimore, on December 16, 1923. Matas wrote "Professor Halsted died without offspring, but nature, as if repentant for her unkindness, endowed him with a brain of prodigious fertility from which has sprung a numerous intellectual family of supermen… He was great in his art. He was great in his science… He was great as the father and founder of a school of surgery which since its existence has stood unsurpassed in surgical scholarship, in surgical craft, and in the obtainment of surgical ideals and achievements. But in none of these was he greater than in the selection of the group of young men (women) in whom he chose to carry on his apostolate and to transmit his teachings." We should all note, as implied by Matas above, isn't one of the most lofty goals of an active surgeon to train the next generation and to train her or him for excellence?

24.6 There Are No Time-Outs

The training of a surgeon can be seen as long, complex, involved, and difficult. There can be no doubt that it is rewarding. After all as noted by Dr. Thirlby in his Top Ten list, "your mother will be proud," and "I love to cut." I am often asked by medical students, about a topic that was never discussed during my training, that is, the topic of work-life balance or the topic of burnout. I consider these difficult questions. I cannot count the number of times where I was "off duty" but was called upon to use my medical skills, use my surgical expertise, and intervene on behalf of a patient. It has happened at restaurants (Heimlich maneuver), on airplanes (applying oxygen to dyspneic patients struggling to breathe in the rarified air), in a movie theater (dealing with an inebriated individual), during a theater performance (intervening on behalf of a patient with a seizure disorder), and even on the little league field (performing CPR on a spectator). I have used my surgical skills on the sidelines of a basketball game, a rugby match, and while traveling through Ireland (at a hurling match). I have witnessed automobile accidents and bicycle-pedestrian encounters and assisted those injured. I am sure all surgeons intervene many times on behalf of patients unknown to them, during their lifetimes. In my mind, there is great truth in the illustration (Fig. 24.7): "Once you put on the white coat there are no substitutions, there are no time outs."

24.7 Atul Gawande

One of my favorite authors is Atul Gawande, who has written about checklists and complications and contributed a wonderful short book entitled *Better: a Surgeon's Notes on Performance* (Fig. 24.8). In this book, Gawande defines what he considers are the three core requirements for success in medicine, those being (1) diligence, the necessity of giving sufficient attention to detail to avoid error and prevail against obstacles; (2) do right, medicine is fundamentally a human profession; and (3) ingenuity, thinking anew, a willingness to recognize failure, and to change.

Furthermore, in *Better*, Gawande provides five suggestions for how to make a worthy difference, that is, how to be a positive deviant in the culture in which you work. What a remarkable theme: how can each of us make a difference among our colleagues? I love these five suggestions:

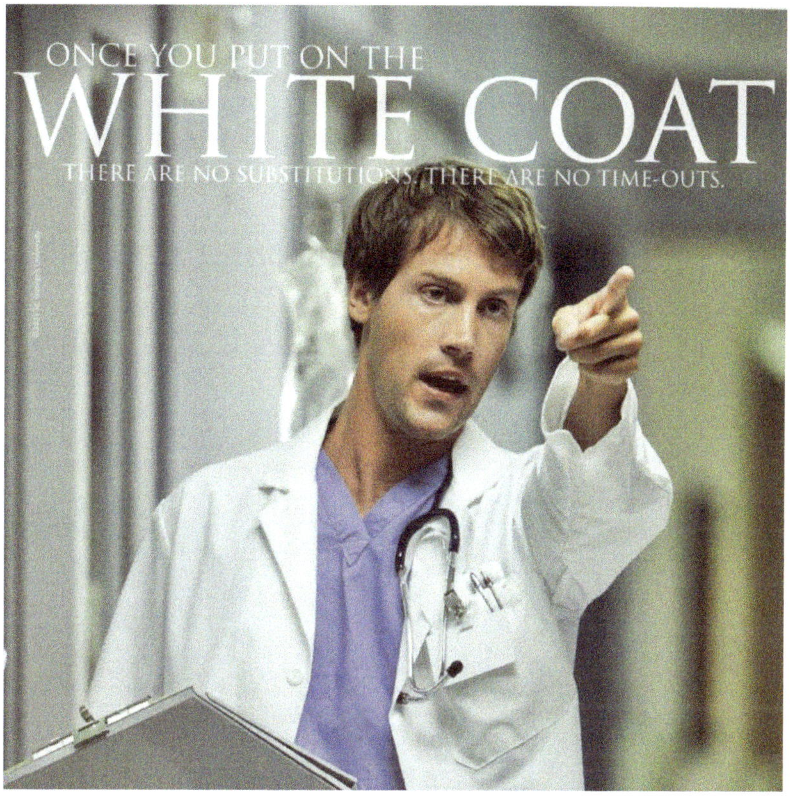

Fig. 24.7 Once you put on the white coat

1. Ask an unscripted question: sometimes you discover the unexpected.
2. Don't complain: resist it; it's boring; it doesn't solve anything: be prepared with something else to discuss.
3. Count something: if you count something you find interesting, you will learn something interesting.
4. Write something: the power of the act of writing or typing.
5. Change—be an early adopter: this is a necessity, with the fast advancement of surgical technology.

24.8 Lessons from a Coach: Part Two

Returning to the basketball theme, John Wooden and his legendary men's basketball team, the UCLA Bruins, won 10 NCAA National Championships, had 4 perfect (undefeated) seasons, and once won 88 straight Division I games (of note, as of this writing, the University of Connecticut women have eclipsed the century mark; 100+ consecutive victories). Much has been written about Coach Wooden—his philosophy, his training schemes, his quotes, his players, and his personality. In my opinion one of his best works is *Wooden on Leadership* (Fig. 24.9), which draws lessons from his private notebooks and focuses on leadership, improving one's performance, exceeding limitations, and achieving "success." The book includes Coach Wooden's "pyramid of success," with the apex of the pyramid (the goal of the pyramid) being "competitive greatness."

With deference to Coach Wooden and with remorse to those who feel that his pyramid is inviolate, I have taken the liberty of modifying his pyramid and have spoken often about what I have termed "the surgery success pyramid," which has been adapted, with apologies, from Coach Wooden (Fig. 24.10). While the five foundational (1st tier) elements remain unchanged (industriousness, friendship, loyalty, cooperation, and enthusiasm), as do the four 2nd tier

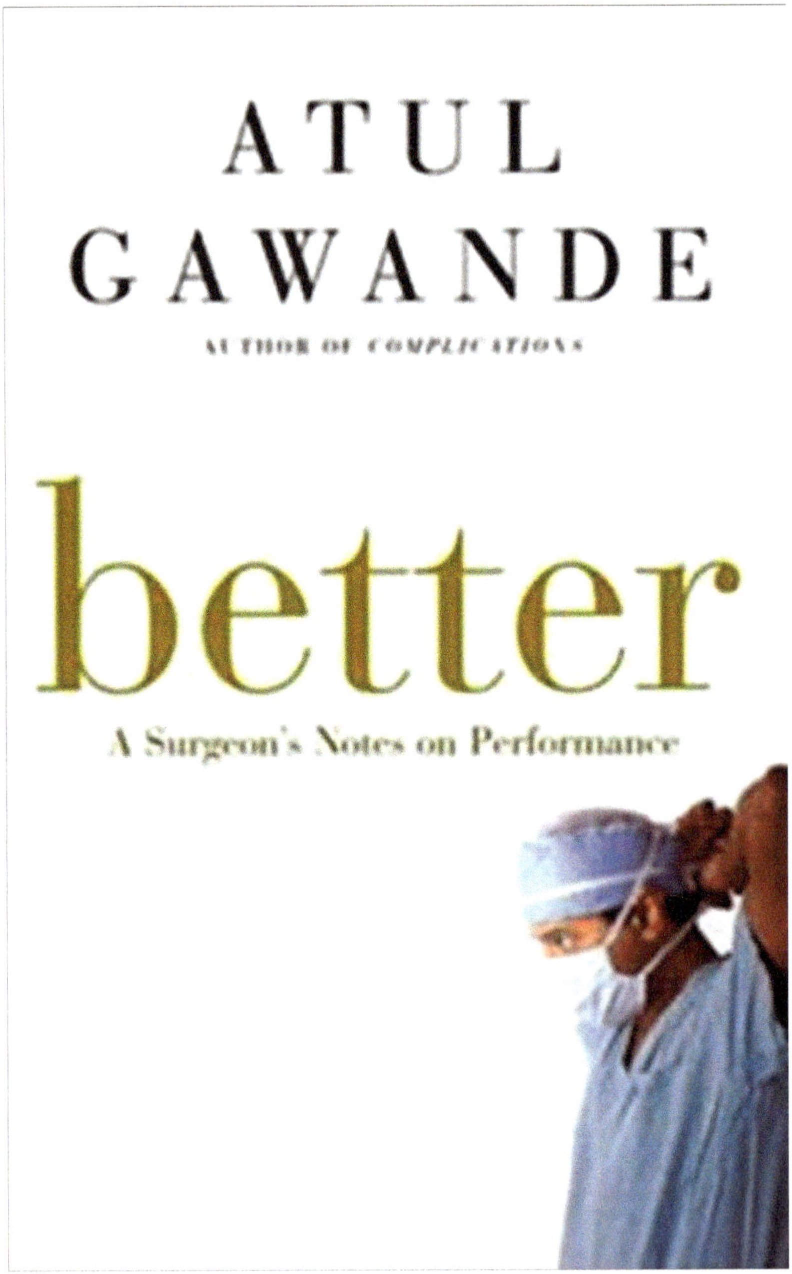

Fig. 24.8 Atul Gawande, *Better: A Surgeon's Notes on Performance*

elements (self-control, alertness, initiative, and intentness), I have modified some of the descriptors within some of the elements to reflect the profession of surgery, as opposed to the activity of basketball.

Take-Home Points

I would like to end with three final concepts, focusing on how to be successful in surgery, either as a medical student or as a surgical resident or as

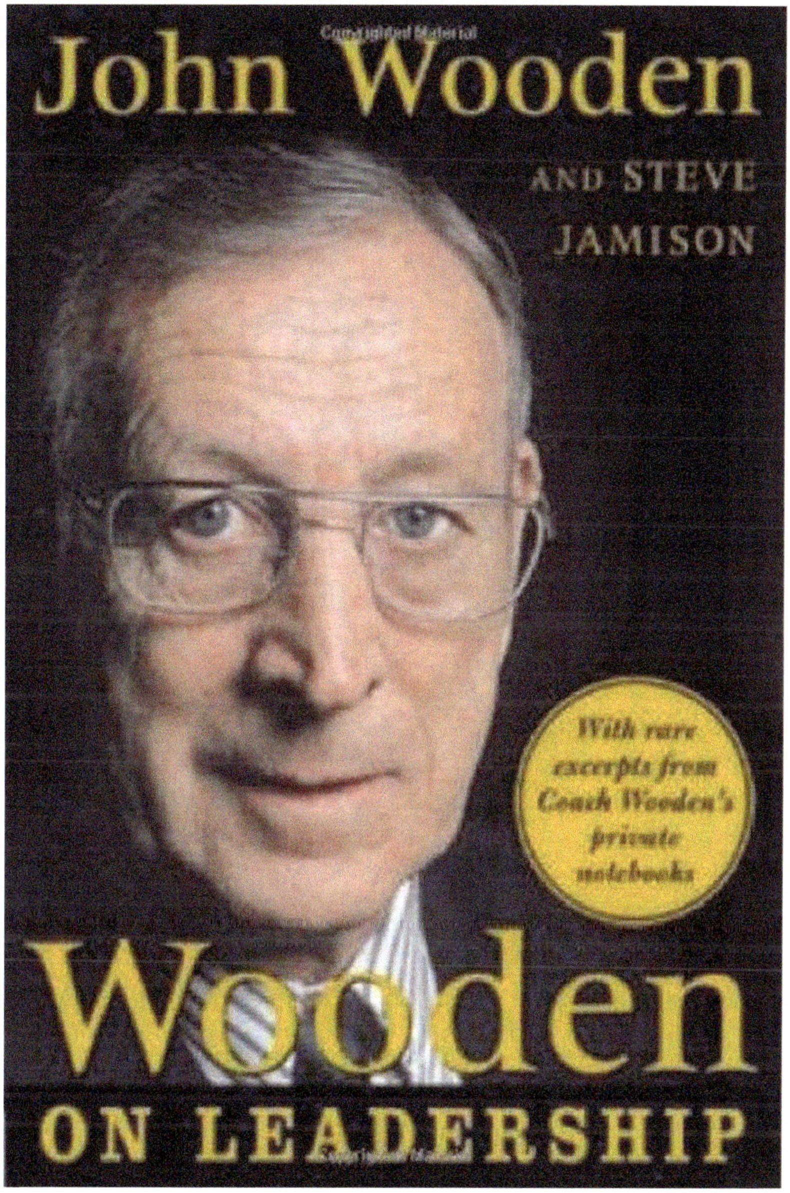

Fig. 24.9 John Wooden: *Wooden on Leadership*

a junior faculty member. I have shown these lists on various occasions, and I am often greeted by wide eye stares, amazement, and hesitancy. Nonetheless, here are my thoughts for how to be a successful medical student (Fig. 24.11), how to be a successful resident (Fig. 24.12), or how to be a successful junior faculty member (Fig. 24.13).

For the medical student, study, practice, or drill 4 h per day on average. No excuses, just do it! Plan to write one paper for the literature per year, perhaps working on case reports or review articles. If you chose to do lab work during medical school, affiliate yourself with a productive laboratory and endeavor to compose a minimum

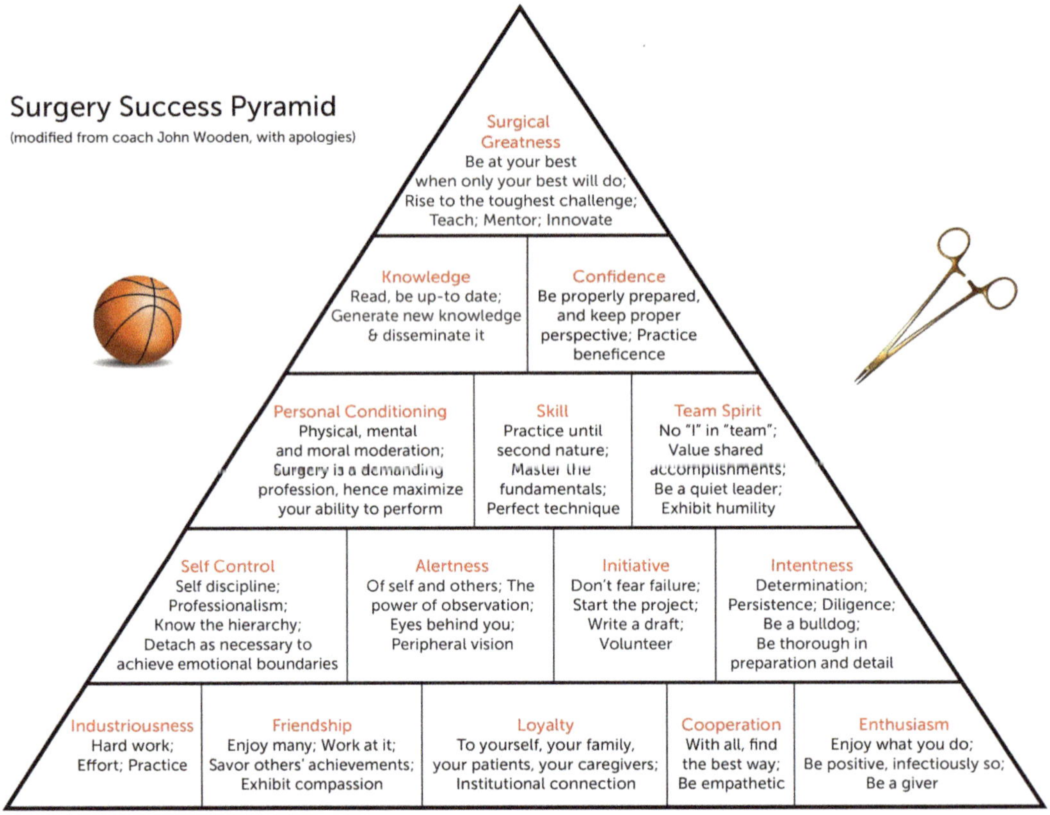

Fig. 24.10 The surgery success pyramid (modified from Coach John Wooden)

Fig. 24.11 How to be a successful student

How to be a successful student

- STUDY/PRACTICE – 4 hours/day; No excuses - period
- Write one paper per year, and a minimum of three per year in the lab (if you choose to do lab work)
- Read journals weekly (NEJM,JAMA) and monthly …
- Grades matter. Be the best medical student you can be!
- Keep a journal or log of all patients, enumerating at least one "item" per case that you learned
- Enjoy your time away from the classroom/hospital, and keep your body fit and in shape
- Do not fall behind on your required tasks: presentations, assignments, case logs, PELS, etc

of three papers per year. Without a doubt, read journals or newsfeeds weekly and monthly. I still get the *New England Journal of Medicine* delivered to my door weekly (old school), and as a medical student, I read *JAMA* at the library each week. With modern technology, this can be accomplished more easily with various news feeds and tables of contents sent directly to your handheld smart phone. Be aware that grades do matter. Try to be the best medical student you can be. Aspire to get elected to the medical honor society, Alpha Omega Alpha. Keep a journal or log of all the patients you see, listing at least one "item" (pearl or oddity) per case that you have learned. Without a doubt enjoy your time away from the hospital or classroom, and exercise, keeping your body fit and in shape. Lastly, do not fall behind on the various required tasks that you have, whether this be presentations, assignments, case logs, patient encounter log system (PELS),

Fig. 24.12 How to be a successful resident

How to be a successful resident

- STUDY/PRACTICE –2 hours/day; No excuses -period
- Write one paper per clinical year, and a minimum of three per year in the lab
- Read journals weekly (NEJM,JAMA) and monthly ...
- Keep a list of processes/ systems/ things that do not work efficiently – will be part of our next White Paper
- Keep a journal or log of all OR cases, enumerating at least one "item" per case that you learned
- Enjoy your time away from the hospital, and keep your body fit and in shape
- Do not fall behind on your required tasks: Work hours, medical records, SCORE, M and M submissions, etc...

Fig. 24.13 How to be a successful junior faculty member

How to be a successful junior faculty member

- Focus on clinical practice and the attainment of mastery level
- Seek out a worthwhile and compatible mentor
- Embark upon new and varied challenges
- Volunteer outside of your comfort zone (say "yes")
- Remember the basics: support stockings (hosiery), maximize retirement benefits and participate in strenuous exercise daily
- Cherish time outside the hospital or clinical setting
- Read: medical and surgical literature and – "great books"
- Teach all comers about the wonders of the human body
- Enjoy the act of writing - contribute to the literature, compose a poem or short story, write a grant, etc.
- Value your colleagues

etc. 4 years of medical school passes in a flash—be the best you can be.

My suggestions for how to be a successful resident are somewhat similar. I am a big fan of deliberate practice and study. Even during residency, one should plan to study or practice at least 2 h a day, on average. Some days this may not be possible, but other days it can be made up for. There should be no excuses for not studying or practicing. In similar fashion to the medical students, plan to write one paper of some form per clinical year and a minimum of three papers per year during your laboratory experience. Also, read journals (weekly and monthly) and take advantage of newsfeeds, etc. Importantly, be a positive deviant. Keep a list of processes, systems, and things that do not work efficiently and pass these on to your residency program director or to your chair of surgery. We rely upon the residents to quickly understand and embrace new technology and innovation, so try to make patient throughput more effective and the surgical experience more satisfying. On every case that you scrub, keep a journal or log, enumerating at least one "item" (clinical pearl, trick, or neat idea) per case that you've learned. It is important to remain active, in shape, and fit. Enjoy your time away from the hospital but make every effort to maintain a high level of physical fitness. Lastly, do not fall behind on the tasks required of your residency: log your work hours, keep up with your assigned medical records, participate in some form of an academic curriculum such as SCORE, submit your M&M lists on time, study for the ABSITE, etc. Residency years similarly pass quickly—you will tell stories of them to others, but you must work hard to launch yourself to the aspirational goal of surgical proficiency and mastery.

For the young faculty member, there certainly are similar suggestions, but the scope of involvement must necessarily be broader and more varied. The young faculty member needs to focus on commencing a practice within the field of their interest and work toward mastery. I would recommend identifying (seeking out) a mentor and working with that individual in some form of a mentee-mentor relationship. It is advisable to take on new and varied challenges (new roles) in the areas of education, research, and administration—the young faculty member should be encouraged to answer in the affirmative (say "yes") when asked to participate in new endeavors, new initiatives, or new challenges. It is quite important to plan ahead for a full career in the field of surgery—hence, (a) wear support stockings or hosiery when faced with long days of standing in the OR,, (b) take advantage of the "miracle" of compound interest and maximize retirement benefits, and (c) develop a regular (daily) strenuous exercise program so as to insure physical fitness. Life outside the hospital or clinical setting is to be valued, promoted, and cherished. I would recommend spending time with family and friends weekly, as being part of a non-medical community is essential. Read the literature—not only in the areas of medicine and surgery but also (broadly defined) "the great books." Do not neglect the responsibility of teaching: find learners in all settings and teach about the human body (anatomy and physiology), the pathology, and the wonders of contemporary surgical techniques. Recognize that you completed university, medical school, and residency by studying the works of others—so enjoy the act of writing: contribute to the literature, compose a poem or short story, write a grant or clinical protocol, etc. Finally, assimilate into your practice setting (hospital, department, practice, division), and value your colleagues—you share a long educational history and a love of surgery. For most of us, there is no more fulfilling life than the life of a surgeon.

Suggested Readings

Carril P, White D. The smart take from the strong. New York: Simon and Schuster; 1997.

Gawande A. Better- a surgeon's notes on performance. New York: Metropolitan Books; 2007.

Gladwell M. Outliers- the story of success. New York: Little, Brown and Co; 2008.

Imber G. Genius on the edge: the bizarre double life of Dr. William Stewart Halsted. New York: Kaplan; 2010.

Wooden J, Jamison S. Wooden on leadership. New York: McGraw-Hill; 2005.

Fundamentals of Managing the Operative Catastrophe

25

Idalid Franco, David L. Hepner, William R. Berry, and Alexander F. Arriaga

25.1 Introduction

There are multiple studies in the literature that suggest management of operative catastrophes is poor, likely because such events are rare to the individual, are associated with a high degree of intensity and uncertainty, and require a high level of coordinated and effective teamwork/crisis resource management [1]. Failure to adhere to best practices during management of an operative catastrophe can be common [2]. Utilizing a structured process in the development and testing of a set of crisis checklists, Arriaga et al. showed a reduction in failure to adhere to critical steps in crisis management and improved team performance during operative catastrophes [3]. As these events are rare and thus difficult to study through randomized clinical trials, studies have tackled these issues through the use of high-fidelity simulation, surveys, and reports of individual clinical case experience. Although other high-stakes fields, such as aviation, have long embraced standardized written procedures as a means to reduce errors and improve performance in critical situations, healthcare has been slower to embrace cognitive aids in high-risk, high-stress situations, possibly due to an ingrained culture which views utilization of such tools as deficiencies in medical competency. Yet, there is growing evidence to support the use of cognitive aids, such as crisis checklists and emergency manuals, to improve clinician and team performance in addition to patient outcomes [4].

The purpose of this chapter is to describe some of the most common operating room catastrophes with supporting evidence on diagnosis and management found in the medical literature for members of the surgical team. It would be impossible to cover all aspects of such a broad topic, for which dedicated books and chapters have been written on regarding individual

I. Franco
Harvard Medical School, Boston, MA, USA

D. L. Hepner
Department of Anesthesiology, Perioperative and Pain Medicine, Harvard Medical School, Brigham and Women's Hospital, Boston, MA, USA

Ariadne Labs, Boston, MA, USA

W. R. Berry
Ariadne Labs, Boston, MA, USA

Center for Surgery and Public Health, Boston, MA, USA

Department of Health Policy and Management, Harvard School of Public Health, Boston, MA, USA

A. F. Arriaga (✉)
Department of Anesthesiology, Perioperative and Pain Medicine, Harvard Medical School, Brigham and Women's Hospital, Boston, MA, USA

Department of Anesthesiology and Critical Care, University of Pennsylvania Health System, Philadelphia, PA, USA
e-mail: aarriaga@post.harvard.edu

F. Palazzo (ed.), *Fundamentals of General Surgery*, https://doi.org/10.1007/978-3-319-75656-1_25

catastrophes and principles of crisis management. Nevertheless, we intend to present high-yield potentially lifesaving information for some of the most common operative catastrophes encountered by surgeons and suggest the reader to become familiar with the availability and use of key resources including crisis checklists (available on www.projectcheck.org/crisis) and emergency manuals (available at www.emergencymanuals.org).

25.2 General Concepts

Before we dive into the specific details for management of individual emergencies, it is essential to discuss the fundamentals that are (nearly) universal to any operative catastrophe. The same initial steps are highlighted in many cognitive aids available for addressing emergency situations, which we hope will become second nature to the reader by the end of this chapter, including calling for help, designating a crisis manager/leader, and requesting additional resources that are needed. These steps should be considered instinctively and without delay to patient care. Of note, the use of a "checklist reader" has been shown in simulated emergency studies to assist the leader in executing all critical steps in a crisis situation by removing the added cognitive burden of reading the checklist and in that way allowing the leader to focus fully on gathering clinical information and effectively managing team communication and coordination [5, 6].

The following section will provide the technical and practice considerations when dealing with an operative catastrophe. These situations, which may present with non-specific signs, pose time-sensitive diagnostic and management decisions to be recalled by even the most experienced clinician. It is therefore our goal to frame the events below in a format that includes a brief introduction, information for clinical diagnosis, and guideline-based treatment recommendations that can be quickly referenced during a crisis situation.

25.3 Technical/Practical Considerations/Safety Precautions

25.3.1 Advanced Cardiovascular Life Support

Advanced cardiovascular life support (ACLS) guidelines are routinely updated by the American Heart Association (AHA). In addition, there are "special circumstances of resuscitation" (e.g., cardiac arrest in pregnancy, cardiac arrest from local anesthetic toxicity). The interested reader is strongly encouraged to review the guidelines that support the popular ACLS "pocket cards" commonly available [7, 8]. It is important to note that knowledge of guidelines alone does not translate to adequate performance during critical events and retention of ACLS knowledge and skills are poor among healthcare providers [9–12]. Yet, even in these studies, those with training had less deviations from protocol illustrating the importance of initial training, periodic reinforcement of skills, and availability of structured guidelines. In this section, we will review some of the most fundamental emergencies specific to advanced cardiovascular life support, namely, unstable bradycardia, unstable tachycardia, and cardiac arrest, providing the surgeon with the skills needed to diagnose and manage these catastrophic operative events through structured, evidence-based guidelines. While the section below is based on the latest guidelines at the time this chapter was written, guidelines such as those from the AHA on ACLS are frequently updated. When a surgeon is integrating the section below together with his/her institution-specific protocols, a quick search for the latest ACLS protocols is prudent.

25.3.1.1 Bradycardia: Unstable

Introduction

There are numerous potential causes of bradycardia, ranging from electrical disturbances (e.g., heart block) medication-related causes (e.g., beta-blocker overdose, side effect from certain anesthetic/analgesic agents) or anatomical reflex manifestations (e.g., carotid sinus reflex, oculocardiac reflex, von Bezold-Jarisch reflex, or other phenomena that may be referred to vaguely as a "vagal response"). Additionally, a lower heart rate can be a common phenomenon in certain populations, including athletes or patients on chronic beta-blocking agents, resulting in baseline heart rates in the 40s–50s, without the symptoms or concerns associated with unstable bradycardia. In the general adult population, however, normal heart rate is generally expected to remain within the range of 60–100 beats per minute (bpm). Given this variability in expected heart rate, in conjunction with the understanding that preoperative patient anxiety can cause tachycardia and anesthetics may cause a degree of bradycardia, patient context should be considered when interpreting the heart rate (i.e., unexplained drop in heart rate more than 20% of the patient's baseline, especially if the resulting rate is below 50 bpm). Unstable bradycardia can be viewed and approached as an operative catastrophe when the low heart rate is coupled with signs and symptoms of hemodynamic instability, such as low blood pressure, acute and otherwise unexplained decline in mental status of an awake patient, or signs of shock and cardiac compromise. In these situations, the surgeon, anesthesiologist, and operating room team must maintain open and coordinated communication to effectively diagnose and treat unstable bradycardia. The American Heart Association guidelines for bradycardia outline detailed and evidence-based steps for management of this condition, and cognitive aids formatted for the operating room are available.

Clinical/Diagnosis

As described above, unstable bradycardia may be considered in the setting of a drop in heart rate to less than 50 bpm, with resulting hemodynamic instability manifested as a drop in blood pressure below normal range (hypotension), signs of shock (resulting in organ hypoperfusion), cardiac compromise (presenting as acute heart failure) or chest discomfort (associated with ischemia), and acute changes in mental status [7, 8]. This definition, which is based on the definition used by the AHA as part of the ACLS guidelines, may not be fully applicable in patients under general anesthesia who are unable to communicate symptoms of ischemic heart pain or acute changes in mental status. In these situations, it is essential for surgeons to communicate with anesthesiologists to (1) gain a full understanding of the clinical signs and symptoms, (2) convey information on what has acutely been done or given that may explain the bradycardia, and (3) promptly address and remove potential causes. The surgeon should keep in mind that placement of abdominal retractors can cause a vagal response, resulting in bradycardia, that can be partially addressed by loosening or removing the retractors until adequate hemodynamics have been restored.

Treatment

The goals of treatment for unstable bradycardia revolve around restoring hemodynamic stability to prevent organ hypoperfusion and cardiovascular collapse. As with any operative catastrophe, an immediate call for help, request of a code cart, and assignment of a crisis manager/leader should all be done without delaying treatment. Depending on the institution, the "code cart" and defibrillator/pacer might not be attached to each other, but the person getting these items should understand that both can be essential to the management of this situation (as well as other ACLS scenarios). The surgeon can also be in constant communication with the anesthesiologist regarding the patient's hemodynamic status and clinical condition including ventilation and oxygenation. The surgeon can stop the surgical stimulation if present (i.e., removing abdominal retractors or desufflation of the abdomen in laparoscopic cases). The anesthesiologist may increase the FiO2 to 100% and ensure the airway is maintained while considering the initial drug of choice. While glycopyrrolate is sometimes given for cases of mild, less concerning bradycardia, the initial drug of choice for severe/unstable bradycardia is atropine. Although certain clinical conditions, such as a complete heart block or recent heart transplant, may not benefit from atropine, this drug has long been listed in ACLS guidelines and in many instances can be an appropriate choice. As this is being done, the nursing team can obtain the code cart and pacer/defibrillator and then connect this device to the patient to allow for transcutaneous pacing. If atropine is not effective, the decision can be made to initiate transcutaneous pacing or utilize alternative drug choices such as an epinephrine or dopamine infusion. Expert consultation should be considered, as transvenous pacing might be necessary. It is also critical that other causes of bradycardia are simultaneously investigated including overdose of beta-blockers or digoxin, both of which have available pharmaceutical treatments. Surgeons are encouraged to familiarize themselves with the defibrillator/pacer of their institution as the device settings differ slightly across different models.

25.3.1.2 Tachycardia: Unstable

Introduction

Similar to bradycardia, there are many potential causes for tachycardia, including pain, fever, hypovolemia, and arrhythmias. It is therefore helpful to put the patient's observed heart rate into the context of the clinical scenario, including the baseline heart rate and potential secondary causes of the tachycardia that would not be addressed by simply returning the patient's heart rate into a normal adult range of 60–100 bpm. An overall clinical evaluation, including assessment of the heart rhythm, is crucial to differentiating the cause of the tachycardia. This distinction is vital in allowing the providers to respond with appropriate and timely treatment. This section will describe the diagnosis and management of unstable tachycardia, described by the AHA as tachycardia with "hypotension, acutely altered mental status, signs of shock, ischemic chest discomfort, and acute heart failure" [7, 8].

Clinical/Diagnosis

In the case of unstable tachycardia, it is important to determine the heart rhythm, in addition to the other patient vital signs including the presence of a palpable pulse, to decide on the best course of action. Determining if there is a narrow versus wide complex and regular versus irregular rhythm can guide appropriate treatment options, and as such providers are encouraged to develop a familiarity with the distinct electrocardiographic features of tachycardia (i.e., sinus tachycardia, narrow-complex supraventricular tachycardia [QRS <0.12 s], and wide-complex tachycardia [QRS ≥ 0.12 s]). In the case of a ventricular fibrillation or ventricular tachycardia without a blood pressure/pulse, the scenario should be managed according to the cardiac arrest guidelines listed in the following section. In other cases of unstable tachycardia, immediate synchronized cardioversion is the initial treatment of choice.

Treatment

As noted above, outside of ventricular fibrillation and pulseless ventricular tachycardia, the treatment for unstable tachycardia is immediate synchronized cardioversion. Synchronized cardioversion is defined as the delivery of a shock on the R-wave of the patient's QRS complex, avoiding the delivery of a shock on the refractory period symbolized by the T-wave of the patient's ECG rhythm, which can cause an "R on T" phenomenon, leading to a potentially lethal arrhythmia. As a surgeon, it is important to familiarize yourself ahead of time with the defibrillator/pacer manufacturer/model being used at your institution. Different machines have different button types to engage the synchronization mode. The time of unstable tachycardia is not the best time to refresh oneself or learn the buttons of the particular machine at your institution. An example of the machine steps, spelled out for the manufacturer/model of a particular institution, can be found on the "tachycardia unstable" entry of the "operating room crisis checklists" for the Brigham and Women's Hospital [13]. A general guideline of biphasic doses is given in the ACLS guidelines for "Adult Tachycardia (with Pulse)," all with increased joules delivered incrementally if prior attempts were unsuccessful [7, 8]. An additional consideration is the use of intravenous adenosine given via the access area closest to the heart in scenarios where the rhythm is narrow complex and regular.

This should only be considered if administration will not delay cardioversion. Communication between the surgeon and the team is critical during management of unstable tachycardia. Potentially reversible causes of the tachycardia can be sought by team members at the same time as stabilizing measures are being done including supplemental oxygen, determining adequate ventilation and oxygen saturation, monitoring blood pressure, and establishing intravenous access. As with any operative catastrophe, immediately calling for help, requesting a code cart with pacer/defibrillator, and assignment of a crisis manager/leader are critical first steps. In addition, a 12-lead ECG can also aid in diagnostics. Expert consultation can be considered to assist the operating room team and can help determine the need for additional antiarrhythmic medications or maneuvers once the patient has been stabilized.

25.3.1.3 Cardiac Arrest

Introduction

An unanticipated cardiac arrest can be an acutely stressful situation for any surgeon and operating room team. This section will focus on unintentional cardiac arrest. Intentional circulatory arrest, such as that which is sometimes needed for certain cardiac or vascular procedures, is beyond the scope of this chapter and will not be discussed. In addition, post-cardiac arrest care and the role of therapeutic hypothermia are ongoing discussions in the literature, and the reader is encouraged to learn about the policies in place for these situations at their individual institution as well as be familiar with the most recent studies on these scenarios.

Frustrations with intraoperative cardiac arrest management have been described for nearly a century, dating back to the 1920s [14]. In a famous 1924 article published in *Anesthesia & Analgesia*, the prominent surgeon Dr. W. Wayne Babcock posed the question "Have you a plan of action so developed that the right thing is always done in the emergency and time is not fritted away with useless or non-essential details?" Dr. Babcock described his personal experiences in the OR and concluded the article by stating "These experiences but emphasize the importance of an efficient routine instantly available for resuscitation in every operating room." Nearly 30 years later, another prominent physician who began his career as a surgical trainee and finished his residency training in anesthesiology, Dr. Peter Safar, became known as the "father of CPR" for his life's work on cardiopulmonary resuscitation [15]. This section will review the key details in the diagnosis and management of cardiac arrest as an operative catastrophe. A key initial consideration for a patient in cardiac arrest is determining whether the patient has a shockable or non-shockable rhythm. Additional considerations on special circumstances of resuscitation are also addressed in the AHA guidelines, including topics on pregnancy and local anesthetic systemic toxicity, which will not be covered in this section [16]. The following is a review of the 2015 American Heart Association guidelines for cardiopulmonary resuscitation and emergency cardiovascular care, which was updated through an in-depth evidence review process and is stratified by the presence of shockable vs. non-shockable heart rhythms.

Clinical/Diagnosis

It is important to look at the heart rhythm in a patient in cardiac arrest, keeping in mind that there are four rhythms that can cause cardiac arrest and can be grouped into shockable and non-shockable rhythms. The first two types of cardiac arrest, asystole and pulseless electrical activity (PEA), are considered together as non-shockable rhythms. Asystole refers to the complete absence of electrical and mechanical activity of the heart, while PEA is the presence of an electrocardiographic rhythm that is unable to sustain the mechanical contractions needed to produce a measurable pulse or blood pressure [7]. Both of these situations result in an inability of the heart to perfuse adequately and can lead to both cerebral and cardiac demise. The shockable rhythms include ventricular fibrillation, a disorganized electrical activity, and pulseless ventricular tachycardia, an organized electrical activity of the ventricles, neither of which is able to generate sufficient forward flow of blood by the heart [7].

As with any emergency situation, a crucial step in the efficient diagnosis and treatment includes an evaluation and removal of potential underlying causes in conjunction with treatment and restoration of hemodynamic stability. In any case of cardiac arrest, the team must consider the "H's and T's" that comprise some potentially reversible causes, including hydrogen ion (acidosis), hypo-/hyperkalemia, hypothermia, hypovolemia, hypoxia, tamponade (i.e., cardiac tamponade), tension pneumothorax, thrombosis (pulmonary, coronary), and toxins. Targeted treatment in each of these cases is essential, and recall of the H's and T's in a stressful environment can be prompted by the use of cognitive aids such as a crisis checklist/emergency manual.

Treatment

AHA guidelines emphasize high-quality CPR as the foundation of successful ACLS, in addition to defibrillation for the shockable rhythms VF and pulseless VT, which can significantly increase the chance of survival to hospital discharge [8]. As with other operative catastrophes, immediately calling for help, requesting a code cart, and assignment of a crisis manager/leader should all be done without delaying treatment. A backboard, placed under the patient in supine position, can be considered to assist with the quality of CPR. Additionally, FiO_2 can be increased to 100% to improve oxygen delivery. In shockable rhythms, an initial shock delivery via the defibrillator is recommended in 2 min intervals with intervening high-quality CPR described as "hard and fast" chest compressions to a depth of 2 in. at 100–120/min while allowing full chest recoil. The person performing chest compressions should be rotated every 2 min to avoid a decrease in quality due to fatigue. While this is occurring, the anesthesiologist or an available team member can monitor the physiological response to CPR delivery, such as the patient's end-tidal CO_2 and/or intra-arterial diastolic pressure. Interruptions of chest compressions must be minimized and excessive ventilation avoided. In either shockable or non-shockable rhythm, epinephrine should be given. In cases of refractory VF or pulseless VT, that is, persistent or recurrent after one's shock, an antiarrhythmic such as amiodarone can be given, which is done to "facilitate the restoration and maintenance of spontaneous perfusing rhythm in concert with the shock termination" [8]. Communication is critical for the successful implementation of all steps, including tasks such as chest compressions, maintenance of the patient's airway, optimization of vascular access, timekeeping, and the other steps noted above. Defibrillator settings differ slightly by model, and the surgeon is encouraged to familiarize themselves with utilization of the devices at their institution prior to an emergency situation. Consistent reevaluation of patient status is recommended, with physiological clues such as a sudden increase of $ETCO_2$ to >40 mmHg potentially indicating a return of spontaneous circulation.

25.3.2 Failed Airway

25.3.2.1 Introduction

Much of the airway management for non-head and neck cases (such as non-tracheostomy, non-otolaryngology cases) falls within the purview of the anesthesiologist. Accordingly, there are guidelines for difficult airway management, most of which involves modalities typically done by an anesthesia provider. The American Society of Anesthesiologists (ASA) has difficult airway guidelines [17], and the Difficult Airway Society has published guidelines on this topic as well [18]. Nevertheless, the surgeon needs to be prepared for the urgent need of a surgical airway. The surgeon should therefore have a basic familiarity with difficult airway guidelines to strengthen their situational awareness of the potentially urgent need for a surgical airway. There is value in a surgeon who knows where the closest difficult airway cart and emergency surgical airway equipment/kits can be found. It is not uncommon for a patient who is difficult to ventilate and intubate to also be a difficult surgical airway. This section will describe the management of a failed airway through a cricothyrotomy. *Cummings Otolaryngology* defines a cricothyrotomy as "the establishment of a surgical opening into the airway through the cricothyroid membrane (CTM) and placement of a tube for ventilation" [19]. The importance of understanding the diagnosis and management of a difficult airway and emergent treatment is critical to the practicing surgeon, as operative catastrophes related to inadequate airway and ventilation have continuously been found to be some of the leading causes of serious and life-threatening intraoperative and perioperative complications [1, 20, 21].

25.3.2.2 Clinical/Diagnosis

ASA practice guidelines acknowledge the variation of definitions of "difficult airway" in the literature and define this term as "the clinical situation in which a conventionally trained anesthesiologist experiences difficulty with facemask ventilation of the upper airway, difficulty with tracheal intubation, or both." They provide a description of a "failed intubation" as "placement of the endotracheal tube fails after multiple attempts." Similarly, one could think of a "failed airway" as the failure to achieve a controlled airway after multiple attempts by an airway expert (or an experienced anesthesiologist). Failed airway, resulting from an inability to intubate and ventilate, has been estimated to occur in the range of 0.01–2 per 10,000 patients with difficult endotracheal intubation ranging between 5 and 35 per 10,000 patients and difficult mask ventilation at an incidence of about 5% [19]. A failed airway can quickly lead to anoxic brain injury and death. The surgeon and operating room team are encouraged to be prepared to quickly and accurately diagnose and address this situation and provide a mechanism for adequate ventilation and oxygenation when less invasive techniques have failed. A key piece of information in the management of a failed airway is whether the patient is able to receive adequate ventilation (such as bag-mask ventilation) while further decisions are being made (ranging from awakening the patient to considering alternative approaches to securing the airway). Below, we will describe and illustrate the necessary steps for management of a failed airway including creating a surgical airway via a cricothyrotomy while understanding that other invasive techniques may also be considered by the team (e.g., needle cricothyroidotomy).

25.3.2.3 Treatment

In a failed airway scenario, immediately calling for help, designating a crisis manager/leader, and requesting a difficult airway cart and video laryngoscope are all essential steps. If ventilation is inadequate and an experienced anesthesiologist has failed to achieve a controlled airway after multiple attempts, the surgeon should communicate with the team and prepare for the possibility that a surgical airway will be urgently needed. While the anesthesiologist continues to attempt to optimize ventilation, possibly through placement of a laryngeal mask airway, alternative supraglottic devices, or other approaches, the surgeon should begin to consider what is available to prep the neck (such as the prep solution available for the surgical case) and how to obtain supplies needed for an urgent surgical airway. Cummings describes a modified "rapid five-step technique" which is "simple to learn and faster in obtaining a surgical airway." This technique is comprised of (1) Identifying landmarks and stabilizing the airway, (2) making a vertical skin incision, (3) making a horizontal incision through the cricothyroid membrane, (4) inserting a clamp to spread and elevate the airway, and (5) inserting a tracheostomy tube or small endotracheal tube. The *Manual of Emergency Airway Management* provides detailed illustrations of the technique used for an emergency cricothyrotomy (Figs. 25.1, 25.2, 25.3, 25.4, 25.5, 25.6, 25.7) [22]. (Used with permission from Walls RM, Murphy MF, editors. Manual of emergency airway management; Fourth Edition. Philadelphia: Lippincott Williams & Wilkins; 2013).

While ventilation status may change over the course of treatment, which alters the acuity of the situation, a surgeon who communicates well and is prepared for the possibility of a surgical airway can be a life-saving member of this critical scenario.

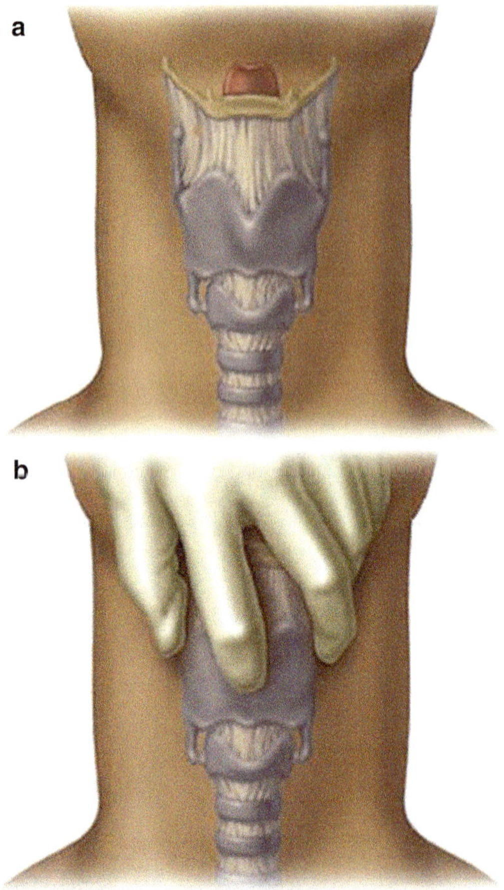

Fig. 25.1 (a) Surface anatomy of the airway. (b) The thumb and long finger immobilize the superior cornua of the larynx; the index finger is used to palpate the cricothyroid membrane. (Used with permission from Walls RM, Murphy MF, editors. Manual of emergency airway management; Fourth Edition. Philadelphia: Lippincott Williams & Wilkins; 2013)

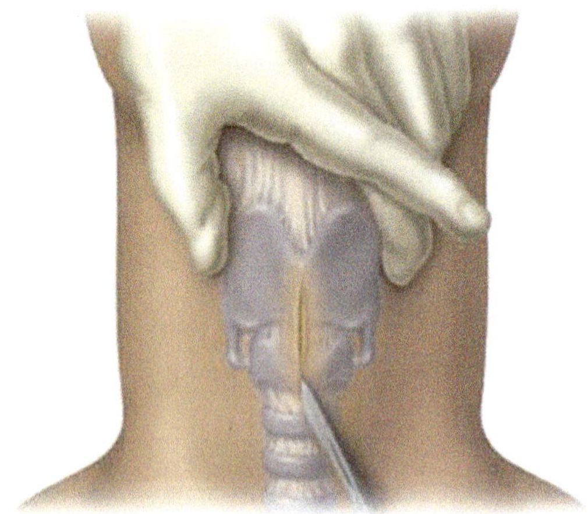

Fig. 25.2 With the index finger moved to the side but continued firm immobilization of the larynx, a vertical midline skin incision is made, down to the depth of the laryngeal structures. (Used with permission from Walls RM, Murphy MF, editors. Manual of emergency airway management; Fourth Edition. Philadelphia: Lippincott Williams & Wilkins; 2013)

25.3.3 Intraoperative Emergencies Where the Diagnosis Is Unclear

25.3.3.1 Hypotension and Hypoxemia

Introduction

Hypotension and hypoxemia present a particularly difficult situation for operating room teams due to their broad differential and subsequent difficulty for accurate and efficient diagnosis and treatment. In these situations, clinical judgment relative to the patient's history, physical exam findings, anesthetics given, and operating room course is key to adequate assessment and optimal treatment. When faced with situations where the diagnosis is unclear, especially when multiple abnormalities in signs and symptoms are observed, it is important to understand the abnormality representing the primary problem as this will prevent unnecessary or invasive procedures that can cause harm to the patient or delay of appropriate treatment. Within the incident reports for 4000 cases of the Australian Incident Monitoring Study (AIMS), 438 reports included the words "hypotension," "cardiovascular collapse," or "cardiac arrest" (~11%), and 706 contained the word "desaturation" (~18%) [23, 24]. In both hypotension and hypoxemia, there were multiple potential causes for the observed abnormality, with other associated signs and symptoms. The use of a structured algorithm was considered to have resulted in a better and/or more prompt resolution in 6% of hypotension cases and 15% of hypoxemic cases. It is known that both of these operative catastrophes have the potential to result in irreversible damage to organs leading to a high degree of morbidity and mortality. Thus, this time-critical need for efficient and

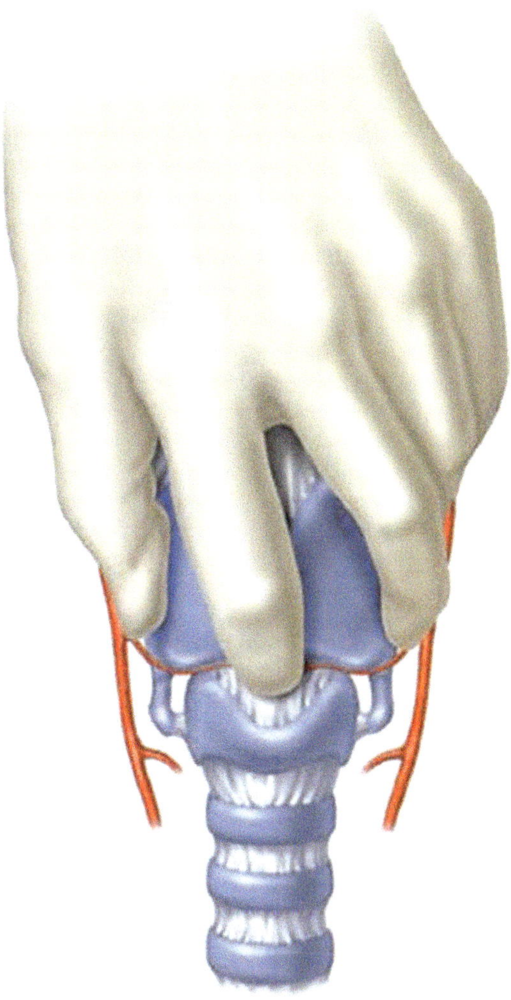

Fig. 25.3 With the skin incised, the index finger can now directly palpate the cricothyroid membrane. (Used with permission from Walls RM, Murphy MF, editors. Manual of emergency airway management; Fourth Edition. Philadelphia: Lippincott Williams & Wilkins; 2013)

effective treatment highlights the importance for the surgeon to have a structured set of key steps to guide the differential diagnosis and treatment management considerations inherent to unclear/sustained hypotension/hypoxemia.

Clinical/Diagnosis and Treatment

Due to the broad differential for these common scenarios, we present this section in the format of crisis checklists that have been adopted by an institution. Figures 25.8 and 25.9 are examples

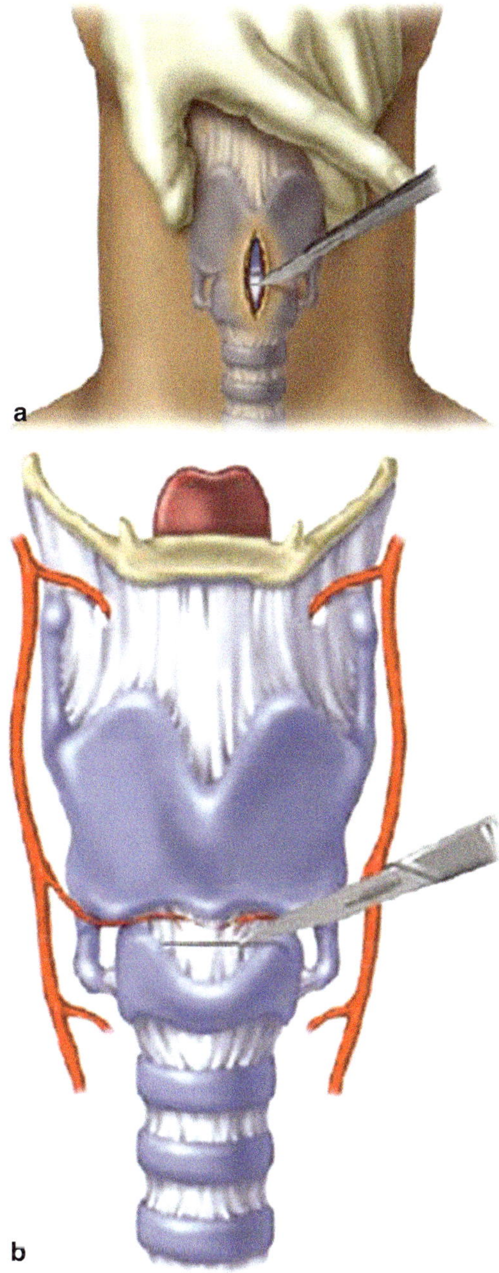

Fig. 25.4 (**a**) A horizontal membrane incision is made near the inferior edge of the cricothyroid membrane. The index finger may be swung aside or may remain in the wound, palpating the inferior edge of the thyroid cartilage, to guide the scalpel to the membrane. (**b**) A low cricothyroid incision avoids the superior cricothyroid vessels, which run transversely near the top of the membrane. (Used with permission from Walls RM, Murphy MF, editors. Manual of emergency airway management; Fourth Edition. Philadelphia: Lippincott Williams & Wilkins; 2013)

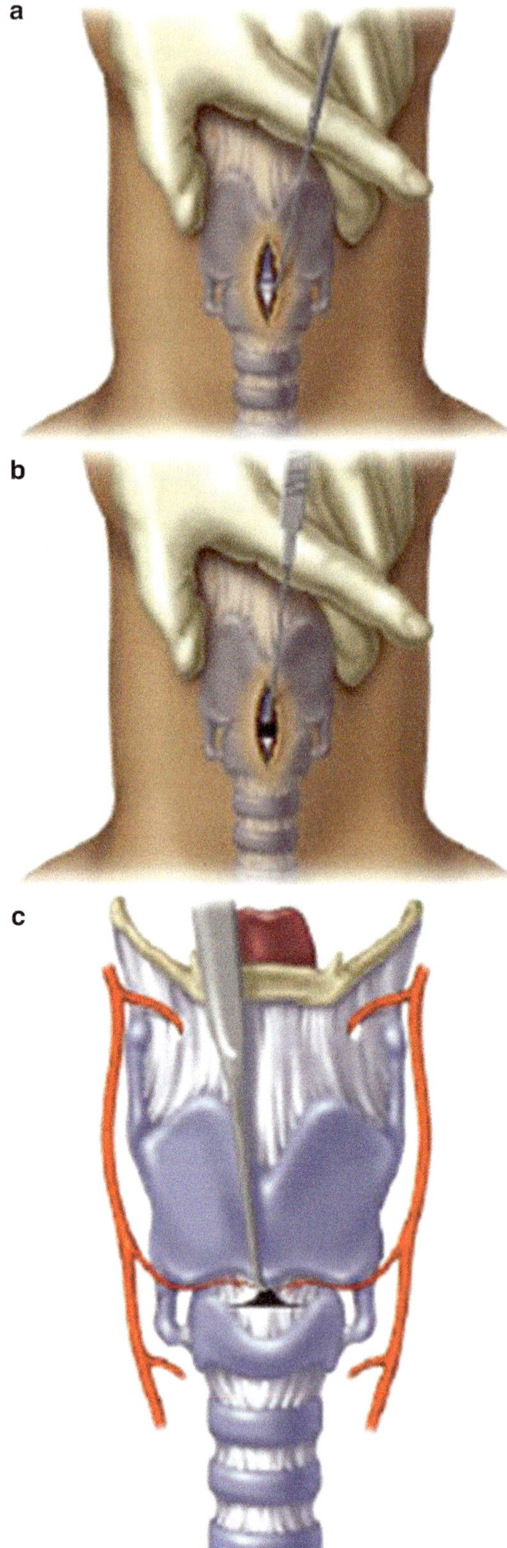

Fig. 25.5 (**a**) The tracheal hook is oriented transversely during insertion. (**b**, **c**) After insertion, cephalad traction is applied to the inferior margin of the thyroid cartilage. (Used with permission from Walls RM, Murphy MF, editors. Manual of emergency airway management; Fourth Edition. Philadelphia: Lippincott Williams & Wilkins; 2013)

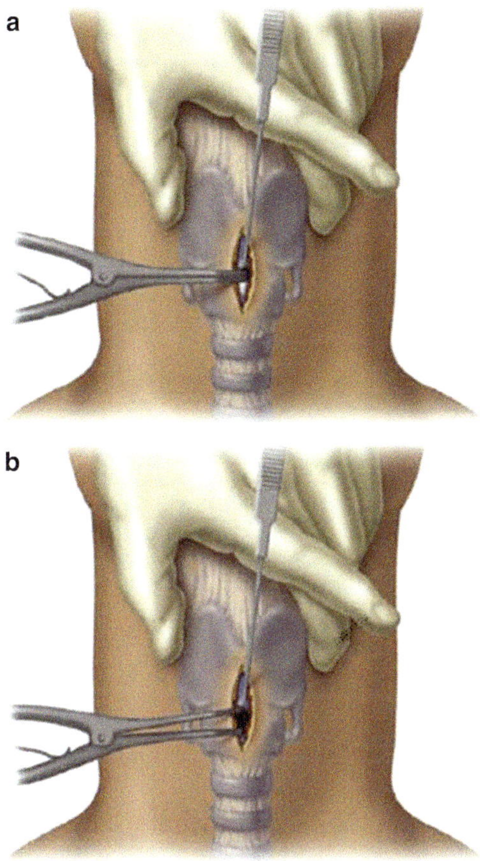

Fig. 25.6 (**a**) The Trousseau dilator is inserted a short distance into the incision. (**b**) In this orientation, the dilator enlarges the opening vertically, the crucial dimension. (Used with permission from Walls RM, Murphy MF, editors. Manual of emergency airway management; Fourth Edition. Philadelphia: Lippincott Williams & Wilkins; 2013)

from (the crisis checklists for structured approaches in the setting of hypotension and hypoxemia (the crisis checklists in their native format are available at www.projectcheck.org/crisis). In both cases, one can see that there are many causes to consider. There can be benefit of a team running through these causes together and attempting to narrow the differential, similar to how one would run though the "H's and T's" in cardiac arrest".

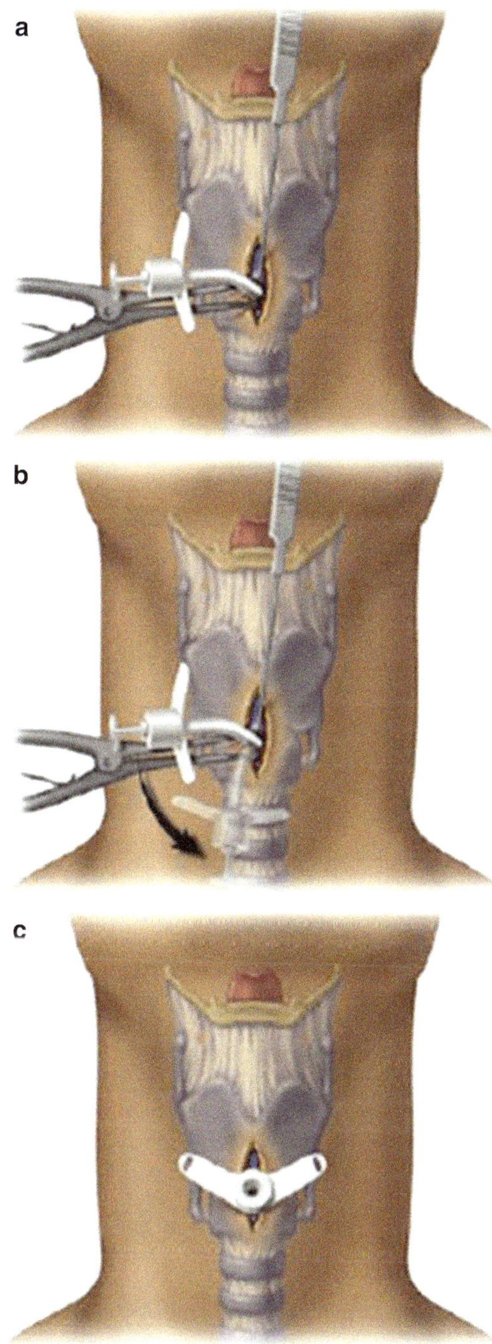

Fig. 25.7 (**a**) Insertion of the tracheostomy tube. (**b**) Rotation of the Trousseau dilator to orient the blades longitudinally in the airway facilitates passage of the tracheostomy tube. (**c**) Tracheostomy tube fully inserted, instruments removed. (Used with permission from Walls RM, Murphy MF, editors. Manual of emergency airway management; Fourth Edition. Philadelphia: Lippincott Williams & Wilkins; 2013)

9 **Hypotension**

Unexplained drop in blood pressure refractory to initial treatment

START

1. **Call for help and a code cart**
   - **Ask:** *"who will be the crisis manager?"*
2. **Check...**
   - Pulse
   - Blood pressure
   - Equipment
   - Heart rate
     - If BRADYCARDIA, *go to* ▷ CHKLST 3
   - Rhythm
     - If VF / VT, *go to* ▷ CHKLST 5
     - If PEA, *go to* ▷ CHKLST 4
3. **Run IV fluids wide open**
4. **Give vasopressors** and titrate to response
   - MILD hypotension: Give ephedrine or phenylephrine
   - SIGNIFICANT/REFRACTORY hypotension: Give epinephrine bolus, consider starting epinephrine infusion
5. **Turn FiO_2 to 100%** and **turn down volatile anesthetics**
6. **Inspect surgical field for bleeding**
   - If BLEEDING, *go to* ▷ CHKLST 8
7. **Consider actions...**
   - Place patient in Trendelenberg position
   - Obtain additional IV access
   - Place arterial line
8. **Consider causes...**

DRUG DOSES and treatments

Ephedrine:	5 – 25 mg IV, repeat as needed
Phenylephrine:	100 – 500 mcg IV,repeat as needed
Epinephrine	BOLUS: 5 – 10 mcg IV INFUSION: 0.1 – 10 mcg/kg/min IV

Operative field
- Mechanical or surgical manipulation
- :Insufflation during laparoscopy
- Retraction
- Vagal stimulation
- Vascular compression

Unaccounted blood loss
- Blood in suction canister
- Bloody sponges
- Blood on the floor
- Internal bleeding

Drugs / Allergy
- Anaphylaxis *go to* ▷ CHKLST 2
- Recent drugs given
- Dose error
- Drugs used on the field (i.e., Intravascular injection of local anesthetic drugs)
- Wrong drug

Breathing
- Increased PEEP
- Hypoventilation
- Hypoxia *go to* ▷ CHKLST 10
- Persistent hyoerventilation
- Pneumothorax
- Pulmonary edema

Circulation
- Air embolism *go to* ▷ CHKLST 1
- Bradycardia *go to* ▷ CHKLST 3
- Malignant hyperthermia *go to* ▷ CHKLST 11
- Tachycardia *go to* ▷ CHKLST 12
- Bone cementing (methylmethacrylate effect)
- Myocardial ischemia
- Emboli (pulmonary, fat, septic, amniotic,CO_2)
- Severe sepsis
- Tamponade

9

All reasonable precautions have been taken to verify the information contained in this publication. The responsibility for the interpretation and use of the materials lies with the reader. Revised July 2013 (072413.1)

Fig. 25.8 Crisis checklist for hypotension. In Ariadne Labs. Operating Room Crisis Checklists. With permission. A version from the Brigham and Women's Hospital is also available at: www.projectcheck.org/crisis. Image compressed to meet publication requirements. For native version, see URL provided. Accessed April 23, 2017

25.3.4 Other Emergencies

As noted above, the goal of this chapter was to familiarize the surgeon with some common operative catastrophes that every surgeon should know. However, we hope that this chapter also encourages the reader to obtain familiarity with other operative emergencies that simply could not be covered due to the space constraints. Hemorrhage, for example, is an operating room emergency that crosses many different disciplines (surgery, obstetrics, anesthesia, nursing, hematology, and potentially trauma, vascular, interventional radiology, and other specialties) and is often presented with dedicated chapters in and of themselves. For this specific emergency, we provide Fig. 25.10, which is an example of the hemorrhage emergency manual entry from the Stanford Cognitive Aid Group (available at www.emergencymanuals.org).

In the suggested reading section, we refer to some essential resources for emergency cognitive aids specific to the O.R. environment. For example, for malignant hyperthermia, an exceptionally rare but life-threatening event, there exist a crisis checklist [13], a critical event checklist geared to the pediatric population [http://www.pedsanesthesia.org/wp-content/uploads/2017/03/Critical_Event_Checklists.pdf], an emergency manual entry [25], posters from the Malignant Hyperthermia Association of the United States (MHAUS) [http://www.mhaus.org/healthcare-professionals/managing-a-crisis], and other resources (www.emergencymanuals.org). We strongly encourage the reader to use these resources to familiarize themselves with opera-

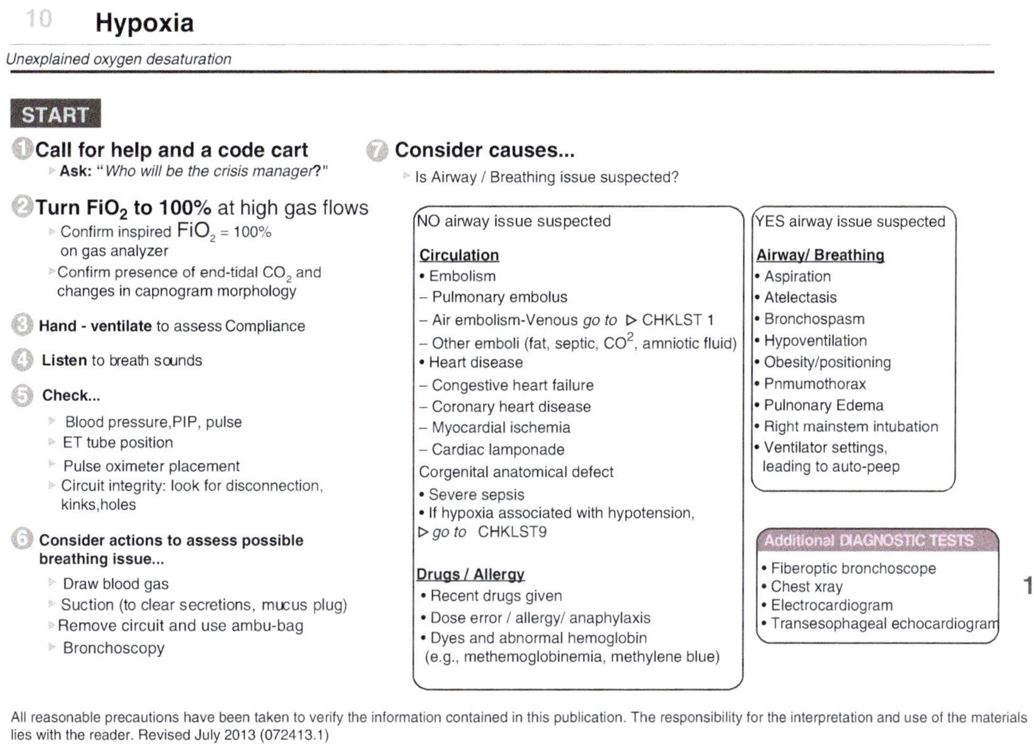

10 **Hypoxia**

Unexplained oxygen desaturation

START

1 **Call for help and a code cart**
- **Ask:** "*Who will be the crisis manager?*"

2 **Turn FiO_2 to 100%** at high gas flows
- Confirm inspired FiO_2 = 100% on gas analyzer
- Confirm presence of end-tidal CO_2 and changes in capnogram morphology

3 **Hand - ventilate** to assess Compliance

4 **Listen** to breath sounds

5 **Check...**
- Blood pressure,PIP, pulse
- ET tube position
- Pulse oximeter placement
- Circuit integrity: look for disconnection, kinks,holes

6 **Consider actions to assess possible breathing issue...**
- Draw blood gas
- Suction (to clear secretions, mucus plug)
- Remove circuit and use ambu-bag
- Bronchoscopy

7 **Consider causes...**
- Is Airway / Breathing issue suspected?

NO airway issue suspected

Circulation
- Embolism
  - Pulmonary embolus
  - Air embolism-Venous *go to* ▷ CHKLST 1
  - Other emboli (fat, septic, CO^2, amniotic fluid)
- Heart disease
  - Congestive heart failure
  - Coronary heart disease
  - Myocardial ischemia
  - Cardiac lamponade

Corgenital anatomical defect
- Severe sepsis
- If hypoxia associated with hypotension, ▷ *go to* CHKLST9

Drugs / Allergy
- Recent drugs given
- Dose error / allergy/ anaphylaxis
- Dyes and abnormal hemoglobin (e.g., methemoglobinemia, methylene blue)

YES airway issue suspected

Airway/ Breathing
- Aspiration
- Atelectasis
- Bronchospasm
- Hypoventilation
- Obesity/positioning
- Pnmumothorax
- Pulnonary Edema
- Right mainstem intubation
- Ventilator settings, leading to auto-peep

Additional DIAGNOSTIC TESTS
- Fiberoptic bronchoscope
- Chest xray
- Electrocardiogram
- Transesophageal echocardiogram

10

All reasonable precautions have been taken to verify the information contained in this publication. The responsibility for the interpretation and use of the materials lies with the reader. Revised July 2013 (072413.1)

Fig. 25.9 Crisis checklist for hypoxemia. In Ariadne Labs. Operating Room Crisis Checklists. With permission. A version from the Brigham and Women's Hospital is also available at: www.projectcheck.org/crisis. Image compressed to meet publication requirements. For native version, see URL provided. Accessed April 23, 2017

tive catastrophes that they are likely to encounter over the course of their practice. The practice patterns of the surgeon and institution are relevant considerations (i.e., certain catastrophes may be more common for the orthopedic surgeon, otolaryngologist, gynecological surgeon, pediatric surgeon, and others).

25.4 Current Controversies/ Future Directions

At present, there are no guidelines mandating crisis checklists or emergency manuals be available or used during patient care [26]. This point is amplified by existing cultural perceptions which attribute the use of cognitive aids to less clinical competence and overall skills by healthcare providers. A survey done at the University of California, San Francisco, found that one potential reason for providers to not use checklists was the "perception of them being less skilled because they needed to use a 'cheat sheet.'" Survey results showed 17% of providers felt uncomfortable using a checklist in front of their team members and only 45% of providers feeling comfortable [27]. Additionally, those reporting uncomfortable feelings were more likely to have fewer years of experience. Addressing these issues necessitates cultural shifts and implementation from leaders within the field to foster a culture that embraces the use of checklists and emergency manuals. To this end the Emergency Manuals Implementation Collaborative (EMIC) was formed to encourage the use of manuals and address barriers to implementation and dissemination by providing free access to multiple versions of emergency aids at www.emergencymanuals.org. Ultimately, these tools must be readily available to be used in cri-

14 HEMORRHAGE

HEMORRHAGE

MASSIVE TRANSFUSION GUIDELINES

By Stanford Anesthesia Cognitive Aid Group

1. CALL FOR HELP.
2. CALL FOR CODE CART?
3. INFORM TEAM.

IMMEDIATE

1. Follow local protocol to order Massive Transfusion Guideline (**MTG**) or equivalent.
2. Increase to **100% O_2**, high flow.
3. **Treat hypotension with IV fluid bolus.**
4. Consider **Trendelenburg** or **elevation of patient's legs**.
5. Use **vasopressor boluses** (ephedrine, phenylephrine, epinephrine) as a temporizing measure. Consider accepting low normal blood pressure until bleeding is controlled.
6. Call for **rapid infuser**.
7. Establish **additional IV access** as needed. Consider intraosseous if needed.
8. Ask surgeon: "Should we page a **vascular surgeon** or other additional help for you?"
9. **Send Type and Cross sample.** TS will provide emergency release Type O PRBC until crossmatched blood is available.
10. **Maintain normothermia.** Use fluid warming devices for IV and blood products. Use forced air warmers.
11. Place **arterial line** as indicated.
12. Follow patient's acid/base status by **ABG as indicator of adequate resuscitation. Monitor for hypocalcemia.**
13. Place **Foley Catheter** when able.
14. Call for **cell-saver** (if non-contaminated, non-malignant case).

Replace products EARLY! until current lab data available:

- If > 1 blood volume of loss expected: give **1 unit FFP for every 1 unit PRBC. Give 1 apheresis unit of platelets** (= old '6-pack') for every 6 units PRBC.
- When labs back: replace factors, platelets, fibrinogen as indicated on next page, but do not wait if blood loss is too rapid.

GO TO NEXT PAGE →

Emergency Manual V3.0 Aug. 2016

Fig. 25.10 (**a**, **b**) Emergency manual entry for hemorrhage. Used with permission from Stanford Anesthesia Cognitive Aid Group. Emergency Manual: Cognitive aids for perioperative critical events. See http://emergencymanual.stanford.edu for latest version. Image compressed to meet publication requirements. For native version, see URL provided. Creative Commons BY-NC-ND. 2016 (Version 3) (http://creativecommons.org/licenses/by-nc-nd/3.0/legalcode) (see Footnote 1)

HEMORRHAGE

MASSIVE TRANFUSION GUIDELINES *continued*

COMPONENTS

PRBC: Give for Hgb <7-10 (CAD? Rate of blood loss?) Each unit PRBC raises Hgb ~ 1g/dL.

PLATELETS: Give for <50,000-100,000 per μL with signs of ongoing bleeding. Each apheresis unit raises platelets ~50,000 per μL.

FRESH FROZEN PLASMA: Give for INR (PT) or PTT >1.5X normal. Give 10-15 cc FFP per kg body weight, then recheck labs and continue with 1:1 FFP:PRBC ratio.

CRYOPRECIPITATE: Give for fibrinogen <80-100 mg/dL. Each 10 units of cryoprecipitate raises fibrinogen ~50 mg/dL.

VOLUMES

$$\text{Est. Blood Loss} = \text{EBV} \times \frac{HCT_{starting} - HCT_{measured}}{HCT_{starting}}$$

Estimated Blood Volume (EBV) ~65-70 ml per kg body weight (~4.5 L for 70 kg)

END

14 HEMORRHAGE

Emergency Manual V3.0 Aug. 2016

Fig. 25.10 (continued)

sis situations and implementation is a key step in ensuring availability and appropriate use. This requires both an awareness of availability and training with the use of crisis checklist and emergency manuals [28].

An additional point of controversy in the use of crisis checklists/emergency manuals suggests that the doctors' use of a cognitive aid may cause providers to become reliant on these cognitive aids, to the point where clinical judgment is no longer used and fixation on one particular course of action can lead to a lack of flexibility and delay in appropriate care [29]. As we have stated throughout this chapter, all clinical signs and symptoms associated with the operative catastrophe must be interpreted in the context of patient history, physical exam, and current patient presentation, such that clinical judgment continues to be a primary driver of ultimate decision-making. In this setting, cognitive aids are implemented as an additional tool in the surgeon's armory, utilized in situations where high stress or high stakes may limit memory and recall of key steps and negatively impact team dynamics.

As with anything else in medicine, there is no "one solution fits all" approach. The recommendations presented in this chapter must be taken in context with the culture and resources of individual institutions and adapted for best use, prior to the occurrence of such events. Surgeons play a unique role in coordinating and executing care for patients in the operating room, as they are tasked with the responsibility of not only the knowledge, clinical expertise, and technical skills to treat patients but must also serve a leadership role in managing and maintaining successful team dynamics, incorporating effective communication skills, assigning appropriate task management, maintaining situational awareness, and ensuring successful team decision-making [30].

Take-Home Points

- Operative catastrophes are rare events that require time-sensitive diagnostic and management decisions to be recalled by even the most experienced clinicians under highly stressful conditions.
- Under stressful circumstances that come from rare life-threatening events, failure to adhere to best practices can be common when relying on memory alone. In these cases, cognitive aids can serve as an additional tool in the surgeon's armory, utilized in situations where high stress or high stakes may limit memory and recall of key steps and negatively impact team dynamics.
- Clinical judgment relative to the patient's history, physical exam findings, anesthetics given, and operating room course is key to adequate assessment and optimal treatment.
- In any operative catastrophe, the first steps should include calling for help, designating a crisis leader/checklist reader, and requesting additional resources needed.
- Crisis checklists and emergency manuals should be adapted to reflect the most up-to-date guidelines available and consistently be evaluated for effectiveness of content, design, and implementation, ensuring that these tools meet the needs of the institution and practicing providers.

As such, we present the topics in this chapter to equip the surgeon with evidence-based guidelines and tools to successfully address operative catastrophes and feel prepared to lead teams in these high-stress and high-stakes situations.

Acknowledgment This work is supported by grants from the University of Pennsylvania, McCabe Fund, and Bach Fund. The authors would like to thank Maryann Henry, CRNA, MS, and Carlene McLaughlin, CRNA, MSN, PhD, for their review of the work and their efforts to advance the principles of crisis management and patient safety. The views expressed in this article are those of the authors and do not necessarily represent the official views of supporting entities.

Suggested Reading

Babcock WW. Resuscitation during anesthesia. Anesth Analg. 1924;3(6):208–13.

Link MS, Berkow LC, Kudenchuk PJ, Halperin HR, Hess EP, Moitra VK, Neumar RW, O'Neil BJ, Paxton JH, Silvers SM, White RD. Part 7: adult advanced cardiovascular life support. Circulation. 2015;132(18 suppl 2):S444–64.

Arriaga AF, Bader AM, Wong JM, Lipsitz SR, Berry WR, Ziewacz JE, Hepner DL, Boorman DJ, Pozner CN, Smink DS, Gawande AA. Simulation-based trial of surgical-crisis checklists. N Engl J Med. 2013;368(3):246–53.

Goldhaber-Fiebert SN, Pollock J, Howard SK, Merrell SB. Emergency manual uses during actual critical events and changes in safety culture from the perspective of anesthesia residents: a pilot study. Anesth Analg. 2016;123(3):641–9.

Bhatti NI. Chapter 6: surgical management of the difficult adult airway. In: Flint PW, et al., editors. Cummings otolaryngology. 6th ed. Philadelphia: Elsevier Saunders; 2014.

References

1. Charuluxananan S, Suraseranivongse S, Jantorn P, Sriraj W, Chanchayanon T, Tanudsintum S, Kusumaphanyo C, Suratsunya T, Poajanasupawun S, Klanarong S, Pulnitiporn A. Multicentered study of model of anesthesia related adverse events in Thailand by incident report (The Thai anesthesia incidents monitoring study): results. J Med Assoc Thai. 2008;91(7):1011.
2. Ziewacz JE, Arriaga AF, Bader AM, Berry WR, Edmondson L, Wong JM, Lipsitz SR, Hepner DL, Peyre S, Nelson S, Boorman DJ. Crisis checklists for the operating room: development and pilot testing. J Am Coll Surg. 2011;213(2):212–7.
3. Arriaga AF, Bader AM, Wong JM, Lipsitz SR, Berry WR, Ziewacz JE, Hepner DL, Boorman DJ, Pozner CN, Smink DS, Gawande AA. Simulation-based trial of surgical-crisis checklists. N Engl J Med. 2013;368(3):246–53.
4. Goldhaber-Fiebert SN, Pollock J, Howard SK, Merrell SB. Emergency manual uses during actual critical events and changes in safety culture from the perspective of anesthesia residents: a pilot study. Anesth Analg. 2016;123(3):641–9.
5. Burden AR, Carr ZJ, Staman GW, Littman JJ, Torjman MC. Does every code need a "reader?" improvement of rare event management with a cognitive aid "reader" during a simulated emergency: a pilot study. Simul Healthc. 2012;7(1):1–9.
6. McEvoy MD, Hand WR, Stoll WD, Furse CM, Nietert PJ. Adherence to guidelines for the management of local anesthetic systemic toxicity is improved by an electronic decision support tool and designated 'reader'. Reg Anesth Pain Med. 2014;39(4):299.
7. Neumar RW, Otto CW, Link MS, Kronick SL, Shuster M, Callaway CW, Kudenchuk PJ, Ornato JP, McNally B, Silvers SM, Passman RS. Part 8: adult advanced cardiovascular life support. Circulation. 2010;122(18 suppl 3):S729–67.
8. Link MS, Berkow LC, Kudenchuk PJ, Halperin HR, Hess EP, Moitra VK, Neumar RW, O'Neil BJ, Paxton JH, Silvers SM, White RD. Part 7: adult advanced cardiovascular life support. Circulation. 2015;132(18 suppl 2):S444–64.
9. Brown TB, Dias JA, Saini D, Shah RC, Cofield SS, Terndrup TE, Kaslow RA, Waterbor JW. Relationship between knowledge of cardiopulmonary resuscitation guidelines and performance. Resuscitation. 2006;69(2):253–61.
10. Semeraro F, Signore L, Cerchiari EL. Retention of CPR performance in anaesthetists. Resuscitation. 2006;68(1):101–8.
11. Kurrck MM, Devitc JH, Cohen M. Cardiac arrest in the OR: how are our ACLS skills? Can J Anaesth. 1998;45(2):130.
12. Yang CW, Yen ZS, McGowan JE, Chen HC, Chiang WC, Mancini ME, Soar J, Lai MS, Ma MH. A systematic review of retention of adult advanced life support knowledge and skills in healthcare providers. Resuscitation. 2012;83(9):1055–60.
13. Operating Room Crisis Checklists. Ariadne Labs, Brigham and Women's Hospital, and Harvard School of Public Health; 2013 (Revised July 2016). http://www.emergencymanuals.org/free-tools.html.
14. Babcock WW. Resuscitation during anesthesia. Anesth Analg. 1924;3(6):208–13.
15. Mitka M. Peter J. Safar, MD: "father of CPR," innovator, teacher, humanist. JAMA. 2003;289(19):2485–6.
16. Lavonas EJ, Drennan IR, Gabrielli A, Heffner AC, Hoyte CO, Orkin AM, Sawyer KN, Donnino MW. Part 10: special circumstances of resuscitation. Circulation. 2015;132(18 suppl 2):S501–18.
17. Apfelbaum JL, Hagberg CA, Caplan RA, Blitt CD, Connis RT, Nickinovich DG, Benumof JL, Berry FA, Bode RH, Cheney FW, Guidry OF. Practice guidelines for management of the difficult airway an updated report by the American society of anesthesiologists task force on management of the difficult airway. Anesth. 2013;118(2):251–70.
18. Frerk C, Mitchell VS, McNarry AF, Mendonca C, Bhagrath R, Patel A, O'sullivan EP, Woodall NM, Ahmad I. Difficult airway society 2015 guidelines for management of unanticipated difficult intubation in adults. Br J Anaesth. 2015;115(6):827–48.
19. Flint PW, Haughey BH, Robbins KT, Thomas JR, Niparko JK, Lund VJ, Lesperance MM. Cummings otolaryngology-head and neck surgery. Amsterdam: Elsevier Health Sciences; 2014.
20. Fasting S, Gisvold SE. Serious intraoperative problems—a five-year review of 83,844 anesthetics. Can J Anesth. 2002;49(6):545–53.

21. Irita K, Kawashima Y, Iwao Y, Seo N, Tsuzaki K, Morita K, Obara H. Annual mortality and morbidity in operating rooms during 2002 and summary of morbidity and mortality between 1999 and 2002 in Japan: a brief review. Masui. 2004;53(3):320–35.
22. Walls RM, Murphy MF, editors. Manual of emergency airway management. 4th ed. Philadelphia: Lippincott Williams & Wilkins; 2013.
23. Morris RW, Watterson LM, Westhorpe RN, Webb RK. Crisis management during anaesthesia: hypotension. Qual Saf Health Care. 2005;14(3):e11.
24. Szekely SM, Runciman WB, Webb RK, Ludbrook GL. Crisis management during anaesthesia: desaturation. Qual Saf Health Care. 2005;14(3):e6.
25. Stanford Anesthesia Cognitive Aid Group.[1] Emergency Manual: Cognitive aids for perioperative critical events. See http://emergencymanual.stanford.edu for latest version. Creative Commons BY-NC-ND. 2016 (Version 3) (http://creativecommons.org/licenses/by-nc-nd/3.0/legalcode).
26. Hepner DL, Arriaga AF, Cooper JB, Goldhaber-Fiebert S, Gaba DM, Berry WR, Boorman DJ, Bader AM. Clinical concepts and commentary: operating room crisis checklists and emergency manuals. Anesthesiology. 2017;127(2):384–92.
27. Krombach JW, Edwards WA, Marks JD, Radke OC. Checklists and other cognitive aids for emergency and routine anesthesia care-a survey on the perception of anesthesia providers from a large academic US institution. Anesth Pain Med. 2015;5(4):e26300.
28. Neily J, DeRosier JM, Mills PD, Bishop MJ, Weeks WB, Bagian JP. Awareness and use of a cognitive aid for anesthesiology. Jt Comm J Qual Patient Saf. 2007;33(8):502–11.
29. Szabo A, August DA, Klainer S, Miller AD, Kaye AD, Raemer DB, Urman RD. The use of emergency manuals in perioperative crisis management: a cautious approach. J Med Pract Manage. 2014;30:8–12.
30. Cima RR, Deschamps C. Role of the surgeon in quality and safety in the operating room environment. Gen Thorac Cardiovasc Surg. 2013;61(1):1–8.

[1] Core contributors in random order: Howard SK, Chu LF, Goldhaber-Fiebert SN, Gaba DM, Harrison TK

Index

F. Palazzo (ed.), *Fundamentals of General Surgery*, https://doi.org/10.1007/978-3-319-75656-1